Lutz's Nutrition *and* Diet Therapy

SEVENTH EDITION

Erin E. Mazur, MSN, RN, FNP-BC
Associate Professor of Nursing
Jackson College
Jackson, Michigan

Nancy A. Litch, MS, RDN
Dietitian, Retired
East Lansing, Michigan

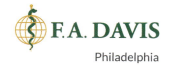

F.A. DAVIS

Philadelphia

F. A. Davis Company
1915 Arch Street
Philadelphia, PA 19103
www.fadavis.com

Printed in the United States of America

Last digit indicates print number: 10 9 8 7 6 5 4 3

Publisher: Megan Klim
Manager of Project and eProject Management: Catherine H. Carroll
Senior Content Project Manager: Christine Abshire
Electronic Project Editor: Samantha Olin
Illustration and Design Manager: Carolyn O'Brien

As new scientific information becomes available through basic and clinical research, recommended treatments and drug therapies undergo changes. The author(s) and publisher have done everything possible to make this book accurate, up-to-date, and in accord with accepted standards at the time of publication. The author(s), editors, and publisher are not responsible for errors or omissions or for consequences from application of the book, and make no warranty, expressed or implied, in regard to the contents of the book. Any practice described in this book should be applied by the reader in accordance with professional standards of care used in regard to the unique circumstances that may apply in each situation. The reader is advised always to check product information (package inserts) for changes and new information regarding dose and contraindications before administering any drug. Caution is especially urged when using new or infrequently ordered drugs.

Library of Congress Cataloging-in-Publication Data

Library of Congress Cataloging-in-Publication Data

Names: Mazur, Erin E., author. | Litch, Nancy A., author. | Preceded by
   (work): Lutz, Carroll A. Nutrition and diet therapy.
Title: Lutz's nutrition and diet therapy / Erin E. Mazur, Nancy A. Litch.
Other titles: Nutrition and diet therapy
Description: Seventh edition. | Philadelphia, PA : F. A. Davis Company,
   [2019] | Preceded by Nutrition and diet therapy / Carroll A. Lutz, Erin E.
   Mazur, Nancy A. Litch. 2015. | Includes bibliographical references and
   index.
Identifiers: LCCN 2018021835 (print) | LCCN 2018022914 (ebook) | ISBN
   9780803689985 () | ISBN 9780803668140 (pbk.)
Subjects: | MESH: Nutritional Physiological Phenomena | Nutrition Therapy
Classification: LCC RM216 (ebook) | LCC RM216 (print) | NLM QU 145 | DDC
   613.2—dc23
LC record available at https://lccn.loc.gov/2018021835

Dedications

Carroll Lutz, thank you for all your years of dedication and hard work to provide six editions of this textbook. Your commitment to providing students with current information regarding nutrition is to be commended. Without your vision and perseverance, this textbook would not be possible.

— Erin E. Mazur and Nancy A. Litch

To my family and friends for the constant support during the writing process, especially Jeff, Spencer, Carter, Mom, and Jen; I'm forever grateful.

— Erin E. Mazur

This is for all the students interested in the facts regarding nutrition and health; never stop seeking knowledge. To my family and friends who have supported me in this process, especially Paul, Evan, and Mom, much love and thanks.

— Nancy A. Litch

Preface

The seventh edition of *Lutz's Nutrition and Diet Therapy* is designed to provide the beginning student with knowledge of the fundamentals of nutrition related to the promotion and maintenance of optimal health. Practical applications and treatment of pathologies with nutritional components are stressed. In addition, basic scientific information is introduced to enable students to begin to understand nutritional issues reported in the mass media. The sequential introduction of material continues to be a unique feature of this text. The authors resist the temptation to introduce concepts and examples of applications before the underlying basic science and vocabulary have been covered. The seventh edition has been extensively streamlined and updated with new information (e.g., the new food label), incorporating updated illustrations and tables. Within the boundaries of a beginning course, specific information is included to enhance understanding of the "why" of nutritional care, not only the "what."

This book was written to meet the educational needs of nursing students, dietetic assistants, diet technicians, and others. Support materials for the student include case studies with examples of care plans, including referrals to other members of the health-care team, followed by Critical Thinking Questions designed to provoke imaginative thought and to foster discussion. Each chapter has review questions and clinical analysis study questions.

As researchers discover new and more effective treatments for nutrition-related disorders and health maintenance, the ability to think critically becomes increasingly important for professional growth and development. Students need not only to grasp the facts but also to apply the information in a clinical environment. This text has been developed to facilitate acquiring these skills.

The text can be used to teach a complete course in nutrition or as a desk reference for practitioners. The student using this book needs no previous grounding in anatomy, physiology, or medical terminology. Subjects are fully supported by diagrams, illustrations, figures, and tables. Depending on the curriculum, chapters may be omitted or presented in a different sequence. We recognize that this text contains an immense amount of data and information. It is our hope that this rich store of information permits instructors to adapt the text to the objectives of their courses while serving as a reference and directory for students, satisfying their curiosities or completing solo or group projects whether in preclinical or in clinical courses.

The content of *Lutz's Nutrition and Diet Therapy*, seventh edition, is organized into three units.

Unit 1, **The Role of Nutrients in the Human Body,** covers basic information on nutrition as a science and how this information is applied to nutritional care. All the essential nutrients are covered, including definitions and descriptions of functions, effects of excesses and deficiencies, and food sources. Nutritional standards, including the Dietary Reference Intakes, are explained and incorporated into discussions of nutrients. Information on the use of food in the body and how the body maintains energy balance completes the unit.

Unit 2, **Family and Community Nutrition,** provides an overview of topics such as nutrition throughout the life cycle, covering pregnancy, lactation, infancy, childhood, adolescence, and adulthood. Lastly, issues in food management are addressed.

Unit 3, **Clinical Nutrition,** focuses on the care of clients with pathologies caused by or causing nutritional impairments. General topics include nutrient delivery via oral, enteral, and parenteral routes, and interactions among foods, nutrients, medications, and supplements. Pathological conditions include diabetes mellitus and hypoglycemia, cardiovascular disease, renal disease, digestive diseases, and cancer. Other pertinent topics include weight control, nutrition in critical care and during stress, diet affecting inflammation and infections, and care of the client with a terminal illness.

Special features are used throughout the text to facilitate the teaching and learning process. Chapters include the following:

Boxes and Tables contain summaries, assessment tools, commonly prescribed diets used in medical nutrition therapy, and research findings.

Clinical Applications stimulate the interest of the beginning student by showing how the information is pertinent to providing health care.

Clinical Calculations isolate and explain many of the mathematical calculations that are used in nutritional science.

Dollars & Sense items focus on costs associated with commonly used foods and supplements. Occasionally, budget-sparing recipes are given to exemplify principles in the chapters.

Genomic Gems highlight links between a person's genetic makeup and utilization of nutrients and dietary substances.

Illustrations reinforce important points in the text or graph statistical data for clarity.

Flowcharts of physiological and pathological processes lead the student to an understanding of the relationship between nutrition and health.

A **Case Study** with a proposed **Care Plan** allows the student to see how the nutrition principles described in the chapter are applied in a specific clinical situation. The case studies were written to incorporate elements that are likely to occur in practice.

Teamwork following the care plan illustrates continuing care of a client by various members of the health-care team.

Chapter Review Questions and **Clinical Analysis Questions** help the student to focus on essential concepts. Answers to these questions are on Davis*Plus*.

Critical Thinking Questions invite the student to think holistically with compassion and creativity. They can be used as a basis for class discussion.

Appendices of Dietary Reference Intakes (Appendix A) serve as a readily available source of information for students in class discussions or group assignments.

A **Glossary** (Appendix B) of more than 1,000 entries assists the reader to recall definitions of terms boldfaced in the text.

The **Bibliography** supports the text with data sources and introduces the student to the scientific literature and is on Davis*Plus*.

Accompanying the text for instructors who adopt it for their classes are:

An **Active Classroom Instructors' Guide** with suggestions for lectures, classroom activities, and student assignments.

PowerPoint Presentations for all the chapters of the book. These presentations provide a ready source of material to select for classroom use.

A **Test Bank** containing over 450 questions, arranged by chapter.

We believe that *Lutz's Nutrition and Diet Therapy,* seventh edition, provides the clinical information necessary for a fuller understanding of the relationship between the knowledge about nutrition and diet and its clinical application. This text balances direct explanations of the underlying science with an introduction to the clinical responsibilities of the health-care professional.

Reviewers

Robin Adams-Weber, DNP, RN, WHNP-BC
Associate Professor of Nursing
Malone University
Canton, Ohio

Debora Boone, MSN, RN
Associate Professor/Health Science ADN Program
Maysville Community and Technical College
Maysville, Kentucky

Stephanie Bruce, MS, RN, ACNS-BC
Assistant Professor
Alverno College
Milwaukee, Wisconsin

Claire Cyriax, DNP, RN, LNC, CAPA
Professor
Bergen Community College
Paramus, New Jersey

Carol Della Ratta, PhD, RN, CCRN
Chair and Clinical Associate Professor
Stony Brook University
Stony Brook, New York

Teresa W. Johnson, DCN, RD
Professor
Troy University
Troy, Alabama

Marina Martinez-Kratz, MS, RN, CNE
Professor of Nursing
Jackson College
Jackson, Michigan

Joseph Molinatti, EdD, RN
Associate Professor
College of Mount Saint Vincent
Riverdale, New York

Rhonda Y. Sims, RN, DNP, MSN, MS, LNC, SANE-A
Professor of Nursing
Maysville Community & Technical College
Maysville, Kentucky

Shantelle L. Wade, MS, RN
Nursing Faculty/Clinical Coordinator
Presentation College
Aberdeen, South Dakota

Acknowledgments

Writing a book, even a seventh edition, is a huge task, requiring the assistance of many people. All of our colleagues and family members contributed to this project, sometimes with information and critiques, sometimes by being supportive, and sometimes just by leaving us alone to work.

We thank all the organizations and publishers that gave permission for the use of their materials for this and previous editions. Our editorial and production staff at F.A. Davis Company, including Megan Klim, Christine Abshire, Daniel Domzalski, and Bob Butler, shared their knowledge and expertise throughout the project. To all of them and the countless others who did not have to deal with us directly go our heartfelt thanks.

Contents

Appendices

Available on Davis*Plus*

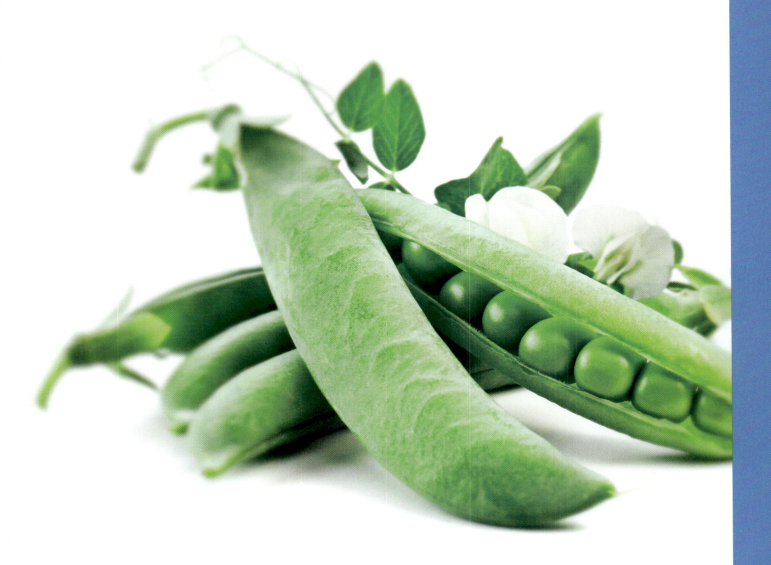

The Role of Nutrients in the Human Body

Nutrition in Human Health

After completing this chapter, the student should be able to:
- Describe the relationship between nutrition and health.
- Identify the six classes of nutrients, their functions, and their essentiality.
- Recognize the possible relationship of genetics to the adequacy of nutrition.
- Compare dietary intakes in the United States with the U.S. Department of Agriculture Dietary Guidelines.
- Discuss issues related to food insecurity.
- List and describe the steps in providing nutritional care.
- Explain the intended use of the Dietary Reference Intakes.
- Give an example of a provider's use of, and respect for, cultural beliefs having a favorable impact on health outcome for a client.
- State the preferences and dietary restrictions of several cultural and religious groups.

Food is essential to life. Choosing food wisely can contribute to a healthy, satisfying life and may prevent and treat various diseases. This chapter introduces concepts and practices that underlie the nourishment of human beings, as well as some barriers to achieving optimal nutrition. Information on the influence of culture on nutrition concludes the chapter.

The Language of Nutrition

Nutrition is the science of food and its relationship to health. Nutrition involves the processes of taking in and utilizing nourishment through natural and artificial feeding.

According to the World Health Organization (WHO), **health** is the state of complete physical, mental, and social well-being and not merely the absence of disease or infirmity. How nutrition influences human health is the subject of this textbook.

Food, or its lack thereof, affects physical health. For example, iron-deficiency **anemia** is, according to WHO, the most prevalent nutritional condition in industrialized countries and affects 30% of children, adolescents, and women in nonindustrialized countries. This may cause slowed growth and development, as well as behavioral issues, in children (Chen et al, 2013; National Institutes of Health, 2014).

Certainly, human beings should take nourishment daily. What an individual chooses to eat may affect his or her health that day but also well into the future.

Disease Prevention

The general prevention of disease is categorized into three levels: primary, secondary, and tertiary. Application of the principles of nutrition can contribute to prevention of disease in each of these levels.

Primary prevention is the implementation of practices that are likely to avert the occurrence of disease. Nutritional changes are essential to prevent medical conditions and diseases caused by nutrient deficiencies, such as iron-deficiency anemia. Excessive body weight is clearly related to heart disease, stroke, type 2 diabetes mellitus, some cancers, joint diseases, and some fertility disorders. The difficulty lies in motivating people to change behavior today for possible benefits in the future. Maintaining a healthy body weight is a primary prevention strategy.

Secondary prevention is the establishment of monitoring techniques to discover diseases early enough to provide the opportunity to control their effects. If a person's risk for diabetes is found in the prediabetes stage by testing blood sugar levels, noninvasive treatments such as weight loss and diet modification can successfully derail or delay the development of the disease.

Tertiary prevention is the use of treatment techniques after a disease has occurred to prevent complications or to promote maximum adaptation. For example, clients with type 2 diabetes who manage their disease well through diet, exercise, and prescribed medications may prevent the development of coronary artery disease (CAD) (see Chapter 18).

Nutrients

Historically, the science of nutrition has been based on the nutrients in food. **Nutrients** are the chemical substances supplied by food that the body needs for growth, maintenance, and repair.

Classes and Essentiality

Nutrients are divided into six classes, each of which is discussed in subsequent chapters:

1. Carbohydrates (often abbreviated as CHO for carbon, hydrogen, and oxygen)
2. Fats (lipids)
3. Proteins
4. Minerals
5. Vitamins
6. Water

Nutrients are considered essential, nonessential, or conditionally essential, depending on whether the body can or cannot manufacture them.

- An **essential nutrient** is the one that the human body requires but cannot manufacture in sufficient amounts to meet bodily needs. Essential nutrients must be supplied by foods in the diet. Vitamin C, vitamin A, and calcium are 3 of the more than 40 essential nutrients.
- **Nonessential nutrients** are not needed in the diet because the body can make them from other substances. For example, the amino acid alanine is a nonessential nutrient because the body can manufacture it from other raw materials.
- **Conditionally essential nutrients** are those that, under most circumstances, a healthy body can manufacture in sufficient quantities. In certain situations of physiological status or disease, the body cannot produce optimal amounts. The amino acid tyrosine is an example of a conditionally essential nutrient (see Chapter 4).

Functions

All nutrients perform one or more of the following functions:

1. Serve as a source of energy or heat
2. Support the growth and maintenance of tissue
3. Aid in the regulation of basic body processes

These three life-sustaining functions collectively are part of **metabolism,** the sum of all physical and chemical changes that take place in the body. Nutrients have specific metabolic functions and interact with one another to maintain the body.

SOURCE OF ENERGY

Energy is defined in the physical sciences as the capacity to do work. Energy exists in a variety of forms, such as electric, thermal (heat), chemical, mechanical, and nuclear.

All food enters the body as chemical energy. The body processes the chemical energy of food and converts it into other energy forms. For example, chemical energy is transformed into electric signals in nerves and into mechanical energy in muscles.

Carbohydrates, fats, and proteins—the nutrients that supply energy—are referred to as the **energy nutrients.** The energy both in foods and in the body is measured in **kilocalories,** abbreviated kcal. Because energy cannot be seen, heard, or felt, it can be a difficult biological concept to understand (see Chapter 5).

GROWTH AND MAINTENANCE OF TISSUES

Some nutrients provide the raw materials for building body structures, and they participate in the continued growth and maintenance of necessary tissues. Water, proteins, fats, and minerals are the nutrient classes that contribute in a major way to building body structures.

REGULATION OF BODY PROCESSES

Some nutrients control or regulate chemical processes in the body. For example, certain minerals and proteins help regulate how water is distributed in the body. Vitamins are necessary in the series of reactions involved in generating energy. Vitamins themselves are not energy sources, but if the body lacks a particular vitamin, it will not produce energy efficiently.

Functional Foods

In addition to the nutrients listed above, foods contain other physiologically active substances from plant (**phytochemical**), animal, and microbial sources, some of which reputedly promote health. Phytochemicals identified thus far number in the tens of thousands, including 8,000 polyphenols, which may stimulate the immune system, prevent cell damage, and reduce inflammation (Gropper & Smith, 2013; American Institute for Cancer Research, 2017). It is small wonder that pinning down the health effect of one component in a food is daunting. Therefore, the amount and quality of evidence for the usefulness of functional foods vary.

Definitions of functional foods are equally varied by source and are not officially recognized as a food category by the U.S. Food and Drug Administration (FDA). The Academy of Nutrition and Dietetics (AND) defines **functional foods** as "whole foods along with fortified, enriched, or enhanced foods that have a potentially beneficial effect on health when consumed as part of a varied diet on a regular basis at effective levels based on significant standards of evidence" (Wolfram, 2017). Functional foods are categorized in Table 1-1. Several examples of functional foods being studied appear in Table 1-2. Bear in mind that a given food may contain thousands of phytochemicals that differ under divergent cultivation and storage methods. The extent to which foods may be labeled with a health claim is discussed in Chapter 15. Specific examples of functional foods with the best **efficacy** are provided as the subject matter dictates in other chapters.

TABLE 1-1 Functional Foods

CATEGORY	SELECTED EXAMPLES
Conventional foods (whole foods)	Blueberries Cranberry juice (see Chapter 21) Cruciferous vegetables: broccoli, cabbage, cauliflower, Brussels sprouts (see Chapter 21) Green tea Mushrooms Some nuts Oatmeal as part of heart-healthy diet Tomatoes (see Chapter 21)
Modified foods, fortified	Omega-3 fatty acids in eggs and margarines (for definition, see Chapter 6)
Synthesized food ingredients	Oligosaccharides functioning as prebiotics (see Chapter 20)

Adapted from Crowe & Francis (2013); Milner, Toner, & Davis (2014).

TABLE 1-2 Selected Functional Foods, Bioactive Components, and Reported Health Benefits

FUNCTIONAL FOODS	BIOACTIVE COMPONENTS UNDER STUDY	REPORTED HEALTH BENEFIT
Apples, tea, onions	Flavonoids	Prevention of cardiovascular disease
Berries	Polyphenols	Protection against cancer through abilities to counteract, reduce, and repair damage from oxidative stress and inflammation
Cruciferous vegetables (broccoli, cauliflower, cabbage)	Isothiocyanates	Reduction of prostate cancer risk
Green Tea	Polyphenols	Inhibition of cancer initiation and blockage of cancer progression
Oats	Beta-glucan (soluble fiber)	Reduction of blood cholesterol levels
Purple grape juice or red wine	Resveratrol	Reduction of heart disease risk by decreasing blood platelet aggregation
Soy products	Isoflavones	Reduction in incidence of hormone-related cancers

Sources: Academy of Nutrition and Dietetics (2013); Kanwar et al (2012); Li et al (2011); Liu, Mao, Cao, & Xie (2012); Majewska-Wierzbicka & Czeczot (2012); Othman, Moghadasian, & Jones (2011); Seeram (2008); Zhang (2012).

Nutritional Genomics

In April 2003, the Human Genome Project announced that the actual sequence of the human genetic code had been completed and published. In simple terms, the genetic code is the human body's internal instructions for manufacturing proteins (see Genomic Gem 1-1). Each of the body's 23 pairs of **chromosomes** contains **genes** that provide the information needed by the body to function and may contain variations that may predispose someone to an increased chance of developing a health condition, such as diabetes or cancer. **Epigenetics** is the process that regulates how and when genes are turned on and off. It may occur in response to internal factors (hormones and enzymes) and external/environmental factors (radiation, chemicals, and diet). Speculation is that, as the price for sequencing the human genome drops, it may become an integral part of medical practice; however, translating the information into clinically significant recommendations for individuals would be required (Academy of Nutrition and Dietetics, 2014).

A subfield of nutritional genomics, **nutrigenetics**, detects gene variants within an individual to identify nutritional factors that trigger dysfunction or disease. Examples of gene variants conveying susceptibility for dysfunction include those for lactose intolerance and celiac disease.

GENOMIC GEM 1-1

Genetic Code as Software

To visualize the relationships among the human body, genetic code, and diet, think of the body as a machine similar to a personal computer. Software provides directions to the computer; a person's genetic code provides instructions to the body. Just as a personal computer cannot operate without software, the human body cannot operate without instructions from the genetic code. Think of data input by the operator as much like food that is taken in or eaten. Computer file storage capacity is measured in megabytes or gigabytes; the body's DNA is comprised of genes and includes information to either express or suppress specific genes.

For years, scientists have studied the effects of nutrients and phytochemicals on our body's hardware, or structure. Only recently have researchers begun the study of nutrients and phytochemicals on the body's software, or genetic code. Almost everyone has software on her or his computer that is never used. The human body also has instructions that are similarly never used.

What causes a software program or gene in the human body to be turned on or expressed? Some scientists are beginning to understand that the activation is partly due to the food we eat or do not eat. The premise underlying nutrigenomics is that diet's influence on health depends on an individual's genetic makeup, thereby suggesting that not all individuals respond identically to a given diet. Thus, one person would be more susceptible to the negative effects of a suboptimal diet than another person would be. More research is needed to identify those who will benefit most from dietary change and those who might be placed at risk because of an adjustment (Riscuta & Dumitrescu, 2012; DeHaan, 2015).

The trigger in lactose intolerance is lactose in dairy products because the body does not make enough lactase to help digest the lactose. This intolerance is more common in individuals of Native American, Asian, African, and South American descent. In celiac disease, it is the gluten in wheat, rye, and barley that causes a chronic inflammatory condition of the small intestine (see Chapter 20) (Pavlidis, Patrinos, & Katsila, 2015).

Another subfield of nutritional genomics is **nutrigenomics,** the study of the interaction between one's diet and his or her genes. These interactions can markedly influence digestion, absorption, and elimination as well as influence their sites of action. A possible application of nutrigenomics in a person susceptible to chronic inflammation is to ensure adequate omega-3 fatty acids intake from food (see Chapter 3) to reduce the expression of genes that may be protective against Crohn disease and may reduce the disease progression in those that have it (Ferguson, 2015).

Body Composition

Nutrient intake can affect body composition, which, in turn, can affect health. The human body is composed of five types of substances:

1. Water
2. Protein
3. Fat
4. Ash (mineral content as in the skeleton)
5. Carbohydrate

Figure 1-1 shows these substances as a percentage of body weight in young adults. Because of its increased muscle, the male body contains more protein than the female

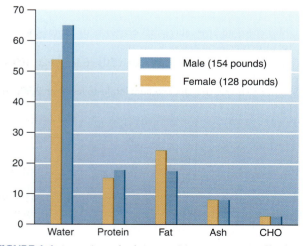

FIGURE 1-1 Approximate body composition as a percent of body weight of a 25-year-old man weighing 154 pounds and woman weighing 128 pounds. Note that the typical woman has more fat and less protein than the man because of differences in muscle. The percentage of ash content is equal in both sexes. The human body has minimal carbohydrate content.

body. With age, body composition typically becomes higher in fat and lower in protein.

Health-care providers are often concerned that their clients retain their muscle, particularly when losing weight (see Chapter 16). When the body loses protein, it is losing muscle tissue, organ mass, the protein stored in body substances, or combinations thereof. Preservation of body protein is necessary for optimal health.

A person's body fat and protein content can be modified by food intake, exercise, or both. Exercise increases body protein content by increasing muscle. Eating too much food increases the fat content of the body because fat is stored for future use as energy. Excessive body fat, both in amount and in location, has health consequences.

Health Promotion and Disease Prevention

Deficiencies of essential nutrients have dramatically decreased, but the rates of chronic diseases (many related to poor diet and physical inactivity) have increased. It is estimated that half of American adults have one or more preventable, diet-related chronic diseases, such as cardiovascular disease (CVD) and type 2 diabetes, and are overweight or obese (https://www.cnpp.usda.gov/2015-2020-dietary-guidelines-americans). Current dietary advice from the U.S. government attempts to remedy that unhealthy state of affairs.

Healthy People 2020

Healthy People 2020 provides science-based national goals designed to improve the health of all people in the United States. Its overarching goals are to help people attain high-quality, longer lives free of preventable diseases through improving the health of all groups throughout all stages of life. There are more than 40 topic overviews available at www.healthypeople.gov to assist in the promotion of health and prevention of disease. Among the topics covered are:

- Nutrition and Weight Status—advocates the consumption of a healthy diet and attainment of a healthy weight. The recommendation for diet is for intake of a wide variety of all food groups, including fruits and vegetables, lean proteins, whole grains, and low-fat dairy. Maintaining a healthy weight helps prevent chronic diseases such as hypertension, hyperlipidemia, osteoarthritis, type 2 diabetes, heart disease, and some cancers.
- Physical Activity—the need for regular exercise is advocated for both children and adults to meet the Physical Activity Guidelines (PAG) for each age range—at least 150 minutes of moderate aerobic exercise each week for adults. The full PAG is available at https://www.healthypeople.gov/. It is estimated that more than 80% of adults do not meet these guidelines. Routine exercise is recommended to help prevent coronary heart disease (CHD), stroke, hypertension, type 2 diabetes, breast and colon cancers, falls, and

depression in adults. Children benefit from regular exercise through improved bone health, cardiorespiratory and muscular fitness, decreased body fat, and reduction in depression symptoms.

Dietary Guidelines

Every five years since 1980, the U.S. Department of Agriculture (USDA) and the U.S. Department of Health and Human Services (HHS) have published the *Dietary Guidelines for Americans* based on the latest scientific and medical information. The *2015-2020 Guidelines* promote a healthy eating pattern and regular physical activity to maintain good health and reduce the risk for major chronic diseases throughout the lifespan. These recommendations accommodate the food preferences, cultural traditions, and economic resources of many diverse groups who live in the United States.

By supporting the *Dietary Guidelines* goals, government policymakers, nutrition educators, and health providers help improve the health of the nation. For example, the *Guidelines* would be used to create menus for school lunch programs, nursing home residents, and prisoners.

The *Dietary Guidelines for Americans, 2015-2020*, recognizes that half of all American adults have one or more preventable, diet-related diseases, including CVD, type 2 diabetes, and overweight and obesity related to poor eating patterns and physical inactivity. This dietary guidance can help maximize the nutritional content of diets. The *2015-2020 Guidelines* focus on the overall eating pattern that should be utilized as a flexible framework based on an individual's personal and cultural choice.

Of note, the guidelines do not apply to individuals who have diseases or conditions that alter normal nutritional requirements. Clinical Application 1-1 summarizes the key recommendations for the general population and certain subsets of the population. Many of the terms may be unfamiliar but will become less so in later chapters.

MyPlate

MyPlate is a USDA program developed to provide simple-to-follow guidelines, and graphics that promote healthy eating patterns (available online at www.choosemyplate.gov). The intent of the MyPlate icon (Fig. 1-2) is to reduce risks for obesity, diabetes, CVD, cancer, and other chronic diseases by helping consumers to eat correct proportions of healthy foods at each meal.

The interactive Web site offers sections for consumers and professionals, sample menus and recipes, tips for vegetarians, and many links to other resources. A page to personalize goals and record progress is located at www.choosemyplate.gov/SuperTracker.

What We Actually Eat

The government periodically surveys food intake of the population to monitor progress toward meeting dietary goals. Information from two such investigations is discussed next.

CLINICAL APPLICATION   1-1

Key Recommendations of *2015-2020 Dietary Guidelines*

FOLLOW A HEALTHY EATING PATTERN THROUGHOUT THE LIFESPAN

Choose a healthy eating pattern at an appropriate caloric level to achieve and maintain a healthy weight, support nutrient adequacy, and reduce the risk of chronic disease. Examples of healthy eating patterns found in the Dietary Guidelines are:

- Healthy U.S. style—based on the types and proportions of foods Americans typically consume in nutrient-dense forms and appropriate amounts
- Mediterranean—similar to the healthy U.S.-style eating pattern, but contains more fruits and seafood and less dairy
- Vegetarian—similar to the healthy U.S.-style eating pattern, but includes more legumes, nuts, seeds, and whole grains but no meats, poultry, or seafood

FOCUS ON VARIETY, NUTRIENT DENSITY, AND AMOUNT

Choose a variety of nutrient-dense foods across and within all food groups in recommended amounts.

- A variety of vegetables, including dark green, red, and orange; legumes; and starchy
- Fruits—especially the whole fruit
- Grains—at least half of which are whole grains

- Fat-free or low-fat dairy and soy
- Lean proteins, including seafood, meats and poultry, eggs, legumes, nuts, and seeds
- Oils

LIMIT CALORIES FROM ADDED SUGARS AND SATURATED FATS, AND REDUCE SODIUM INTAKE

- Reduce added sugars and saturated fats to less than 10% of calories per day
- Shift food choices to reduce sodium intake to less than 2,300 mg of sodium per day
- If alcohol is consumed, it should be consumed in moderation—up to one drink per day for women and two drinks per day for men

SHIFT TO HEALTHIER FOOD AND BEVERAGE CHOICES

Choose nutrient-dense foods while honoring cultural and personal preferences to make healthy changes more easily sustainable.

Consume more whole fruits and vegetables—eliminate more processed foods and replace with the whole food (an apple in place of applesauce or a fruit snack bar)

- Half of all grains consumed should be whole grains—consume less refined grains (brown rice in place of white rice)
- Substitute nutrient-dense snacks in place of high-calorie snacks (unsalted nuts in place of candy or chips)

Continued

CLINICAL APPLICATION—cont'd   1-1

- Replace sugar-sweetened beverages (fruit drinks, sweetened carbonated beverages) with unsweetened (low-fat dairy, unsweetened tea, water)
- Increase variety of lean-protein food choices to more nutrient-dense foods (chicken breast, fish, legumes, tofu) in place of higher-fat meats (beef, sausage, processed meats)
- Replace saturated fats (butter, margarine, coconut oil) with unsaturated oils (olive, canola)

SUPPORT HEALTHY EATING PATTERNS FOR ALL

Across all population groups in the United States, the vast majority of individuals do not meet these recommendations. Everyone has a role in supporting these goals. Targeting change in the community, school, and retail settings can assist the individual in meeting goals. If the goal is to reduce sodium in the diet, the following strategies could be enacted:

- Individual education to discuss changes to eating patterns
- Working with restaurants and schools to prepare lower-sodium foods, and providing the sodium content of foods on the menu
- Conduct public health campaigns to promote the importance of reducing sodium in the diet

SOURCE: *Dietary Guidelines for Americans, 2015-2020.* Available at http://health.gov/dietaryguidelines/2015/guidelines/

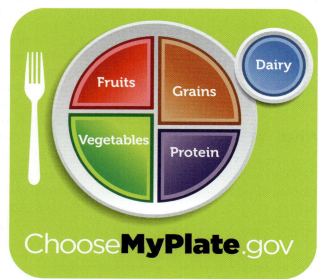

FIGURE 1-2 The MyPlate icon shows relative proportions of five food groups to permit consumers to more easily visualize an ideal meal. The ChooseMyPlate.gov interactive Web site offers dietary assessment tools, nutrition education resources, and clear actionable information about how to make better food choices. *(From U.S. Department of Agriculture, 2011, with permission.)*

The "What We Eat in America" Survey

Each year, more than 5,000 U.S. residents are interviewed about what they ate and drank for 24-hour periods on 2 nonconsecutive days. The data are part of the HHS National Health and Examination Survey (**NHANES**) that also includes physical examinations (Centers for Disease Control and Prevention, 2015).

Americans consume the following:

1. Most people reported eating 1 ounce or less of whole grains per day compared with the 1.5 to 5 ounces recommended according to age and gender.
2. Refined grains (white bread, bagels, white rice, cereals, desserts [cake, cookies, pies, sweet rolls, pastries, donuts], etc.) are eaten at a high rate. When averaged together, Americans are eating in the recommended range for grain consumption (3 to 8 ounce equivalents based on age and gender), but at a disproportional rate for refined grains. A 1 ounce equivalent is 1 regular slice of bread. A bagel is up to 4 ounce equivalents.
3. The only age group that meets its recommended target for the intake of dairy (2 to 2.5 cup equivalents) is children 1 to 3 years of age. Children 4 to 18 years of age, although below their recommendations of 2.5 to 3 cup equivalents, are only slightly below. Adults have the largest drop-off in dairy consumption as they age. The recommendation for adults is to consume 3 cup equivalents of dairy each day. From age 19 to 71, intake drops from 2 to 1.5 cup equivalents of dairy daily.
4. Added sugars account for an average of 270 calories, or more than 13% of daily calories in the United States. The major source (47%) of added sugars in the typical U.S. diet is from beverages (soft drinks, fruit drinks, sweetened coffee and tea, "energy" drinks, alcoholic beverages, and flavored waters). The other major sources of added sugars are snacks and sweets (grain-based desserts [cakes, pies, cookies, etc.], ice cream and other frozen desserts, candies, sugars, jams, syrups, and sweet toppings). Together beverages, snacks, and sweets make up approximately 75% of added sugars in the U.S. diet.
5. Sodium intake in the United States averages 3440 mg per day, with adult men averaging 4240 mg and adult women averaging 2980. Most sodium consumed in the United States comes from salts added during commercial food processing and preparation (http://health.gov/dietaryguidelines/2015/guidelines).

Eating healthier foods to maintain a healthy weight is still an unachieved goal for most Americans. Much more information on this topic appears in Chapter 16.

State-Specific Trends in Fruit and Vegetable Consumption

Reflecting the importance of fruit and vegetable intake to a healthy diet (encompassing one-half of the MyPlate graphic), the Centers for Disease Control and Prevention

(CDC) monitors dietary intake through a telephone survey. Results show that much behavior change is needed to increase the consumption of fruits and vegetables. In the 2013 survey (https://www.cdc.gov/nutrition/downloads/state-indicator-report-fruits-vegetables-2013.pdf):

1. An estimated 37.7% of U.S. adults consumed less than 1 serving of fruit per day, but overall adults consumed 1.1 servings of fruit per day. The highest consumption of fruit, 1.3 servings per day, was found in Washington, DC, California, Connecticut, New Hampshire, and Vermont. The lowest consumption of fruit, an average of 0.9 servings per day, was found in Oklahoma and Mississippi.
2. Nationally, an estimated 22.6% of adults consumed vegetables less than 1 time per day, with an average of 1.6 servings per day. The highest number of servings was in Oregon (1.9 per day). The lowest number of servings per day, 1.4, was reported in South Dakota, North Dakota, Mississippi, Louisiana, and Iowa.

To increase the consumption of fruits and vegetables, the CDC recommends that states and communities:

- Improve access to and affordability of fruits and vegetables in stores and use a farm-to-consumer approach
- Support the percentage of farmers' markets accepting Supplemental Nutrition Assistance Program (SNAP) and Women, Infants, and Children (WIC) Food and Nutrition Service vouchers/coupons
- Increase the number of schools providing fruits and vegetables, which are low in added fats and sugar
- Support the consumption of fruits and vegetables in regulations governing child care

Unbalanced Nutrition

Ingesting too much or too little of a nutrient can interfere with health and well-being. Each nutrient has a beneficial range of intake; an intake below or above that range is incompatible with optimal health.

Malnutrition

Malnutrition can be caused by inadequate or unbalanced intake of food or nutrients or by ineffective processing by the body due to malfunction or disease. The body requires adequate calories, protein, and other nutrients in order to maintain and repair tissue (Hand et al, 2016).

Ideally, a person should consume a diet marked by balance, moderation, and variety.

1. Balance is displayed in the MyPlate icon that shows the proportions of foods in a meal.
2. Moderation is exemplified by judicious portion sizes such as those used on the Nutrition Facts labels found on many food items (see Chapter 13).
3. Variety is characterized by selection of many different foods rather than always eating one's favorites or those easiest to prepare.

If those three qualities of a good diet are consistently absent, health may suffer and recovery from illness may be prolonged. It is estimated that approximately one-third of individuals admitted to a hospital in developed countries are malnourished, and if not corrected, two-thirds of those individuals will have a further decline in their nutrition status. Of the well-nourished clients admitted to a hospital, approximately one-third may become malnourished during hospitalization. Hospitalized individuals who are not well-nourished experience more complications; a length of stay (LOS) estimated to be three times that of well-nourished individuals, resulting in approximately three times the cost of the stay; and are more likely to be readmitted within 30 days of discharge (Guenter et al, 2015).

Malnutrition involving protein is addressed in Chapter 4. Vitamin- and mineral-deficiency diseases are discussed in Chapters 6 and 7. Effects of other nutritional imbalances are considered in other chapters as appropriate.

Food Insecurity

Food insecurity is the limited or uncertain availability of nutritionally adequate and safe foods or doubtful ability to acquire food, whether some of the time or always. Food insecurity, often associated with poverty and low income, has important implications for the health and nutrition of individuals and the nation.

In the United States

The *2015-2020 Dietary Guidelines for Americans* acknowledged the extent of food insecurity in the country. One objective of the *Guidelines* was to assist residents with limited resources to maximize the nutritional content of their meals.

EXTENT OF THE PROBLEM

The USDA (September 2017) estimates that 12.3% (15.6 million) of American households were food insecure in 2016, down from 14% in 2014. These households had limited or uncertain access to nutritionally adequate and safe food.

Rates of food insecurity are higher for households with children (16.5%) than those without children (10.5%). Among households with children, married-couple families had the lowest rate of food insecurity (9.9%). Single women with children have a greater rate of food insecurity (31.6%) than those headed by a single man (21.7%) with children. There is marked imbalance in the rates of food insecurity among different races/ethnicities. Black, non-Hispanic households (22.5%) have a higher rate than Hispanic households (18.5%); white households have a rate of 9.3%.

The prevalence of food insecurity was highest for households located in nonmetropolitan areas (15.0%), intermediate for those in principal cities of metropolitan areas (14.2%), and lowest in suburban and other metropolitan areas outside principal cities (9.5%). Regionally, the food insecurity rate was higher in the south (13.5%) than in the northeast (10.8%) and west (11.5%). The food insecurity rate in the Midwest (12.2%) was not statistically different from the other regions. See Figure 1-3 to compare the percentages of the household groups categorized as food insecure. It is apparent that a household fits into several of the subgroups simultaneously. For instance, a single Hispanic mother living in a metropolitan area in the south below the federal poverty line is at risk on all those levels. The degree of compounded risk is not discernible from these statistics.

FOOD COSTS AND RESOURCES

Low-income households with incomes below 185% of the poverty threshold (31.6%) are at a high risk of food insecurity. The Federal poverty line was an annual income of $24,036 for a family of four in 2015.

In 2010, all U.S. households spent a **median** of $43.75 per week per person on food. Households with low food security and very low food security spent $34.00 per week per person (Coleman-Jensen, Nord, Andrews, & Carlson, 2011). The USDA estimates the cost of providing a thrifty nutritious diet in the home can cost $36.83 per week per person, based on a family of four. The weekly cost for a senior (>71 years of age) ranges from $36.20 per week for a woman to $39.00 for a man (U.S. Department of Agriculture, 2017). Figure 1-4

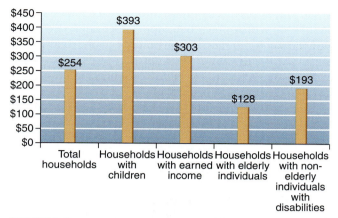

FIGURE 1-4 Average monthly SNAP benefits by household in dollars. *(Data from U.S. Department of Agriculture [USDA]: Characteristics of Supplemental Nutrition Assistance Program Households: Fiscal Year 2015.)*

provides the average financial assistance provided by household type. Individuals relying solely on Supplemental Nutrition Assistance Program (SNAP) benefits receive funds to cover a thrifty nutritious diet.

The SNAP participation rate among eligible individuals rose from 69% in 2007 to 83% in 2014, the most recent year for which USDA estimates are available (Center on Budget and Policy Priorities, 2016).

1. SNAP provided benefits to 46 million individuals overall in 2011 to over 44 million in 2016, a decrease of 4.4% (www.fns.usda.gov). SNAP serves vulnerable families with almost 90% of participants in a household with children, an elderly (≥60 years old), or disabled adult (Center on Budget and Policy Priorities, 2017).
2. Over 30 million children received free (66.6%) or reduced cost lunches in fiscal year 2016 (www.fns.usda.gov).
3. Approximately 7.7 million people received food vouchers from the **Women, Infants, and Children's** program (WIC) in 2016 at a cost of almost 4 million dollars (www.fns.usda.gov).

Lowering the cost of fruits and vegetables can increase consumption. A pilot project that gave random SNAP recipients 30 cents in added benefits for every dollar spent on certain fruits and vegetables saw a 26% increase in consumption of those foods daily (Center on Budget and Policy Priorities, 2016).

Despite that assistance, food intake for people with low incomes tends to be concentrated in inexpensive, high-kilocalorie food of low nutritional quality. Low-cost, high-kilocalorie foods containing added sugar and fat comprise almost 40% of the daily kilocalorie intake of people with low resources because their communities offer little else. The lack of full-service supermarkets with fresh produce and low-fat dairy products led to the descriptor of *food deserts* for such neighborhoods.

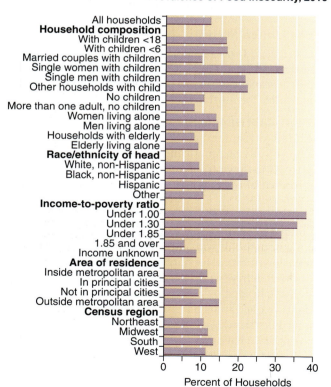

FIGURE 1-3 Percentage of household groups of the U.S. population experiencing food security. *(From U.S. Department of Agriculture [USDA], Economic Research Service, using data from the December 2016 Current Population Survey Food Security Supplement in USDA: Key Statistics and Graphics. Updated September 2017. Available at https://www.ers.usda.gov/topics/food-nutrition-assistance/food-security-in-the-us/key-statistics-graphics.aspx.)*

Nutritional Care

Nutritional status refers to the body's condition related to the intake and use of nutrients. All members of the health-care team have roles in the effective evaluation of a client's nutritional status. See Team Work 1-1.

Dietary status describes what a client has been eating. Although a client's dietary status may be adequate, his or her nutritional status may be poor. An evaluation of a client's dietary status can help to determine the reason for this poor nutritional status, or it may rule out poor diet as the source of the client's problem.

Providing nutrition care usually involves several health-care providers to conduct the four steps of the process: assessment, analysis/diagnosis, planning/intervention, and monitoring/evaluation. Fictional case studies throughout this book integrate the steps to provide nutritional care for the described clients with commonly encountered problems.

Assessment

Initiation of nutrition assessment in a timely manner is a requirement of accrediting and licensing agencies. Because of the increased risk of complications and negative outcomes of hospitalized individuals discussed in the section of malnutrition, it is imperative that early assessment take place to identify and take action on those at nutritional risk. Normally nutritional screening is required within 24 hours for individuals admitted to a health-care facility (Guenter et al, 2015). Two levels of methodology are commonly used to identify clients at nutritional risk. Institutions are likely to select a screening technique expected to identify nutritional problems

---

TEAMWORK 1-1

HEALTH-CARE PROVIDERS IN NUTRITION DELIVERY

A client's health-care team may include many members. The following are the respective titles and responsibilities of the major members of the health-care team.

Registered nurses (RNs) are often the first team members to interview a client, and they communicate important nutritional information such as a client's response to food, including intake and tolerance, to other team members. In addition, they identify and refer clients at nutritional risk to other team members, and they provide some nutritional information to clients.

Licensed practical nurses/licensed vocational nurses (LPNs/LVNs), supervised by RNs, feed clients, monitor food consumption, measure intake and output, and record data.

Registered dietitians (RDs) and physicians are responsible for meeting clients' nutritional needs. Dietitians may recommend an appropriate diet for the physician to order in terms of clients' food habits and food choices, calculate clients' nutritional requirements, evaluate clients' response to therapeutic diets, recommend the best route for nutrient administration, **enteral** or **parenteral**, and provide in-depth nutrition education and counseling to clients. Among team members, the registered dietitian has the most education and training in the nutritional sciences.

Dietetic technicians (DTs) assist dietitians by taking nutrition histories and body measurements, reviewing records, and monitoring clients' food intake. They are often responsible for screening clients for nutritional risk and referring clients at risk to the registered dietitian.

Physicians are responsible for the diagnosis and treatment of medical conditions. They manage medical care, order laboratory tests, and prescribe medications and diets. Physicians are responsible for communicating the diagnosis and explaining treatment options to clients. Treatment options should always be presented to clients at the same time they are given bad news. Only the physician or the designee can order diagnostic tests, medications, and other treatments.

Medical assistants are responsible for taking vital signs and measuring a client's height and weight. When this information is not available, a complete nutritional assessment is not possible.

Clinical pharmacists (RPhs) prepare, preserve, and compound medicines and **parenteral nutrition** preparations and dispense them according to the prescriptions of physicians, normally in collaboration with the dietician. They function as valuable resources for all team members and may also counsel clients about food–drug and drug–drug interactions.

Speech pathologists diagnose and treat swallowing disorders along with other non–nutrition-related disorders. Diagnosis involves determining the type of **dysphagia** the client manifests (see Chapter 9). Treatment for swallowing disorders may include exercises, positions, and strategies such as changing food and liquid textures for easier and safer swallowing.

Occupational therapists recommend strategies to assist clients with disabilities attain maximum functioning in activities of daily living; regarding nutrition, they may provide assistive feeding devices or help modify food preparation areas.

Social workers assess the family support system and link clients with services to help with care; they also provide assistance with financial concerns related to health care and with obtaining appropriate levels of care. They will help clients with food insecurity identify programs in their area such as food pantries and assistance programs, such as SNAP and Meals on Wheels.

Other health-care personnel who may be involved in client care include medical technologists, nurse practitioners, and psychologists. Many health-care personnel have advanced training and certification in one specific area. For example, both RNs and RDs may elect to obtain Certified Diabetes Educator (CDE) certification.

Identifying a problem but having insufficient resources to address it is more likely than having too much assistance from other team members. Many functions of health-care personnel overlap to avoid missing a client's problem (see Dollars & Sense 1-1).

Dollars & Sense 1-1

All health-care workers' roles are interconnected. Often coworkers cannot function efficiently unless someone else has completed his or her assigned duties in a timely fashion. For example, the dietitian cannot accurately estimate a client's nutritional needs without knowing the accurate height of the client. The physician is hesitant to order a tube feeding without the dietitian's recommendations, and the pharmacist will not mix a solution without knowing the client's weight. Delays in obtaining such information can have a significant impact on the cost of health care.

TABLE 1-3   Sample Subjective and Objective Nutritional Data

SUBJECTIVE	OBJECTIVE
Usual diet and fluid intake	Measured height and weight
Number of meals per day	**Edema,** severity, location
Last meal: time, foods, beverages, and amounts	Skin **turgor** and/or dryness
Food and nutrient supplements	Condition of teeth and gums
Appetite	Hair quantity and quality (brittle, easily plucked)
Problems with digestion and/or elimination	Body fat measurements
Allergies or food intolerances	Complete blood count
Usual alcohol consumption	Serum **albumin** (often of limited value)
Chewing and swallowing problems	Serum **electrolytes**
Use of dentures	Test results, such as swallow studies
Usual weight and recent changes	
Food likes and dislikes	

common in their clientele. Although no nutritional screening tool is considered the gold standard for identifying nutritional risk, a comparison of four such tools found that each identified such clients at risk.

A nutritional screening should be brief enough that the information can be gathered quickly because time is limited and there is a great deal of information that needs to be gathered. If found to be at nutritional risk, the client is referred to a dietitian.

More comprehensive than screening, a **nutritional assessment** is the second level of methodology. It is an evaluation of a client's nutritional status (nutrient stores) based on a physical examination, **anthropometric measurements,** laboratory data, and food intake information. Many members of the health-care team are involved in a comprehensive nutritional assessment, including the physician, dietitian, nurse, social worker, and laboratory staff.

Because it requires considerable resources, this second level of nutritional assessment is usually completed only in the cases of clients at high nutritional risk. For example, a surgeon may order a comprehensive nutritional assessment before surgery to determine whether the client could tolerate a procedure better after nutritional rehabilitation.

Assessment involves an organized and systematic search for pertinent subjective (what the client reports) and objective (what the health-care provider measures) data. (See samples in Table 1-3.) Note the difference between a client's reported height and weight as subjective data and the health-care provider's measured height and weight as objective data. Sometimes they may be identical, but not always. A conscientious search for accurate data creates a sound foundation on which to build nutritional care.

Subjective Data

Subjective data as they relate to nutrition include the client's history from an interview, questionnaire, or food diary. Information from the five techniques listed in Table 1-4 may be used. Some of the advantages and disadvantages of each are listed in the table. Of special concern are the food frequency questionnaires, food records, and dietary recalls, which are based on self-reported data. Though there can be substantial underreporting of intake in an individual's self-report dietary information, the practice is valuable for practitioners and to inform public health policy. The *2015-2020*

Dietary Guidelines used dietary surveillance data self-reported from NHANES to adjust recommendations to promote healthy patterns of eating, including limiting sugar to less than 10% of total caloric intake. Medical practitioners can review self-reported dietary information to obtain insight into an individual's food intake and eating patterns, but not necessarily an accurate estimate of caloric intake. However, the overall self-reported dietary intake data can be used to help guide the individual in how to eat more healthfully (Subar et al, 2015).

Neither reported dietary intake nor any other item of assessment data is suitable to use as the sole criterion of nutritional status.

Objective Data

A physical examination can include general appearance, anthropomorphic measurements, and laboratory or other diagnostic tests.

GENERAL APPEARANCE

Well-nourished people generally look healthy and usually have an optimistic perspective. Table 1-5 compares the appearance of a well-nourished individual with that of an individual who is less well-nourished. A person need not display all of the abnormal signs listed to be regarded as malnourished.

ANTHROPOMETRIC DATA

For clinical purposes, body size, weight, and proportions are determined by **anthropometry,** the science of measuring

TABLE 1-4   Commonly Used Techniques to Obtain Food Intake Information

TECHNIQUE	ADVANTAGES	DISADVANTAGES
Comparison With the MyPlate Model Health-care provider asks client what he or she eats and compares this reported food intake with MyPlate Model.	Can be used to screen many clients quickly. Requires a minimally trained interviewer.	Is not comprehensive. May overlook some clients who would benefit from nutritional care.
Food Frequency Questionnaire Health-care provider requests client fill out a questionnaire asking about **usual food intake** during specified times, such as, "What do you usually eat for breakfast?"	Questionnaire can be tailored to particular nutrients of interest (e.g., lactose, gluten). May assess food usage for any length of time: day, week, month, weekends versus weekdays, summer versus winter, etc. Initial client contact does not require a highly trained interviewer.	May require special resources (e.g., computerized database) to evaluate the information collected. Provides limited information on a client's food behaviors such as shopping and preparation, meal spacing, length of usual mealtime, etc.
Food Records Health-care provider asks client to record his or her food intake for a specified length of time (1, 3, or 7 days).	A motivated client will provide reasonably accurate information. Research shows that some clients will change their food habits while keeping a food record; therefore, this technique works well when a behavior change is desired.	A less highly motivated client will "forget to keep" part or all of the food record or record questionable amounts. Thus, this technique could yield inaccurate data to determine a client's actual dietary and/or nutritional status. May require special resources (e.g., a computerized database) to evaluate the information obtained. Requires a follow-up visit to review the evaluated food records. Analysis of data is time-consuming.
24-Hour Dietary Recall Health-care provider asks client what he or she has eaten during the previous 24 hours.	Technique is fairly simple. Interviewer should be trained not to ask leading questions.	Yields limited information. The previous 24 hours may not have been usual for the client. Typically, clients may not remember what they ate and the amounts they ate. Estimates of amounts are frequently inaccurate.
Diet History Health-care provider conducts an in-depth interview to obtain information about usual food intake, drug and medication usage, alcohol and tobacco use, financial and physical ability to obtain food, special dietary needs, food allergies and intolerances, weight history, cultural and religious preferences that may influence food selection, ability to chew and swallow foods, previous dietary instructions received, client knowledge about nutrition, and elimination patterns.	Technique is comprehensive. Requires a highly trained interviewer, usually a dietitian. An analysis of the results obtained can usually be provided on the same day the information is collected. Is a good technique for high-risk clients when information is needed to evaluate the need for nutritional support and the likelihood of dietary prescriptions being implemented.	Is highly dependent on the willingness of the client to reveal information to the interviewer. Client must be a good historian. Technique is time-consuming.

the body. Such measurements are used to determine growth, body composition, and nutritional status. The body's energy and protein stores also can be derived from these measurements. Underwater weighing and dual-energy x-ray absorptiometry (DEXA) are considered the gold standards for body composition assessment (Wang, Lim, & Caballero, 2014).

The collection of anthropometric data on height and weight—triceps skinfold, midarm circumference, abdominal circumference, waist measurements, and body density measures—is described briefly in the following sections. Other measurements may also be selected.

HEIGHT AND WEIGHT. These are the most widely used anthropometric measurements, and their derivative, the **body mass index,** is the most commonly used indirect indicator of obesity and body adiposity (Wang et al, 2014). Height may be measured in inches or centimeters. Adults and older children are measured standing with head erect; infants and young children are measured lying on a firm, flat surface.

TABLE 1-5   General Appearance as an Indicator of Nutritional Status

	NORMAL	ABNORMAL
Demeanor	Alert, responsive Positive outlook	Lethargic Negative attitude
Weight	Reasonable for build	Underweight Overweight, obese
Hair	Glossy, full, firmly rooted Uniform color	Dull, sparse; easily, painlessly plucked
Eyes	Bright, clear, shiny	Pale conjunctiva Redness, dryness
Lips	Smooth	Chapped, red, swollen
Tongue	Deep red Slightly rough One longitudinal furrow	Bright red, purple Swollen or shrunken Several longitudinal furrows
Teeth	Bright, painless	Painful, mottled, or missing, **dental caries**
Gums	Pink, firm	Spongy, bleeding, receding
Skin	Clear, smooth, firm, slightly moist	Rashes, swelling Light or dark spots Dry, cracked
Nails	Pink, firm	Spoon shaped or ridged Spongy bases
Mobility	Erect posture Good muscle tone Walks without pain or difficulty	Muscle wasting Skeletal deformities Loss of balance

Weight may be recorded in pounds or kilograms. The agency policy regarding calibration of the scale should be followed. Each time the client is weighed, it should be on the same scale at the same time of the day, and the client should be wearing the same kind of clothing.

TRICEPS SKINFOLD. Because skin is typically only 0.5 to 2 millimeters thick, skinfolds can be used as a measure of underlying fat. For this site, the tissue over the triceps muscle in the back of the upper arm is measured with calibrated calipers (Gropper & Smith, 2013). The **triceps skinfold** measurement helps to differentiate between a person who is heavy because of muscle mass and one who is heavy because of excess fat.

Dietitians usually take skinfold measurements, a skill requiring much practice. All measurements should be repeated two or three times with the average recorded as the skinfold value. A skilled provider may achieve accuracy within 5% (Gropper & Smith, 2013). Body areas other than the triceps can also be used to measure skinfolds. When measuring extremities, if U.S. survey data are the standard of comparison, the right side of the body is used. In the United Kingdom and some other locales, the left side is used (Gropper & Smith, 2013).

MIDARM CIRCUMFERENCE. Because 50% of the body's protein stores are located in muscle tissue, the circumference (the outside edge of a circle) of the midarm provides information about body protein stores. The upper arm is measured between the shoulder and the elbow. The **midarm circumference** measurement is easily obtained and can be used to monitor a client's nutritional progress.

WAIST MEASUREMENTS. A standard procedure should be used for waist measurements that are recorded in inches or centimeters according to agency procedure. In general, with the person standing, the waist is measured at the narrowest site. The tissue should not be compressed.

Abdominal circumference or girth is also used to monitor growth of a fetus or of body fat distribution within the abdomen. The measure is also valuable when an individual is accumulating fluid in the abdominal cavity, a condition called **ascites.**

BODY DENSITY MEASURES. Muscle and fat tissue have different rates of metabolism. Therefore, the proportions of each in the body influence whether a person is overweight. These proportions can be determined by several techniques, including underwater weighing, dual-energy x-ray absorptiometry (DXA), and bioelectrical impedance analysis (BIA).

Underwater weighing compares the person's scale weight with his or her weight underwater. After correcting for lung volume, the examiner calculates the proportion of body fat. Underwater weighing provides the most accurate assessment of the amount of fat in the body. It is not easily determined, however. Even in research studies, several measurements must be taken and averaged to obtain a value that minimizes error. Because the technique is cumbersome, is time-consuming, and requires special equipment, its main use is in research.

In **DXA,** two x-ray beams are passed through the body. The amount of energy detected after the beams pass through the body varies with bone, fat, and muscle tissue, and the percentage of those tissues in the body can be calculated. The x-ray exposure is relatively low: 1% to 10% of that used for a chest x-ray (Gropper & Smith, 2013). Unlike bioelectrical impedance, discussed next, DXA is not affected by the client's hydration status (Moran, Lavado-Garcia, & Pedrera-Zamorano, 2011). However, the test is resource intensive.

In clinical practice, DXA is used to measure bone mineral density as an indicator of conditions marked by bone loss, such as **osteopenia** and **osteoporosis** (see Chapter 7). A screening test to determine a person's level of risk for those conditions can be conducted with an **ultrasound bone densitometer** that involves no radiation exposure.

In the **bioelectrical impedance test,** electrodes on the extremities are stimulated with a small amount of electrical current, which is then measured at the exit electrodes. Muscle tissue, organs, and blood, rich in water and **electrolytes,** allow an electrical current to pass with greater ease than does denser fat tissue. The greater electrolyte content and conductivity of the body's **fat-free mass** is compared with that of fat. Currents are not painful and usually are not felt because of the small amount of current used.

Body composition is predicted from equations developed on specific populations and may not be valid for tests performed on other groups. The client's fat-free mass is predicted, and his or her percentage of body fat is determined by comparing body weight with the predicted fat-free mass. The three measurements obtained are percentages of the following:

1. Body water
2. **Lean body mass**
3. Body fat

Because bioelectrical impedance is based on total body water, any factors disturbing water balance may alter the results. Examples are diuretic use, excessive sweating, hemodialysis, premenstrual edema, and alcohol consumption within the 24 hours before the test.

This technology is the basis for the bathroom scales and handheld devices that measure body fat percentages (Buzzell & Pintauro, 2012).

LABORATORY TESTS

Laboratory tests analyze body fluids and excretions. These data include results from blood, urine, and stool tests. From these tests, much information can be obtained concerning what a person has eaten, what his or her body has stored, and how the body is using nutrients.

Blood can be analyzed for glucose, protein, or fat content. Vitamin and mineral status can be determined directly by examining the blood or indirectly by examining enzymes related to the vitamin or mineral. Many experts doubt, however, that vitamin or mineral body stores can be accurately determined by blood samples. The uncertainty lies in whether the nutrient in the blood reflects body stores, a transport form of the nutrient, or the amount in one specific body compartment.

Also circulating in the blood are **metabolites** that are formed in and by the body as it processes food and nutrients. An international project documented 84% of the human **serum** metabolites and electronically published a catalog of 4,229 of them for the use of scientists. In the future, a person's metabolic fingerprint might reliably evaluate his or her health and risk for certain diseases (Wood, 2012), fine-tuning present-day measures of cholesterol, for instance, which is an imperfect predictor of health or illness.

Good clinical judgment must be used in selecting tests and interpreting results. Reliance on a single test or single reading is not recommended.

Analysis/Diagnosis

The health-care provider uses subjective data, objective data, or both to identify the level of the client's wellness regarding nutrition. The client's physical findings are compared with standard nutritional parameters. His or her dietary intake is compared with that recommended for his or her age and activity level.

Physical Standards

The data gathered for a client are compared with expected results for similar clients. Commonly used standards include body mass index and waist measurements.

BODY MASS INDEX

The BMI, also known as the **Quetelet Index,** is derived from weight and height calculation to determine a person's weight status compared to an ideal weight. The BMI is non-invasive, is easily assessed at low cost, and has a strong association with body fat and health risks. There are many free BMI calculators available online (https://www.cdc.gov/healthyweight/assessing/bmi/) and for smart phones through the Google and Apple App stores.

The CDC states that BMI correlates fairly strongly as an indicator of "body fatness," but two individuals with the same BMI may have different amounts of fat. The BMI fails to distinguish **adipose tissue** from muscle or water weight. For very athletic individuals, BMI charts may falsely indicate obesity when the major body mass is not fat but muscle. In general, the difference in body fat at the same BMI can be categorized as follows: women have more than men; blacks less than whites, and Asians more than whites; older people more than younger people; and athletes less than nonathletes (Centers for Disease Control and Prevention, 2015).

Clinical Calculation 1-1 shows the calculations using metric and American measurements. Although not identical, the results are close when calculated without rounding until the final result at three decimal places. For an approximate value using whole numbers, see Table 16-2.

Having derived a value for BMI, what meaning does it have for one's health? In general, the following classifications are used:

- BMI below 18.5: Underweight
- BMI of 18.5 to 24.9: Normal
- BMI of 25 to 29.9: Overweight
- BMI of 30 to 39.9: Obese
- BMI of 40 or greater: Morbidly obese

WAIST CIRCUMFERENCE

Waist circumference of more than 40 inches in men and 35 inches in women is indicative of an android (apple) shape body and is related to increased risks of type 2 diabetes, CVDs, and all-cause mortality. This measure should be used in conjunction with other anthropometric measures to assist with the assessment of nutrition status (Harvard School of Public Health, 2017).

Dietary Intake

A client's reported or recorded food intake can be grouped according to the food classifications in MyPlate, meal patterns containing the various food groups outlined in the *2015-2020 Dietary Guidelines*, or individual foods/meals can be analyzed using a computerized diet analysis program.

CLINICAL CALCULATION 1-1

Body Mass Index

Consider a person 5 feet 10 inches tall who weighs 170 pounds.

To calculate the body mass index using metric measures:

$$BMI = \text{weight in kilograms}/(\text{height in meters})^2$$

1. Convert 70 inches to meters:
   Divide 70 by 39.37 (inches/meter) = 1.778 meters
2. Convert pounds to kilograms:
   Divide 170 by 2.2 (pounds/kilogram) = 77.273 kg
3. Insert values into BMI formula:

$$BMI = \text{weight in kilograms}/(\text{height in meters})^2$$
$$77.273/(1.778 \times 1.778)$$
$$77.273/3.161 = 24.446$$

Using the same values in an alternative American measures formula:

Weight in pounds × 705; divide by height (in inches); divide result by height in inches
$$170 \times 705 = 119,850/70 = 1712.143/70 = 24.459$$

ANALYSIS BY FOOD GROUPS

A simple method of comparing a client's reported intake with that recommended for him or her is to focus on the food groups found in MyPlate. Online calculation is available at www.choosemyplate.gov/supertracker-tools/super-tracker.html. Omitting entire food groups raises serious concerns about the adequacy of dietary intake and merits further investigation.

Remember the phrase "Garbage In, Garbage Out" pertaining to computer user fallibility; the same can be applied to dietary intake—errors are likely if amounts consumed are estimated rather than measured.

ANALYSIS OF NUTRIENTS

More detailed information can be obtained by examining foods for their component nutrients and comparing the client's data to Dietary Reference Intakes (described later). This process can be performed manually or electronically, but is normally calculated by a dietitian. In an inpatient setting, nursing staff document the client's intake of all foods at each meal and any supplements, if a more exacting calculation of intake is ordered by the health-care provider. The dietitian calculates the nutrient intake.

The USDA publishes *National Nutrient Database for Standard Reference* and updates it annually. It contains data on nearly 8,000 food items and up to 146 food components. It serves as the foundation for most food composition databases in use such as those in ChooseMyPlate.gov, commercial weight-loss firms, and apps for mobile handheld devices. Search for nutrient content of individual foods at http://ndb.nal.usda.gov.

Whether analyzed manually or electronically, care must be taken when selecting food items. For example, selection of "orange juice concentrate" instead of "orange juice" will skew the analysis badly.

Regardless of the process used, the data accumulated need correct interpretation. The only scientifically correct statement justified when intake falls short of recommended levels is that the intake for a given period does not meet whatever standard is being used as a measuring stick. It is inappropriate to base a judgment of nutritional or dietary status solely on one piece of information.

Planning/Intervention

The next step in providing nutritional care is to plan a strategy that addresses identified problems to treat or strengths to reinforce. All members of the client's health-care team should use **Motivational Interviewing (MI)** with the client. It helps determine what the client is feeling about identified issues. Then the team can determine how best to approach issues from a client-centered prospective. If a client is ambivalent about making changes to improve health, MI may help him or her discover what his or her interests in health and diet are to facilitate change and strengthen commitment (https://www.centerforebp.case.edu/practices/mi). Depending on the availability of resources and the desires of the client, the strategy for dietary intervention involves referral to a dietitian.

Prioritizing Problems

To be successful in initiating behavior change, the health-care provider, together with the client, must prioritize the problems and select acceptable interventions. Making one or two changes may be easier for the client to sustain than overhauling the client's entire diet. For that reason, selecting the interventions most likely to make a major difference in the client's health status is important.

Except for providing basic nutritional informational handouts (such as recommended eating patterns), a nurse should refer the client to a dietitian. Nurses with advanced training and certification in nutrition, such as Certified Diabetes Educators, may assume the responsibility for a client's nutrition as part of comprehensive care. Referral to a dietitian has two functions:

1. Ensuring comprehensive care.
2. Increasing the client's awareness of the need for and benefits of nutritional services.

Using Dietary Reference Intakes

To focus care more finely than the broad approach using food groups, a client's dietary intake can be compared with **Dietary Reference Intakes (DRIs).**

The DRIs are composed of five nutrient-based reference values that can be used for assessing and planning diets according to life stage and gender. The DRIs are intended to apply to the healthy general population and refer to average daily intakes for 1 or more weeks. The components of the DRIs are as follows:

- **Estimated Average Requirements (EARs):** Intake that meets the estimated nutrient needs of 50% of the individuals in the defined group. EAR is used to set the recommended dietary allowance (RDA) and to assess or plan the intake of groups.

- **Recommended Dietary Allowances (RDAs):** Intake that meets the needs of 97% to 98% of individuals in the defined group. RDA is intended for use as a goal for daily intake by individuals, not for assessing the adequacy of an individual's nutrient intake.
- **Adequate Intakes (AIs):** Average observed or experimentally determined intake that appears sufficient to meet individuals in the stated group. AI is used if an EAR or RDA cannot be set because of lack of information.
- **Acceptable Macronutrient Distribution Range (AMDR):** Percentage of kilocalories (see Chapter 5 for information on kilocalories) from carbohydrate, fat, and protein associated with reduced risk of chronic disease while still providing sufficient intake of essential nutrients.
- **Tolerable Upper Intake Levels (ULs):** Highest average daily intake by an individual that is unlikely to pose risks of adverse health effects in 97% to 98% of individuals in the defined group. Ordinarily the UL refers to intake from food, fortified food, water, and supplements; exceptions are footnoted in the table in Appendix A. The UL is designed for the general population and may be exceeded under medical supervision in clients with special needs.

Because the RDAs and AIs represent the quantities of nutrients found in typical diets in the United States and Canada, caregivers must adjust their planning for clients who take supplements or follow unusual diets. Table 1-6 compares and gives examples of these components of the DRIs. The DRIs, except the EARs, are listed in Appendix A.

Implementation

After assessment, diagnosis, and planning, the next step is implementation. It may take time and patience to select appropriate interventions for an individual client or family. Eating wisely or unwisely involves choices every day, several times a day, that affect the budget as well as health (see Dollars & Sense 1-2).

Dollars & Sense 1-2

Choosing Snacks Wisely

Veggies as snacks are not only healthier than salty munchies but also less costly and less kilocalorie dense.

Item	Price	Serving Size	Kilocalories/ Fiber	Cost/ Serving
Potato chips, national brand	$3.98/ 13.5 oz	1 oz, about 12 chips	160/1 gram	$0.30
Baby cut carrots, store brand	$1. 34/lb	2 oz, about 6 carrots	25/2 grams	$0.17

Encouraging and supporting healthy changes in a client's diet may be accomplished in various ways, but the client needs simple and flexible options to empower him or her to make healthy choices a way of life. Two straightforward, food-based (as opposed to nutrient-based) interventions include (1) ChooseMyPlate and (2) Healthy US-Style Food Pattern.

ChooseMyPlate

Much assistance, including budget advice, tips for choosing healthy foods, menus, recipes, games and activities for children, as well as guidance for parents appear on this Web site. For clients who wish to use it, the USDA interactive Web site offers a personalized nutrition and physical activity plan that also permits tracking of a person's progress at www.choosemyplate.gov/SuperTracker.

Healthy U.S.-Style Food Pattern

The *2015-2020 Dietary Guidelines* provide suggestions for different healthy meal patterns on their Web site https://www.cnpp.usda.gov/USDAFoodPatterns. The food patterns use the food group approach, ensuring that a variety of foods are chosen across and within the food groups to promote

TABLE 1-6 Dietary Reference Intake (DRI) Components

DRI	PERCENTAGE OF HEALTHY POPULATION INCLUDED	USE	EXAMPLES
EAR	50	Set RDAs Assess/plan for groups	Not applicable to individuals
RDA	97–98	Goal for individual daily intake	290 mcg of iodine for lactating women
AI	Unknown	Goal for individuals Tentative goals for groups	Vitamin K amounts for all ages Most nutrients for infants
UL	97–98	Monitor potential excesses	45 mg of iron for all older than 14 years
AMDR	Not specified	Suggested allocation of kilocalories to optimize health	Protein should contribute 10%–35% of daily kilocalories for adults

AI, adequate intake; AMDR, acceptable macronutrient distribution range; EAR, estimated average requirement; RDA, recommended dietary allowance; UL, tolerable upper intake level.

optimal consumption of high-quality, nutrient-dense food choices. Using this type of meal pattern, a 2,000-calorie-level diet would contain:

Fruit	2 cups
Vegetables	2½ cups
Grains	6 ounces (at least 3 ounces should be whole grains)
Protein	5½ ounces
Dairy	3 cups

Table 1-7 provides 3 different suggested meal patterns.

Evaluation and Documentation

After implementing a nutritional plan, the health-care provider and the client decide to what extent the objective has been met. If progress has been unsatisfactory, they explore the reasons, such as

1. Unrealistic expectations and/or client ambivalent over need to change.
2. Insufficient time allotted.
3. Interventions not appropriate.
4. Interventions incorrectly implemented or not implemented.

Documentation of services provided is a basic requirement for all health-care providers. Nurses may use the Nursing Process, and dietitians the Nutrition Care Process. The employing agency dictates the format for documentation.

One system was designed for use by several disciplines. Employing such a universal format facilitates communication among providers. An example is the system using SOAP notes. The letters stand for:

S: Subjective data (explained earlier)
O: Objective data (explained earlier)
A: Analysis or diagnosis based on S and O data
P: Plan of action or treatment

Within an agency, the client's problems may be numbered sequentially, and each SOAP note is numbered to correspond to a specific problem. In other systems, each encounter with the client is treated separately.

The Teamwork Notes following the Case Studies in this text are written in the SOAP format even though that may not be the required documentation format in the clinical facilities used by students studying nutrition. SOAP notes have the advantage of simplicity and focus on problems that should assist the student to begin to think critically as well as to see the potential for comprehensive nutritional care.

Impact of Culture on Nutrition

Culture refers to all the socially transmitted behavior patterns (attitudes, beliefs, and customs) shared by most members of a particular group that guide their thoughts and actions. Nation of origin, ethnic identity, and religious affiliation are prime examples of culture.

TABLE 1-7 Sample Meal Patterns for the Healthy U.S.-Style Food Pattern at the 2,000 Calorie Level

Meal and Snack Plans A, B, and C are examples that show just a few ways to combine meals and snacks to meet daily food group intake targets. For the 2,000-calorie-level food pattern, these targets are:
Fruits 2 cups
Vegetables 2½ cups
Grains 6 ounces (at least 3 ounces whole grains)
Protein Foods 5½ ounces
Dairy 3 cups

MEAL AND SNACK PLAN A	MEAL AND SNACK PLAN B	MEAL AND SNACK PLAN C
Breakfast 1 ounce Grains	**Breakfast** 1 ounce Grains	**Breakfast** 1 cup Fruit
½ cup Fruit	1 cup Dairy	1 cup Dairy
½ cup Dairy	1½ ounces Protein Foods	
Morning Snack 1 ounce Grains	**Morning Snack** 1 cup Fruit	**Morning Snack** 1 ounce Grains
1 cup Fruit	½ cup Dairy	½ cup Dairy
		1½ ounces Protein Foods
Lunch 2 ounces Grains	**Lunch** 2 ounces Grains	**Lunch** 2 ounces Grains
1 cup Vegetables	1 cup Vegetables	1 cup Vegetables
½ cup Fruit	½ cup Dairy	1 cup Dairy
1 cup Dairy	2 ounces Protein Foods	
2½ ounces Protein Foods		
Afternoon Snack ½ cup Vegetables	**Afternoon Snack** 1 ounce Grains	**Afternoon Snack** 1 ounce Grains
½ cup Dairy	½ cup Vegetables	½ cup Vegetables
		½ cup Dairy
		2 ounces Protein Foods
Dinner 2 ounces Grains	**Dinner** 2 ounces Grains	**Dinner** 2 ounces Grains
1 cup Vegetable	1 cup Vegetables	1 cup Vegetables
1 cup Dairy	1 cup Fruit	1 cup Fruit
3 ounces Protein Foods	1 cup Dairy	2 ounces Protein Foods
	2 ounces Protein Foods	

From cnpp.usda.gov/USDAFoodPatterns.

Health practices draw together people of similar habits, such as athletes or vegetarians. Some aspects of culture are passed on from birth, but other aspects are voluntarily selected. All aspects of culture, including the family's food ways, ethnicity, and religion, may influence an individual's food choices.

Even among individuals of similar cultural heritage, differences exist. Dietary preferences, for example, differ among people of Hispanic descent from such diverse places as Cuba, Puerto Rico, and Mexico. Just because a person belongs to a certain ethnic or religious group does not mean that he or she has adopted its traditional lifestyle and practices.

Caution is advised before replacing traditional food preparation techniques that have succeeded for generations; changes can sometimes foster disease. For example, botulism outbreaks were traced to substituting plastic bags for clay pots in preparing a Native American dish in Alaska and to swapping similar bags for waxed paper and wooden crates to ship smoked fish in Michigan. The plastic bags excluded air and permitted the botulism organism to produce its toxin. Another example is mad cow disease spreading widely after changes in feed production in England.

Relation to Longevity

Life expectancy is the prospect of a certain mean length of life at a specified age based on current **mortality** rates in the population being considered. In 2014, the life expectancy at birth was 78.8 years. Life expectancy in the United States in 2014 narrowed to 4.8 years higher for women since 1978 when they lived 7.8 years longer than men. As shown in Figure 1-5, life expectancy at birth has risen for whites and blacks in the United States since 1970, but not equally for all. The difference in Hispanic and non-Hispanic white populations' life expectancy increased by 0.3 years, from 2.7 years in 2013 to 3 years in 2014 (Kochanek et al, 2016).

The number of Americans aged 100 and above increased 43.6% from 2000 to 2014 (Xu, 2016). Certain groups display exceptional longevity that relates to nutrition. Although a single dietary pattern promoting longevity has not been recognized, kilocalorie restriction may play a role in persons surviving to the age of 100 years. Populations with an unusually high prevalence of centenarians all tended to be (or were) physically active, nonobese, and small in stature (Hausman, Fischer, & Johnson, 2011). An NIH-supported 2-year clinical trial found that calorie restriction in normal and moderately overweight individuals modified the risk factors for age-related disease. Keeping these risk factors—blood pressure, cholesterol, and insulin resistance—within normal parameters is associated with a longer life spans.

Basic Terminology

To provide sensitive health-care services to people different from oneself requires some introspection as to one's own values and attitudes. Knowledge of a few terms from the study of culture will help to arrive at a level of self-understanding and perhaps increased respect for others.

Ethnocentrism

The belief that one's own group's view of the world is superior to that of others is **ethnocentrism.** Especially in health care, providers must be sensitive and honor the cultural values of different people. Never assume that an experience with one person of a certain ethnic background can be exactly translated to another. It is very important to speak with clients to determine foods, customs, preparation techniques, and so on important to him or her. Many people are of different ethnic backgrounds, and there may be a blending of different cultures into family traditions.

Health-care providers have tried, often unsuccessfully, to deliver their own version of health care to clients without regard to the clients' cultures. Hence, clients who failed to achieve goals imposed on them were labeled "noncompliant" when in fact there was a lack of clarity in expectations due to care not being correctly focused on the client's needs.

Acculturation

The process of adopting the values, attitudes, and behavior of another culture, **acculturation,** often encourages less-desirable health behaviors than were previously practiced. An adverse effect of acculturation is the increase in various diseases in native populations. A major disease affecting widely scattered indigenous populations undergoing acculturation is type 2 diabetes mellitus. Before the 20th century, diabetes was virtually unknown among native people, but by 1987, most indigenous people had diabetes prevalence and mortality rates several times higher than comparable Caucasian populations (Ely, Zavaskis, & Wilson, 2011). The Pima Indians in Arizona currently have the highest recorded prevalence of diabetes in the world. On average, American Indian and Alaska Native adults are 2.6 times more likely to have diabetes than non-Hispanic whites of similar age (Centers for Disease Control and Prevention, 2011).

Acculturation can have positive as well as negative effects on dietary patterns; it can lead to increased awareness and knowledge of healthy foods, increased consumption of fruits and vegetables, and increased knowledge of healthy

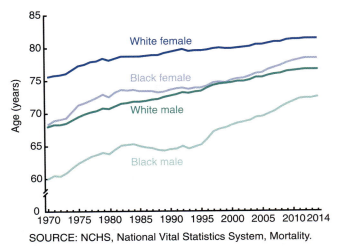

SOURCE: NCHS, National Vital Statistics System, Mortality.

FIGURE 1-5 Life expectancy at birth for U.S. blacks and whites, 1970–2014. Although all segments of the population gained some expected years of life, the ascent is steadier overall for whites than for blacks. *(From Kochanek KD, Murphy SL, Xu JQ, Tejada-Vera B. Deaths: Final Data for 2014. National Vital Statistics Reports; vol 65 no 4. Hyattsville, MD: National Center for Health Statistics. 2016. Updated April 2017. Figure 5. Available at https://www.cdc.gov/nchs/data/nvsr/nvsr65/nvsr65_04.pdf.)*

food preparation practices (Rosenmoller, Gasevic, Seidell, & Lear, 2011).

Culturally Competent Care

Knowledge and acceptance of and respect for other cultures underpin culturally competent care, which is a willingness and ability to deliver culturally congruent and acceptable care to clients. Employing institutions can assist health-care providers by attending to demographic, cultural, and epidemiological characteristics of their service areas to plan for and implement services appropriate for the cultural and language needs of their clients (U.S. Department of Health and Human Services, 2007).

Even though health-care providers cannot be experts on every cultural group they encounter, they can develop openness to learning the client's perspective. The goal is a treatment plan that successfully blends the client's cultural beliefs with the practices of modern medicine.

KEYSTONES

- Health is a state of complete physical, mental, and social well-being, not just the absence of disease or infirmity. Optimal health is not possible with an inferior diet.

- The six classes of nutrients are carbohydrates, fats (lipids), proteins, vitamins, minerals, and water. Nutrients provide fuel, support tissue growth and maintenance, and regulate body processes. Essential nutrients are those that must be supplied by the diet or artificially because the body cannot manufacture sufficient amounts for health.

- New genetic knowledge offers the potential to personalize nutrition prescriptions to avoid interactions between one's diet and his or her genes, which can adversely affect the body's use of nutrients.

- According to the USDA *Dietary Guidelines*, most people do not consume enough whole grains, milk, or fruit and ingest too many solid fats and added sugars in grain-based desserts and snacks.

- Food insecurity in the United States, affecting certain demographic groups, is addressed with information measures and market strategies with a mixed record of success.

- Nutritional care begins with assessment followed by analysis, planning, implementation, and evaluation. Assessment compiles subjective and objective data that are then analyzed to identify strengths and weaknesses. Planning with the client is essential to maximize the possibility of effective implementation and a favorable evaluation.

- The Dietary Reference Intakes (DRIs) encompass five nutrient-based reference values that can be used for assessing and planning diets for groups according to life stage and gender. The DRIs are intended to apply to the healthy general population and refer to average daily intakes for 1 or more weeks, not to judge adequacy of an individual's intake that necessitates a broader perspective.

CASE STUDY 1-1

A student in a beginning nutrition course is showing a friend the textbook. "You could help me improve my diet," the friend says. "I know I am not eating right." At the time, the friend was eating a chocolate bar. She described herself as 18 years old and sedentary. The student asks the friend to list what she had eaten during the past 24 hours. From the friend's list, the student gathers the following data:

Breakfast: 8 ounces of reconstituted frozen orange juice, 2 cups of black coffee
Lunch: 6 ounces of low-fat fruit yogurt and 6 square graham crackers
Midafternoon snack: Mr. Goodbar, 1.2 ounces
Dinner: 1 medium baked pork chop, lean only eaten, 2 cups of green salad, 2 tablespoons reduced-calorie French dressing, 12 ounces of Diet Coke

Opening a profile on ChooseMyPlate.gov, and inserting the friend's height and weight (5 ft 4 in., 163 lbs), the student finds that her friend's BMI is 28.0 (overweight) and her 1-day intake compares with the recommended 1800 kilocalorie intake as follows:

	Friend's Intake	ChooseMyPlate
Oils	3 tsp	5 tsp
Milk	¾ cup	3 cups
Meat and beans	4 oz	5 oz
Vegetables	1 cup	2½ cups
Fruits	1 cup	1½ cups
Grains	1½ oz	6 oz
Discretionary kilocalorie allowance	327	161

In this situation, the student probably would not formalize a nutritional care plan for the friend, but the following plan illustrates the thought process involved in developing a care plan for this case.

CARE PLAN

Subjective Data
Expressed need for instruction in healthy diet. Twenty-four-hour recall shows less than the recommended ChooseMyPlate intake for all food groups but excessive discretionary kilocalories.
Overweight from reported height and weight

Objective Data
Observed eating a chocolate bar at 3 p.m.

Analysis
Self-reported need to improve nutrition

Plan

DESIRED OUTCOMES EVALUATION CRITERIA	ACTIONS/ INTERVENTIONS	RATIONALE
Friend will keep a food record for 3 days.	Instruct friend to list everything she eats or drinks for 3 days.	Food record will gather facts about the friend's food intake to use as an instructional tool.
Friend will read the section on ChooseMyPlate in student's textbook by this evening.	Lend friend textbook to read.	Providing literature uses expert opinion to reinforce student's teaching. Reading and seeing illustrations elicits active participation and employs senses other than hearing.
Friend will meet with student in 4 days to compare food record to ChooseMyPlate profile and design a plan of action.	Meet with friend in 4 days to sort and analyze food record data. Provide apples at meeting to model healthy snack food.	Setting follow-up visit just after food record is completed will maintain the friend's interest. Modeling desirable behavior is a technique to encourage change.

After 4 days, the two friends met in the college library to access ChooseMyPlate on the Internet. The friend says that she has not been keeping the requested food diary. "I'm hopeless. I'll never be able to change," she moans. They sat outdoors and ate the apples that the nutrition student provided, but her friend washed hers down with another Mr. Goodbar. At that point, thinking that her friend required more professional help than her friendship could provide, the student recommended the free clinic run by the college's nursing department. They walked to the clinic together so that the friend could make an appointment.

TEAMWORK 1-2

CLINIC'S NOTES

The following Clinic's Notes are representative of the documentation found in a client's medical record.

Subjective: Requesting assistance with diet planning. Shared dietary recall from last week. Not inclined to keep food diary. Denies chronic illness. Has attempted weight control on her own with little success due to splurging on sweets. Recognizes need for lifestyle changes as well as dietary improvement. Unsure of social support for lifestyle changes.

Objective: Ht 5 ft 4 in. Wt 163 lbs. BMI 28.0. VS WNL (vital signs within normal limits)

Analysis: Overweight due to unbalanced diet and sedentary lifestyle.

Plan: Instruct in basic nutrition. Suggest private use of ChooseMyPlate.gov site to track diet and activity, or downloading an app to her smart phone to track diet and activity. Recommend participation in daily walking group that meets in the Physical Education Department to achieve 150 minutes of physical activity weekly along with the possibility of social support from fellow walkers. Follow-up visit in 1 week.

CRITICAL THINKING QUESTIONS

1. The 24-hour dietary recall in Case Study 1-1 tallies just 987 of the 1800 kilocalories recommended for the individual, yet she has been unsuccessful with weight control. What possible factors might explain the discrepancy?

2. When the nutrition student met with the friend after 4 days, what other options might have been chosen instead of referral to the nursing clinic?

3. You have a friend or relative who displays food intake similar to that described in Case Study 1-1. You care deeply for this person. How might you approach the subject of healthy eating if the person does not ask for assistance?

CHAPTER REVIEW

1. Which of the following is an energy nutrient? Select all that apply.
   1. Phytochemicals
   2. Fats
   3. Vitamins
   4. Minerals
   5. Carbohydrates

2. Which of the following techniques is used to estimate the body's protein stores?
   1. Weighing the person under water
   2. Measuring midarm circumference
   3. Calculating the body mass index
   4. Determining triceps skinfolds

3. Intake that meets the needs of 97% to 98% of individuals in a defined group is called:
   1. Acceptable macronutrient distribution range
   2. Adequate intakes
   3. Estimated average requirements
   4. Recommended dietary allowances

4. Most individuals in the United States eat all of the following *except*: (Select all that apply.)
   1. A healthy U.S.-style diet
   2. Too much sodium and simple sugars
   3. Too little fiber
   4. Too few fruits and vegetables
   5. Not enough servings of dairy

5. The important, supportive role nurses have in obtaining a client's accurate nutritional assessment includes: (Select all that apply.)
   1. Obtaining an accurate height and weight
   2. Documenting what the client states about recent food intake
   3. Documenting that the client states that he has had nausea and vomiting for the past 2 days
   4. Obtaining client's cultural and/or religious food preferences

CLINICAL ANALYSIS

1. Ms. G has just been found to have type 2 diabetes. Which of the following actions by the nurse shows respect for Ms. G?

   a. Instructing her to increase her intake of vegetables
   b. Telling her to lose weight and avoid alcohol and fast-food restaurants
   c. Giving Ms. G an instruction sheet based on MyPlate
   d. Asking Ms. G what her interests are in respect to learning about a healthy lifestyle related to diabetes

2. Mr. P is a 65-year-old man, recently widowed, whose physician is recommending weight loss. Mr. P has had little experience with grocery shopping or cooking. Which of the following systems for instructing Mr. P would the nurse select to offer the best chance of success?

   a. A computerized diet analysis program
   b. ChooseMyPlate
   c. Exchange lists
   d. The RDA/AI tables

3. Ms. E attended a community health fair where she entered her recalled intake for the previous 24 hours into a computer for analysis. On the basis of the printout she was given, she now thinks that she should begin taking vitamin and mineral supplements. A friend who is a nurse correctly bases her advice on the following:

   a. A 1-day diet recall offers inadequate data on which to base supplementation.
   b. A hand recalculation should be done to verify the accuracy of the computer printout.
   c. The RDAs on which computer programs are based are intended for only the 50% of the population who are obsessed with health.
   d. Undoubtedly, the operators of the computer at the fair had a product to sell: "Let the buyer beware."

CHAPTER 2

Carbohydrates

LEARNING OBJECTIVES

After completing this chapter, the student should be able to:

- Describe the types of carbohydrates, identify food sources of each, and indicate their functions in the body.
- List the major functions of carbohydrates and methods through which the body stores them.
- Discuss dietary fiber and list its functions.

- Describe the relationship between carbohydrates and dental health.
- List the carbohydrate content (in grams) of each appropriate food group.
- Discuss dietary recommendations related to fiber, added sugar, and total carbohydrate intake.

Carbohydrates, fats, and proteins all meet the body's basic energy needs. Carbohydrates are the major source of energy because they break down rapidly and are readily available for use. This chapter defines basic terminology related to carbohydrates and discusses the body's use of carbohydrates and the way carbohydrates relate to the other energy nutrients.

Green plants manufacture carbohydrates during a complex process called **photosynthesis.** In this process, carbon dioxide from the air and water from the soil are transformed into sugars and **starches.** Sunlight and the green pigment **chlorophyll** are necessary for this conversion. All the food we eat is a product of photosynthesis. If this process did not occur, the whole food chain would collapse, and life would cease. Figure 2-1 illustrates this process.

On the basis of their chemical structure, carbohydrates are divided into two major groups: sugars and starches. Sugars have a simple structure; starches are more complex. Therefore, sugars are often called **simple carbohydrates,** and starches are called **complex carbohydrates.**

Composition of Carbohydrates

Understanding the composition of carbohydrates involves understanding three structures: molecule, element, and atom:

1. A **molecule** is the smallest quantity in which a substance may be divided without loss of its characteristics. For example, the chemical formula for water is H_2O. If the hydrogen atoms are pulled from the oxygen atom, the resulting products are hydrogen and oxygen, which bear no resemblance to water. Molecules are made of elements. In the case of water, H_2O, the elements are hydrogen and oxygen.

2. An **element** is a substance that cannot be separated into simpler parts by ordinary means.
3. An **atom** is the smallest particle of an element that retains its physical characteristics.

Basic Terminology

Carbohydrates are composed of the elements carbon, hydrogen, and oxygen. The ratio of hydrogen to oxygen is the same as that for water: two parts of hydrogen to one part of oxygen. The simplest carbohydrates have the formula $C_6H_{12}O_6$. Carbohydrates are frequently abbreviated CHO.

Simple carbohydrates (sugars) include monosaccharides and disaccharides (*mono* means one, *di* means two, and *saccharide* means sweet). Starches are called **polysaccharides.**

Simple Carbohydrates

Simple carbohydrates are of two types: monosaccharides and disaccharides.

1. A **monosaccharide** contains one molecule of $C_6H_{12}O_6$.
2. A **disaccharide** is composed of two molecules of $C_6H_{12}O_6$ joined together (minus one unit of H_2O).

When the body joins two monosaccharide molecules, a molecule of water is released in the process.

Monosaccharides

Monosaccharides are the building blocks of all other carbohydrates. The three monosaccharides of importance in human nutrition are glucose, fructose, and galactose. Note the *ose* ending in the name of each of these sugars. All monosaccharides and disaccharides end with the letters *ose*.

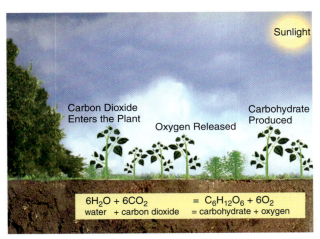

FIGURE 2-1 Photosynthesis is a vital process that transforms carbon dioxide and water into carbohydrates.

$$6H_2O + 6CO_2 = C_6H_{12}O_6 + 6O_2$$
water + carbon dioxide = carbohydrate + oxygen

Glucose

The monosaccharide glucose in the body is commonly called blood sugar. It is the major form of sugar in the blood. Normal **fasting blood sugar (FBS)** is 70 to 100 milligrams per 100 milliliters of serum or plasma. **Impaired fasting glucose (IFG)** is 100 to 125 milligrams per 100 milliliters of serum or plasma (https://www.niddk.nih.gov/health-information/diabetes/overview/what-is-diabetes/prediabetes-insulin-resistance). Regardless of the form of sugar consumed, the body readily converts it to glucose.

Another name for glucose is **dextrose** (abbreviated D). Clients in health-care facilities often receive intravenous feedings. **Intravenous** means within or into a vein. The most common intravenous feeding is D_5W (5% dextrose in water), used primarily to deliver fluids to the client.

Fructose

Fructose is found in fruits and honey. It is the sweetest of all the monosaccharides. Fructose is used extensively in soft drinks, canned foods, and various other processed foods. High-fructose corn syrup (HFCS) is very sweet because the cornstarch has been treated with an enzyme that converts some of the naturally present glucose to the sweeter fructose. The human body readily converts fructose to glucose. HFCS has been used by the food industry because it is a cheaper sweetener for beverages than sugar. Sweetened beverages account for 47% of added sugars in the U.S. population, age 2 and older. The *Dietary Guidelines* recommend that added sugars should comprise less than 10% of total daily calories. It is estimated that Americans consume more than 13% of added sugars in their daily diet (https://health.gov/dietaryguidelines/2015/guidelines/). The increased calories from sweetened beverages may contribute to the incidence of overweight and obese individuals, which increases the chances of developing diabetes and cardiovascular disease.

Galactose

The monosaccharide galactose comes mainly from the breakdown of the milk sugar lactose. Yogurt and unaged cheese may contain free galactose. It is the least sweet of all the monosaccharides. The body converts galactose into glucose after ingestion.

Disaccharides

When two monosaccharides are linked, a disaccharide is formed. The three important disaccharides are:

1. Sucrose
2. Lactose
3. Maltose

Sucrose

The most prevalent disaccharide, sucrose, is ordinary white table sugar made commercially from sugar beets and sugar cane. Brown, granulated, and powdered sugars are all forms of sucrose. Sucrose is also found in molasses, maple syrup, fruits, and vegetables. The two monosaccharides joined to form sucrose are glucose and fructose. See Box 2-1 for more information on sugar in the U.S. diet.

Lactose

Because lactose occurs naturally only in milk, it is commonly referred to as milk sugar. Lactose is the least sweet of the disaccharides. The two monosaccharides that make up lactose are glucose and galactose.

Maltose

Maltose is a double sugar that occurs primarily during starch digestion. The disaccharide maltose is produced when the body breaks starches into simpler units. Smaller amounts

---

BOX 2-1 ■ Added Sugar in the U.S. Diet

Added sugars contribute to dental caries, reduce the intake of essential micronutrients when sugar in the diet displaces more nutritious items such as milk, and may lead to an increased incidence of cognitive impairment in the elderly.

The increased consumption of added sugars is linked to a decreased intake of essential micronutrients and an increase in body weight. Data from the National Health and Nutrition Examination Survey, 2005–2010, indicate that children and adolescents obtain approximately 16% of their total kilocalories from added sugars, and adults 13% (Ervin & Ogden, 2013; https://health.gov/dietaryguidelines/2015/guidelines/).

What is an appropriate amount of added sugar in a healthful diet? According to the American Heart Association, no more than 100 kilocalories for women and 150 kilocalories for men should consist of added sugars per day (American Heart Association, 2017).

Currently, the largest contributor of added sugar in the diet is sweetened beverages (sweetened soft, fruit, sport, and energy drinks), which provide 47% of added sugars. The second largest contributor is snacks and sweets at 31% (https://health.gov/dietaryguidelines/2015/guidelines/).

of this disaccharide are present in malt, malt products, beer, some infant formulas, and sprouting seeds. Maltose consists of two units of glucose.

Sugar in Foods

The amount of sugar that is in a food product can be found on its label. The total amount of sugar in grams can be found on the Nutrition Facts portion of the label. The Food and Drug Administration (FDA) has mandated that by 2020 manufacturers will have to use a new food label, shown in Figure 2-2, which discloses the total amount of added sugar in a product. Sugar is present naturally in foods and added to foods. The definition of added sugars includes sugars that are either added during the processing of foods or are packaged as such (https://www.fda.gov/Food/GuidanceRegulation/Guidance-DocumentsRegulatoryInformation/LabelingNutrition/ucm513734.htm#AddedSugars).

The federal government regulates the use of the terms such as *sugar-free*, *reduced sugar*, and *less sugar* for food products that have added sugar. Terms such as these can be located anywhere on the package's label. Table 2-1 lists the standards, or definitions, for legally defined label descriptors.

TABLE 2-1   Approved Definitions for Food Label Terms

TERM	STANDARD
Sugar-free	Contains less than one-half gram of sugars per serving
Reduced sugar or less sugar	At least 25% less sugar or sugars per serving than a standard serving size of a traditional food
No added sugar or without added sugar	No sugars added during processing or packing, including ingredients that contain sugar, such as juice or dry fruit
Low sugar	May not be used as a claim on a food label

From Food and Drug Administration (2017).

Sugar Alcohols

Some food products contain **sugar alcohols.** Sugar alcohols have various names, such as sugar replacers, polyols, nutritive sweeteners, and bulk sweeteners. Lactitol, maltitol, isomalt, sorbitol, xylitol, and mannitol are all sugar alcohols and currently are approved for use in the United States.

Sugar alcohols are commonly used on a one-for-one replacement basis for sugars in recipes. For example, one cup of sugar would be replaced with one cup of isomalt in a recipe. Sugar alcohols add not only sweetness but also bulk to recipes. Sugar alcohols have the following characteristics:

- Generally do not promote tooth decay.
- Commonly have a cooling effect on the tongue.
- Are slowly and incompletely absorbed from the intestine into the blood.
- May have a laxative effect for some people if consumed in excess.

Nonnutrative Sweeteners

Nonnutrative sweeteners (NNS) are sugar substitutes that provide intense sweetness. Unlike sugar replacers, NNS do not add bulk or volume to a food product; they add only sweetness. They are 150 to 500 times as sweet as sugar and are mostly artificial, or synthetic. There are eight NNS approved for use in the United States, shown in Table 2-2 (Food and Drug Administration, 2015).

Complex Carbohydrates

Chemically complex carbohydrates are called polysaccharides. *Poly* means many, and polysaccharides consist of many molecules of $C_6H_{12}O_6$ joined and many molecules of water released in the process. Polysaccharides can be composed of various numbers of monosaccharides and disaccharides. The three types of complex carbohydrates of nutritional importance are starch, glycogen, and fiber. Table 2-3 summarizes the composition of carbohydrates.

Nutrition Facts

8 servings per container
Serving size   2/3 cup (55g)

Amount per serving
Calories   **230**

	% Daily Value*
Total Fat 8g	**10%**
Saturated Fat 1g	**5%**
Trans Fat 0g	
Cholesterol 0mg	**0%**
Sodium 160mg	**7%**
Total Carbohydrate 37g	**13%**
Dietary Fiber 4g	**14%**
Total Sugars 12g	
Includes 10g Added Sugars	**20%**
Protein 3g	
Vitamin D 2mcg	10%
Calcium 260mg	20%
Iron 8mg	45%
Potassium 235mg	6%

* The % Daily Value (DV) tells you how much a nutrient in a serving of food contributes to a daily diet. 2,000 calories a day is used for general nutrition advice.

FIGURE 2-2 New food label showing total added sugar. *(From https://www.fda.gov/Food/GuidanceRegulation/GuidanceDocumentsRegulatoryInformation/LabelingNutrition/ucm385663.htm#QA, accessed on Nov. 27, 2017.)*

TABLE 2-2 Nonnutritive Sweeteners

ARTIFICIAL SWEETENER	TRADE NAME	COMMENTS
Acesulfame potassium (Ace-K)	Sweet One Sunett	Used as a sweetener and flavor enhancer in foods in general, excluding meat and poultry
Advantame		Used to sweeten dairy drinks, frozen desserts, beverages, and chewing gum
Aspartame	Nutrasweet	Used in sweetened products such as puddings, gelatins, frozen desserts, yogurt, hot cocoa mixes, powdered soft drinks, carbonated beverages, teas, breath mints, chewing gums, some vitamins, and cold preparations. Also used as a tabletop sweetener. Reviewed by regulatory agencies such as the Centers for Disease Control and FDA and found to be safe. Should not be used by individuals with a rare genetic disease called phenylketonuria (www.aspartame.org).
Neotame	Newtame	Used as a sweetener and flavor enhancer in foods in general, excluding meat and poultry
Saccharin	Equal Sweet'N Low Sugar Twin	Artificial sweetener Carbonated beverages, toothpaste, cold remedies, dietetic puddings, cakes, cookies Saccharin was banned in Canada in 1977. The U.S. FDA also proposed a ban on saccharin, but Congress passed a moratorium on the ban. Although high doses of saccharin were shown to cause bladder cancer in male rats, numerous human studies have shown no association between saccharin and cancer at human levels of consumption.
Sucralose	Splenda	The only noncaloric sweetener made from sugar. Approved for use by the FDA.
Steviol glycosides	Truvia PureVia Enliten	Only the forms listed have been granted approval by the FDA, not whole stevia leaves (which are sold as dietary supplements).
Siraitia grosvenorii Swingle (Luo Han Guo) fruit extracts (SGFE)	Nectresse Monk Fruit in the Raw PureLo	

Adapted from https://www.fda.gov/Food/IngredientsPackagingLabeling/FoodAdditivesIngredients/ucm397725.htm#Advantame (2015).

TABLE 2-3 Composition of Carbohydrates

Elements	C (carbon) H (hydrogen) O (oxygen)
Molecule	$C_6H_{12}O_6$
Monosaccharide (simple)	One unit of $C_6H_{12}O_6$
Disaccharide (simple)	Two units of $C_6H_{12}O_6$ minus one unit of H_2O
Polysaccharide (complex)	Many units of $C_6H_{12}O_6$ minus many units of H_2O

BOX 2-2 ■ Legumes

Legumes include these dried peas and beans:

- Black beans
- Pinto beans
- Kidney beans
- Navy beans
- Soybeans
- Black-eyed peas
- Split peas
- Yellow peas
- Chick peas (garbanzo)
- Lentils

Starch

Starch, the major source of carbohydrate in the diet, is found primarily in grains, starchy vegetables, legumes, and in foods made from grains—cereals, breads, and pasta. Box 2-2 lists different kinds of legumes. Strictly speaking, all starches yield simple sugars on digestion; starchy foods are mostly low in fat and high in carbohydrates, and some starchy foods have the advantage of containing much fiber.

Glycogen

Glycogen represents the body's carbohydrate stores. Glucose is stored in liver and muscle tissue as the polysaccharide **glycogen.** Glycogen is crucial to the function of the human body. During intense physical activity, the body uses blood glucose for energy. When blood glucose is depleted, muscle glycogen is broken down to provide immediate fuel in the form of glucose. Glycogen is built up and stored in muscle and the liver when blood glucose levels are high after infusion from the diet. Liver glycogen helps sustain blood glucose levels during sleep.

The typical human body has an available store of glucose in the form of glycogen for about 1 day's energy needs. Because the body's ability to store carbohydrates in the form of glycogen is limited, an adequate intake of dietary carbohydrates is essential. When glycogen is stored, water is also stored. Each glycogen molecule attracts many molecules of water because of the way the elements are arranged. When glycogen stores are completely filled, the average person weighs about 4 lb more than when glycogen stores are empty.

Dietary Fiber

Dietary fiber refers to foods, mostly from plants, that the human body cannot break down to digest and is eliminated in intestinal waste. Sometimes called roughage or bulk, fiber adds almost no fuel or energy value to the diet, but it does add volume. Bulk fills the stomach, and most experts believe that a full stomach contributes to a feeling of **satiety,** and so further eating ceases. The *2015-2020 Dietary Guidelines* recommend that at least half of grains consumed are whole grain, to help attain the goal of increasing fiber in the diet. The recommended daily **adequate intake (AI)** for fiber is based on 14 grams of fiber per 1,000 kcalories consumed or:

- Males (age): grams per day
  - (9 to 13): 31
  - (14 to 50): 38
  - (51 to >70): 30
- Females (age): grams per day
  - (9 to 18): 26
  - (19 to 50): 25
  - (51 to >70): 21

In the United States, the average person consumes less than the recommended amount of dietary fiber, and few people consume the recommended levels. The U.S. Department of Agriculture (USDA) estimates that men consume 18 grams and women 15 grams of fiber each day (U.S. Department of Agriculture, 2014). Whole grains are an excellent source of dietary fiber. Dollars & Sense 2-1 provides a recipe for an economical, easy-to-prepare vegetable soup.

Eating too much fiber can cause problems. Evidence suggests that eating more than 50 grams of fiber a day can interfere with mineral absorption, which can lead to conditions such as anemia and osteoporosis. Healthy people should achieve a desirable fiber intake by consuming fiber-rich fruits, vegetables, legumes, and whole-grain cereals, which also provide minerals, vitamins, and **phytochemicals,** instead of adding fiber concentrates (such as psyllium) to their diet.

Fiber is classified as either soluble or insoluble. **Solubility** is the ability of one substance to dissolve in another. For example, oil does not dissolve in water, and so oil is insoluble in water. Insoluble fiber does not dissolve in water, whereas soluble fiber does. Soluble fiber and insoluble fiber react differently in the body and are needed for different reasons.

Dollars & Sense 2-1
Vegetable Soup

Plan your meals around whole grains. Start with whole-wheat pasta, precooked brown rice, and beans (kidney, chick peas, white, etc.) and add other ingredients (leftover meats, seafood, quinoa, tofu, etc.) as your budget allows.

Pack several containers, freezing some as desired, of this economical, easy-to-fix lunch or dinner for those super busy times.

16-ounce can beans (any kind—kidney, chick peas, white, etc.), drained
2 fifteen-ounce cans tomatoes, stewed, low sodium
28 ounces vegetable broth, low sodium
16 ounces vegetables, mixed, frozen (any kind—plain, no sauce)
1 cup whole-wheat pasta, quinoa, precooked brown rice (frozen or packaged)
½ cup onion, chopped
1 teaspoon olive oil
2 cloves garlic, to taste (optional)
dash pepper, to taste (optional)
dash cayenne pepper or red pepper flakes, to taste (optional)

1. Sauté onion in olive oil for approximately 5 minutes or until slightly soft.
2. Combine all ingredients, except the whole-wheat pasta or precooked brown rice.
3. Bring to a boil.
4. Add whole-wheat pasta or precooked brown rice (along with optional ingredients, if desired) to the pot and simmer, covered, for approximately 10 minutes or until the pasta (if using) and/or vegetables are tender.

Makes approximately 6 servings.

Soluble Fiber

Sources of soluble fibers include beans, oatmeal, barley, broccoli, and citrus fruits; oat bran is a particularly good source of soluble fiber. Soluble fibers dissolve in water and thicken to form gels. Reported health benefits of soluble fibers include reduced cholesterol levels, regulated blood sugar levels, and weight loss (by helping dieters feel full).

Insoluble Fiber

Examples of sources of insoluble fibers include the woody or structural parts of plants, such as fruit and vegetable skins, and the outer coating (bran) of wheat kernels. Insoluble fibers have been reported to promote regularity of bowel movements and reduce the risk of diverticular disease and some forms of cancer. The mechanism of these effects for insoluble fiber is due to decreased intestinal transit time and decreased intestinal pressure. Table 2-4 lists the food sources of each type of fiber and their reported health benefits.

Functions of Carbohydrates

Carbohydrates play the following roles in the body:

- Provide fuel
- Spare body protein

TABLE 2-4 **Foods and Reported Benefits of Fiber**

	INSOLUBLE FIBER	SOLUBLE FIBER
Solubility	Does not dissolve in water	Dissolves in water
Food sources	Wheat bran Corn bran Vegetables Nuts Fruit skins Some dry beans*	Oatmeal Oat bran, barley Some fruits, such as apples, oranges Broccoli Some dry beans*
Benefit	Promotes regularity May help reduce risk of some forms of cancer May reduce risk of diverticular disease	May help reduce cholesterol levels May assist in regulating blood sugar levels May promote weight loss by increasing satiety†

*Current laboratory methods to assay soluble fiber content of individual foods are imprecise. This is the subject of much research.
†Satiety is defined as the sensation of fullness after eating.

- Help prevent ketosis
- Enhance learning and memory processes

Provide Fuel

Carbohydrates, fats, and proteins provide the body's energy needs. **Energy** is the capacity to do work. To understand the concept of energy, think of the human body as a machine. Just as gasoline is a car's fuel, carbohydrates, proteins, and fats are the human machine's fuel. Without fuel, a car powered by gas ceases to operate. Without fuel sources over an extended time, the human machine dies from starvation. Just as a person cannot efficiently substitute something other than gasoline to fuel a car with a gasoline engine, a person cannot efficiently substitute something other than carbohydrate, protein, or fat for fuel in the human body.

Carbohydrate is a primary source of fuel for all cells in the body. The brain is a carbohydrate-dependent organ and must have an uninterrupted, ongoing source. The recommended dietary allowance (RDA) for carbohydrate is 130 grams per day for adults and children based on the minimum amount of glucose used by the brain. The diet should be composed of 45% to 65% carbohydrates (National Academies of Sciences, 2016).

Spare Body Protein

A continuous supply of glucose is required for all cells to function, particularly those of the central nervous system. Body glycogen stores are limited, and after they are depleted, the body can convert protein to glucose. The body will break down internal protein stores (muscle tissue) before fat stores if carbohydrate intake is inadequate. An adequate supply of dietary carbohydrates spares body protein stores from being partially converted into glucose and

allows protein to be used for growth and repair of body tissue. This principle has important ramifications, which are discussed throughout the text.

Help Prevent Ketosis

A balanced intake of energy nutrients is vital. If carbohydrate intake is too low, the body will break down both stored fat and internal protein to meet its fuel needs. The body cannot handle the excessive breakdown of stored fat because the body lacks the necessary equipment. As a result, partially broken-down fats accumulate in the blood in the form of ketones, and the person is said to be in a state of **ketosis.** Survival is possible on a very low carbohydrate diet, but good health is not.

Fatigue, nausea, and lack of appetite are some of the undesirable consequences of ketosis. Coma and death have occurred in severe cases. The presence of ketosis is easily determined by testing for the presence of acetone or diacetic acid in the urine. **Acetone** and **diacetic acid** are ketone bodies. The American Diabetes Association (ADA) recommends 130 grams of carbohydrate per day as the minimum intake. A very low carbohydrate diet, which is ketogenic, is defined as 20 to 50 grams per day. It is recognized that between individuals and even the same individual over time the level of carbohydrate to induce ketosis may vary (Feinman et al, 2015).

Enhance Learning and Memory

Considerable evidence exists that blood glucose concentrations regulate neural and behavioral processes. Glucose enhances learning and memory in humans throughout the life cycle. Performance in school improves for children who consume breakfast with regular frequency. Children who eat breakfast have a higher intake of fiber, total carbohydrate, and lower fat and cholesterol. Those who eat breakfast were also found more likely to have a normal body mass index (Adolphus, 2013). Diets that are high in fats and sugars have been found to cause impairment of cognition and mood and dysregulation of appetite control, a vicious cycle that leads to obesity (Beilharz, Maniam, & Morris, 2015).

Health and Carbohydrates

The kinds of carbohydrates eaten are important to health. Epidemiological data support the association between a high intake of vegetables and fruits and low risk of chronic disease. Legumes are low in fat and are excellent sources of protein, fiber, micronutrients, and phytochemicals. Studies have linked regular consumption of whole grains with a lower risk of certain cancers and heart disease. Many nutrition experts attribute these health benefits to the fiber contained in whole grains.

Sugary foods also often displace other more nutritious foods in the diet. For example, carbonated beverages may be consumed instead of milk and fruit juices. The *2015-2020 Dietary Guidelines for Americans* recommends reducing the calories consumed from added sugars. The American Heart

Association (AHA) recommends that women should eat or drink no more than 100 calories per day from added sugars (25 grams or 6 teaspoons) and men 150 calories per day (38 grams or 10 teaspoons) (American Heart Association, 2017). Clinical Calculation 2-1 provides information on converting grams of sugar into teaspoons of sugar.

Consumption Patterns

Most of the world's population subsists primarily on carbohydrates. Foods rich in carbohydrates are easily grown in most climates, low in cost, and easily stored. Many carbohydrates do not require refrigeration or electricity, and their shelf life (the time a product can remain in storage without deterioration) may stretch to years. In Asia, where rice is a dietary staple, carbohydrates provide as much as 80% of the fuel in the diet. The *Dietary Guidelines* recommend that no more than 10% of total calories should come from added sugars. In the United States, added sugar is 13% of total calories, with the highest consumption in beverages, which accounts for 47% of intake. Adults average only one serving per day of whole grains, and three-fourths of the population has an eating pattern low in vegetables, fruits, and dairy (https://health.gov/dietaryguidelines/2015/guidelines/).

The *2015-2020 Dietary Guidelines for Americans* recommend shifts in meal patterns to include foods from across and within all food groups in correct portions to assist in maintaining a healthy weight. Nutrient density recommendations include consuming:

- A variety of vegetables
- Whole fruits
- Grains, at least half should be whole grains
- Fat-free or low-fat dairy (milk, yogurt, cheese), and soy products
- Legumes as a good plant-based source of protein and fiber

Dental Caries

Several studies have shown a relationship between carbohydrate consumption and dental caries (see Clinical Application 2-1). Dental caries is the gradual decay of the teeth. A dental cavity is a hole in a tooth caused by dental caries. Dental caries results from the interaction of four factors: a genetically susceptible tooth, bacteria, carbohydrate, and time. All four must occur simultaneously for a cavity to form, as Figure 2-3 illustrates. Some people are more genetically susceptible to caries than other people, as Genomic Gem 2-1 discusses.

CLINICAL APPLICATION   2-1

Nursing-Bottle Syndrome

Nursing-bottle syndrome is a dental condition caused by the frequent and prolonged exposure of an infant's or young child's teeth to liquids containing sugars. Milk, formula, fruit juice, and other sweetened drinks can all cause rampant dental cavities.

Typically, nursing-bottle syndrome occurs when a caretaker habitually puts a baby to bed with a bottle of milk, juice, or other sweetened liquid. During sleep, the flow of saliva decreases, which allows liquids from the nursing bottle to pool around the teeth, undiluted for extended periods. Parents need to be cautioned against this practice.

The main ways to maintain oral health include these steps:

- Reduce consumption and especially frequency of food and drink containing sugar.
- Consume sugar only as part of a meal.
- Snacks and drinks should be sugar-free.
- Avoid frequent consumption of acidic drinks.

CLINICAL CALCULATION   2-1

Converting Grams of Sugar Into Teaspoons of Sugar

An added sugar intake of 60 grams does not mean much to average American consumers, because most Americans are not familiar with the metric system. Food labels use the metric system to list the nutritional content of a product. To enhance understanding of label reading, let us convert grams of sugar into teaspoons. One teaspoon of sugar contains 4 grams of carbohydrates. Therefore, 60 grams of sugar is equal to 15 teaspoons.

Distinguished from the natural sugars, such as lactose in milk and fructose in fruits, added sugars are those incorporated into foods and beverages during production. Major sources of added sugar include the following:

- Candy
- Soft drinks
- Fruit drinks
- "Energy" and sports drinks
- Grain-based desserts, such as cookies, cakes, and pastries

In the *2015-2020 Dietary Guidelines*, the U.S. Department of Agriculture estimates that most Americans consume a diet of 13% added sugars. This contributes to a diet high in calories and low in nutrients.

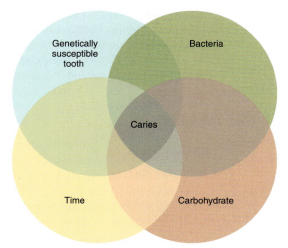

FIGURE 2-3 Interactions necessary for dental cavity formation.

GENOMIC GEM 2-1

Caries

Genetic susceptibility is an individual's likelihood of developing a given trait as determined by heredity. We cannot control our genetic susceptibility for cavities, and bacteria are always present in our mouths and difficult to eliminate. However, we can control the length of time carbohydrate-containing foods are in our mouths and the kinds of carbohydrates we eat.

Risk Factors for Cavity Formation

Bacteria, carbohydrate-containing foods, and the length of time that teeth are exposed to sugars influence cavity formation. Bacteria that normally present in the mouth interact with dietary carbohydrates and produce acids. The acids, not the sugar, cause decay. All types of sugars can promote cavity formation, including fructose, glucose, maltose, lactose, and sucrose.

A strong relationship exists between the length of time sugars are present in the mouth and the development of caries. For example, sticky foods such as caramels and raisins, which adhere to the tooth surface for long periods, are more likely than other foods to lead to tooth decay in susceptible people. Sipping sweetened beverages continually throughout the day can lead to tooth decay.

Eating Right to Prevent Cavities

Certain foods may help counteract the effects of the acids produced by oral bacteria. Aged cheese (cheddar, Swiss, blue, Monterey jack, brie, gouda), as well as processed American cheese, may inhibit tooth decay. Cheese stimulates the production of saliva. Chewing fibrous foods such as apples or celery stimulates the production of generous amounts of saliva. Saliva helps clear the mouth of food and counteracts acid production. Because saliva production is increased during a meal, sugars eaten with a meal are less likely to cause decay than those eaten between meals.

Food Sources

Carbohydrates fall into two general groups: sugars and starches. All starches contain fiber; however, all starches do not provide equal amounts of fiber.

Sugars

Table sugar contains approximately 4 grams of carbohydrate per teaspoon. When determining a person's sugar consumption, consider not only the simple sugars, such as honey, jam, and jelly, but also the sugars present in sweet foods and drinks, such as carbonated beverages, ice cream, sherbet, cakes, pies, cookies, and donuts. Sugar alcohols contain on average about 2 grams of carbohydrate per teaspoon.

Starches

Starches are complex carbohydrates and are important sources of fiber and other nutrients. Figure 2-4 illustrates a typical cereal grain. Its main parts are the germ, bran, and endosperm. Most of the nutrients in cereal are in the bran and germ.

Whole grains are more nutritious than refined grains, in which nutrients are removed during the **milling** process. During the milling of grain, the germ and bran are removed from the grain kernel. White flour results from the milling of wheat and white rice from the milling of rice. Oat products are not normally milled. The nutritive value of cereal depends on the amount of bran and germ retained during the milling process. For this reason, the use of whole grains should be encouraged whenever possible. Examples of whole grains include the following:

- Cornbread made from whole ground cornmeal
- Ground cornmeal
- Cracked wheat bread
- Oatmeal and oatmeal bread
- Pumpernickel bread (when made from whole-grain flours)
- Rye bread (when made from whole-grain flours)
- Whole-wheat bread
- Breads made from bran
- Barley
- Graham crackers

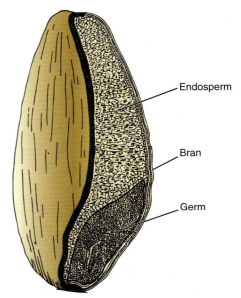

FIGURE 2-4 The most nutritious parts of wheat germ are the bran and endosperm, which are removed during the milling of grain.

Endosperm

Bran

Germ

Carbohydrate Counting

In health care, carbohydrate counting helps teach clients about the carbohydrate content of foods and healthful portion sizes, which helps manage blood glucose levels. A serving is not the amount commonly eaten but a defined amount of a particular food according to nutrition experts. One serving of dairy, fruit, grain, cereal, bread, or starchy vegetable is considered to be 15 grams of carbohydrate (American Diabetes Association, 2015). Eating 45 to 60 grams of carbohydrate at each meal is recommended as a starting point for managing diabetes (Diabetes.org). Eating too much of any of the energy nutrients can result in unhealthful weight gain and uncontrolled blood glucose. Portion sizes are important to know for the success of carbohydrate counting. Food labels, which list the grams of carbohydrate per serving, must be used along with correct portion size of foods. If the label indicates that a serving size of rice is ½ cup of cooked rice, the rice must be measured before consumption. If a nutrition label indicates that a package of a prepared food, such as pretzels, contains 2½ servings, the consumer must portion the number of pretzels per serving (which is listed on the label) and count out the pretzels to have the correct amount of carbohydrate per serving.

Food Groups

For a well-balanced diet, it is important to consume a variety of foods from within and across all the food groups each day. The following are examples of portion sizes for common foods within the food groups equaling one portion of carbohydrate, which would be used in carbohydrate counting (https://ndb.nal.usda.gov/ndb/search/list?).

Grains

Grains can be important contributors to meeting recommendations for fiber intake in the diet, if the food contains whole grains. One serving from the grain food group is 15 grams of carbohydrate.

- ¾ cup ready-to-eat cereal, unsweetened
- ½ cup cooked cereal, unsweetened
- 1, one-ounce slice whole-wheat bread

Vegetables

Raw and cooked vegetables are also good sources of carbohydrates. Vegetables contain between 2 and 3 grams of fiber per serving. One serving of vegetable contains approximately 5 grams of carbohydrate. One-half cup of cooked vegetables or one cup of raw vegetables equals one serving. Vegetables also contribute vitamins and minerals to the diet.

Starchy vegetables contain 15 grams of carbohydrates per serving.

- ½ cup starchy vegetable (corn, peas)
- 3 ounces potato (baked, boiled)

Fruits

Fruits are another source of carbohydrates. One serving of fruit contains approximately 15 grams of carbohydrates. Many fruits are excellent sources of fiber and contain vitamins and minerals.

- 1, four-ounce raw apple
- ½ cup applesauce, unsweetened
- ½ small banana (4 ounce)
- ¾ cup blueberries
- ½ cup unsweetened 100% juice (orange, grapefruit, pineapple)

Dairy

Milk, with its lactose content, is an important source of carbohydrates. One cup of milk contains 12 grams of carbohydrates. Skim, whole, and 2% milk all contain approximately the same amount of carbohydrates.

- 1 cup milk (cow's, soy, rice)
- 6 ounces yogurt (plain or artificially sweetened)

Protein

Plant-based proteins are significant sources of protein, fiber, vitamins, and minerals. One serving of beans or lentils contains 15 grams of carbohydrate.

- ½ cup cooked legumes (beans: black, garbanzo, kidney, lima, navy, pinto white, soy; lentils: brown, yellow, green, red)

Dietary Recommendations

The Food and Nutrition Board of the National Academy of Sciences, Institute of Medicine, issued dietary recommendations for carbohydrates in 2005 (Food and Nutrition Board, 2005). To meet the body's daily energy and nutritional needs, while minimizing risk for chronic disease, adults should get 45% to 65% of their calories from carbohydrates.

The committee reasoned that because carbohydrates, fat, and protein all serve as energy sources and can substitute for one another to some extent to meet caloric needs, the recommended ranges for consuming energy nutrients should be useful and flexible for dietary planning—hence the wide 45% to 65% range. The ranges for children are similar to those for adults in respect to carbohydrates.

The RDA for children older than 1 year and most adults younger than 70 years is 130 grams of carbohydrates per day. The RDA is 175 grams of carbohydrates per day for pregnant women and 210 grams per day for lactating women. According to the *2015-2020 Dietary Guidelines for Americans,* no more than 10% of total calories eaten should comprise added sugars (https://health.gov/dietaryguidelines/2015/guidelines/). The emphasis in these guidelines is to ensure that nutrient-dense foods are consumed across and within the food groups, ensuring adequate intake of all nutrients required for good health.

KEYSTONES

- Carbohydrates are composed of sugars and starches.
- The average American's intake of sugars is considered excessive, whereas the intake of starches is considered low.
- Many Americans would benefit from increasing their fiber intake through the consumption of more whole-grain starches, fruits, and vegetables.
- Dietary carbohydrates promote tooth decay in susceptible individuals.
- Strong evidence exists that a minimum of 130 grams of carbohydrates per day is necessary for adequate brain and body function.
- When there is no or little carbohydrate in the diet and the body uses protein or fat as a fuel source, the body in effect cannibalizes itself for glucose. Muscle and organ mass is lost in the process.
- The RDA for carbohydrates is 130 grams of carbohydrates a day. Pregnant and lactating women have a higher RDA for carbohydrates.

CASE STUDY 2-1

K.L. is a 19-year-old college student. He is interested in bodybuilding and spends much of his time on strength conditioning. He lifts weights or uses an elliptical machine daily. He is 6 feet tall and weighs 175 lb. For the past 3 weeks, he has been drinking a powdered protein supplement (that contains no carbohydrate) instead of eating the dorm food, which he states "isn't any good anyway." He also takes a high-stress vitamin and mineral tablet. He arrived at the clinic today with complaints of fatigue, nausea, a lack of appetite, lightheadedness, and memory loss. His urine tested positive for ketones. The client is willing to talk to a registered dietitian.

CARE PLAN

Subjective Data
The client has chosen not to eat any foods that contain carbohydrates for approximately 3 weeks.

Objective Data
Urine positive for ketones.

Analysis
Inadequate intake of carbohydrates, related to erroneous ideas about healthy eating as evidenced by verbal statements that he has not been eating carbohydrate-containing foods and by urine positive for ketones.

Plan

DESIRED OUTCOMES EVALUATION CRITERIA	ACTIONS/ INTERVENTIONS	RATIONALE
Client will state one reason why he needs carbohydrates by the end of the appointment.	Encourage client to consume foods from MyPlate, including milk, starches, fruits, and vegetables. Refer to the dietitian for instruction on normal nutrition and protein needs for athletes.	Explaining why carbohydrates are necessary in the diet may motivate the client to eat carbohydrates. Milk, vegetables, fruits, and starches are all good sources of carbohydrates. The nurse may need to educate the client about dietary sources of carbohydrates.
Schedule the client for a return visit in 1 week. Client will keep a food record for the dietitian.	On next visit, ask client to demonstrate knowledge gained. (For example, "How many servings of starch, fruits, and vegetables do you need daily?") Test the urine for ketones at the next visit.	

TEAMWORK 2-1

DIETITIAN'S NOTE

The following Dietitian's Notes are representative of the documentation found in a client's medical record.

Subjective: *Client states that he wants to be able to lift more weight. Food records for 4 days show an average daily intake of 18 meats, 12 fats, 1 starch, 1 fruit, 1 vegetable, and 1 low-fat milk. Client states that he has just recently added starch, fruit, and milk to his diet per nurse's recommendation. Client continues to complain of fatigue and constipation. He finds it difficult to concentrate and study.*

Objective: *Ketones in urine, weight 175 lb (79.54 kg), height: 6 ft*

Analysis: *Ideal body weight 178 ± 10%; estimated protein needs 81–97 grams. Estimated kcal need based on 79.54 kg and 25–35 kcal/kg = 1989–2784. Food records show an approximate intake of 2111 kcal and 25% protein, 66% fat, and 8% carbohydrate.*

Inadequate carbohydrate intake related to food and nutrition–related knowledge deficit as evidenced by ketone smell on breath, complaints of fatigue and difficulty concentrating, and food records.

Client appears open to learning and prefers written and oral instructions.

Plan:
1. *Client to substitute carbohydrates kcal for fat kcal by eliminating bacon, olives, soy nuts, and fatty meats from diet.*
2. *Client agreed to try adding 3 cups low-fat milk, 4 vegetables, 3 fruits, and 6 whole grains to diet.*
3. *Appointment scheduled for follow-up in 1 week.*
4. *Copy of MyPlate given to client.*

CRITICAL THINKING QUESTIONS

1. At the client's next visit, what would you do if the food records showed a recorded carbohydrate intake of only 30 grams for most days? What if the client said, "I don't want to eat any more because I feel better"?

2. At the next client visit, what would you do if the food records showed that the client ate only sugar to increase his carbohydrate intake because "Sugar is a quick energy food"?

3. At the next client visit, what would you do if he made no changes to his diet?

CHAPTER REVIEW

1. Which of the following is a disaccharide?
   1. Glucose
   2. Lactose
   3. Fructose
   4. Galactose

2. A healthy adult needs ____ grams of fiber each day.
   1. 5 to 11
   2. 12 to 20
   3. 21 to 38
   4. More than 50

3. Twelve grams of simple carbohydrate is equal to ____ teaspoon(s) of sugar.
   1. 1
   2. 2
   3. 3
   4. 8

4. The average American doesn't consume enough: (Select all that apply.)
   1. Fiber
   2. Simple carbohydrate
   3. Fruit and vegetables
   4. Energy drinks

5. Carbohydrates have the following roles in the body *except*: (Select all that apply.)
   1. Promotes ketosis
   2. Spares body protein
   3. Provides fuel
   4. Impact learning and memory
   5. Promotes tooth decay

6. The average American consumes: (Select all that apply.)
   1. 46% added sugars each day
   2. Enough whole grains
   3. 15 to 18 grams of fiber
   4. 15 grams of carbohydrate
   5. 13% added sugars

CLINICAL ANALYSIS

1. Ms. C is concerned about the dangers associated with the consumption of artificial sweeteners and wants to know if they are safe. As a health-care worker, it is appropriate for you to:

   a. Ignore Ms. C's comments because you think that she is overly concerned.
   b. Assure her that the government would not allow a food or herbal product to be sold if it was hazardous to her health.
   c. Explain to her that no food is guaranteed to be 100% safe, and it is best to avoid artificial sweeteners if she is not comfortable with these products.
   d. Refer her to the local health food store.

2. Mr. J claims that he is trying to lose weight, and his urinalysis shows that his urine contains ketones (ketonuria). You should ask him:

   a. When he ate last
   b. How much milk, fruit, and starch he usually eats
   c. What else he usually eats
   d. All of the above

3. Mr. P complains of constipation. As his nurse, you would like to teach him to eat more insoluble fiber to help alleviate his discomfort. You should encourage the intake of:

   a. Wheat and corn bran, nuts, fruit skins, and dried beans
   b. Eggs, cheese, and chicken
   c. Milk, yogurt, and ice cream
   d. Oatmeal, barley, and broccoli

CHAPTER 3

Fats

After completing this chapter, the student should be able to:
- Identify how fats are classified.
- List the major functions of fats both in the diet and in the body.
- Discuss the relationships to health of cholesterol, saturated fat, polyunsaturated fat, *trans*-fatty acids, and monounsaturated fat.

- List three current recommendations of the Food and Nutrition Board of the National Research Council that pertain to fat.

This chapter presents an introduction to lipids for students without a chemistry background. Chapter 18 expands on this chapter and discusses clinical nutrition in more detail. The descriptive name for fats of all kinds, *lipids*, is used in clients' medical records. **Lipids** include true fats and oils as well as related fatlike compounds such as **lipoids** and **sterols.** Fats are a major source of fuel for the body. Dietary fat is found in both animal and plant products. Animal fats, which consist of a larger content of saturated fats, tend to have a higher melting point and are solid at room temperature. Plant-derived fats are normally in the form of oils, having a lower melting point and comprising more unsaturated fats than animal products.

Lipids are **insoluble** in water and are greasy to the touch. When two insoluble substances are mixed together, such as vinegar and oil, they separate readily. You can shake the vinegar and oil combination repeatedly, but it will still separate after the agitation stops.

Basic Terminology

Lipids are composed of the elements carbon, hydrogen, and oxygen. These are the same three elements that make up carbohydrates, but the proportion of oxygen to carbon and hydrogen is lower in fats. The basic structural unit of a true fat is one molecule of **glycerol** joined to one, two, or three fatty acid molecules. Glycerol is the backbone of a fat molecule.

A **fatty acid** is composed of a chain of carbon atoms with hydrogen and a few oxygen atoms attached. The fatty acid chains joined to the glycerol molecule vary in length (depending on the number of carbon atoms present) and composition. The different taste, smell, and physical appearance of each fat results from the variety of fatty acids and their physical arrangement in the fat molecules. Beef fat

tastes, smells, and looks different from that of chicken mostly because of the difference in fatty acid composition. All fats contain fatty acids.

A fat can have from one to three fatty acids, and the number of fatty acids a fat contains has important implications for both diet and health.

Monoglycerides and Diglycerides

When a single fatty acid is joined to a glycerol molecule, the resulting fat is called a **monoglyceride.** When two fatty acids are joined to a glycerol molecule, the fat is called a **diglyceride.** The terms *monoglyceride* and *diglyceride* are commonly seen on food labels.

Triglycerides

When three fatty acids are joined to a glycerol molecule, a **triglyceride** is formed. Most of the fat found in our diets and in the body is in the form of triglycerides. Excess triglycerides are stored in the specialized **adipose cells** that make up adipose tissue. The human body has a virtually unlimited capacity to store fat. Figure 3-1 illustrates the structure of monoglycerides, diglycerides, and triglycerides.

Length of Fatty Acid Chain

Fatty acids vary in the length of their fatty acid chains: Each chain is determined by the number of carbon atoms present, which can vary from 2 to 24. The length of the chain determines how the body transports the fat in the body; fatty acid chains of short length (<6 carbon atoms) and medium length (8 to 12 carbon atoms) are processed differently compared with longer chains. The chain length has dietary implications in many diseases. For example, in certain diseases

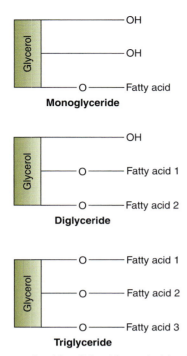

Monoglyceride

Diglyceride

Triglyceride

FIGURE 3-1 Monoglycerides, diglycerides, and triglycerides. A monoglyceride has one fatty acid attached to the glycerol molecule, a diglyceride has two fatty acids attached to the glycerol molecule, and a triglyceride has three fatty acids attached to the glycerol molecule.

of malabsorption, the client cannot tolerate foods with long-chain fatty acids. This problem is discussed in more detail in Chapter 20.

Degree of Saturation

The terms *saturated,* trans *fats, unsaturated, monounsaturated,* and *polyunsaturated* have become household words. Consumers and clients ask sophisticated questions about fats and expect health-care professionals to define and explain the terminology. Technically, all of these terms refer to the chemical structure of fatty acids, based on the degree or nature of the hydrogen atom saturation.

The degree of saturation of a fatty acid depends on the extent to which hydrogen is joined to the carbon atoms present. A **saturated fatty acid** is filled with as many hydrogen atoms as the carbon atoms can bond with and has no double bonds between carbons. In this case, a **double bond** describes the type of chemical connection between two neighboring carbon atoms, each lacking one hydrogen atom. In an **unsaturated fatty acid,** the carbon atoms are joined together by one or more of such double bonds.

Wherever a double bond occurs, another hydrogen atom could potentially join the chain. In other words, the fatty acid chain is lacking hydrogen atoms and is thus less saturated than a chain that is completely filled. A fatty acid with only one carbon-to-carbon double bond is **monounsaturated.** A fatty acid with more than one carbon-to-carbon bond is **polyunsaturated.** In addition to the fats in the

body, the fats found in foods are combinations of saturated and unsaturated fatty acids. They are designated as follows:

- Saturated fat: Composed mostly of saturated fatty acids
- Unsaturated fat: Composed mostly of unsaturated fatty acids
- Monounsaturated fat: Composed mostly of monounsaturated fatty acids (MUFA)
- Polyunsaturated fat: Composed mostly of polyunsaturated fatty acids (PUFA)
- *Trans*-fatty acids: Composed of partially hydrogenated fatty acids

Figure 3-2 shows the types of fatty acids in common dietary fats and oils.

Physical Properties and Food Sources

Terms such as *saturated fats, unsaturated fats,* and *hydrogenation* are commonly used. This section introduces these terms and discusses food sources.

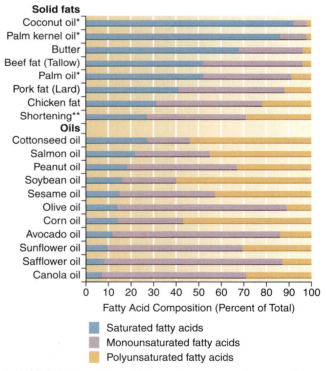

FIGURE 3-2 Comparison of fatty acid composition of common fats and oils. The oil with the highest monounsaturated fat content is olive oil. The oil with the lowest saturated fat content is canola. *Coconut, palm kernel, and palm oil are called oils because they come from plants. However, they are solid or semi-solid at room temperature due to their high content of short-chain saturated fatty acids. They are considered solid fats for nutritional purposes. **Shortening may be made from partially hydrogenated vegetable oil, which contains trans fatty acids. *(From U.S. Department of Agriculture and U.S. Department of Health and Human Services: Dietary Guidelines for Americans, ed 8. December 2015. Available at http://health.gov/dietaryguidelines/2015/guidelines/. Data from U.S. Department of Agriculture, Agricultural Research Service, Nutrition Data Laboratory. USDA National Nutrient Database for Standard Reference. Release 27, 2015. Available at http://ndb.nal.usda.gov/. Accessed August 31, 2015.)*

Saturated Fats

Saturated fats, which are likely to be solid at room temperature, are usually found in animal products such as meat, poultry, and whole milk. The exceptions are tropical coconut and palm-kernel oils and cocoa butter, which are vegetable sources of saturated fat. See Tables 3-1 and 3-2 for a more complete list of foods containing saturated fat.

Saturated fats are more chemically stable than unsaturated fats. For this reason, saturated fats become **rancid** slowly because the chemical bond between carbon and hydrogen is stable. A rancid fat has an offensive odor and taste caused by the partial chemical breakdown of the fat's molecular structure. Consumers usually discard rancid foods because of the highly offensive odor.

Products made with saturated fats have a fairly long shelf life because the fat in the product is fairly stable. However, saturated fats have been targeted for reduction in the average American's diet by health authorities because these fats have unhealthful effects when ingested in excess of the body's needs.

Unsaturated Fats

Unsaturated fats are likely to be liquid at room temperature and of plant origin; they tend to become rancid more quickly than saturated fats. The double carbon bonds in unsaturated fatty acids are unstable and therefore easily broken. For this reason, many convenience products have traditionally been made with saturated fats to lengthen their shelf life. The food industry is changing this practice; increasingly, more convenience products are made with unsaturated fats. Examples of unsaturated fats are corn, cottonseed, safflower, soybean, and sunflower oils. See Table 3-3 for a more complete list of unsaturated fats.

Hydrogenation

Commercial food processing frequently involves hydrogenation—adding hydrogen to a fat of vegetable origin (unsaturated) either to extend the fat's shelf life or make the fat harder. This process of adding hydrogen to a fat is called **hydrogenation.** If only some of the fat's double bonds are broken by the hydrogenation, the product becomes partially hydrogenated. If all of the double bonds are broken, the product becomes completely hydrogenated.

Completely hydrogenated fats are highly saturated fats; that is, they have no carbon-to-carbon double bonds. For example, a completely hydrogenated corn oil is closer to lard in saturation than a partially hydrogenated corn oil. All vegetable spreads, such as corn oil margarine, have been hydrogenated to some extent. If these spreads had not been hydrogenated, they would be liquids (except for the saturated tropical oils). Clients are usually advised to avoid products that contain completely hydrogenated

TABLE 3-1   Food Sources of Saturated Fats

Meat products	Visible fat and marbling in beef, pork, and lamb, especially in prime-grade and ground meats, lard, suet, salt pork
Processed meats	Frankfurters Luncheon meats, such as bologna, corned beef, liverwurst, pastrami, and salami Bacon and sausage
Poultry and fowl	Chicken and turkey (mostly beneath the skin), Cornish hens, duck, and goose
Whole milk and whole-milk products	Cheeses made with whole milk or cream, condensed milk, ice cream, whole-milk yogurt, all creams (sour, half-and-half, whipped)
Plant products	Coconut oil, palm-kernel oil, cocoa butter
Miscellaneous	Fully hydrogenated shortening and margarine, many cakes, pies, cookies, and mixes

TABLE 3-2   Selected Foods High in Cholesterol and/or Saturated Fat

FOOD	AMOUNT	CHOLESTEROL (mg)	SATURATED FAT (mg)
Liver	3 oz	410	2.4
Cream puff	1	228	10.0
Baked custard	1 cup	213	7.0
Egg, hard cooked	1	215	5.0
Waffles, homemade	2	204	8.0
Coconut custard pie	1 piece	183	8.0
Cheesecake	3.25 oz	170	10.0
Shrimp, boiled	6 large	167	0.2
Eggnog, commercial	1 cup	149	11.0
Bread pudding/raisins	1 cup	142	4.5
Whole milk	1 cup	124	5.0
Ground beef, 21% fat	3 oz cooked	76	7.0

TABLE 3-3 Food Sources of Unsaturated Fats

FOODS HIGH IN MONOUNSATURATED FATTY ACIDS	FOODS HIGH IN POLYUNSATURATED FATTY ACIDS
Canola, olive, peanut oils	Corn, cottonseed, mustard seed, safflower, sesame, soybean, and sunflower seed oils
Almonds, avocados, cashews, filberts, olives, and peanuts	Halibut, herring, mackerel, salmon, sardines, fresh tuna, trout, whitefish

fats when the therapeutic goal is to decrease saturated fat intake.

A health consequence of hydrogenation is the formation of *trans*-**fatty acids.** *Trans*-fatty acids are produced by the partial hydrogenation of unsaturated vegetable oils. The Food and Drug Administration (FDA) has determined that partially hydrogenated fats are not generally recognized as safe (GRAS). Beginning in June 2018, manufacturers were required to stop using these fats in foods (FDA.gov).

During hydrogenation, many of the fatty acids are converted into *trans* fats. Evidence indicates that the *trans* fats are detrimental to health. If the dietary goal is to decrease consumption of *trans*-fatty acids, the client must decrease consumption of hydrogenated foods. Foods that may be high in *trans*-fatty acids may include the following:

- Commercially baked goods
- Fried foods in restaurants
- Hard margarines and shortenings
- Crackers
- Biscuit and some cake mixes
- Some candy
- Animal crackers and cookies
- Frozen waffles and pancakes
- Microwave popcorn

The food industry has reformulated many of these products to decrease their *trans*-fatty acid content in anticipation of the FDA ban. It is important for clients to read nutrition labels on foods to ensure that ingestion of *trans* fats is avoided or greatly limited.

Functions of Fats

Lipids are important in the diet and serve many functions in the human body.

Fats in Food

Fats serve several functions in food, including serving as a fuel source and acting as a vehicle for fat-soluble vitamins.

Fuel Source

Fats are the major dietary source of fuel. Because fats have proportionately more carbon and hydrogen and less oxygen than carbohydrates, fats have a greater potential for the release of energy. In practical terms, this means that fats are a concentrated source of fuel or kilocalories.

Fats furnish more than twice as many kilocalories, gram for gram, as carbohydrates. Each gram of fat yields 9 kilocalories, so 1 teaspoon of fat, which is equivalent to 5 grams of fat, yields 45 kilocalories. Compare these numbers with those for carbohydrates, each gram of which yields only 4 kilocalories. A teaspoon of sugar contains 4 grams of carbohydrates and therefore yields only 16 kilocalories.

Vehicle for Fat-Soluble Vitamins

In foods, fats act as a vehicle for vitamins A, D, E, and K.

Satiety Value

Fats also contribute flavor, satiety value, and palatability to the diet. They supply texture to food, trap and intensify its flavor, and enhance its odor. Satiety is a person's feeling of fullness and satisfaction after eating. Fat contributes to the sensation of satisfaction because it leaves the stomach more slowly than carbohydrates.

Consider for a moment the sensations felt when eating 2 cups of ice cream versus 2 cups of chopped apples. Ice cream has a high fat content, and apples have no fat. An individual may feel full after eating 2 cups of apples but complain of a bloated feeling and a lack of gratification. Satiety is feeling full and completely satisfied, and that enough or too much food has been eaten.

Sources of Essential Fatty Acids

An essential nutrient is one that must be supplied by the diet because the body cannot manufacture it in sufficient amounts to prevent disease. Fat contains the essential fatty acids linoleic, arachidonic, and linolenic. Linolenic acid is subdivided into two groups, alpha and gamma. Figure 3-3 shows the pathways of these fatty acids.

Although the body can manufacture gamma-linoleic (linolenic) acid and arachidonic acid from linoleic acid, all three of these fatty acids are considered essential. Linoleic is called an omega-6 fatty acid. Omega is the last letter in the Greek alphabet and is used by chemists for naming fatty acid classes by their chemical structure. The six designation means that the first double bond is located six carbons down the chain (counting from the omega end).

Linoleic acid strengthens cell membranes and has a major role in the transport and metabolism of cholesterol. The omega-6 fatty acids together prolong blood-clotting time, hasten fibrolytic activity, and are involved in the development of the brain. **Prostaglandins,** compounds with extensive **hormone**-like actions, require arachidonic acid for synthesis.

Another name for alpha-linolenic fatty acid (ALA) is omega-3 PUFA. The omega-3 PUFA has a variety of biological effects that may influence the risk of cardiovascular disease. Eicosapentaenoic acid (EPA) and docosahexaenoic acid (DHA) are inefficiently converted from ALA. The recommendation is to obtain these fatty acids from foods

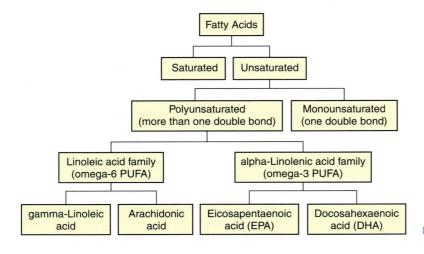

FIGURE 3-3 Classification of fatty acids.

due to their anti-inflammatory role. The AHA recommends two servings of seafood per week to increase omega-3 PUFA in the diet, which has been demonstrated to reduce the incidence of cardiovascular disease when consumed through food, but not supplements (Jump, 2014; American Heart Association, 2017).

The clinical signs of essential fatty acid deficiency are manifested in dry scaly skin, decreased growth in infants and children, increased susceptibility to infection, and poor wound healing (Jump, 2014).

Linoleic acid deficiency was observed in the early 1970s in hospitalized clients fed exclusively with intravenous fluids containing no fat. Symptoms included scaly skin, hair loss, impaired wound healing, increased susceptibility to infection, and immune dysfunction. When lipids were introduced into intravenous feedings, such symptoms ceased.

Fats in the Body

The major functions of fat in the human body include the following:

1. Supply fuel to most tissues
2. Function as an energy reserve
3. Insulate the body
4. Support and protect vital organs
5. Lubricate body tissues
6. Form an integral part of cell membranes
7. Carrier for the absorption of fat soluble vitamins

Fuel Supply

Fat serves as a fuel that supplies body tissues with needed energy.

Fuel Reserve

Fat also functions as the body's main fuel or energy reserve. Excess kilocalories consumed are stored in specialized cells called adipose cells. When an individual does not eat enough food to meet the energy demands of the body, the adipose cells release fat for fuel.

Lubrication

Fats also lubricate body tissue. The human body manufactures oil in structures called sebaceous glands. Secretions from the sebaceous glands lubricate the skin to retard loss of body water to the outside environment.

Organ Protection

Fatty tissue cushions and protects vital organs by providing a supportive fat pad that absorbs mechanical shocks. Examples of organs supported by fat are the eyes and kidneys.

Insulation

The subcutaneous layer of fat beneath the skin helps to insulate the body by protecting it from excessive heat or cold. A sheath of fatty tissue surrounding nerve fibers provides insulation to help transmit nerve impulses.

Cell Membrane Structure

Fat serves as an integral part of cell membranes and in this capacity plays a vital role in drug, nutrient, and metabolite transport and provides a barrier against water-soluble substances.

Carrier for Fat-Soluble Vitamins

Fat is a carrier of the fat-soluble vitamins A, D, E, and K and carotenoids so that they may be adsorbed by the body.

Cholesterol

Cholesterol is not a true fat but belongs to a group called sterols. Cholesterol is a component of many of the foods in our diet. In addition, the human body manufactures about 1,000 milligrams of cholesterol a day, mainly in the liver. The liver also filters out excess cholesterol and helps eliminate it from the body. See Genomic Gem 3-1.

Functions

Cholesterol has several important functions. It is:

1. A component of bile salts that aid digestion
2. An essential component of all cell membranes

GENOMIC GEM 3-1

Familial Hypercholesterolemia

Familial hypercholesterolemia (FH) is a genetic disorder that causes severely elevated LDL cholesterol and a 90-fold increase in atherosclerotic cardiovascular disease (ASCVD) mortality in young adults if left untreated. Early intervention with statins is essential in reducing ASCVD mortality. It has previously been thought to be present in 1 out of 500 people. Recent analysis has estimated the figure to be closer to 1 out of every 250 people or approximately 1.5 million people in the United States (de Ferranti et al, 2016).

3. Found in brain and nerve tissue and in the blood
4. A precursor for the production of steroid hormones

Cholesterol is necessary for the production of several hormones, including:

- Cortisone
- Adrenaline
- Estrogen
- Testosterone

A **hormone** is a substance produced by the endocrine glands and secreted directly into the bloodstream. Hormones stimulate functional activity of organs and cells or stimulate secretion of other hormones to do so.

Food Sources

Cholesterol is present only in animal foods. When animal products are ingested, one also ingests the cholesterol the animal made. The *2015-2020 Dietary Guidelines for Americans* recommends a healthy eating pattern that limits the amount of saturated fat to less than 10% of total calories and therefore a decreased level of cholesterol (from 100 to 300 mg per day based on the calorie level followed). According to the *2015-2020 Dietary Guidelines for Americans*, evidence suggests that a lower intake of dietary cholesterol is associated with a reduced risk of cardiovascular disease. However, eating patterns consist of multiple food components that may interact. The relationship to health exists for the overall pattern and not necessarily one component. The *Dietary Guidelines* no longer make a specific quantitative guideline for cholesterol, citing the need for more evidence. Some foods, such as eggs and shellfish, are higher in cholesterol but not saturated fats and may be consumed with a variety of other foods as part of a healthy eating pattern. See Table 3-2 for a list of selected foods high in cholesterol.

Most nutrition experts evaluate the total diet for risk prevention. An overall healthy eating pattern that includes fruits, vegetables, and whole grains is important for risk reduction. No one food, even if it contains cholesterol, is unhealthy if eaten in appropriate amounts.

Dietary Recommendations Concerning Fat

The National Academy of Science report on Dietary Reference Intakes for Macronutrients issued guidelines pertaining to fats in 2005 (Food and Nutrition Board, Institute of Medicine, 2005). These remain the current guidelines. Box 3-1 discusses the acceptable macronutrient distribution range (AMDR) for fats.

Before this recommendation, most government health authorities and professional groups recommended that the fat content of the U.S. diet should not exceed 30% of caloric intake. The rationale for the change is that carbohydrates, fat, and protein all serve as fuel sources and can substitute for one another to some extent to meet fuel needs. Therefore, the recommended ranges for consuming these nutrients should be useful and flexible for dietary planning (Food and Nutrition Board, Institute of Medicine, 2005). Table 3-4 lists the recommended ranges in grams of fat for various calorie levels. See Clinical Calculation 3-1 as well.

The Food and Nutrition Board of the Institute of Medicine stated that saturated fat and cholesterol provide no known beneficial role in preventing chronic diseases and are not required at any level in the diet. However, the complete elimination of saturated fat and cholesterol from the diet would make it difficult to meet other nutritional guidelines. The *2015-2020 Dietary Guidelines* recommend that individuals reduce the intake of calories from solid fats, and limit *trans* fats as much as possible in the diet because they are not essential in the diet and may be linked to increasing

BOX 3-1 ■ Acceptable Macronutrient Distribution Range for Fats

A range of intake for a particular energy source that is associated with a reduced risk of chronic disease and that provides adequate intakes of essential nutrients is called the acceptable macronutrient distribution range (AMDR). The AMDR for adults is 25%-35% of kilocalories from fat. The AMDR for children aged 1-3 is 30%-40% of kilocalories from fat.

TABLE 3-4 Recommended Range of Fat Intake at Selected Kilocalorie Levels

KILOCALORIE LEVEL	TOTAL FAT (GRAMS)
1200	26–46
1500	33–58
1600	35–62
1800	40–70
2000	44–78
2200	49–85
2400	53–93
2500	55–97

CLINICAL CALCULATION   3-1

Percent of Kilocalories from Fat

The following formula can be used to determine the percentage of kilocalories from fat in many packaged foods:

Kilocalories from fat per serving/kilocalories* $\times$ 100 = percent kilocalories from fat per serving

Example: kilocalories from fat = 30
Kilocalories per serving = 90
% kilocalories from fat = 30%

*Food labeling regulations require manufacturers to list both the number of kilocalories in a serving and the number of kilocalories from fat.

Dietary Fat

A diet that has an appropriate balance of fat and carbohydrate is important for optimal health. Chronic consumption of either a low-fat/high-carbohydrate or a high-fat/low-carbohydrate diet may result in the inadequate intake of nutrients. A diet too low in fat not only lacks satiety and palatability but may also lack adequate levels of the essential fatty acids, zinc, and certain B vitamins. Excessive dietary fat has been associated with an increased risk of cardiovascular disease, the development of obesity and diabetes, and an increased risk of certain cancers (U.S. Department of Agriculture, 2015).

Studies have concluded that by replacing 5% of total calories from saturated fatty acids with PUFA and MUFA, there is a 13% lower risk of coronary events and a 26% lower risk of coronary death. It is estimated that for each 5% energy increase in PUFA (with a concurrent reduction in saturated fatty acids) there is a 10% reduction in coronary heart disease (Jump, 2014).

The USDA reports that 11% of calories in the American diet are composed of saturated fatty acids, which it recommended be reduced to less than 10% of total calories. Only 29% of Americans limit saturated fatty acids to the recommended level. The AHA advocates lowering this percentage to 5% to 6%. The top foods consumed by Americans that contribute to the high saturated fatty acids intake are pizza, grain-based desserts, dairy desserts, chicken and chicken-mixed dishes, and beef and beef-mixed dishes (Jump, 2014; U.S. Department of Agriculture, 2015).

the risk of cardiovascular disease. The American Heart Association's Nutrition Committee recommends that *trans* fats should constitute less than 1% of the diet (www.heart.org).

Some MUFA and PUFA are required to provide the essential fatty acids. See Box 3-2 and Dollars & Sense 3-1.

Dietary Fat Intake and Health

Fat plays a key role in diet and health. A diet too low in fat not only lacks satiety and palatability but may also lack adequate levels of the essential fatty acids; a diet with excessive fat may result in increased risk of disease.

BOX 3-2 ■ Essential Fatty Acids

AI for Essential Fatty Acids for Adults 19–51 Years Old*	Kind	Food Sources
Men: 17 grams Women: 12 grams	Omega-6 fatty acids Linoleic acid	■ Vegetable oils, such as safflower, corn, soybean, cottonseed ■ Poultry fat ■ Nuts and seeds
Men: 1.6 grams Women: 1.1 grams	Omega-3 fatty acids Linolenic acid	■ Human milk ■ Fatty fish ■ Vegetable oils, such as soybean, flax, canola ■ Wheat germ ■ Soybeans

AI, adequate intake.
*Refer to dietary reference intakes tables for other age groups.

Dollars & Sense 3-1

Dietary Guidelines for Fat

The *Dietary Guidelines for Americans 2015-2020,* American Heart Association, and the National Heart, Lung, and Blood Institute (NHLBI) recommend that most dietary fats come from sources of polyunsaturated and monounsaturated fatty acids. One way to obtain these fats is to incorporate nuts in the diet.

Nuts also provide other essential nutrients, such as linolenic acid, vitamins A and E, magnesium, dietary fiber, copper, and zinc. Many nuts are also high in phytonutrients.

The *2015-2020 Dietary Guidelines* recommend an increase in consumption of nuts, seeds, and soy products. The best method of incorporating nuts into the diet is to practice good portion control. Based upon a 2,000-kilocalorie diet, the recommendation is for five 1-ounce equivalents each week. One ounce of nuts contains about 170 kilocalories. Unsalted and raw or roasted without oil is the healthiest option for consumption.

Monounsaturated Fats

Monounsaturated fats are a form of unsaturated fat. Health educators recommend increasing intake of monounsaturated fats while decreasing intake of saturated fats. Evidence suggests that individuals with a higher intake of monounsaturated and polyunsaturated fats, a low intake of saturated fats, and a low total fat intake may have a decreased risk of coronary heart disease.

Monounsaturated fats are found in nuts, avocado, canola, olive, and peanut oil. Nutrition experts advocate the consumption of fats derived from plant sources, such as those shown in Figure 3-4, because those foods also contribute fiber, antioxidants, and phytochemicals to the diet.

Polyunsaturated Fats

Polyunsaturated fats come in the form of omega-6 and omega-3 PUFA. Food sources of omega-6 PUFA include nuts and vegetable oils, such as soybean, safflower, and corn. Good food sources of omega-3 PUFA include walnuts, flaxseeds, fatty fish, and some oils, including soybean, canola, flax, and fish.

Body Fat

Both the amount of body fat a person carries and its distribution on the body are related to health risk. Many experts believe that the ratio of body fat to total weight is more important than total weight. Healthy ranges for body fat are 15% to 19% for men and 18% to 22% for women. A high percentage of body fat has been associated with increased risk of disease, even when total body weight is normal.

The location of excess body fat is also important. Excessive fat on the lower body, specifically on the hips and thighs, seems to be less dangerous than excessive fat on the abdomen and upper body, which is associated with a much higher risk of diseases such as cancer, heart disease, and diabetes. The food groups in the next section can be used to assist in planning meals low in fat and teach clients about food composition.

Food Groups

Food groups can be used to learn food composition and portion control and assist in planning lower-fat meals. For example, many people do not know that sugar and fruit

contain no fat, and oil contains no carbohydrate. Food groups that include fat are dairy, protein, and fat. The amount of fat in one serving of protein or dairy varies within the group. The composition of foods can be found on many food calculators, such as the USDA food composition tables (https://ndb.nal.usda.gov/ndb/), smart phone apps, and by reviewing food labels (see Box 3-3).

Dairy

The fat content of milk varies according to the type of milk—whole, 2%, 1%, or nonfat. Table 3-5 shows the grams of fat and percentage of kilocalories from fat in one serving of milk for each kind of milk. Although whole milk and 2% milk contain saturated fat and cholesterol, the protein, carbohydrate, vitamin, and mineral contents of whole, 2%, 1%, and nonfat milk are comparable. Nonfat milk contains only a trace of fat and is thus a nutritional bargain.

Protein

Table 3-6 lists selected food examples and portions from the protein food group. A lean protein contains 0 to 3 grams of fat, medium-fat protein contains 4 to 7 grams of fat, and high-fat protein contains 8 or more grams of fat per ounce or equivalent of food.

Many clients have misconceptions about meat. Some clients avoid all red meat because they think that it contains

---

BOX 3-3 ■ Food Label Terms

Food labeling regulations spell out what terms may be used to describe the level of fat in a food and how the labels can be used. These are the terms:

- *Fat-free* on a food label means that the food contains no more than 0.5 grams of fat per serving. Synonyms for *free* include *without*, *no*, and *zero*. *Nonfat* is another synonym for *fat-free*. These terms legally can be used on a food label only if the product contains no amount of—or only trivial or "physiologically inconsequential" amounts of—fat, saturated fat, and cholesterol.
- *Low-fat* is legally defined as a food that contains no more than 3 grams of fat in a serving.
- *Low saturated fat* is legally defined as a food that contains no more than 1 gram of saturated fat per serving.
- *Low cholesterol* is defined as a food that contains less than 20 milligrams of cholesterol per serving. Synonyms for *low* include *little*, *few*, and *low source of*.

In addition, serving sizes listed on food labels are standardized to make nutritional comparisons of similar products easier.

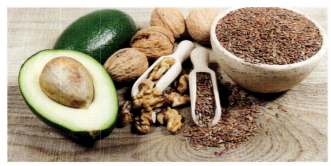

FIGURE 3-4 Plant sources of fats include avocado, nuts, and some seeds, such as sesame and flax.

TABLE 3-5   Grams of Fat in One Serving of Dairy

TYPE	FAT (GRAMS)	PERCENTAGE OF KILOCALORIES FROM FAT
Whole milk	8	48
2% (low fat)	5	38
Nonfat milk	Trace	<1

TABLE 3-6   Examples of Lean, Medium-Fat, and High-Fat Proteins

Each of the following is a lean protein and contains less than 1 gram of fat:		
Poultry	Chicken or turkey (white meat, no skin)	1 oz
Fish	Fresh or frozen cod, flounder, haddock	1 oz
Game	Venison	1 oz
Cheese	Nonfat cottage cheese	¼ cup
	Fat-free cheese	1 oz
Other	Egg whites	2
	Hot dogs with less than 1 g of fat	1 oz
	Egg substitute	¼ cup
Each of the following is a lean protein and contains 3 grams of fat:		
Beef	Round, sirloin, or flank steak	1 oz
Fish	Salmon (fresh or frozen)	1 oz
Pork	Tenderloin	1 oz
Veal	Lean chop or roast	1 oz
Poultry	Chicken, dark meat, no skin	1 oz
Game	Goose, no skin	1 oz
Cheese	4.5% fat cottage cheese	¼ cup
	Cheeses with less than 3 g of fat per oz	1 oz
Other	Hot dogs with less than 3 g of fat per oz	1 oz
	Processed lunch meat with less than 3 g of fat per oz	1 oz
Each of the following is a medium-fat protein and contains 5 grams of fat:		
Beef	Ground beef, corned beef	1 oz
Pork	Chops	1 oz
Poultry	Chicken, dark meat, with skin	1 oz
Fish	Any fried fish product	1 oz
Cheese	Mozzarella	1 oz
Other	Egg (high in cholesterol)	1
	Tofu	¼ cup
Each of the following is a high-fat protein and contains 8 grams of fat:		
Pork	Spareribs, pork sausage	1 oz
Cheese	All regular cheeses, such as cheddar, Swiss, and American	1 oz
Other	Bologna	1 oz
	Knockwurst, bratwurst	1 oz

excessive fat. In fact, some beef and pork products are not excessively high in fat. Many consumers are not aware of the lean cuts of beef or pork. Conversely, not all fish and poultry items are lean proteins. Nurses and other health educators can help clients by providing correct information about meats.

Different methods of food preparation can greatly influence the fat content of meats. Those that are baked, broiled, grilled, or roasted contain fewer kilocalories than fried versions. Some clients have the misconception that if they eat only lean meats, they can eat large quantities prepared in any manner, but preparation really does count. For example, a 3-ounce breaded fried chicken breast contains more fat than the same size grilled hamburger patty.

A portion of meat is 3 ounces, about half a chicken breast. Typically, Americans eat large amounts of meats such as prime rib (from 6-ounce to 16-ounce servings). Therefore, teaching clients about meat portion sizes is usually

indicated when the goal is to decrease fat intake and decrease total kilocalorie intake.

When a portion of meat is calculated, it is based on the following assumptions:

- Visible fat on meat is not consumed.
- Meat is weighed after cooking.
- Meat is cooked by a low-fat method—baked, boiled, broiled, grilled, or roasted (unless otherwise indicated).

Since 1994, food-labeling regulations have allowed two definitions for the fat content labeling of meat, poultry, seafood, and game meats: *lean* and *extra lean*.

- *Lean* can be used on meat, poultry, seafood, or game meat products only if the product contains less than 10 grams of fat, less than 4.5 grams of saturated fat, and less than 95 milligrams of cholesterol per 100-gram serving (3.5 ounces).

- *Extra lean* can be used only if the product contains less than 5 grams of fat, less than 2 grams of saturated fat and *trans* fat combined, and less than 95 milligrams of cholesterol per serving and per 100 grams (3.5 ounces).

Some clients may choose not to eat animal products. Health-care workers should always accommodate their client's religious, ecological, and ethical beliefs and values. See Appendix A for brief food group information, which includes some meat substitutes. Many low-fat meat substitutes, including dried beans, peas, and lentils, are not derived from animals. Vegetarian protein sources include soymilk, tempeh, and tofu. Peanut butter contains 8 grams of fat per portion (2 tablespoons).

Fats

The fat food group is comprised of foods high in PUFA, MUFA, and saturated fatty acids. Table 3-7 lists selected foods and portions from each group.

Additional Food Sources of Fat

It is important to advise clients that snack foods, including crackers, cakes, pies, donuts, and cookies, may be high in both total fat and *trans*-fatty acids. Often, potato chips, gravies, cream sauces, soups, pizza, tacos, and spaghetti are high in fat. Microwave popcorn is higher in fat than air-popped popcorn (without added fat).

Consumers who desire low-fat foods need not avoid eating out, but they do need to make wise food choices, especially if they eat most meals in restaurants. Many of the specialty fast-food hamburgers are high in fat; therefore, a small hamburger is the best burger choice. A small side salad with low-fat dressing is a better low-fat choice than French fries. Nonfat milk is lower in fat than either a milkshake or whole milk. A grilled chicken breast salad with a fat-free dressing is also a good choice.

TABLE 3-7 Examples of Monounsaturated, Polyunsaturated, and Saturated Fats

Each of the following is a fat portion high in monounsaturated fatty acids and contains 5 g of total fat:

Olives	5 large
Canola oil	1 tsp
Peanut butter	2 tsp
Pecans	4 halves

Each of the following is a fat portion high in polyunsaturated fatty acids and contains 5 grams of total fat:

Margarine, stick or tub	1 tsp
Mayo, regular	1 tsp
Corn oil	1 tsp
English walnuts	4 halves

Each of the following is a fat portion high in saturated fatty acids and contains 5 grams of total fat:

Bacon	1 slice (20 slices/lb)
Butter, stick	1 tsp
Cream cheese, regular	1 tbsp (½ oz)
Cream cheese, reduced-fat	2 tbsp (1 oz)
Sour cream, regular	2 tbsp
Sour cream, reduced-fat	3 tbsp

Plant Stanols and Sterols

Plant stanols and sterols are found in the membranes of plants. They are substances which resemble the chemical structure of cholesterol and are present in small quantities in fruits, vegetables, nuts, seeds, cereals, legumes, and vegetable oils. They have been shown to reduce blood cholesterol levels. Plant sterols and stanols work by blocking dietary cholesterol's entrance into the body. Foods that contain plant stanols and sterols may not be eaten in enough quantity each day to affect a change in cholesterol. Therefore, some foods have stanols and sterols added to them, including margarine spreads, salad dressings, and fruit juice (www.foodinsight.org).

KEYSTONES

- The group name for all fats is *lipids*.
- Hydrogen, oxygen, and carbon are the primary elements in fats.
- Gram for gram, fats contain more than twice the kilocalories of carbohydrates.
- Fats are labeled according to the amount and type of fatty acids they contain as saturated, unsaturated, monounsaturated, polyunsaturated, and *trans*-fatty acids.
- Fats serve many important functions in our diets and our bodies.
- A balanced intake of carbohydrate and fat is essential for optimal health. Excess fats in our diets are associated with cardiovascular disease, obesity, diabetes, and some types of cancer.
- Cholesterol is a fatlike substance that is present in animal food sources and produced by the human body.
- Many Americans would benefit from decreasing their intake of cholesterol, *trans*-fatty acids, and saturated fat.
- The National Academies of Science current Dietary Reference Intakes for Macronutrients recommends that adults consume between 20% and 35% of their kilocalories from fat (Food and Nutrition Board, 2005).
- *Dietary Guidelines for Americans* recommends a saturated fat intake of less than 10% of kilocalories and dietary cholesterol intake of 100–300 mg per day based upon the calorie level consumed in a healthy eating pattern each day.

CASE STUDY 3-1

Mr. D had a physical examination by his family physician, who also treated the client's brother and his father. His father had died of a stroke, and his 35-year-old brother recently had a myocardial infarction (heart attack). The physician noted several xanthomas (fat buildup under the skin) around his eyes. His height was 5 feet 6 inches, and his weight was 160 lb. The client reported consuming frequent or large portions of high-fat foods. The client agreed to speak with the student nurse directly after the appointment. The student is doing a practicum in the doctor's office. The registered nurse supervising the student nurse (Mike) requested that he do the following:

1. Schedule the client for follow-up with the physician.
2. Develop a nursing care plan that addresses the client's nursing problem to complement the medical diagnosis.

Because the student was assigned only one client, he had the time to complete his assigned tasks in greater detail than a nurse normally would. The student did not have a computer data program available, so it took him several hours to complete this assignment.

Mike, the student nurse, scheduled the follow-up appointment with the physician for 2 days later (just before the client was leaving for a cruise). Mr. D was instructed by the student to write down all food he consumed, or log it on his smart phone app, for 1 day before the appointment. The client was advised to choose a typical day to record his food intake to provide a more accurate analysis of his usual diet.

Two Days Later

Mr. D arrived on the appropriate day and showed his food record to the student for review. Mike calculated the grams of fat in Mr. D's food record based on a combination of food groups and a table of food composition. Mr. D's food record and Mike's calculations follow.

The physician has just seen the client at his follow-up appointment and reviewed Mr. D's food record and Mike's calculations. Mr. D's total cholesterol was 350 mg/dL (normal for laboratory test is <200 mg/dL). His low-density lipoprotein (LDL) cholesterol was elevated to 150 mg/dL (normal for laboratory test is <100 mg/dL).

Mr. D told the doctor, "I cannot understand why my cholesterol is elevated. My weight is stable. I always select the salad bar for lunch, avoid sweets, and drink low-fat milk." The client agreed to meet with the dietitian after his cruise.

11:00 a.m.	
Food	*Grams of Fat*
Salad bar	
Assorted vegetables and lettuce	0
4 tbsp blue cheese dressing (cup)	20
4 oz shredded cheese	32
1 oz diced ham	3
1 cup potato salad	14
Dinner roll	0
4 tsp butter	20
1 cup clam chowder	7

7:00 p.m. Restaurant	
Food	*Grams of Fat*
4 oz hamburger, checked weight	20
2 oz cheese	16
2 tbsp mayo	30
Bun	0
6 onion rings	15
Tossed salad	0
4 tbsp blue cheese dressing	20

11:00 p.m. Home	
Food	*Grams of Fat*
1 cup 2% milk	5
1 orange	0
Total fat for the day	202 g of fat

CARE PLAN

Subjective Data
Admitted knowledge deficit. Food record for 1 day contained 202 grams of fat.

Objective Data
Cholesterol level: 350 mg/dL and LDL level was 150; height: 5 ft 6 in.; weight: 160 lb

Analysis
Client's dietary intake of cholesterol is related to elevated blood cholesterol levels.

Plan

DESIRED OUTCOMES EVALUATION CRITERIA	ACTIONS/ INTERVENTIONS	RATIONALE
Client will keep a food record for 1 day.	Instruct the client on the recording of his food intake.	Keeping food records will remind the client of the importance of decreasing his or her fat intake. If done on his smart phone app, it will provide immediate feedback to client regarding food composition. Reviewing them with the client permits positive reinforcement and correction of misperceptions.
Client will decrease his fat intake by 50%.	Encourage client to first cut the major sources of fat in his diet: salad dressings and cheese.	50% of client's fat intake is from cheese, mayo, and salad dressings.
Encourage the client to meet with the dietitian after his cruise.	Offer the client a referral to the dietitian so that his estimated nutritional needs can be calculated and determine client's motivation and goals to help obtain long-term compliance.	A student nurse cannot be expected to follow client long-term.
	Tell the client to call the nurse if he is having trouble interpreting dietary instructions at home.	Offers the client support between visits.

TEAMWORK 3-1

DIETITIAN'S NOTE

The following dietitian's notes are representative of the type of documentation found in the narrative portion of a client's medical record.

Six Weeks Later

Subjective: *Met with the client and his significant other. Although the client has made a recent change to substitute fat-free mayo and salad dressings for regular dressings, he was not able to give up cheese. Admits to sedentary lifestyle. The 24-hour dietary recall cross-checked with a food frequency showed a three-meal-per-day pattern with a salad for lunch and the evening meal in a restaurant.*

Objective: *Most recent cholesterol was 330 mg/dL, and LDL was 142 mg/dL. Height: 5 ft 6 in.; weight 158 lb.*

Analysis: *Ideal body weight at 106 lb for the first 5 ft and 6 lb for each additional inch = 128–156. Estimated caloric need at 10–11 kilocalories/lb at 156 lb (maximum body weight) = 1560–1760 kilocalories. Maximum recommended kilocalories from fat at 35% of total kilocalories = 546–616 kilocalories and 60–68 grams. Client's estimated fat intake from 24-hour recall and food frequency showed an intake of 110–115 grams of fat.*

Excessive fat intake as evidenced by food- and nutrition-related knowledge and elevated cholesterol (330) and LDL (142) and reported food intake.

Plan: *After discussing client's interest in making lifestyle changes, it was agreed that he would:*

1. *Attend group class "Healthy Heart."*
2. *Monitor weight and blood lipid levels.*
3. *Substitute low-fat cheese for regular cheese and consider packing his lunch.*
4. *Record his food intake 3 days per week using his smart phone app, sharing information with provider at next visit.*
5. *Provide contact information to schedule follow-up, prn.*

CRITICAL THINKING QUESTIONS

1. Do you think that this client will respond to diet therapy? What would you do if after 3 months a client's food diary shows greatly reduced dietary fat but his or her cholesterol has not dropped? The physician would probably decide to prescribe medication to lower the cholesterol. How would you explain this therapy to the client?

2. What would you do if, at the following visit, the food diary shows that the client has returned to his former eating habits, thinking fat consumption no longer matters because he is taking medication?

CHAPTER REVIEW

1. Monoglycerides and diglycerides are names of lipids commonly seen:
   1. In clients' medical records
   2. On laboratory reports
   3. On food labels
   4. On clients' skin

2. Cholesterol is found:
   1. Only in saturated fats
   2. Only in foods of animal origin
   3. Mostly in eggs
   4. Only in triglycerides

3. Saturated fats are not: (Select all that apply.)
   1. Liquid at room temperature and of vegetable origin
   2. More likely to become rancid than other types of fats
   3. Primarily of animal origin
   4. Comprise over 10% of the average American's diet

4. According to most health authorities, the average American would benefit by increasing his or her intake of which of the following fats while decreasing intake of other fats?
   1. Corn oil
   2. Olive oil
   3. Safflower oil
   4. Lard

5. To lower your risk of coronary heart disease, the average person should: (Select all that apply.)
   1. Take 3 g of purified fish oil supplement daily
   2. Consume no more than 11% saturated fatty acids
   3. Eat 2 servings of fish per week based upon a 2,000-kilocalorie diet
   4. Consume no more than 5%–6% saturated fatty acids (AHA guidelines)
   5. Consume less than 10% saturated fatty acids (*Dietary Guidelines for Americans*)

6. The average adult should consume the following percent range of fat in the diet:
   1. 20–30
   2. 0–15
   3. 35–45
   4. 25–35

CLINICAL ANALYSIS

1. Mrs. S, 50 years old, has a cholesterol level of 233 mg/dL. She weighs 125 lb and is 5 ft 5 in. tall. The dietitian has estimated her body fat content to be 35%. When taking a nursing history, the nurse asks Mrs. S if she eats any foods that may be related to her elevated cholesterol level. Which of the following groups of foods are most related to an elevated cholesterol level?

   a. Vegetable oils, such as corn, cottonseed, and soybean
   b. Fruits and vegetables
   c. Starches, such as bread, potatoes, rice, and pasta
   d. Animal fats, such as butter, meats, lard, and bacon

2. Mr. B buys as many low-fat foods as possible. He eats fat-free muffins for breakfast, eats low-fat brownies or cookies for lunch each day, uses only fat-free ice cream, and buys fat-free salad dressings. He eats little meat and chooses fat-free dairy products. He wonders why he hasn't lost more weight. The best advice is to encourage him to:

   a. Consider the amount of sugar he consumes especially by consuming low-fat baked goods and desserts
   b. Eat even less meat
   c. Consume fewer dairy products
   d. Quit trying to lose weight

3. When Mrs. L describes her regular intake of foods, you observe that her diet is especially low in monounsaturated fats. Which of the following oils would you recommend be used in place of corn oil to increase her intake of monounsaturated fats?

   a. Sunflower seed
   b. Soybean
   c. Olive
   d. Cottonseed

CHAPTER 4

Protein

LEARNING OBJECTIVES

After completing this chapter, the student should be able to:

- Distinguish protein from the other energy nutrients.
- Contrast essential and nonessential amino acids.
- Define and give two examples of conditionally essential amino acids.
- Relate nitrogen balance to conditions in which anabolism or catabolism predominate.
- Explain the difference between complete and incomplete proteins and give examples of food sources of each.
- Identify plant-based protein sources.
- Describe how protein is essential to circulation.
- Explain the principle of complementation and its application to meal planning.

Along with carbohydrate and fat, protein is an energy nutrient, but in many ways, it is paramount. Even the term *protein,* which is derived from the Greek *proteos,* means primary or taking first place. Protein makes unique contributions to the body's health that cannot be duplicated by carbohydrate or fat. This chapter covers the functions, composition, and dietary sources of protein.

Protein can be used as an auxiliary source of energy if kilocaloric intake is inadequate. As is true of carbohydrates and fats, protein eaten in excess can contribute to body fat stores.

Composition of Proteins

To understand the functions of protein in the body, it is necessary first to comprehend their basic structure: their chemical **elements** and the arrangement of those elements.

Proteins are composed of four elements:

1. Carbon
2. Hydrogen
3. Oxygen
4. Nitrogen

These elements are arranged in building blocks called amino acids. Nitrogen is the element that distinguishes the structure of proteins from that of carbohydrates and fats as described in previous chapters. Sometimes sulfur and other elements also form part of the protein **molecule.**

Amino Acids

Amino acids are linked by **peptide bonds** in an exact order to make a particular protein. A chain of two or more amino acids joined together by peptide bonds is called a **polypeptide**. A single protein may consist of a polypeptide comprising from 50 to thousands of amino acids. Scientists have estimated that the human body contains up to 50,000 proteins, of which only about 1,000 have been identified. Thus, an enormous variety of combinations is possible.

Animal and vegetable proteins that we eat are disassembled in the digestive process into component amino acids. They are absorbed in the small intestine and used to synthesize enzymes and structural proteins essential for growth and repair of tissue (Tabers.com). Descriptions of some of the tissues composed of protein appear in Box 4-1.

Twenty-three amino acids have been identified as important to the body's metabolism. These amino acids are classified as essential, conditionally (or acquired) essential, and nonessential.

Essential Amino Acids

An amino acid is classified as essential if the body is unable to make it in sufficient amounts to meet metabolic needs. All **essential amino acids** must be available in the body simultaneously and in sufficient quantity for the synthesis of body proteins (Fig. 4-1). These amino acids may come from recently ingested food or from the body's own cells as they age and are broken down and replaced. The liver regulates the amount of amino acids available for protein synthesis at any given time. This is referred to as the amino acid pool. Amino acids that are in excess of needs are broken down by the body and converted to carbohydrate for energy needs (Tabers.com).

Conditionally (Acquired) Essential Amino Acids

Other amino acids are conditionally essential or can become essential, depending on the biochemical needs of the body and the health of its organs due to illness or stress. For example, cysteine and proline are indispensable for premature

49

BOX 4-1 ■ Examples of Proteins in the Human Body

People need a steady intake of protein for normal body maintenance because most cells require periodic replacement. Even bone tissue undergoes change and renewal in healthy adults. When a person is growing, or has diseased or injured tissue to repair, the need for protein is even greater than usual.

Scar Tissue

Wound healing requires proteins. Many blood-clotting factors, such as the protein prothrombin, form a blood clot. The fibrin threads that form the mesh to hold the scar tissue in place are composed of protein. Wound-healing requires much energy that is usually released from body energy stores and protein reserves, a major challenge for undernourished and malnourished clients (Wild et al, 2010).

Hair

Hair cells are dead. Hence, haircuts are not painful. The new growth of hair does require protein building blocks, however. One sign of malnutrition is hair that can be easily and painlessly plucked.

Blood Albumin

Albumin is a transport protein that carries nutrients or elements. In addition to carrying substances to body cells, albumin has functions relating to water balance (see Chapter 8) and plays a significant role in medication absorption and metabolism (see Chapter 15).

Hemoglobin

Another transport protein, **hemoglobin,** is the oxygen-carrying part of the red blood cell. The **globin** part of this molecule is a simple protein.

infants. Cysteine becomes essential in clients with **cirrhosis** of the liver (Gropper & Smith, 2013).

Nonessential Amino Acids

Nonessential amino acids are those that the body ordinarily can build in sufficient quantities to meet its needs. Typically, they are derived from other amino acids. Nonessential amino acids are necessary for good health, but under normal conditions, adults do not have to obtain them from food. Table 4-1 lists the amino acids that have been classified as essential, conditionally and/or acquired essential, and nonessential.

Functions of Proteins in the Body

Protein serves six major functions in the body, as shown in Table 4-2.

Provision of Structure

Proteins provide much of the body's mass. Contractile proteins, actin and myosin, are found in skeletal, smooth, and cardiac muscles. Fibrous proteins, such as **collagen,** elastin, and keratin, are found in blood vessels, bone, cartilage, hair, nails, tendons, skin, and teeth.

Maintenance and Growth

Because protein is a part of every cell (half the dry weight), adults as well as growing children require adequate protein intake. As cells of the body wear out, they must be replaced.

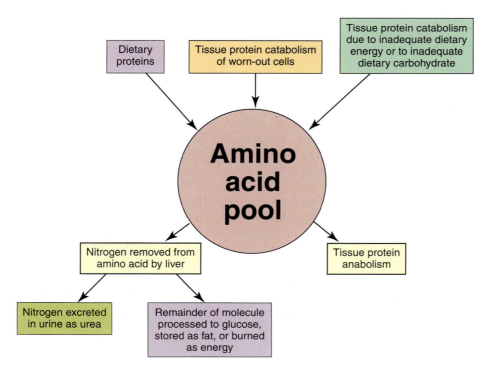

FIGURE 4-1 Anabolism/catabolism of protein. The body obtains amino acids from dietary protein and the catabolism of body tissue, enzymes, and secretions. The body uses amino acids to build new tissue or for immediate or future energy use. Every meal or snack does not have to contain every essential amino acid to permit anabolism. To maximize an adult's health, all essential amino acids should be supplied in adequate amounts by diet daily or at least every 2–3 days.

TABLE 4-1   Essential, Conditionally and/or Acquired Essential, and Nonessential Amino Acids

ESSENTIAL	CONDITIONALLY AND/OR ACQUIRED ESSENTIAL	NONESSENTIAL
Histidine	Glutamine	Alanine
Isoleucine		Arginine
Leucine		Aspartic acid
Lysine		Citruline
Methionine		Glutamic acid
Cysteine		Glycine
Phenylalanine		Hydroxyglutamic acid
Tyrosine		Hydroxyproline
Threonine		Norleucine
Tryptophan		Proline
Valine		Serine

www.tabers.com

TABLE 4-2   Functions of Protein

FUNCTION	EXAMPLE
Provide structure	Muscle mass
Maintain and build cells	Hair growth
Regulate body processes	**Glucagon** (actions opposite those of insulin)
Produce immunity	Antibodies
Substitute as fuel	If adequate carbohydrate and fat are lacking
Maintain blood volume and pressure	**Albumin** draws fluid back into capillaries from interstitial (between the cells) spaces

Anabolism and Catabolism

Anabolism is the building up of tissues as occurs in growth or healing. **Catabolism** is the breaking down of tissues into simpler substances that the body can reuse or eliminate.

Both processes occur simultaneously in the body. For example, tissue proteins are constantly being broken down into amino acids, which are then reused for building new tissue and repairing old tissue. Anabolism and catabolism, however, are not always in balance; at times, one process may dominate the other.

Nitrogen Balance

Foods or artificial feedings containing protein are the body's only external sources of nitrogen. Nitrogen is excreted in the urine, feces, and sweat; nitrogen is also sometimes lost through bleeding or vomiting. A person is in nitrogen equilibrium or nitrogen balance when the amount of nitrogen taken in equals the amount excreted

(Clinical Calculation 4-1). A healthy adult at a stable body weight is usually in nitrogen equilibrium. Under certain circumstances, however, nitrogen balance may be either positive or negative.

POSITIVE NITROGEN BALANCE

A person consuming more nitrogen than he or she excretes is in positive **nitrogen balance.** The body is building more tissue than it is breaking down, a normal state during periods of growth such as infancy, childhood, adolescence, and pregnancy.

NEGATIVE NITROGEN BALANCE

A person consuming less nitrogen than he or she excretes is in negative nitrogen balance. Such a person is receiving insufficient protein and/or the body is breaking down more tissue than it is building. Situations marked by negative nitrogen balance include undernutrition, illness, and trauma.

Beginning at age 55, the average person begins to have a decline in muscle mass. Evidence exists that older individuals with *sarcopenia*, or muscle loss, have a greater negative response to critical illness than younger individuals. There is greater mortality and morbidity in older individuals who are in a **catabolic** state. Therefore it is important to determine the level of muscle loss, through nitrogen balance studies and a nutrition-focused physical examination, which looks at grip strength and physical signs of muscle wasting. This is typically evaluated by a dietitian. Higher intakes of protein are recommended of 1 to 1.25 grams of protein per kilogram of body weight to help prevent catabolism of muscle (Dickerson, 2016). In the critical care setting, protein is the most important macronutrient to support wound healing, supporting the immune function, and maintaining lean body mass. An intake of 1.2 to 2.0 g/kg/day is recommended in the critical care setting, especially if nitrogen balance studies are not available to assess the client's protein state. Serum protein markers are not a valid indicator of protein intake (McClave et al, 2016).

CLINICAL CALCULATION   4-1

Nitrogen Balance Studies

To calculate a client's nitrogen balance, the dietitian compares the amount of nitrogen in the foods the client consumes with the amount of nitrogen excreted in the urine. Other potential losses are estimated.

Nitrogen balance is calculated using the following formula:

$$\text{Nitrogen balance} = \text{total protein intake (grams)}/6.25 - (\text{UUN} + 4 \text{ grams})$$

where 6.25 = 6.25 grams of protein per gram of nitrogen, UUN = grams of nitrogen excreted in the urine over a 24-hour period, 4 = 4 grams of nitrogen lost each day as "insensible losses" via the skin and gastrointestinal tract (http://www.surgicalcriticalcare. net/Resources/nitrogen.php).

BED REST. One of the most consistent effects of prolonged bed rest is an increase in nitrogen excretion derived from skeletal muscle. Prolonged bed rest for multiple conditions results in decreased muscle mass, strength, and function predominantly caused by decreased muscle protein synthesis. Muscle mass wasting is seen within 10 days in healthy older individuals on bedrest. Up to 40% loss of muscle strength can occur within the first week. Further compounding the muscle loss is critical illness, which causes more muscle wasting and weakness due to immobility and inflammation. This catabolism is not appreciably stopped even with adequate protein intake. Up to 30% muscle loss can occur within 10 days of an intensive care unit (ICU) admission. Studies are being done to examine the possible benefits to muscle in the ICU in the use of assistive technologies such as supine cycle ergometry and muscle stimulation. Definitive conclusions cannot be made regarding benefits, if any, to muscle (Parry & Puthucheary, 2015).

MALNUTRITION. Clients who receive inadequate food, sometimes for days, because of food insecurity, medical treatments, or diagnostic tests are at risk for malnutrition. Nursing staff are critical in assisting in the identification and prevention of malnutrition. Nurses obtain information from clients and perform simple nutritional screening, which focuses on the client's recent food consumption, changes in weight, and overall health. This screening may trigger a consult with a dietitian. Institutionalized clients are susceptible to malnutrition when they are unable to feed themselves, their meal schedule is interrupted by tests, or their illness prevents or inhibits eating (i.e., cancers and/or treatments may cause anorexia). Malnutrition is often accompanied by a loss of **lean body mass,** chiefly skeletal and visceral (internal organs) muscle, which is evaluated in the diagnosis of malnutrition. Hand grip strength is measured as an indicator of muscle strength. Dietitians evaluate subcutaneous fat loss, muscle loss, and edema to determine if a client may be malnourished.

The importance of ensuring feeding of even critically ill individuals is recognized by the American Society of Parenteral and Enteral Nutrition (ASPEN). Their 2016 guidelines recommend early enteral feeding for critical care clients within 24 to 48 hours of admission as a way to reduce infection, complications, and mortality. Protein is considered the most important macronutrient for wound healing, supporting the immune function, and maintaining lean body mass. There is a higher-than-normal protein requirement in these clients. The recommendation is to use a weight-based formula of 1.2 to 2.0 grams per kilogram per day (McClave et al, 2016).

Regulation of Body Processes

Protein contributes to the regulation of body processes. Hormones and enzymes are prime examples. Table 4-3 lists some of these regulators and gives examples of each. Nucleoproteins, also containing protein, are essential to normal body functioning.

Hormones

Hormones are chemicals secreted by various organs to regulate body processes. Hormones are secreted directly into the bloodstream rather than into a duct or an organ. **Insulin** and **glucagon** are two important hormones that help control glucose metabolism. Growth hormone regulates cell division and protein synthesis. The hormone **melatonin** that influences sleep–wake cycles is produced in the brain from the amino acid tryptophan.

Enzymes

Enzymes are crucial to many body processes, such as digestion. The breakdown of foods in the stomach and small intestine involves enzymes, which act as **catalysts** (chemicals that influence the speed at which a chemical reaction takes place but do not actually enter into the reaction). Chapter 9 details the enzymes listed in Table 4-3. Without the aid of enzymes, many of the processes in the body would proceed too slowly to be effective.

An enzyme provides a place (its surface) for two substances to meet and react with each other. The new substance is then released, and the enzyme catalyzes a new reaction. If it were not for enzymes, the two substances would be less likely to encounter one another, and basic body functioning would be impossible.

Nucleoproteins

Nucleoproteins are regulatory complexes that include proteins. These complexes are located in the cell nucleus, where they direct the maintenance and reproduction of the

TABLE 4-3   Examples of Regulators of Body Processes

REGULATOR	EXAMPLES	SOURCE	ACTION
Hormones	Growth hormone	Anterior pituitary	Increases transport of amino acids into cells Increases rate of protein synthesis
	Glucagon	Pancreas	Raises blood glucose by stimulating its release from liver glycogen
	Insulin	Pancreas	Lowers blood glucose by increasing its uptake by cells
Enzymes	Lipase	Pancreas	Breaks down emulsified fats into fatty acids and glycerol
	Peptidase	Small intestine	Splits polypeptides into amino acids
	Sucrase	Small intestine	Splits sucrose into glucose and fructose

cell. **Deoxyribonucleic acid (DNA)** and **ribonucleic acid (RNA)** are nucleoproteins that control the protein synthesis in the cell.

A **gene** is a part of the DNA that carries the code to direct the synthesis of a single protein. The kinds of proteins the cell makes vary with the nature of the cell—for example, whether an intestinal or skin cell or an ovum or sperm cell.

Immunity

A protein called an **antibody** is produced in the body in response to the presence of a foreign substance or a substance that the body senses to be foreign. Antibodies provide **immunity** to certain diseases and other toxic conditions. A specific antibody is created for each foreign substance.

If a person is exposed to a certain kind of disease-producing organism, the body designs an antibody that neutralizes the harmful effects of only that particular species or strain of organism. For some diseases, once the body has produced many copies of a given antibody, it can respond quickly to another attack, making the individual immune to that disease.

Circulation

The main protein in blood is albumin. It helps to maintain blood volume by drawing fluid back into the veins from body tissues. It plays a major role in maintaining blood pressure. In addition, some proteins aid in maintaining the body's acid–base balance. This buffering action is described in Chapter 8.

Some proteins in cell membranes carry nutrients into and out of cells. Proteins also attach to fats to become **lipoproteins** for moving lipids in the bloodstream. Drugs bind with albumin in the bloodstream. The term *protein-bound* refers to the portion of a drug dose that is inactive because it is attached to albumin. Chapter 15 elaborates on this process and its implications.

Energy Source

Glucose is the most efficiently used source of energy, but fat and protein can be adapted as backup sources. Most other body systems use fat for energy more readily than the nervous system does. The brain is rich in neurons and is the most energy demanding organ in the body, and uses glucose as an energy source, using one half of all the sugar energy in the body (Mahoney, 2017). When the body has insufficient glucose available for nervous system energy needs (as in a carbohydrate dietary deficit of longer than 12 hours, for instance, in an overnight fast), the body will use body protein tissue to meet the energy needs of the brain and spinal cord.

Adequate carbohydrate and overall caloric intake is necessary to:

1. Spare protein for its unique contribution to tissue building
2. Avoid the undesirable consequences—**ketosis** and muscle loss—of obtaining energy from the less efficient sources: fat and protein

Once liver glycogen stores are depleted, less than 24 hours into a fast, the glucose needs of the brain are derived by **gluconeogenesis** by sacrificing amino acids from protein. Without a change in the process, the use of the body's protein for glucose production would cause death within days. Fortunately within a week of the onset of starvation, the muscles use free fatty acids and the brain uses ketone bodies for energy (Matthews, 2014).

The amount of energy obtained from a gram of protein is the same as the amount obtained from a gram of carbohydrate: 4 kilocalories. Loss of more than about 30% of body protein is likely to be fatal due to reduced muscle strength for breathing, impaired immune function, and decreased organ function (Matthews, 2014).

Classification of Food Protein

Few foods are composed solely of protein. The white of an egg comes close, with 92% of its kilocalories derived from protein. Most foods contain various combinations of protein, fat, and carbohydrates. Some foods, however, are better sources of protein than others.

Protein foods are classified by the number and kinds of amino acids they contain:

- **Complete proteins** are foods that supply all nine essential amino acids in sufficient quantity to maintain tissue and support growth.
- **Incomplete proteins** lack one or more of the essential amino acids.

Complete Protein

With few exceptions, single foods containing complete protein come from animal sources such as meat, poultry, fish, eggs, milk, and cheese. Based on the absorption of amino acids, animal protein foods are 90% to 99% digestible. Of the dairy group, butter contains no protein; sour cream and cream cheese contain only 1 gram per serving. Although gelatin is an animal product, it is an incomplete protein because it lacks the essential amino acid tryptophan. Soybeans are one plant source of complete protein that is processed into several products. Compared with milk protein at 100, soybean's protein digestibility corrected amino acid score is 94 (Gropper & Smith, 2013).

Meat and most milk products are both good sources of complete protein. An adult requiring 2,000 kilocalories per day following MyPlate guidelines (Table 4-4) would consume the equivalent of 5 to 6½ ounces from the meat group and 3 cups of milk daily. Table 4-5 lists the foods and portion sizes within the protein food group. Dollars & Sense 4-1 illustrates a means to stretch meat resources and to bolster protein content in sauces with readily available products.

Incomplete Protein

Most plant foods that contain protein lack the amounts of one or more essential amino acids necessary to maintain tissue and support growth. Therefore, the protein of plants

TABLE 4-4 Daily Protein Recommendations*

Children	2–3 years old	2 ounce equivalents
	4–8 years old	4 ounce equivalents
Girls	9–13 years old	5 ounce equivalents
	14–18 years old	5 ounce equivalents
Boys	9–13 years old	5 ounce equivalents
	14–18 years old	6½ ounce equivalents
Women	19–30 years old	5½ ounce equivalents
	31–50 years old	5 ounce equivalents
	51+ years old	5 ounce equivalents
Men	19–30 years old	6½ ounce equivalents
	31–50 years old	6 ounce equivalents
	51+ years old	5½ ounce equivalents

*These amounts are appropriate for individuals who get less than 30 minutes per day of moderate physical activity, beyond normal daily activities. Those who are more physically active may be able to consume more while staying within calorie needs. Source: ChooseMyPlate.gov. Retrieved from https://www.choosemyplate.gov/protein-foods on April 20, 2017.

is called *incomplete*, but the term does not mean that these foods are undesirable. Different types of plant foods can be combined to provide all the essential amino acids. Grains, vegetables, legumes, nuts, and seeds contain incomplete protein and are 70% to 90% digestible (Gropper & Smith, 2013).

Limiting Amino Acids and Complementation

Plants are classified as incomplete protein sources because they lack one or more essential amino acids. This

Dollars & Sense 4-1
Stretching the Meat Budget

Here is a suggestion to stretch leftover (or planned-over or deli) cooked chicken with a new look. Adding dry powdered milk boosts the protein content of the sauce and can be used in other similar sauces or puddings.

Curried Chicken
If using raw rice, prepare first. Note suggested method in
  Chapter 7 under arsenic.
Brown rice, 1.5 servings/person
  Prepare as above or substitute quick rice after making sauce.
3 tablespoons canola, olive, or peanut oil
1 teaspoon curry powder
  Sauté.
3 tablespoons flour
¼ teaspoon pepper
  Add. Cook 1 minute. Remove from heat.
2 cups milk
⅓ cup powdered dry milk
  Add. Cook over low heat, stirring until thick.
2 cups (more or less, about 10 oz) cooked diced chicken
  Add. Heat. Serve over rice.
4 tablespoons chopped, slivered, or sliced almonds
  Top each serving.
  4 servings, 34 grams protein each
Total cost, assuming that oil, flour, and pepper are available in pantry and a bottle of curry powder had to be purchased and charged to this meal = $4.29, which amounts to $1.072 per serving.

TABLE 4-5 Ounce-Equivalent of Protein Foods

	AMOUNT THAT COUNTS AS 1 OUNCE-EQUIVALENT IN THE PROTEIN FOODS GROUP	COMMON PORTIONS AND OUNCE-EQUIVALENTS
Meats	1 ounce cooked lean beef	1 small steak (eye of round, filet) = 3½–4 ounce-equivalents
	1 ounce cooked lean pork or ham	1 small lean hamburger = 2–3 ounce-equivalents
Poultry	1 ounce cooked chicken or turkey, without skin	1 small chicken breast half = 3 ounce-equivalents
	1 sandwich slice of turkey (4½" × 2½" × ⅛")	½ Cornish game hen = 4 ounce-equivalents
Seafood	1 ounce cooked fish or shell fish	1 can of tuna, drained = 3–4 ounce-equivalents
		1 salmon steak = 4–6 ounce-equivalents
		1 small trout = 3 ounce-equivalents
Eggs	1 egg	3 egg whites = 2 ounce-equivalents
		3 egg yolks = 1 ounce-equivalent
Nuts and seeds	½ ounce of nuts (12 almonds, 24 pistachios, 7 walnut halves)	1 ounce of nuts or seeds = 2 ounce-equivalents
	½ ounce of seeds (pumpkin, sunflower, or squash seeds, hulled, roasted)	
	1 Tablespoon of peanut butter or almond butter	
Beans and peas	¼ cup of cooked beans (such as black, kidney, pinto, or white beans)	1 cup split pea soup = 2 ounce-equivalents
	¼ cup of cooked peas (such as chickpeas, cowpeas, lentils, or split peas)	1 cup lentil soup = 2 ounce-equivalents
	¼ cup of baked beans, refried beans	1 cup bean soup = 2 ounce-equivalents
	¼ cup (about 2 ounces) of tofu	1 soy or bean burger patty = 2 ounce-equivalents
	1 oz tempeh, cooked	
	¼ cup roasted soybeans	
	1 falafel patty (2¼", 4 ounces)	
	2 Tablespoons hummus	

Source: ChooseMyPlate.gov. Retrieved from https://www.choosemyplate.gov/protein-foods on April 20, 2017.

undersupplied amino acid is called the **limiting amino acid.** In cereal grains, the limiting amino acid is **lysine;** in legumes, the limiting amino acids are **methionine** and **cysteine** (Gropper & Smith, 2013).

On the basis of animal studies, the principle of **complementation** was promoted, recommending every meal contain a combination of plant foods that provide all the essential amino acids. Later human studies showed that adults are adequately nourished by consuming assorted plant proteins throughout the day. As shown in Figure 4-1 supplying the amino acid pool is a dynamic process, not completely dependent on diet. **Endogenous** protein sources from the digestive tract include shed mucosal cells yielding about 50 grams and enzymes and glycoproteins delivering about 17 grams of protein daily (Gropper & Smith, 2013).

Vegetable Sources of Protein

For vegetarians or other individuals who limit their intake of animal foods, **legumes** are an important protein source. Legumes are plants having roots containing **nitrogen-fixing bacteria** that lock nitrogen into the plant's structure, thus increasing its nitrogen content.

Commonly consumed legumes are peas, beans, lentils, and peanuts. Not all peas and beans are legumes. Figure 4-2 compares the protein content of peas, beans, and nuts. Many legumes are not only low in fat but also high in fiber. Instructions at ChooseMyPlate.gov for people who seldom eat meat, poultry, or fish permit counting some peas and beans as part of the protein group, ¼ cup cooked equaling 1-ounce equivalent of protein.

Vegetarianism

There are many degrees of vegetarianism, depending on the beliefs of the individual or family. Some reasons frequently offered include long-term health benefits, religious convictions, environmental concerns, and economic necessity. Some vegetarians eat fish or poultry occasionally. Clinical Application 4-1 distinguishes various vegetarian diets. The more restrictive the diet, the more care is required to ensure adequate nutrition.

Pregnant women, infants, children, and elderly people who are vegetarians may need special assessment and instruction in the use of fortified foods and supplements. A well-balanced lacto-ovo–vegetarian diet, including eggs and

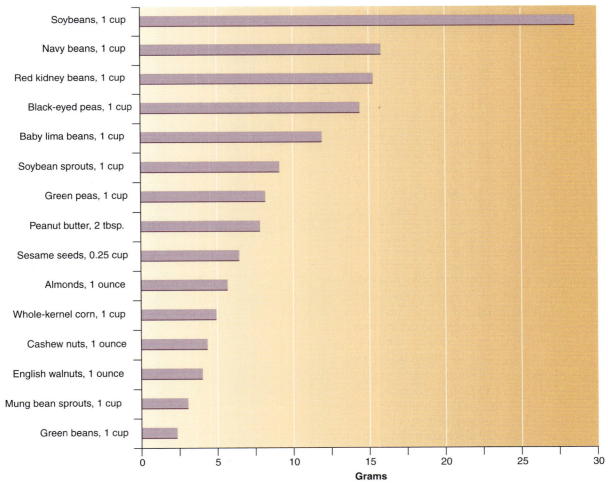

FIGURE 4-2 Protein content of selected plant foods. Notice that all foods named *peas* or *beans* are not legumes. Green beans offer just 2 grams of protein, whereas navy beans contain 16 grams.

CLINICAL APPLICATION 4-1

Vegetarian Diets

Vegetarians practice different degrees of strictness. From most liberal to most restrictive, the vegetarian diets are ovolactovegetarian, lactovegetarian, ovovegetarian, pescatarian, and or vegan. The prefixes *ovo* and *lacto* mean eggs and milk, respectively. Pescatarians consume seafood in addition to one of the other vegetarian diets. Persons following macrobiotic diets consume unrefined/unprocessed grains; small amounts of fruits, vegetables, and legumes; and sometimes milk products. A fruitarian consumes only raw fruits, nuts, seeds, and berries.

Foods Chosen in the Various Vegetarian Diets

	MEAT, SEAFOOD, POULTRY	DAIRY	EGGS
Ovolactovegetarian	No	Yes	Yes
Lactovegetarian	No	Yes	No
Ovovegetarian	No	No	Yes
Pescatarian	Seafood	Maybe	Maybe
Vegan	No	No	No

Nutrients Vegetarians May Need to Obtain From Supplements or Designated Food Sources

NUTRIENT	SITUATION TO CONSIDER SUPPLEMENTATION
Vitamin B$_{12}$	Individuals consuming few or no animal products; infants of vegan mothers
Vitamin D	Individuals consuming few or no animal products, living in northern latitudes, and those with dark skin or limited sun exposure; vitamin D$_2$ may be preferred source (see Chapter 6)
Calcium	Individuals not consuming dairy products
Iron	Individuals consuming few or no animal products
Omega-3 fatty acid	Adequate sources of linolenic acid (flaxseed and canola acids—oils, walnuts, and soy) provide the precursor to **DHA** and **EPA** (see Chapter 18)

Source: Amit, 2010.

---

dairy products, can satisfy all nutritional needs of the growing child. In contrast, a vegan diet, excluding all animal food sources, at least has to be supplemented with vitamin B$_{12}$, with special attention to adequate sources of vitamin D, calcium, zinc, and energy-dense foods containing enough high-quality protein for young children. Embracing a healthful vegetarian lifestyle encompasses more than just eliminating foods derived from animals. It is necessary to find appropriate substitutes for the nutrient-dense animal products. Many traditional regional or ethnic dishes combine a grain with a legume, with each supplying the other's limiting amino acid, for example:

- Peanut butter and whole wheat bread
- Baked beans with brown bread
- A bean burrito

Similarly, eliminating meat does not necessarily decrease fat intake. Vegetable oils and cheeses used in sauces to enhance flavor are high in fat.

Usually a hospital or care facility can provide balanced vegetarian diets. Rather than expecting the client to select acceptable items from a general menu, it is better to inform the dietitian of the client's wishes. Dollars & Sense 4-2 offers an easily made, economical vegetarian main dish using readily available grocery items.

Dietary Reference Intakes

Dietary reference intakes are provided in Appendix A. On the basis of body weight (grams per kilogram of body weight per day), infants synthesize more than twice the whole-body protein that adults do. Infants less than 6 months of age are given an adequate intake based on mean intake of healthy full-term breastfed infants because protein deficiencies have not been reported in such infants. Individuals older than 6 months have assigned recommended dietary intakes (RDAs) (Clinical Calculation 4-2).

Dollars & Sense 4-2

Pantry Vegetarian Chili

This easy suggestion provides a satisfying meatless entrée, high in fiber and protein, and low in fat. Although it specifies dried seasonings to be consistent with the pantry theme, fresh ones could be substituted if available. About four times the amount of fresh ingredients should substitute well for dried ones. The chili could be cooked and stirred in a large pot, but the slow cooker may be more convenient.

Pantry Vegetarian Chili
Place all ingredients in 3-quart electric slow cooker. Cook on low about 8 hours.
1 qt unsalted vegetable broth
1 can (15.5 oz) drained reduced sodium black beans
1 can (15.5 oz) drained reduced sodium kidney beans
1 can (15.5 oz) drained reduced sodium pinto beans
1 can (15 oz) drained no added salt whole kernel corn
1 can (14.5 oz) no-added-salt diced tomatoes
2 tablespoons dried onion
3 tablespoons chili powder
1 teaspoon oregano
1 teaspoon coriander or caraway seeds
Hot Sauce or chili powder/flakes to taste (optional)
1 teaspoon garlic powder
¼ teaspoon black pepper
2 tablespoons dark chocolate chips
1 tablespoon dried orange peel
¼ cup corn meal
Makes 12 cups, 7.3 g protein/cup
Six 2-cup servings, 14.6 g protein/serving
Total cost if all the ingredients except pepper must be purchased = $8.08. Cost per 2 cup serving = $1.47. If chili is made using low-fat ground beef, it would add $5.00 per recipe or $13.08 per recipe and $2.18 per serving. A 2-cup serving equals 4 ounce-equivalents from the protein group, providing an economical way of obtaining most of the day's required protein (see Table 4-4).

CLINICAL CALCULATION 4-2

Individualized Protein Requirement

The standard on which the adult RDA is based is 0.8 grams of protein per kilogram of body weight.

Weight in pounds is converted to kilograms by dividing by 2.2.

$$154 \text{ lb} = 70 \text{ kg} \times 0.8 = 56 \text{ grams of protein}$$

The RDAs for protein assume adequate intake of the other energy nutrients to avoid the use of protein for energy. The acceptable macronutrient distribution range (AMDR) of 10% to 35% of kilocalories offers a broad goal for protein intake, but severely restricting kilocalorie intake as well as choosing the 10% value as a benchmark for protein energy intake would not be sufficient to maintain nitrogen balance in an adult (Gropper & Smith, 2013). See Appendix A. Higher intakes may be prescribed for elderly clients and athletes (see Chapters 12 and 15).

Wise Protein Choices

Some protein foods are much less expensive than others. Dollars & Sense 4-3 lists equivalent sources of 10 grams of protein by price. Typical regular prices of store brands were used, lessening the cost.

Whether high-protein diets are detrimental to health is controversial but no tolerable upper intake level has been established for protein. Concerns focus on the following:

- Risk of dehydration because the kidneys must excrete large amounts of nitrogenous waste products
- Risk to bones from acidity produced by protein metabolism and consequent leeching of minerals from bone to **buffer** the acid if adequate sources of **bicarbonate,** mostly from fruits and vegetables, are unavailable

Dehydration is avoidable with adequate fluid intake. Little evidence supports the hazard of high protein intake in healthy individuals. When there is adequate ingestion of calcium, potassium, and magnesium in the diet (through dairy, fruits, and vegetables), no negative effects are consistently demonstrated. More studies of the effect of a high-protein diet on bone health are needed, but the recommendation is to consume protein based on the Dietary Reference Intakes (Kohn, 2015).

Amino acid supplements are not recommended for the following reasons:

- Potential imbalanced absorption caused by competition for common carrier systems
- Nitrogen assimilation from protein-containing foods is superior to that from free amino acids
- Expense
- Unpalatability
- Possible gastrointestinal distress (Gropper & Smith, 2013)

Environmentally and socially conscious consumers may choose to decrease the amounts of animal proteins they ingest to conserve resources. Because meat production requires many pounds of plant protein per pound of meat obtained, these consumers believe that such plant protein could be better used to feed people directly.

Dollars & Sense 4-3

Comparative Sources of 10 Grams of Protein

Prices listed are based on food prices choosing store brands from a large, discount grocery. Prices will vary depending on store and many market considerations such as area of the country and cost of transportation.

Food	Portion	kcalories	Price/ Amount	Cost/10 grams of Protein
Bean soup, canned	0.6 cups	204	$1.58/ 11.5 oz	$0.08
1% milk	1¼ cups	128	$1.98/gal	$0.155
Large egg	1.6	124	$1.18/doz	$0.157
Whole-wheat bread	2.5 slices	202	$1.50/18 sl loaf	$0.208
Bologna	3.15 oz	240	$ .98/12 oz	$0.257
Tuna, canned in water	1.4 oz	46	$1.00/5 oz	$0.28
Cheese, reduced-fat cheddar	1.5 oz	74	$1.54/8 oz	$0.289
Peanut butter	2.75 tbsp	263	$2.24/ 16.3 oz	$0.378
Cottage cheese, 1% low fat	3 oz	61	$3.18/ 24 oz	$0.398
Beef, ground, lean	1.75 oz	75	$5.00/lb	$0.547

KEYSTONES

- All three energy nutrients contain carbon, hydrogen, and oxygen, but protein also contains nitrogen and sometimes sulfur and uniquely serves to build and maintain tissue.

- Essential amino acids must be obtained externally because the body cannot produce a sufficient supply to meet metabolic needs. Nonessential amino acids can usually be manufactured by the body from other amino acids.

- Conditionally essential amino acids are nonessential amino acids that must be obtained externally because of the disease or condition of the client.

- Someone who is building tissue for growth and obtaining more than sufficient protein for those needs is in positive nitrogen balance. Someone in negative nitrogen balance is not receiving enough protein to replace tissue that is being broken down because of malnutrition or illness.

- Complete protein foods are those that supply all essential amino acids in sufficient quantities to maintain tissue and support growth. Animal products, except gelatin, are complete protein foods. Most plant foods lack one or more essential amino acids but can still be part of a healthy diet.

- The major protein in the blood, albumin, aids the return of fluid from the cells and tissues to the bloodstream to maintain blood volume and pressure.

- The complementation principle relates to balancing the intake of plant foods lacking a particular amino acid with foods providing it but lacking another amino acid.

- Although not regarded as crucial for people consuming animal foods, complementation may play a role in planning vegetarian diets.

CASE STUDY 4-1

Mrs. F is a 72-year-old widow who eats independently in her family home. Her usual meals are tea and toast for breakfast, canned fruit and a muffin for lunch, and frozen potpie or canned hash for dinner. She complains that she has been having trouble chewing with her old dentures and has not been eating as much food as she usually does. She does not like milk.

CARE PLAN

Subjective Data

Food deficit as evidenced by usual food intake information ■ Has trouble chewing. ■ Does not like milk.

Objective Data

Height: 5 ft 4 in. ■ Weight: 103 lb ■ Loose-fitting dentures

Analysis

Inadequate intake of protein and kilocalories, related to difficulty chewing, as evidenced by stated usual intake of 28–32 grams of protein per day and body mass index of 17.73, classified as underweight.

Plan

DESIRED OUTCOMES EVALUATION CRITERIA	ACTIONS/ INTERVENTIONS	RATIONALE
Client will gain 1 lb per week during the next 2 weeks.	Encourage easily chewed sources of complete protein: cottage cheese, eggs, ground meat, and fish.	Complete protein foods contain all essential amino acids necessary for tissue building.
Client will increase her total protein intake by 14–18 grams per day by 2-week follow-up.	Create a model meal plan with Mrs. F using food groups or MyPlate.	Mrs. F's RDA is 46 grams of protein. The meal plan she described in her history contains only 28–32 grams depending on dinner selection.
Client will call for dental appointment within next 2 weeks.	Refer to social worker for client to obtain information regarding available financial assistance.	Better-fitting dentures would permit Mrs. F a wider variety of foods.

When following up after 2 weeks, the nurse finds that Mrs. F has gained one-half pound instead of 2 as set in the desired outcome. She has increased her intake of eggs and cheese on occasion but says she feels full before finishing her meal.

TEAMWORK **4-1**

SOCIAL WORKER'S NOTES

The following Social Worker's Notes are representative of the documentation found in a client's medical record.

Subjective: *Client's resources are mainly Social Security payments. She does not have dental insurance.*

Objective: *Demonstrable ill-fitting dentures.*

Analysis: *Financial issues preclude private dental care.*

Plan: *Refer to Family Health Center dental clinic.*

CRITICAL THINKING QUESTIONS

1. What other food groups or nutrients are lacking in Mrs. F's usual diet? Would you have given any of them a higher priority than protein? Why or why not?

2. Speculate on the reasons why Mrs. F has developed her present meal pattern. What additions could you make to the care plan to take those reasons into consideration?

3. If Mrs. F added one egg and one ounce of Swiss cheese per day without changing the other components of her meal plans, to what extent would she have met her protein needs? What additional interventions would you suggest?

CHAPTER REVIEW

1. For which of the following functions of protein can other nutrients be substituted?
   1. Energy source
   2. Immunity
   3. Maintenance and growth
   4. Regulation of body processes

2. The following foods are incomplete proteins, except?
   1. Baked beans
   2. Broccoli
   3. Beef kabobs
   4. Bread sticks

3. If a person has difficulty purchasing meat to serve every day, which of the following foods should the nurse suggest as offering the best source of protein?
   1. Bran muffins with raisins
   2. Red beans and rice
   3. Green bean, onion, and mushroom casserole
   4. Sweet potatoes and cornbread

4. How much protein would a person receive from a glass of milk?
   1. 7 grams
   2. 8 grams
   3. 14 grams
   4. 21 grams

5. Which of the following people would the nurse regard as being in a catabolic state?
   1. Adolescent boy who is into bodybuilding
   2. Lactating mother
   3. Pregnant woman in the second trimester
   4. Surgical client, first day after a stomach resection

CLINICAL ANALYSIS

1. Mr. P, a 65-year-old man, widowed for 6 months, has been referred to your home health agency for weight loss. He has lost 10 pounds over the past 6 months. A physical examination within the past month revealed no disease processes requiring treatment. In assessing Mr. P, which of the following data would the nurse gather first?

   a. List of current medications the client takes
   b. Blood protein levels analyzed during the recent physical examination
   c. A description of the procedure Mr. P uses to weigh himself
   d. Dietary recall of Mr. P's food and fluid intake

2. Which of the following plans would be most appropriate to increase Mr. P's protein consumption immediately?

   a. Refer client to nutrition education program.
   b. Have Mr. P apply for home-delivered meals.
   c. Recommend that Mr. P supplement his meals with one of the milk-based liquid breakfast products.
   d. Suggest to Mr. P that he sign up for cooking lessons at the local high school or community college.

3. Which of the following outcomes would indicate achievement of the nutritional objective for Mr. P?

   a. A gain in weight of 2 pounds in 2 weeks
   b. An invitation to the nurse to join him for a dinner he has learned to cook
   c. A report by Mr. P that he is eating better
   d. A visual inspection of Mr. P's refrigerator revealing fresh meat and milk products in abundance

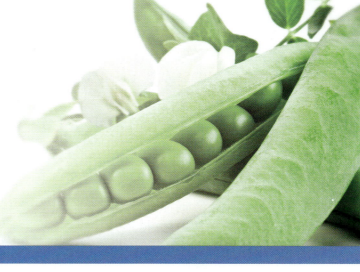

CHAPTER 5

Energy Balance

LEARNING OBJECTIVES

After completing this chapter, the student should be able to:

- Describe energy homeostasis. List two reasons the body needs energy.
- Describe how energy is measured both in foods and in the human body.
- Discuss the effect of body composition on energy output.
- Name the energy nutrient that has the highest kilocalorie density and identify two substances usually found in foods with a low kilocalorie density.

A complete understanding of the human body's energy balance system eludes experts. In approximately 40% of the U.S. population, the human body regulates energy intake and expenditure automatically to maintain an **energy balance.** This balance occurs even when the amount of energy needed varies and food intake is erratic. The body can also compensate during food restriction or starvation by conserving energy. Maintenance of a reduced or elevated body weight is associated with compensatory changes in energy expenditure, which oppose the maintenance of a body weight that is different from the usual body weight.

A basic understanding of what is known about energy balance is necessary for understanding energy imbalance. This chapter therefore focuses on energy balance (Chapter 16 on weight management focuses on energy imbalance), and in particular on the effects of energy intake and expenditure on energy balance. Topics include the following:

- Energy measurements
- Factors influencing the body's energy need
- Energy consumption patterns
- The kilocaloric content and nutrient density of foods
- Energy allowances
- Current recommendations concerning energy consumption

Homeostasis and Survival

The human body seeks homeostasis—that is, equilibrium, or balance. Homeostasis, in terms of energy balance, occurs when the number of kilocalories eaten equals the number used to produce energy. An individual who maintains a stable body weight is usually in energy balance.

However, the human body has developed biological mechanisms allowing it to survive at the cost of maintaining energy balance. Throughout human history, periods of feast or famine were common. The human body developed numerous redundant systems to safeguard against death by starvation. In the event that one metabolic pathway malfunctioned, another evolved to compensate. However, in modern times—when food is often plentiful—these evolutionary survival mechanisms have proved to be a detriment for many people. This disadvantage is evident by the increasing number of people who are overweight or obese. Obesity has nearly doubled worldwide since 1980 (World Health Organization, 2016).

Energy Intake

The typical adult eats 500,000 to 850,000 kilocalories per year. Eating an excess of only 1% or 15 extra kilocalories per day would result in a weight gain of 1.5 pounds per year—the kilocalories in $1/3$ teaspoonful of butter or a quarter of a small apple. Individuals at a stable, healthy weight give little thought to the amount of food that they eat each day, yet their body weight remains constant.

Eating appears to be a voluntary act influenced by the external environment, but it is regulated internally as well. The internal regulation of energy balance involves the gastrointestinal tract, the endocrine system, the brain, and body fat stores. Physiologic regulation is evidenced by the constancy of body weight in adults and the fact that, after weight gain or loss, this constant body weight is reestablished. Over the long-term, food energy intake is regulated to balance energy expenditure. See Box 5-1 for a discussion on appetite and hunger.

BOX 5-1 ■ Appetite versus Hunger

Appetite is different from hunger.

Appetite is a strong desire for food or a pleasant sensation, based on previous experience, that causes one to seek food for taste and enjoyment.

Hunger is a sensation that results from a lack of food, characterized by a dull or acute pain around the lower part of the chest. A truly hungry person will most likely eat anything and take drastic action to acquire food.

Unfortunately, eating is not always the result of hunger. People eat or do not eat in response to stress, time of day, boredom, physical activity, and other reasons. In short, people can override the internal biological signals for eating.

Energy Expenditure

Energy expenditure, which varies daily, is measured by the number of kilocalories used to meet the body's demand for fuel. A person uses many more kilocalories to run a marathon than to sleep.

Adaptive Thermogenesis

Energy expenditure frequently adapts to large increases or decreases in food intake of several days' duration by means of a process called **adaptive thermogenesis**. Adaptive thermogenesis is one example of how the human body evolved to cope with feast-or-famine conditions. Energy expenditure decreases during food restriction or starvation. Kilocalories are burned more efficiently. Adaptive thermogenesis causes an individual trying to lose weight either to lose at a slower rate or to stop losing weight. As a result, losing weight is difficult for many people but not impossible.

Measuring Energy

Both the energy (fuel) foods contain and the amount of energy the body uses can be measured. The methods used to measure energy are fairly universal.

Units of Measure

The energy content of food is measured in calories and, increasingly, in joules.

A **calorie** is the amount of energy required to raise or lower the temperature of 1 kilogram of water to 1°C. In chemistry, a calorie is the amount of heat required to raise the temperature of 1 gram of water to 1°C. One kilocalorie, as used in the nutritional sciences, contains 1,000 times as much energy as 1 calorie used in chemistry. In summary, one calorie, as used in chemistry, is equal to 1,000 calories or 1 kilocalorie. Understanding the difference is important. *Kilocalorie* (abbreviated *kcalorie* or *kcal*) and *Calorie* are the terms used throughout this text because these terms are used in the medical literature, including clients' medical records.

Using kcalories for nutritional measurement eliminates the large numbers that using the chemical term would necessitate.

Energy Nutrient Values

The energy nutrients are carbohydrates, fat, and protein. Alcohol (ethanol) also yields energy. A food's kcalorie value is determined by its content of protein, fat, carbohydrates, and alcohol.

- 1 gram of carbohydrate equals 4 kilocalories
- 1 gram of protein equals 4 kilocalories
- 1 gram of fat equals 9 kilocalories
- 1 gram of alcohol equals 7 kilocalories

Water, fiber, vitamins, and minerals do not provide kilocalories. Clinical Calculation 5-1 demonstrates how to determine the energy content of a food item.

Determining Energy Values

Energy, whether in foods or in the body, is measured as a form of heat.

Foods

The energy content of individual foods is measured by a device called a bomb calorimeter. A bomb calorimeter is

CLINICAL CALCULATION 5-1

Calculating the Energy Content of a Food Item

If you know the carbohydrate, fat, and protein content of a food item, you can readily calculate the food's kcalorie content. Two examples are shown here. One starch serving contains 3 grams of protein and 15 grams of carbohydrate. Adding the protein and carbohydrate content in the starch serving equals 18.

	CARBOHYDRATE (GRAMS)		PROTEIN (GRAMS)		FAT (GRAMS)		TOTAL (GRAMS)
One starch serving	15	+	3	+	0	=	18

Each gram of carbohydrate and protein has 4 kcal, and so to obtain the kcalorie content of the starch serving, multiply 4 by 18. Thus, one starch serving has 72 kcal.

One fat serving contains 5 grams of fat.

	CARBOHYDRATE (GRAMS)		PROTEIN (GRAMS)		FAT (GRAMS)		TOTAL (GRAMS)
One fat serving	0	+	0	+	5	=	5

A gram of fat has 9 kcal. To obtain the kilocaloric content of one fat serving, multiply 5 by 9. Thus, one fat serving contains 45 kcal.

an insulated container that has a chamber in which food is burned. The amount of heat (kcalories) produced by the burning of the food is determined by the change in the temperature of a measured amount of water that surrounds the chamber. All energy in food is in the form of chemical energy. In a bomb calorimeter, the chemical energy stored in the food sample is transformed into heat energy. The following equation may facilitate understanding of this concept:

Protein + oxygen = heat energy + water + carbon dioxide

(Carbohydrate or fat may be substituted for protein in the equation.)

The Human Body

A process similar to the combustion of food in the bomb calorimeter occurs in the body. The amount of energy the human body uses can be measured directly or indirectly.

Direct measurement of energy used by the human body requires expensive equipment that is used only in scientific research. Energy is measured directly by placing a person in an insulated heat-sensitive chamber and measuring the heat emitted by the body.

Indirect measurement of energy (also called indirect calorimetry) is discussed in Clinical Application 5-1.

In clinical practice an estimation of the resting energy expenditure (REE) can be made using formulas such as the Harris-Benedict equation (see Table 5-1). REE is estimated on the basis of the height, weight, age, and sex of the individual. There are separate formulas for men and women.

CLINICAL APPLICATION   5-1

Measurement of Resting Energy Expenditure by Indirect Calorimetry

The process of measuring resting energy expenditure (REE) with indirect calorimetry is the preferred measurement of REE measurement (Kruizenga, Hofsteenge, & Weijs, 2016). Indirect involves measuring oxygen and carbon dioxide concentrations in expired air during a prescribed period. The amount of oxygen that is used and the amount of carbon dioxide produced are entered into a scientific formula that will calculate energy expenditure. This method can be used with spontaneous breathing or with a mechanically ventilated individual, such as a client in an intensive care unit.

TABLE 5-1   Harris-Benedict Equation to Calculate REE

To convert weight in pounds to kilograms (kg): 1 kg = 2.2 pounds; divide body weight in pounds by 2.2.

To convert height in inches to centimeters (cm): 1 inch = 2.54 cm; multiply height in inches by 2.54.
- REE for men: 66.5 + (13.8 × weight in kg) + (5 × height in cm) – (6.8 × age in years)
- REE for women: 655 + (9.6 × weight in kg) + (1.8 × height in cm) – (4.7 × age in years)

Components of Energy Expenditure

The human body requires energy to meet its REE needs, satisfy its physical activity requirements, and process nutrients. REE, which includes all involuntary activities, is the kcalories a person burns under controlled conditions and lying comfortably. Voluntary physical activity includes the energy needed for voluntary activities—which are consciously controlled, such as running, walking, and swimming. The third component of energy expenditure is the energy expended to digest, absorb, transport, and use nutrients.

Resting Energy Expenditure

REE represents the energy expended or used by a person at rest. In most people, REE requires more total kcalories than physical activity. Clinical Application 5-1 discusses the measurement of REE in clients. The term *REE* is generally associated with the use of a respirometer or a device that measures oxygen consumption. The kcalories necessary to support the following contribute to REE:

- Contraction of the heart
- Maintenance of body temperature
- Repair of the internal organs
- Maintenance of cellular processes
- Muscle and nerve coordination
- Respiration (breathing)

REE accounts for 45% to 80% of total energy expenditure. Body composition influences REE. Individuals of similar age, sex, height, and weight with a higher percentage of muscle (lean body mass) have a higher REE than those with less muscle. It takes more energy, or kcalories, to support lean body mass (protein) than to support body fat. Muscle tissue requires more kcalories than does fat tissue, even when muscle tissue is resting. Therefore, the higher a person's body protein content, the more kcalories he or she can eat and still maintain a stable body weight.

Age

REE varies with lean body mass, which varies with age. The highest rates of energy expenditure per pound of body weight occur during infancy and childhood. In adults, REE declines about 1% to 2% per decade after age 20 because of a decline in lean body mass. The result is a reduced need for kcalories. Individuals can slow the decline in lean body mass somewhat by increasing their exercise. An individual who fails either to decrease kilocaloric intake to compensate for this reduced need or to increase physical activity may experience a slow weight gain.

Sex

Differences in body composition between men and women occur as early as the first few months of life. The differences are relatively small until the child reaches age 10. During adolescence, body composition changes radically. Men develop proportionately greater lean muscle mass than women, who deposit fat as they mature. Consequently, REE differs by as much as 10% between men and women.

Growth

Human growth is most pronounced during the growth spurts that take place before birth and during infancy and puberty. Kcalories required per kilogram of body weight are highest during these growth spurts because the kilocaloric cost of anabolism is greater than the kilocaloric cost of catabolism.

Body Size

People with large bodies require proportionately more energy than smaller ones. A tall individual uses more energy because he or she has a greater skin surface through which heat is lost than does a shorter person. A shorter person also has less muscle tissue or lean body mass than a taller person.

Most health-care professionals are surprised at the large volume of food needed to maintain a tall male's body weight (greater than 6 feet tall) and how small a volume of food is needed to maintain weight in a short female (less than 5 feet tall). In proportion to total body weight, the infant has a large surface area, loses more heat through the skin, and therefore has a proportionately high REE.

Climate

Climate affects REE because kcalories are needed to maintain body temperature. This fact pertains to extreme differences in external temperatures, whether cold or hot. In the United States and Canada, most people do not need to eat more kcalories during colder months, because most living environments range from 68°F (20°C) to 77°F (25°C). Outside, people usually protect themselves from extreme cold and shivering, which causes an increase in REE, by wearing warm clothes.

Genetics

REE is strongly influenced by individual genetic patterns; see Genomic Gem 5-1.

Thermic Effect of Food

The heat produced by the body after a meal is called the **thermic effect of food**. An older term for this energy cost is *specific dynamic action*. Energy is needed to chew, swallow, digest, absorb, and transport nutrients. Metabolism increases after eating. As metabolism increases, more kcalories are used.

The consumption of protein and carbohydrates results in a larger thermic effect than the consumption of fat. Fat is metabolized efficiently as compared with glucose. Protein requires the most energy to digest, followed by carbohydrate, with fats requiring the least amount of energy. It is estimated that for every 100 kcalories of protein consumed it requires up to 30 kcalories to digest, whereas fat would require only a maximum of 3 kcalories per 100 kcalories consumed to digest. If an individual eats as many kcalories from carbohydrate or protein as from fat, he or she will store fewer of the nonfat kcalories as body fat.

Kcalories do count, however, regardless of the source. Consumers need to read food labels carefully. Sometimes a regular version of a food may actually contain fewer kcalories than the fat-free or reduced-fat version. For example, a regular fig cookie contains 50 kcalories, and one fat-free version contains 70 kcalories. One-half cup of regular ice cream contains 180 calories, and the same amount of one kind of reduced-fat ice cream contains 190 kcalories. Sometimes consumers are under the illusion that because the food they are eating is low fat, they can eat unrestricted amounts and maintain body weight (Dollars & Sense 5-1).

Physical Activity

For most of the world's population, physical activity uses fewer kcalories than those required for REE. Physical activity accounts for 25% to 50% of human energy expenditure (Walpole et al, 2012). Very few people are active enough to burn more kcalories as a result of physical activity than as a result of their REE; however, some very active individuals do expend more kcalories as a result of physical activity (Fig. 5-1). For example, professional athletes may burn a

GENOMIC GEM 5-1

Resting Energy Expenditure

REE is strongly influenced by individual genetic patterns. Each person appears to be programmed with a need to burn a certain number of kcalories to maintain energy balance. This fact becomes apparent to health-care workers when counseling two very similar clients. Both clients may be of the same sex, of equal weight, perform similar types of physical activity, and have about the same body fat content. Yet each client may need to eat a different number of kcalories to maintain a stable body weight. Many individuals have little control over the number of kcalories required to meet the needs of REE.

Dollars & Sense 5-1
Kcalorie Control

Kcalorie control = Portion control = Fewer dollars spent at the grocery store.

Here's why: Some nutrients are needed daily because the body is unable to store them. Vitamin C is one example. Orange juice is high in vitamin C and is best consumed in 1/2 cup serving sizes to meet the daily need for vitamin C. If a food purchaser drinks an entire quart of orange juice daily, he or she will need to buy this item frequently.

Because fruits and fruit juices are becoming increasingly more expensive, think of expensive food items primarily as sources of nutrients to be eaten in recommended serving sizes.

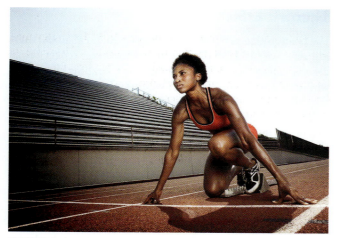

FIGURE 5-1 A trained athlete may burn more kcalories as a result of physical activity than as a result of resting energy expenditure.

large number of kcalories as a result of training and engaging in competition.

As Table 5-2 shows, the intensity and duration of any physical activity enormously influences kcalorie expenditure. For example, a 154-pound man who trains by running vigorously at a speed of 5 miles per hour will expend almost 600 kcalories in a 1-hour training session. The energy cost of physical activity is frequently referred to as the thermic effect of exercise.

Nonexercise Activity Thermogenesis

Nonexercise activity thermogenesis (NEAT) refers to the activities of daily living that burn kcalories, such as fidgeting, cleaning, standing, and hygiene practices. Clients with higher NEAT tend to stay leaner throughout their lifespan due to burning more kcalories during the day (Clark, 2015). The benefits of NEAT have demonstrated an increase in daily kcalories burned and a decrease in the occurrence of metabolic syndrome and cardiovascular events (Villablanca et al, 2015).

Daily fluctuations in physical activity can greatly influence an individual's energy requirements (Table 5-3). For example, a 38-year-old man of normal weight may require only 2,400 kcalories on a sedentary day and as many as 3,000 kcalories on a very active day. A 38-year-old woman of normal body weight may require only 1,800 kcalories on a sedentary day and as many as 2,200 kcalories on a very active day.

TABLE 5-2 Kcalories Expended in 30 Minutes and 1 Hour

ACTIVITY	KCALORIES EXPENDED BY A 154-POUND MAN IN 30 MINUTES	KCALORIES EXPENDED BY A 154-POUND MAN IN 60 MINUTES
Moderate Activity		
Walking (3½ miles per hour)	140	280
Light gardening/yard work	165	330
Golf (walking and carrying clubs	165	330
Dancing	165	330
Vigorous Activity		
Running/jogging (5 miles per hour)	295	590
Cycling (more than 10 miles per hour)	295	590
Walking (4½ miles per hour)	230	510
Swimming (slow freestyle laps)	255	510

Source: United States Department of Agriculture, https://www.choosemyplate.gov/physical-activity-calories-burn

TABLE 5-3 Energy Needs Based on Age and Activity

ENERGY NEEDS IN KCALORIES BASED ON ACTIVITY LEVEL

	Sedentary*	Moderately Active**	Active***
18-year-old males	2,400	2,800	3,200
18-year-old females	1,800	2,000	2,400
26–30-year-old males	2,400	2,600	3,000
26–30-year-old females	1,800	2,000	2,400
31–40-year-old males	2,400	2,600	3,000
31–40-year-old females	1,800	2,000	2,200
51–55-year-old males	2,200	2,400	2,800
51–55-year-old females	1,600	1,800	2,000
76+-year-old males	2,000	2,200	2,400
76+-year-old females	1,600	1,800	2,000

Male reference is 5 ft 10 in. tall and weighs 154 pounds and female reference is 5 ft 4 in. tall and weighs 126 pounds.
* Sedentary is defined as lifestyle that includes only the physical activities of independent daily living.
** Moderately active is defined as activity that includes walking 1.5–3 miles per day at 3–4 miles per hour, in addition to activities of independent living.
*** Active is defined as lifestyle that includes physical activity that includes walking more than 3 miles per day at 3–4 miles per hour, in addition to activities of independent living.
Source: Adapted from U.S. Department of Health and Human Services and U.S. Department of Agriculture (2015), https://health.gov/dietaryguidelines/2015/guidelines/

The Institute of Medicine of the National Academies (2006) put together a report on Dietary Reference Intakes that describes a method to estimate energy needs that includes both those needed for REE and activity (https://www.nal.usda.gov/fnic/dri-nutrient-reports). This method to estimate kcaloric need is often used in wellness programs to give clients some idea of their approximate energy need. The most accurate method for determining a client's kcalorie requirement is to monitor both food intake and body weight over time. Sometimes in clinical settings, obtaining weight and food intake information is impossible during a client's assessment. In Chapter 22, we provide a formula that takes into account age, sex, weight, and height for estimating kcal need.

Thermic Effect of Exercise

Energy expended during exercise is only a portion of the total energy cost of physical activity. Exercise may also affect both REE and the thermic effect of exercise. Some clients' REE increases for up to 48 hours after exercise. Although the exact reason for this increase is unknown, the most plausible explanation is that glycogen stores need to be refilled. Because exercise depletes glycogen stores, energy is used to provide glycogen stores pre-exercise and to refill these stores during the postexercise periods.

Adaptive Response to Exercise

An individual with well-developed muscles performs more efficiently—uses fewer kcalories to perform a given amount of physical work—than an individual with less well-developed muscles. As exercise is repeated, the body learns how to get the job done with the least effort (the body's adaptive response to exercise). If an individual has a weight loss due to increased exercise, he or she will eventually use fewer kcalories to do a specific activity. This is the reason body builders need to continually increase the amount of weight lifted to achieve maximum results. Lighter people require fewer kcalories for a given amount of exercise than heavier people do; it takes fewer kcalories to move a smaller mass than a larger one.

Although heavier people, who move more weight, burn more kcalories than lighter people when they exercise, a heavy body is a disincentive for movement and physical activity. Heavier people tend to do fewer energy-demanding activities.

Exercise and Appetite

Many exercise researchers think that exercise decreases appetite—that is, a person may be satisfied with less food after exercise. Exercise at a sufficient intensity and duration releases a chemical in the brain called beta-endorphin and leads to increased circulating concentrations of serotonin (Bostani & Ranjbar, 2014). Beta-endorphin has an effect similar to that of natural morphine; it produces a state of relaxation. In effect, exercise can be a safe substitute for overeating in some individuals who eat to decrease stress and tension. However, an individual with a severe eating disorder may exercise compulsively to relax.

Aerobic Exercise

Aerobic exercise is any activity during which the energy metabolism needed is supported by the amount of increase in oxygen inspired. Aerobic exercises increase physical fitness and involve large muscle groups. Vigorous workouts that last at least 30 minutes require an increase in the amount of oxygen inspired. Walking is a low-impact, moderate-intensity aerobic exercise that is the most popular exercise of Americans (Hosler, Gallant, Riley-Jacome, & Rajulu, 2014). Box 5-2 provides examples of aerobic exercise. Aerobic exercise provides many health benefits, including the following:

- Decreased risk of cardiovascular disease
- Improved blood sugar control for people with diabetes
- Decreased risk of obesity
- Reversal or prevention of varicose veins
- Decreased risk of osteoporosis
- Improved quality of sleep
- Improved hypertension control

Anaerobic Exercise

Exercise during which energy is provided without an increase in the use of inspired oxygen is **anaerobic exercise.** Short bursts of vigorous activity, such as resistance or muscle strength training (e.g., weight lifting), are forms of anaerobic exercise. Anaerobic exercise allows for:

- Muscle toning
- The building of muscular strength and endurance
- Building of bone mass

This kind of training provides added strength and toughness, which help to reduce injury during aerobic exercise, prevents lower back problems, and allows for a more muscular appearance.

Balance and Stretching

Balance and stretching exercises such as yoga, t'ai chi, and martial arts promote:

- Increased physical stability
- Increased flexibility
- Decreased risk of injury

BOX 5-2 ■ Examples of Aerobic Exercise

These are some popular forms of aerobic exercise:

Fast walking
Cycling
Swimming
Skating
Jumping rope
Dancing
Hiking
Jogging
Rowing

Bone strengthening

Exercises that place force on the bone, such as jumping rope and running, will promote growth and strength of bone. This form of exercise is recommended to be included in the weekly exercise program of children.

Diet and Activity

A healthy lifestyle depends on much more than diet. Physical activity makes a vital contribution to health, function, and performance. The greatest benefit derived from physical activity is gained when a person moves from sedentary to moderate levels of activity. The combination of a balanced diet and regular physical activity has a stronger effect on energy balance than either strategy alone.

The Centers for Disease Control and Prevention (CDC) and the World Health Organization (2015) currently recommend the following minimum activity guidelines for adults aged 18 to 65 years:

- 150 minutes of moderate-intensity aerobic activity every week and muscle-strengthening activities on 2 or more days a week, or
- 75 minutes of vigorous-intensity aerobic activity every week and muscle-strengthening activities on 2 or more days per week, or
- A combination of moderate- and vigorous-intensity aerobic activities and muscle-strengthening activities on 2 or more days a week. One minute of vigorous-intensity activity is equivalent to about 2 minutes of moderate-intensity activity (Centers for Disease Control and Prevention, 2015).

For additional health benefits, adults should increase their moderate-intensity aerobic activities to 300 minutes per week or engage in 150 minutes of vigorous-intensity aerobic physical activities per week, or an equivalent combination of moderate- and vigorous-intensity activities. Muscle-strengthening activities should include all major muscle groups—legs, hips, back, abdomen, chest, shoulders, and arms. The activity need not be continuous but may be broken up into short sessions. For example, six brisk 10-minute walks would meet the minimum requirement. A 154-pound man performing this activity for 60 minutes expends 280 total kcalories. In general, the more time a person spends exercising each week will increase the total number of kcalories expended and increase overall health benefits. For complete activity guidelines visit https://www.cdc.gov/physicalactivity/basics/adults/.

Energy Intake

Between 2013 and 2014, the mean reported energy intake for men aged 20 to 59 was 2,493 to 2,704 kcalories per day (U.S. Department of Agriculture [USDA], 2016). The mean reported energy intake for women aged 20 to 59 was between 1,779 and 1,933 kcalories per day (USDA, 2016). The average reported intakes for women are of special concern because of the difficulty of incorporating all nutrients at recommended levels in a diet so low in kcalories. The average woman's need to increase energy output or physical activity is well documented.

Many experts attribute increased obesity to decreased energy expenditure. America is becoming an increasingly sedentary society. The current recommendation is that the average person increase physical activity rather than decrease kcalorie intake below their estimated energy requirements (EER) to achieve energy balance. If the average reported intakes for both sexes are compared with the EER, the need for more physical activity in most people becomes clear. For specifics, refer to the dietary reference intakes in Appendix A.

Kilocaloric Density of Foods

Some foods are more kilocalorically dense than other foods. Density is the quantity per unit volume of a substance. **Kilocaloric density** refers to the kcalories contained in a given volume of a food, generally the number of kcalories in a gram. Foods with a high water and fiber content tend to have a lower kcaloric density. Fruits and vegetables such as lettuce, watermelon, and celery are high in water content and low in kcalories. A given volume of grapes has fewer kcalories than an equal volume of raisins because grapes contain more water than raisins.

Fats or foods high in fat have the highest kcaloric density (see Fig. 5-2). Whole-milk products; high-fat animal food items such as meat, cheese, and eggs; and foods made with these ingredients all contain appreciable amounts of fat. Box 5-3 lists several tips for decreasing the kcaloric density of a diet.

Studies have demonstrated that diets with high energy density have been associated with obesity, and low-energy-density diets encourage weight maintenance and weight loss (Hebestreit et al, 2014).

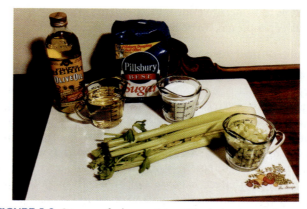

FIGURE 5-2 One cup of celery contains 17 kcalories, 1 cup of sugar contains 770 kcalories, and 1 cup of oil contains 1,925 kcalories. Celery is the least kcalorically dense of the foods pictured, and oil is the most dense. Sugar is between celery and oil in kcaloric density.

BOX 5-3 ■ Tips for Decreasing the Kilocaloric Density of a Diet

- Use low-fat or nonfat dairy products, including skim milk, cheese, and yogurt.
- Brown meats by broiling or cooking in nonstick pans with little or no fat. Avoid fried foods.
- Chill soups, stews, sauces, and broths. Lift off and discard hardened fat.
- Add extra vegetables to casseroles, chili, lasagna, or other hot dishes.
- Trim all visible fat from meat before cooking.
- Use water-packed, canned foods such as fruits and tuna.
- Use fresh fruits and vegetables often. Try to eat at least 2½ cups of these foods each day.
- Use low-kcalorie salad dressings.
- When you eat out, do not look at the menu. Instead, have an idea of what you would like to eat before you arrive at the restaurant. Explain to the waitress or waiter what you would like to eat.
- Eat smaller portion sizes of all foods, but particularly sandwiches.
- Limit consumption of sweetened carbonated beverages and other empty kcalorie foods.

Nutrient Density of Foods

Kilocaloric content alone should not be the criterion to decide whether to include a food in one's diet. The nutrient density of a food—the concentration of nutrients in a food compared with the food's kilocaloric content—is also an important consideration. If a food is high in kcalories and low in nutrients, the nutrient density of the food is low. **Empty kcalories** means that the food contains kcalories and almost no nutrients; table sugar is an example of such a food. If a food is low in kcalories and high in nutrients, the nutrient density of the food is high.

Cantaloupe is an example of a food with a high nutrient density—it is low in kcalories and high in vitamin C and contains a moderate amount of vitamin A. Skim milk and whole milk are similar in nutrient content; both types of milk contain about the same amounts of protein, calcium, vitamin D, and riboflavin. Eight ounces of skim milk provides about 90 kcalories compared with 150 kcalories in 8 ounces of whole milk. Skim milk thus has a higher nutrient density than whole milk.

Portion Size

Portion size varies from serving size. Serving size is the amount listed on a product's nutritional facts, and portion size is the amount a person chooses to consume (National Institutes of Health, 2016). Portion sizes have demonstrated an increase over the past decades with a correlation in the rise of obesity in America. The increase in portion sizes has caused people to no longer recognize what a recommended portion is; this is referred to as "portion distortion" (Vermeer, Steenhuis, & Poelman, 2014). Table 5-4 and Figure 5-3 demonstrate the increase in portion sizes over the years.

TABLE 5-4   Portion Size

	20 YEARS AGO		TODAY	
	Portion Size	Calories	Portion Size	Calories
Bagel	3″ diameter	140	6″ diameter	350
Soda	6.5 ounces	82	20 ounces	250
Blueberry muffin	1.5 ounces	210	5 ounces	500

Source: National Institutes of Health: National Heart, Lung, and Blood Institute: Serving sizes and portions. Reviewed September 30, 2013. Accessed on April 13, 2017. Available at https://www.nhlbi.nih.gov/health/educational/wecan/eat-right/distortion.htm

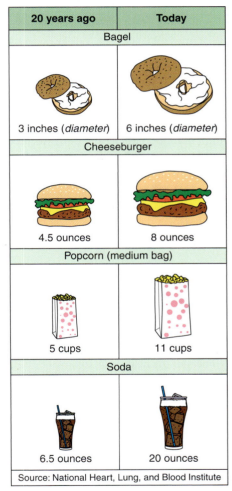

Portion Distortion

20 years ago	Today
Bagel	
3 inches (*diameter*)	6 inches (*diameter*)
Cheeseburger	
4.5 ounces	8 ounces
Popcorn (medium bag)	
5 cups	11 cups
Soda	
6.5 ounces	20 ounces

Source: National Heart, Lung, and Blood Institute

FIGURE 5-3 Portion sizes have grown over the past 20 years. *(From National Heart, Lung, and Blood Institute, https://www.nhlbi.nih.gov/health/educational/wecan/news-events/matte1.htm. Accessed on November 30, 2017.)*

Dietary Recommendations

All the major national health organizations recommend that individuals maintain a healthy body weight. The American Heart Association recommends maintaining a healthy body weight to decrease the risk of heart and circulatory diseases. The American Cancer Society cites numerous studies suggesting that lower kilocaloric intake may lower an individual's risk of cancer. Most individuals would benefit by monitoring their weight and increasing their energy expenditure or decreasing their energy intake as necessary to maintain a healthy body weight.

Current guidelines for the distribution of macronutrients and daily caloric intake for adults, aged 19 years and older, are:

- Carbohydrate 45% to 65%
- Protein 10% to 35%
- Fat 20% to 35%

KEYSTONES

- Energy balance exists when energy intake equals energy output. A person whose body weight remains stable is usually in energy balance.

- A person's appetite can overrule the body's ability to maintain homeostasis.

- A hungry person will most often be willing to eat almost anything.

- When an individual is not in energy balance, he or she is gaining or losing weight.

- The most accurate method for determining kcalorie need is to monitor both food intake and body weight over time.

- Foods high in water and fiber (fruits and vegetables) are low in kilocaloric density.

- Foods high in fat (fatty meats, oils, spreads, salad dressings, and food made with those ingredients) are high in kilocaloric density.

- Foods that are low in kcalories and contain substantial amounts of one or more nutrients are high in nutrient density.

- Most Americans are not following recommended portion sizes.

- The recommended range of energy nutrient intake is:
  - 45% to 65% for carbohydrate
  - 20% to 35% for fat
  - 10% to 35% for protein

- The current recommendation is that individuals who gain weight while consuming their energy EER should increase their activity to maintain energy balance.

- Most Americans are eating too much of one, two, or three of the energy nutrients to maintain energy balance.

CASE STUDY 5-1

The Fairview Nursing Home holds a weekly client care conference. Nursing care plans for all of the facility's residents are reviewed on a rotating basis, with each client's nursing care plan reviewed once every 3 months. All members of the health-care team are often present at the conference. Team members include the administrator, the physician, the director of nursing, the staff nurse, the nursing assistant, the activities director, the social worker, the dietitian, and the client or a family member representing the client.

Mr. G has been experiencing a slow weight gain. His weight history follows:

2/08	169 lb (77 kg)
6/08	172 lb (78 kg)
9/08	175 lb (80 kg)
12/08	180 lb (82 kg)
03/09	183 lb (83 kg)

Mr. G is 5 ft 8 in. tall and 79 years old. He is alert, feeds himself, and has normal bowel and bladder function. Mr. G walks to the dining room three times a day. His favorite activity is watching television. He has good dentition and is on a regular diet. According to the appetite records kept by the nurse's aide, Mr. G's intake is good to excellent. He accepts all of the major food groups. He admits to overeating at social activities, especially those sponsored by the facility in the evenings. Mr. G is concerned with his slow weight gain but claims that he does not know what to do. To address the slow weight gain problem, the health-care team and Mr. G developed the following nursing care plan.

CARE PLAN

Subjective Data
Client expressed concern about his slow weight gain.

Objective Data
Height is 5 ft 8 in. Weight: 2/08, 169 lb (BMI 25.7) ■ 03/09, 183 lb (BMI 27.8)

Analysis
Weight gain related to sedentary activity level and eating in response to external cues.

Plan

DESIRED OUTCOMES EVALUATION CRITERIA	ACTIONS/ INTERVENTIONS	RATIONALE
Client will select fresh fruits at social activities.	Request that Foods and Nutrition Department serve fresh fruit at social functions.	Replacing kilocalorically dense cakes, pies, and cookies with fresh fruit will promote weight maintenance.
Refer client to registered dietitian (RD).	Reinforce dietitian's teaching.	The dietitian will generally be able to spend more time with client than the floor nurse.
Refer client to activities director.	Reinforce activities director's teaching.	The activities director will be able to discuss opportunities to exercise with client as well as order appropriate foods for activities.

TEAMWORK 5-1

DIETITIAN'S NOTES

The following Dietitian's Notes are representative of the documentation found in a client's medical record.

Subjective: *Client states that he would like to lose weight but can't resist treats served at social functions. Loves cakes, pie, donuts, and cookies and admits to lack of self-control. Client would appreciate having more healthful snacks available at social functions. Admits to being unaware of what he actually eats every day. Admits that he avoids body movement.*

Objective: *Height 5 ft 8 in. 02/08 weight 169 lb (BMI 25.7), 03/09 weight 183 lb (BMI 27.8). Appetite records show a food intake of 100% of all food served plus second portions.*

Analysis: *Ideal body weight 148–180 lb (BMI 18.5–24.9)*

Estimated kcal needs at 12 kcal/pound = 2,280 (between sedentary and moderately active).

Excessive energy intake related to failure to adjust for lifestyle changes and decreased metabolism as evidenced by body weight and client history. Client expressed verbal desire to manage his weight.

Plan:
1. *Client will keep a food record for 3 of every 7 days to enable him to be more conscious of food choices (self-monitor behavior). Will evaluate food records for 2 weeks.*
2. *Client's goal is to maintain weight and perhaps lose a few pounds.*
3. *Will encourage activities director to order fresh fruit at facility functions and evaluate client for physical activity opportunities.*

TEAMWORK 5-2

ACTIVITY DIRECTOR'S NOTE

The following Activities Director's Notes are representative of the documentation found in a client's medical record.

Met with client and discussed activities calendar, including those with an exercise component. Will order a fresh fruit option at social activities that serve food.

CRITICAL THINKING QUESTIONS

1. What would you do at the next client care conference if Mr. G changed his mind about weight control and said, "All I have left in life is food. I don't want to lose weight"?

2. What would you do at the next client care conference if Mr. G had done everything asked but only managed to maintain his weight.

3. What types of exercise would be appropriate to suggest to Mr. G?

CHAPTER REVIEW

1. The components of energy expenditure are:
   1. Mental activity and physical activity
   2. Thermic effects of exercise and foods
   3. Resting energy expenditure, physical activity, and, to a lesser extent, the thermic effect of foods
   4. Thermic effect of foods, physical activity, and thermic effect of exercise

2. Energy homeostasis exists when:
   1. Kcalories from food intake equal kcalories used for energy expenditure.
   2. Kcalories used for physical activity equal kcalories used for energy expenditure.
   3. An individual is gaining weight.
   4. Kcalories from food intake equal kcalories used for resting energy expenditure.

3. A kilocalorie is used to measure both:
   1. Weight and percentage body fat
   2. Height and weight
   3. The units of energy used in the body and contained in foods
   4. Leanness and body-fat content

4. Kilocalories required per kilogram of body weight are highest during:
   1. Starvation
   2. Growth
   3. Weight loss
   4. Old age

5. Which of the following foods has the highest kilocalorie density?
   1. 1 cup of sugar
   2. 1 cup of celery
   3. 1 cup of skim milk
   4. 1 cup of margarine

CLINICAL ANALYSIS

1. Monitoring a resident's weight is a government requirement in long-term care facilities. The goal is to prevent a slow weight loss, which, over time, can have health consequences. Mr. I has been experiencing an undesirable slow weight loss. His weight history is as follows:

Feb	180 lb (82 kg)
June	175 lb (80 kg)
Oct	170 lb (77 kg)

   As Mr. I's nurse, you should first:

   a. Encourage Mr. I to eat only twice a day
   b. Call the doctor
   c. Wait for the next client care conference to act on this problem
   d. Monitor Mr. I's food intake and physical activity

2. A teacher noticed that many students in her fifth-grade class were overweight. As a school project, the class kept food records for 3 days. A computer software program analyzed the records. Many students were eating less than their recommended dietary allowance for kcalories but gaining weight nonetheless (a common problem among our nation's young). The teacher asked the class by a show of hands what they did after school and on weekends. Many of the same children who were overweight raised their hands when asked if they played mostly video games and watched television when not in school. The teacher shared this information with the school nurse and asked her to speak to the class. The school nurse correctly decided that:

   a. The teacher is overly concerned because the percentage of overweight students approximates the percentage of overweight adults in the community.
   b. The computer program must be in error.
   c. All the students need to increase their total intake, including foods from the major food groups.
   d. Many students would benefit from an increase in physical activity.

3. A client appears to be totally concerned with the kilocaloric density of foods and not at all concerned with the nutrient density of foods. You need to encourage the consumption of both types of foods. Which of the following behaviors do you need to discourage?

   a. The substitution of skim milk for 2% milk
   b. The avoidance of all meat, fish, and poultry
   c. The inclusion of dark green and yellow fruits and vegetables in the diet
   d. The inclusion of whole grains in the diet

CHAPTER 6

Vitamins

LEARNING OBJECTIVES

After completing this chapter, the student should be able to:

- Define vitamins.
- Differentiate between fat- and water-soluble vitamins.
- Describe Dietary Reference Intake for Americans.
- Describe the diseases caused by deficiencies of vitamins A and D.
- List four diseases caused by specific water-soluble vitamin deficiencies.
- Identify two vitamins with food sources limited to the fruit and vegetable group.
- Differentiate enrichment from fortification.
- Distinguish two vitamins with associated toxicities from natural or fortified foods, emphasizing persons with increased risk.
- Name three food sources of provitamin A and vitamin C.
- Describe the prudent use of vitamin supplements.
- Relate two large population groups for whom supplements or fortified foods are recommended to the specified vitamin for each group.

The importance of vitamins was first recognized by the effects of their absence. Some deficiency diseases have been known for centuries, but it was not until the early 20th century that vitamins were isolated in the laboratory. This chapter considers the importance of vitamins in the body and diet, the general functions of vitamins, the classification of vitamins, and the use of vitamin supplements. It also includes information on metabolism, functions, sources, deficiencies, toxicities, and factors affecting stability.

The Nature of Vitamins

Vitamins are organic substances needed by the body in small amounts for normal metabolism, growth, and maintenance. Organic substances are derived from living matter and contain carbon. Vitamins are not sources of energy nor do they become part of the structure of the body. Vitamins act as regulators or adjusters of metabolic processes and as **coenzymes** (substances that activate enzymes) in enzymatic systems.

Specific Functions

Vitamin functions are specific. With few exceptions, bodily processes do not permit substitutes. Thus, vitamins are similar to keys in a lock. All the notches in a key have to fit the lock, or the key will not turn. Overall, one vitamin cannot perform the functions of another. If a person does not consume enough vitamin C, for instance, taking vitamin D will not correct the deficiency. Vitamin D is the wrong key for that lock.

Classification

A major distinguishing characteristic of vitamins is their solubility in either fat or water (Table 6-1). This physical property is used to classify vitamins and is also significant for storage and processing of foods that contain vitamins and for the utilization of the vitamins in the body. Vitamins A, E, D, and K are fat soluble. The eight B-complex vitamins and vitamin C are water soluble.

Dietary Reference Intakes

Dietary Reference Intakes (DRI) is the general term for a set of reference values used to plan and assess nutrient intakes of healthy people and include Recommended Dietary Allowance (RDA), Adequate Intake (AI), and Tolerable Upper Intake Level (UL) (National Institutes of Health, 2016). The amounts of vitamins recommended in the United States to meet the needs of almost all healthy individuals are listed by age and physiological status in Appendix A. Recommended amounts vary in other countries.

Vitamins A, D, and E historically have been measured in **International Units (IUs),** a dosage amount that still appears on some labels. The RDAs and AIs, however, are listed using the metric system: **micrograms** and milligrams. There are no generic units that can be converted directly to the metric system. The amount designated by a unit is specific for each vitamin. The principles used to convert IUs to the metric system are given in Clinical Calculation 6-1.

TABLE 6-1   Classification of Vitamins

FAT SOLUBLE	WATER SOLUBLE
Vitamin A	Vitamin C
Vitamin D	Thiamin
Vitamin E	Riboflavin
Vitamin K	Niacin
	Vitamin B$_6$
	Folic acid
	Vitamin B$_{12}$
	Biotin
	Pantothenic acid

CLINICAL CALCULATION   6-1

The Elusive International Unit

Formerly, fat-soluble vitamins were measured in international units (IUs), as defined by the International Conference for Unification of Formulae. *A unit of vitamin A is not an equal measure of vitamin D or of vitamin E.* Because that system still appears in laws, on labels, and in research reports, the principles used to convert IUs to metric measures are given here. These equivalents incorporate recent changes in the calculation of provitamin A using **retinol activity equivalents (RAEs)** to compensate for varying amounts of vitamin A obtainable from animal versus plant sources and beta-carotene versus other plant-based carotenoids.

VITAMIN A
Animal foods: 1 IU = 0.3 microgram of retinol
Plant foods: 1 IU = 3.6 micrograms of beta-carotene

Fat-Soluble Vitamins

More or less of a vitamin may be retained in a food, depending on the methods of processing and storing. Water-soluble vitamins, for example, are more unstable than fat-soluble vitamins during processing.

Sources of the fat-soluble vitamins with examples of foods containing the RDA/AI of each are listed in Table 6-2. Fat-soluble vitamins are absorbed from the intestine in the same way as fats, and like fats, they can be stored in the body for varying lengths of time, giving the potential for health problems due to excessive intake. Toxicity from vitamins A and D can be fatal.

Vitamin A

For DRIs, see Appendix A. For food and other sources, see Table 6-2. To investigate the vitamin content of a particular item, go to http://ndb.nal.usda.gov or to http://nutritiondata. self.com.

Vitamin A comes in two forms: preformed vitamin A (**retinol**) and **provitamin A** (found in **beta-carotene** and other **carotenoids**). A **preformed vitamin** is already in a complete state in ingested foods, whereas a **provitamin** requires conversion in the body to be in a complete state. Provitamin A is converted to retinol mainly in the intestine. The term *precursor* is often used interchangeably with the term *provitamin*. A **precursor** is a substance from which another substance is derived.

Absorption, Metabolism, and Excretion

Retinol absorption is relatively unregulated, even when intake is very high (Ross, 2014). Of preformed vitamin A, 70% to 90% is absorbed if consumed with at least 10 grams

TABLE 6-2   Fat-Soluble Vitamins

VITAMIN	ADULT RDA/ AI AND FOOD PORTION CONTAINING IT*	FUNCTIONS	DEFICIENCY DISEASE	SIGNS AND SYMPTOMS OF DEFICIENCY	SOURCES
A	700–900 mcg 0.5–0.8 cups cooked sliced carrots	Dim light vision Differentiation of epithelial cells	Night blindness Xerophthalmia	Night blindness Dry and thick outer covering of eye Blindness Growth retardation Increased susceptibility to infections Increased intracranial pressure Infertility	*Preformed:* Liver Egg yolk Fortified milk Fish *Provitamin:* Carrots Sweet potatoes Squash Apricots Cantaloupe Spinach Collards Broccoli Cabbage
D	15–20 mcg (600–800 IU) 5.2–6.9 cups 1% fortified milk	Increases intestinal absorption of calcium	Rickets Osteomalacia	Bowlegs, knock- knees, misshapen skull Tetany in infants	Sunlight on skin Fortified milk Cod liver oil Salmon

TABLE 6-2 Fat-Soluble Vitamins (Continued)

VITAMIN	ADULT RDA/ AI AND FOOD PORTION CONTAINING IT*	FUNCTIONS	DEFICIENCY DISEASE	SIGNS AND SYMPTOMS OF DEFICIENCY	SOURCES
		Stimulates bone production Decreases urinary excretion of calcium		Soft fragile bones, especially of spine, pelvis, lower extremities	Herring Tuna Eggs Liver Fortified cereals
E	15 mg 3.3 tbsp safflower oil	Antioxidant Protects polyunsaturated fatty acids in red blood cell membranes from oxidation in lungs	No specific term	Muscle pain and weakness Hemolytic anemia Degenerative neurological problems (peripheral neuropathy, **ataxia**) Anemia in premature infants	Sunflower, safflower, and canola oils Almonds, hazelnuts, and peanuts Broccoli, cooked spinach Fortified ready-to-eat cereals
K	90–120 mcg 0.6–0.8 cup raw chopped spinach	Used in synthesis of several clotting factors, including prothrombin Assists vitamin D to synthesize a regulatory bone protein	No specific term	Prolonged clotting time	Collards Spinach Brussels sprouts Cabbage Broccoli Soybean and canola oils Synthesis in intestine

AI, Adequate Intake; RDA, Recommended Dietary Allowances.
*Example; not suggested as sole source of the vitamin.

of fat. Retinol transport in the blood requires a retinol-binding protein and prealbumin, both of which are synthesized in the liver. Consequently, poor nutritional protein status interferes with the transportation and usage of vitamin A. The kidneys are responsible for the excretion of vitamin A.

Up to a year's supply of retinol is stored in the liver. Excessive carotene, which is apparently harmless for most people, is stored in adipose tissue, giving fat a yellowish tint. (See Hypervitaminosis A in this chapter for information on exceptional situations.)

Functions

Several crucial body functions depend on vitamin A, or retinol: vision, bone growth, and maintenance of epithelial tissue. In addition, provitamin A serves as an antioxidant (see Vitamin E in this chapter).

VISION

In many ways, a camera mimics the eye: both have a dark layer to keep out excess light, a lens to focus light, and a light sensor. In the eye, the sensor is a light-sensitive layer at the back of the eye, called the **retina.** In the retina, light rays are changed into electrical impulses that travel along the **optic nerve** to the back of the brain. The vitamin A metabolite **retinal** is part of a chemical in the retina responsible for this electrical conversion. The body can synthesize this retinal chemical, **rhodopsin** (or visual purple), only if it has an appropriate supply of vitamin A.

MAINTAINING EPITHELIAL TISSUE

Epithelial tissue covers the body and lines the organs and passageways that open to the outside of the body. Skin is epithelial tissue, as are the surface of the eye and the lining of the gastrointestinal tract. Epithelial tissue has a protective function, often producing mucus to wash out foreign materials. Vitamin A helps to keep epithelial tissue healthy by aiding the differentiation of specialty cells. This function, control of gene expression, has led some scientists to believe that vitamin A may play a role in cancer prevention. See Clinical Application 6-1 for more information on vitamin A and cancer.

CLINICAL APPLICATION 6-1

Vitamin A and Cancer

Cancers begin with abnormal differentiation and rampant proliferation of cells. Vitamin A plays a hormone-like role in normal cell differentiation throughout the body. In studies of populations, lower intakes of vitamin A have been associated with higher risk of certain cancers, particularly those of epithelial origin. In experimental animals, vitamin A deficiency increased tumor incidence and susceptibility to chemical **carcinogens.**

The provitamin also functions as an antioxidant to neutralize **free radicals.** These highly reactive **atoms** or **molecules** can damage **DNA,** with resultant abnormal cell growth. Intervention studies using beta-carotene were not protective, however, but actually resulted in increased cancers in susceptible individuals.

Evidence does not support a benefit for consuming more than the RDA for vitamin A (Ross, 2014). See dietary supplements in Chapter 15.

OTHER FUNCTIONS

Vitamin A participates in bone metabolism in an undefined manner in that deficiency causes excessive deposition of bone by **osteoblasts** and reduced bone degradation by **osteoclasts.** Vitamin A is recognized as an important regulator in several types of immune cells (Ross, 2014). Vitamin A also contributes to blood formation and to normal reproduction, but less is understood about the physiology involved in those areas.

Deficiency

Even though vitamin A is effectively stored in a healthy body when intake is adequate, deficiencies can occur. Vitamin A deficiency (VAD) is a public health problem in more than 100 countries, especially in low-income countries in Africa and Southeast Asia, affecting mostly pregnant women and young children (Iskakova, Karbyshev, Piskunov, & Rochette-Egly, 2015). Worldwide, more than 250 million preschool-aged children are estimated to be vitamin A deficient, and nearly 250,000 to 500,000 of these children will become blind every year and nearly half will die within the year as the result of this deficiency (World Health Organization [WHO], 2017).

Vitamin A deficiency in the United States is most often due to disease. For example, clients with long-lasting infectious disease, fat absorption problems, or liver disease are at risk of vitamin A deficiency.

SIGNS AND SYMPTOMS

Lack of vitamin A in retinol form causes night blindness. In this condition, the resynthesis of rhodopsin is too slow to allow quick adaptation to dim light.

All epithelial tissue suffers because of vitamin A deficiency. The most serious effect is the thickening of the epithelial tissue covering the eye. **Xerophthalmia,** an abnormal thickening and drying of the outer surface of the eye, is the leading cause of preventable childhood blindness (Akhtar et al, 2013).

Vitamin A deficiency has also been associated with degenerative diseases, respiratory and intestinal disorders, cardiovascular disease, and some types of cancer (Tomlekova, White, Thompson, Penchev, & Nielen, 2017).

TREATMENT AND PREVENTION

Providing vitamin A by any of the following strategies is the treatment for vitamin A deficiency.

Active corneal xerophthalmia is a medical emergency demanding high-dose vitamin A orally. If vomiting or diarrhea precludes oral dosing, a water-miscible injection is given, a form that can also be used to provide adequate vitamin A to individuals with fat absorption disorders. Supplements of vitamin A palmitate are used in vitamin A deficiency and require clients to have regular monitoring of serum vitamin A levels and liver function tests.

Prevention of vitamin A deficiency involves multiple strategies:

- Breastfeeding
- Vitamin A supplementation
- Fortification of foods
- Diet diversification
- Nutritional education

Sources

Preformed vitamin A is found in animal foods, with the highest levels occurring naturally in liver, fish liver oils, and other organ meats. Good sources include egg yolk, fish, and fortified milk products.

The body converts the provitamin A carotenoids present in fruits and vegetables to retinol. The best-utilized sources are yellow, orange, and red brightly colored fruits and cooked yellow tubers, followed by dark green leafy vegetables.

Carotene, a yellow pigment found mostly in fruits and vegetables, is readily visible in yellow and orange foods, such as carrots, sweet potatoes, squash, apricots, and cantaloupe. Although not as noticeable because chlorophyll masks the yellow color, carotene is also present in dark leafy green vegetables, including spinach, collards, broccoli, and cabbage.

Carotene content of a species of vegetable can vary with the vegetable's maturity, handling, and preparation. Carrots packaged in plastic bags are better protected from light and air than the bouquets secured by a rubber band. **Beta-carotene** is more available to the body in carrots cooked with a small amount of fat than in raw carrots, an exception to the general rule that cooking depletes vitamins.

Individuals with higher-than-normal requirements for vitamin A include those with:

- Chronic kidney disease
- Acute protein deficiency
- Type 1 and type 2 diabetes

Toxicity

Fetal malformations can be caused by either deficiency or excess of vitamin A. Although most other vitamin toxicities are a result of supplementation, hypervitaminosis A can be caused by foods. For instance, liver contains 27,720 micrograms of retinol (91,476 IU) in a 3-ounce serving. Even when intake is high, about 70% of dietary vitamin A is absorbed.

In addition, vitamin A derivatives are often prescribed to control severe acne, which presents a threat to unborn children. The risk of fetal malformations was significantly higher among women who consumed more than 3,000 micrograms (10,000 IU) of retinol in early pregnancy. See also Chapter 10.

CAROTENEMIA

Beta-carotene is recognized by the Food and Drug Administration (FDA) as Generally Recognized as Safe (**GRAS**) as a dietary supplement and a colorant. Nevertheless, carotene can be consumed to excess, causing **carotenemia.** The person's skin becomes yellow, similar to that shown in jaundice; but with carotenemia, the palms of the hands and the soles of the feet are also affected. Also in contrast to jaundice, the whites of the eyes do not become yellow in carotenemia. A common cause of carotenemia in infants is consumption of too much squash and carrots. The skin returns to normal within 2 to 6 weeks after stopping the excessive intake.

HYPERVITAMINOSIS A

Vitamin A toxicity is called **hypervitaminosis A.** An acute case can result from even a single dose of 50,000 IU of vitamin A. Clients with renal failure are also at a risk of vitamin toxicity due to the decrease in the kidney's ability to excrete waste products, including excess vitamins (Manickavasagar et al, 2015). Symptoms of hypervitaminosis A can include **ataxia,** pain in the bones and joints, liver failure, dry skin, and poor appetite.

Vitamin D

For DRIs, see Appendix A. For food and other sources, see Table 6-2. To investigate the vitamin content of a particular item, go to http://ndb.nal.usda.gov.

Vitamin D deficiency diseases were recognized by Dutch and English physicians in the 17th century. By the turn of the 20th century, rickets reached almost epidemic proportions in the industrialized cities of Northern Europe because of air pollution and long indoor working hours.

Vitamin D is not a true vitamin because there are sources other than diet. Instead, this key nutrient is a prohormone. **Vitamin D,** long known to be essential for bone growth, targets more than 200 human genes in a wide variety of tissues. Vitamin D receptors have been found in almost every tissue and cell in the body, including the brain, heart, skin, and immune cells (Jasinski, 2012).

Absorption, Metabolism, and Excretion

Two forms of vitamin D are metabolically active. Vitamin D_2, **ergocalciferol,** is formed when ergosterol (provitamin) in plants is irradiated by sunlight. Vitamin D_3, **cholecalciferol,** is formed when 7-dehydrocholesterol (another provitamin) in the skin of animals or humans is irradiated by ultraviolet light or sunlight.

Both forms are absorbed into the blood. Vitamin D_3 is absorbed primarily in the duodenum of the small intestine with the assistance of gastric juices, bile, and pancreatic enzymes. Intestinal absorption of vitamin D decreases with age, as does the capacity of the skin to synthesize cholecalciferol. Like other fat-soluble vitamins, it is transported in the blood bound to protein. The liver alters the vitamin to **calcidiol,** an inactive form of vitamin D. By enzyme action, the kidney converts the calcidiol to calcitriol, the active form of vitamin D. Figure 6-1 diagrams the path of these processes.

Functions

Vitamin D has long been recognized as essential to proper bone metabolism. Recent findings suggest a role in the prevention and treatment of a wide range of chronic diseases, such as cancer, type II diabetes, and hypertension.

BONE METABOLISM

Vitamin D promotes normal bone mineralization by stimulating:

- DNA to produce transport proteins to increase intestinal absorption of calcium and phosphorus
- Bone cells to build and maintain bone tissue with calcium and phosphorus
- The kidneys to return calcium to the bloodstream rather than excreting it in the urine

An opposite effect is caused by **parathyroid hormone** that is secreted in response to a low serum calcium level. Parathyroid hormone causes the **catabolism** of bone to raise the serum calcium level. The body's priority goal is maintenance of correct serum calcium for blood clotting, nerve function, and muscle contraction. Without this mechanism to sustain vital functions, a person would not live long enough to develop rickets, the bone disease of vitamin D deficiency.

Emerging research is finding correlation with vitamin D and chronic disease.

- Fibromyalgia pain is shown to be increased in the presence of vitamin D deficiency (Vaidya, Nakarmi, Chaudhary, Batajoo, & Rajbhandari, 2014).
- Low levels of vitamin D have been associated with increased insulin resistance in adults and adolescence (Datchinamoorthi, Vanaja, & Rajagopalan, 2016).
- Lower vitamin D has been associated with metabolic syndrome and cardiovascular disease (Chailurkit, Aekplakorn, Srijaruskul, & Ongphiphadhanakul, 2016).

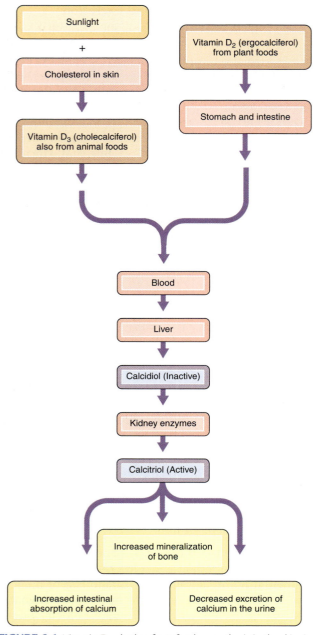

FIGURE 6-1 Vitamin D, whether from food or synthesis in the skin, is metabolized by the liver and the kidneys to its active form.

- Clients with obstructive sleep apnea and hypopnea syndrome (OSAHS) have been found to have lower serum vitamin D levels (Toujani et al, 2017).

Ongoing research is needed to completely understand the actions vitamin D has in cell differentiation and immune system function in the treatment and prevention of disease. See Genomic Gem 6-1.

Deficiency

One difficulty with setting an RDA for vitamin D is the multiple sources of the vitamin. Some people, particularly outdoor workers, may achieve optimal serum levels without

GENOMIC GEM 6-1

Vitamin D and Tuberculosis

Tuberculosis (TB), caused by infection with *Mycobacterium tuberculosis*, is one of the major bacterial infections worldwide resulting in approximately 2 billion persons becoming infected annually (Iftikhar et al, 2013). Among racial and ethnic groups born in the United States, the greatest racial disparity in TB rates occurred among non-Hispanic blacks, whose rate was eight times the rate for non-Hispanic whites (Centers for Disease Control and Prevention, October 27, 2016).

Vitamin D has a role in the production of *cathelicidin*, an antimicrobial protein that provides defense against bacterial infections. Vitamin D has also been shown to have a role in macrophage activation and suppressing the growth of *M. tuberculosis* (Iftikhar et al, 2013).

Although not the only mechanisms at work in resisting microbes, **polymorphisms** in vitamin D receptors may contribute to susceptibility to tuberculosis. Investigators have hypothesized that increased risk of tuberculosis is associated with a lack of appropriate vitamin D receptor–dependent antimycobacterial activity (Tang, Smit, & Semba, 2014).

supplements. Overall, skin synthesis of vitamin D contributes somewhat to the body's supply because serum vitamin D levels are generally higher than would be predicted on the basis of vitamin D intakes alone. In contrast, homebound or institutionalized individuals, women who wear long robes and head coverings for religious reasons, and people with occupations that limit sun exposure are unlikely to obtain adequate vitamin D from sunlight (National Institutes of Health, February 11, 2016).

A body mass index of 30 or greater is associated with lower serum vitamin D levels compared with nonobese individuals. Obesity does not affect the skin's capacity to synthesize vitamin D, but greater amounts of subcutaneous fat sequester more of the vitamin and alter its release into the circulation. Obese individuals who have undergone gastric bypass surgery may become vitamin D deficient over time without a sufficient intake of this nutrient from food or supplements because part of the upper small intestine where vitamin D is absorbed is bypassed. Any vitamin D mobilized into the serum from fat stores may not compensate over time (National Institutes of Health, February 11, 2016).

A varying percentage of the population is vitamin D deficient, at any time, during any season, at any latitude, although the percentage is higher in the

- Winter
- Aged
- Obese
- Sun deprived
- Dark skinned
- Long-term use of anticonvulsants

- Renal disease
- Liver disease

Besides lack of sunshine, low vitamin D intake, fat malabsorption disorders, chronic liver or kidney disease, and rare genetic disorders cause vitamin D deficiency. Vitamin D–deficient diets are associated with milk allergy, lactose intolerance, ovo-vegetarianism, and veganism (National Institutes of Health, February 11, 2016). Children whose bones are still growing are most vulnerable to this deficiency.

RICKETS

Vitamin D deficiency in children results in a disease called **rickets,** which causes soft bones and skeletal deformities. Although nutritional rickets is preventable, it still occurs in developed countries. Rickets is more likely to develop in infants who are strictly breast-fed without proper vitamin D supplementation, during winter months, and in ethnic groups who have darker skin tones, such as Hispanics and African Americans (Lindley, Farmakis, & Tanios, 2017). Many infants with rickets will present with growth patterns that are abnormal. To prevent such deficiency diseases or to diagnose them early, health-care providers should assess the client's total situation and not just focus on the immediate reason for the visit.

Rickets can occur without vitamin D deficiency. Studies have demonstrated a form of rickets in Africa and Asia, where children had sufficient serum vitamin D, but they had elevated urinary excretion of phosphorus (Prentice, 2013).

OSTEOMALACIA

Vitamin D deficiency in adults is called **osteomalacia.** This deficiency disease occurs most often in women who have insufficient calcium intake and little sunlight exposure. It occurs frequently among those who are pregnant or lactating.

Environmental causes for osteomalacia are similar to those for rickets. People with low exposure to sunlight are at increased risk—for example, office workers, residents of smoggy areas, and institutionalized elderly people.

Because of the complex processes involved in vitamin D metabolism, liver or kidney disease can lead to bone deterioration. Chronic kidney failure has caused osteomalacia because of the inability of the kidneys to convert vitamin D to its active form. Clients with kidney disease are commonly prescribed pharmaceutical vitamin D supplements.

SIGNS AND SYMPTOMS

Children with rickets have soft, fragile bones. Classic deformities include bowlegs, knock knees, and misshapen skulls due to decreased mineralization at the growth plate. Vitamin D deficiency may cause **tetany** in infants due to low levels of blood calcium.

Adults with osteomalacia also have increasing softness of the bones, causing deformities due to loss of calcium. The bones most commonly affected are those of the spine, pelvis, and lower extremities.

DRIs and Sources

In 2010, because of increased information on which to base recommendations, the Institute of Medicine revised the DRIs for vitamin D. The AIs for infants were doubled. The AIs for all other age groups were upgraded to RDAs: the amounts tripled for those up to the age of 50 and increased by smaller amounts for those older than 50 years. ULs were also increased except for infants younger than 6 months. For sources of vitamin D, see Table 6-3. Two sources are readily available to most people: synthesis by the skin and fortified milk, which is widely available in the United States.

SKIN SYNTHESIS

A major source of vitamin D is the body itself. Vitamin D is manufactured in the skin. Children with low dietary intakes may escape rickets if their exposure to sunlight is adequate. Some researchers suggest that approximately 5 to 30 minutes of sun exposure between 10 a.m. and 3 p.m. at least twice a week to the face, arms, legs, or back without sunscreen usually leads to sufficient vitamin D synthesis. Complete cloud cover reduces ultraviolet (UV) energy by 50%; shade (including that produced by severe pollution) by 60%, and window glass by 100%. Sunscreens with a sun protection factor (SPF) of 8 or more appear to block vitamin D–producing UV rays, although in practice people generally do not apply sufficient amounts, cover all sun-exposed skin, or reapply sunscreen regularly. Therefore, skin likely synthesizes some vitamin D even when protected by sunscreen as typically applied (National Institutes of Health, February 11, 2016).

Aging significantly decreases the skin's ability to synthesize vitamin D_3 (Azmathullah et al, 2016). Exposure of the face is not recommended at any age because precancerous *actinic keratoses* are related to sun exposure. The body regulates skin synthesis of vitamin D to avoid overdosing from this source.

TABLE 6-3 Selected Food Sources of Vitamin D

FOOD AND PORTION	IUs	MICROGRAMS
Swordfish, cooked, dry heat, 3 ounces	566	14.2
Salmon, pink, canned, total contents, 3 ounces	465	11.6
Salmon (sockeye), cooked, 3 ounces	447	11.2
Tuna fish, canned in water, drained, 3 ounces	154	3.9
Milk, nonfat, reduced fat, and whole, vitamin D fortified, 1 cup	100	2.5
Liver, beef, cooked, 3 ounces	42	1.1
Egg, one large (vitamin D is found in yolk)	41	1.0
Shitake mushrooms, ½ cup, cooked	20	0.5

Sources: National Institutes of Health, Office of Dietary Supplements: Fact Sheet for Health Professionals: Vitamin D. Reviewed February 11, 2016. Accessed March 21, 2017. Available at https://ods.od.nih.gov/factsheets/VitaminD-HealthProfessional/

FOOD

For people not exposed to sunshine, food sources of vitamin D become increasingly important.

Few commonly consumed foods naturally provide vitamin D. The flesh of fatty fish, such as swordfish, salmon, and tuna, are among the best sources. Smaller amounts of vitamin D are found in beef liver and egg yolks. Vitamin D in these foods is primarily in the form of vitamin D_3. Some mushrooms provide vitamin D_2 in variable amounts, and mushrooms with enhanced levels of vitamin D_2 from being exposed to UV light under controlled conditions are also available. Food labels, however, are not required to list vitamin D content unless a food has been fortified with this nutrient (National Institutes of Health, February 11, 2016).

Fortified foods provide most of the vitamin D in the American diet. In the United States, the major food source of vitamin D is fortified milk. Milk is the ideal food to link with vitamin D because it also contains calcium and phosphorus, which are necessary for bone **anabolism.** Almost all of the U.S. milk supply is voluntarily fortified with 100 IU (2.5 micrograms) per cup. Other dairy products made from milk, such as cheese and ice cream, are generally not fortified. Ready-to-eat breakfast cereals often contain added vitamin D, as do some brands of orange juice, yogurt, margarine, and other food products.

In Canada, milk is fortified by law with 35 to 40 IU/100 mL, as is margarine at 530 IU/100 grams or higher. Both the United States and Canada mandate the fortification of infant formula with vitamin D: 40 to 100 IU/100 kcal in the United States and 40 to 80 IU/100 kcal in Canada (National Institutes of Health, February 11, 2016).

See Box 6-1 and Clinical Application 6-2 on the **fortification** of foods. For other food sources, see Table 6-2 and Table 6-3.

BOX 6-1 ■ Enrichment and Fortification

Enrichment is the replacing of nutrients lost in processing or during storage. Enriched flour is an example. Not all the nutrients are replaced; therefore, whole-grain products are recommended.

Fortification is the addition of nutrients not normally present in a given food to increase its nutritional value, for example, vitamins A and D in milk.

CLINICAL APPLICATION 6-2

Fortification of Foods: Use and Misuse

Fortification is the addition of nutrients to foods in amounts greater than normally present. Many cereals are fortified with vitamins and minerals not normally found in grains. Occasionally, intentions are better than practices. Experts are concerned that voluntary fortification of multiple foods by the producers could lead to excessive intakes along with the increase in consumers utilizing multivitamins. Currently, foods permitted to be fortified with vitamin D include milk products, cereals, and fruit juices. Maximum levels of added vitamin D are specified by law.

SUPPLEMENTS

Historically, the means to obtain vitamin D was cod liver oil, which contains 453 IU (11.3 micrograms) of vitamin D_3 per teaspoonful. Although a natural product, cod liver oil is a supplement, not a food. In various forms, vitamin D supplements are used by 37% of the U.S. population (National Institutes of Health, February 11, 2016). The form that many vegans prefer is vitamin D_2 because of its plant origin. Intake from multiple fortified and supplemental sources should be monitored to avoid toxicity.

Interfering Factors

Little special handling of foods is necessary but a high-fiber diet interferes with the vitamin's absorption. Abnormalities of absorption such as diarrhea, fat malabsorption, and biliary obstruction also may lead to vitamin D deficiency. See Chapter 15 for drug–nutrient interactions.

Toxicity

Although excessive sun exposure is a risk factor for skin cancer, it does not result in acute vitamin D toxicity.

Intake of vitamin D from foods that are high enough to cause toxicity is unlikely. Toxicity is much more likely to occur from high intakes of dietary supplements containing vitamin D (National Institutes of Health, February 11, 2016).

DOSAGE

More than any other vitamin, a high consumption of vitamin D supplements is likely to cause toxicity from excess. The use of supplements of both calcium (1,000 mg/day) and vitamin D (400 IU) by postmenopausal women was associated with a 17% increase in the risk of kidney stones over 7 years in the Women's Health Initiative (National Institutes of Health, February 11, 2016).

SIGNS AND SYMPTOMS

Clinical manifestations of hypervitaminosis D include loss of appetite, nausea, vomiting, polyuria, muscular weakness, and constipation. More serious consequences of vitamin D overdose result from calcium deposits in the heart, kidneys, and brain.

Vitamin E

For DRIs, see Appendix A. For food and other sources, see Table 6-2. To investigate the vitamin content of a particular item, go to http://ndb.nal.usda.gov or to http://nutritiondata.self.com.

Absorption, Metabolism, and Excretion

The primary site of absorption of vitamin E is the **jejunum,** where fat and bile are required for optimal uptake. The liver is responsible for excretion via bile in the feces.

Functions

The major function of vitamin E is to protect the integrity of cell membranes. To do this, vitamin E serves as an **antioxidant** by accepting oxygen instead of allowing other molecules to become unstable. In this role, vitamin E protects provitamin A and unsaturated fatty acids from **oxidation**. It also preserves the stability of the polyunsaturated fatty acids in the red blood cell membranes, protecting them from oxidation in the lungs. The vitamin E in lung cell membranes provides an important barrier against air pollution.

Deficiency

No particular disease is caused by vitamin E deficiency. Vitamin E deficiency is rare, virtually never resulting from dietary deficiency, but rather is usually related to lipid metabolism disorders. Premature infants are at risk because of impaired fat utilization. Diseases characterized by fat malabsorption, such as cystic fibrosis and hepatobiliary diseases, can lead to deficiencies.

Signs and symptoms include peripheral **neuropathy,** ataxia, skeletal myopathy, retinopathy, and impairment of the immune response (National Institutes of Health, November 3, 2016).

Premature infants with inadequate reserves of vitamin E develop anemia. Without sufficient vitamin E, the membranes of the red blood cells break down easily when exposed to oxygen or an oxidizing agent.

Sources, Stability, and Interfering Factors

The best sources of vitamin E are vegetable oils and nuts. Selected food sources of vitamin E are listed in Table 6-4. All vegetable oils are not equal in vitamin E content. Those highest in alpha-tocopherol are sunflower and safflower oils. In contrast, corn and soybean oils have a greater proportion of gamma-tocopherol, which no longer is counted as contributing to vitamin E intake (see Table 6-2 for other good resources).

Vitamin E and selenium (see Chapter 7) have a complementary relationship. Higher concentrations of one can compensate for lower concentrations of the other.

TABLE 6-4 Selected Sources of Vitamin E

	MG
Wheat germ oil, 1 tablespoon	20.3
Sunflower seeds, dry roasted, unsalted, 1 ounce	7.4
Almonds, dry roasted, 1 ounce (22 kernels)	6.8
Sunflower oil, 1 tablespoon	5.6
Safflower oil, 1 tablespoon	4.6
Hazelnuts, 1 ounce	4.3
Peanut butter, smooth, 2 tablespoons	2.9
Canola oil, 1 tablespoon	2.4
Peanuts, 1 ounce	2.2

Sources: National Institutes of Health: Office of Dietary Supplements: Fact Sheet for Health Professionals: Vitamin E. Reviewed November 3, 2016. Accessed March 27, 2017. Available at https://ods.od.nih.gov/factsheets/VitaminE-HealthProfessional/

Vitamin E is stable to acid, but heat and light lead to destruction. Thus, roasting of nuts reduces their vitamin E content. Persons who limit fat in their diets are likely limiting their vitamin E intake also.

Toxicity

Toxicity from natural vitamin E from food is unknown. Excessive supplemental vitamin E can cause gastrointestinal symptoms, muscle weakness, double vision, and increased bleeding tendencies. Thus clients taking anticoagulant drugs should not exceed the UL for vitamin E. Clinical Application 6-3 describes a client with vitamin E toxicity.

Vitamin K

For DRIs, see Appendix A. For food and other sources, see Table 6-2. To investigate the vitamin content of a particular item, go to http://ndb.nal.usda.gov or to http://nutritiondata.self.com.

Vitamin K is frequently prescribed as a medication. Its intake has an impact on the effectiveness of the commonly prescribed anticoagulant **warfarin,** which interferes with the synthesis of vitamin K. Vitamin K can also serve as an antidote for warfarin overdose. Instructions regarding food intake for clients taking warfarin are given in Chapter 15.

Absorption, Metabolism, and Excretion

Two naturally occurring forms of vitamin K can meet the body's needs. Vitamin K_1, or **phylloquinone,** is found in plant foods. Vitamin K_2, or **menaquinone,** is synthesized by intestinal bacteria. A synthetic, water-soluble pharmaceutical form of vitamin K_1, **phytonadione,** can be administered orally or by injection. An aqueous oral preparation is available for people with fat malabsorption disorders.

CLINICAL APPLICATION 6-3

Vitamin E Toxicity

A client was admitted to the hospital for **narcolepsy,** a disorder characterized by recurrent, uncontrollable, brief periods of sleep from which the individual is easily awakened. This client would fall asleep while driving his car.

Narcolepsy can be a sign of uremia, hypoglycemia, diabetes, hypothyroidism, increased intracranial pressure, tumors of the brain stem or hypothalamus, or absence **epilepsy.** If all of these causes are ruled out, the medical diagnosis is either classical or independent narcolepsy.

During her assessment, the dietitian discovered one unusual nutritional practice: After a clerk in a health foods store had recommended vitamin E, the client had begun and continued to take this supplement. The dietitian investigated vitamin E's adverse effects and suggested to the physician that the narcolepsy could be caused by excessive vitamin E. After the client discontinued taking vitamin E, the narcolepsy disappeared.

In this case, a thorough nutritional assessment and an inquiring attitude eliminated the need for extensive diagnostic tests.

Phylloquinone is absorbed primarily in the jejunum, and menaquinone is absorbed in the distal small intestine and the colon. Absorption and utilization of menaquinone vary considerably from person to person. Within the body, vitamin K is stored primarily in cell membranes of the lungs, kidneys, bone marrow, and adrenals. The total amount in the body is estimated to be only 50 to 100 milligrams. Turnover of vitamin K in the body occurs about every 1.5 days. Vitamin K is excreted in urine and feces via bile.

Functions

The actions of vitamin K in blood clotting have been known since 1941, when its discoverers received the Nobel Prize in medicine. A vitamin K–dependent protein in bone that helps regulate serum calcium levels requires both vitamin K and vitamin D for synthesis. Vitamin K is present in the liver and other body tissues, including the brain, heart, pancreas, and bone (National Institutes of Health, February 11, 2016).

BLOOD CLOTTING

Vitamin K is necessary for the liver to make factors II (**prothrombin**), VII, IX, and X. Four additional coagulation proteins are vitamin K dependent. These factors and proteins plus calcium are key links in the chain of events producing a blood clot.

BONE METABOLISM

Two vitamin K–dependent proteins have been identified in bone and cartilage. Vitamin K is converted to K_2 within the femur, which increases **osteocalcin** production (Verna, Hemlata, & Kusum, 2013).

Deficiency

Individuals at risk of vitamin K deficiency include newborn infants as well as adults who avoid green leafy vegetables or are undergoing long-term antibiotic therapy. Clients with fat malabsorption syndromes are also at risk. Careful assessment of dietary factors in these clients is warranted.

Infants are at risk because inadequate amounts of vitamin K cross the placenta and because the intestinal tract of a newborn infant is sterile. For this reason, the baby is unable to produce vitamin K until the intestine is colonized with bacteria from the environment, usually within 24 hours, when the baby can begin to synthesize vitamin K. To prevent vitamin K deficiency bleeding of the newborn, the American Academy of Pediatrics (2015) recommends an intramuscular dose of vitamin K be administered to the baby immediately after birth.

Deficiencies, uncommon in healthy adults, have been associated with disease and with drug therapy. For example, fat absorption problems from gastrointestinal diseases may hinder vitamin K absorption, resulting in prolonged blood clotting time. In addition, antibiotics, which kill normal bacteria—some of which produce vitamin K—along with the infectious organisms can cause low levels of vitamin K.

Sources

The human body is capable of manufacturing some vitamin K, and many common foods contain adequate amounts.

INTESTINAL SYNTHESIS

The amount of bacterially produced vitamin K that is absorbed and utilized varies from one individual to another. Bacterial synthesis alone will not satisfy the RDA for vitamin K.

FOOD

Green leafy vegetables and vegetables of the cabbage family are the best sources of vitamin K (see Table 6-2). Limited studies suggest that phylloquinone from vegetable sources has a **bioavailability** that is about 15% to 20% of that from a supplement (Suttie, 2014). With two vegetables, lesser bioavailability would be no problem, but preparation mode has an impact:

- Cooked spinach has 889 micrograms per cup, but raw 145 mcg.
- Cooked collards have 836 micrograms per cup, but raw 184 mcg.

In some situations, that rich a source would be problematic. Controlling intake of vitamin K is part of the treatment plan for clients receiving a common anticoagulant drug, warfarin (see Chapter 15).

Stability and Interfering Factors

Vitamin K is susceptible to significant destruction by light and heat and is unstable in the presence of oxygen, alkalis, and strong acids. In addition, overconsumption of vitamins A and E can interfere with the absorption of vitamin K, and excess vitamin E may also interfere with vitamin K's metabolism, affecting coagulation (Linus Pauling Institute, 2014). The anticoagulant warfarin interferes with the liver's use of vitamin K, but that is the desired effect of the medication.

Toxicity

The naturally occurring forms of vitamins K_1 and K_2 have not been associated with adverse effects, but caution is warranted, particularly if high doses are taken. Phytonadione, the pharmaceutical preparation of vitamin K_1, causes fewer adverse effects than earlier, stronger formulations, but because of life-threatening reactions, intravenous administration is not recommended except in emergencies. As always, special care must be taken when administering any medication, including vitamin K, to infants.

Table 6-2 summarizes the fat-soluble vitamins. See Clinical Application 6-4 for a description of two conditions that mimic deficiencies of fat-soluble vitamins.

Water-Soluble Vitamins

Vitamins that dissolve in water are vitamin C, or **ascorbic acid**, and the B vitamins (**thiamin, riboflavin, niacin,** vitamin B_6, **folate,** vitamin B_{12}), as well as **pantothenic**

CLINICAL APPLICATION   6-4

Conditions Mimicking Fat-Soluble Vitamin Deficiencies

PROTEIN DEFICIENCY

Water and fat do not mix. To circulate fats in the water-based blood, the liver attaches fat-soluble vitamins to protein carriers. Sometimes a protein deficiency hinders the use of the fat-soluble vitamins.

ZINC DEFICIENCY

A zinc-containing protein carries vitamin A from storage in the liver to tissues. Zinc deficiency can affect vitamin A metabolism through its involvement with protein synthesis and cellular enzyme function. For this reason, a zinc deficiency can mimic a vitamin A deficiency.

acid, **biotin,** and choline—the last, strictly speaking, not a vitamin.

Vitamin C

For DRIs, see Appendix A. For food and other sources, see Table 6-5. To investigate the vitamin content of a particular item, go to http://ndb.nal.usda.gov or to http://nutritiondata. self.com.

Scurvy, the deficiency disease caused by lack of vitamin C, was described by the Egyptians in 3,000 B.C. In 1753, James Lind proved that citrus fruits cured scurvy, but not until 1795 did the Royal Navy mandate issuing citrus juice to sailors after 2 weeks at sea, leading to the term "limey" for a British sailor. Diffusion of the citrus mandate to

TABLE 6-5   Water-Soluble Vitamins

VITAMIN	ADULT RDA AND FOOD PORTION CONTAINING IT*	FUNCTIONS	DEFICIENCY DISEASE	SIGNS AND SYMPTOMS OF DEFICIENCY	SOURCES
C (ascorbic acid)	75–90 mg 0.8–0.9 cup of orange juice, prepared from frozen concentrate	Formation of collagen Antioxidant Facilitation of iron absorption	Scurvy	Bleeding mucous membranes Poor wound healing or reopening of scars Softened ends of long bones Teeth loosen, may fall out Death probably due to internal bleeding	Citrus fruit and juice Broccoli, Brussels sprouts Green and red peppers Cantaloupe, strawberries Kiwi fruit Papayas
B$_1$ (thiamin)	1.1–1.2 mg 4.1–4.5 oz pork loin, roasted, lean only	Coenzyme in CHO and amino acid metabolism	Beriberi	Anorexia, weight loss Muscle weakness and wasting Peripheral neuropathy Right heart failure Wernicke encephalopathy	Pork Beef liver Salmon Black beans Wheat germ Fortified cereals
B$_2$ (riboflavin)	1.1–1.3 mg 2.2–2.6 cups 1% milk	Coenzyme in protein metabolism; need increases as protein needs increase	Ariboflavinosis	Lesions on lips and in mouth Seborrheic dermatitis Normochromic, normocytic anemia	Milk and dairy products Eggs Meats, especially liver Fortified cereals
B$_3$ (niacin)	14–16 mg niacin equivalents 3.8–4.3 oz water-packed light tuna	Coenzyme in energy production Participant in synthesis of fatty acids and steroid hormones	Pellagra	Bilaterally symmetrical dermatitis on face, neck, hands, and feet Diarrhea Dementia	Liver Tuna Meats, fish, poultry Whole, enriched, or fortified grains Coffee Tea
B$_6$ (pyridoxine)	1.3–1.7 mg 2.2–2.8 cups sliced banana	Coenzyme in metabolism of amino acids	No specific term	Mouth lesions Peripheral neuropathy Confusion Hypochromic, microcytic anemia Convulsions in infants	Sirloin steak Salmon Chicken breast Whole grains, fortified cereals Bananas

(continued)

TABLE 6-5   Water-Soluble Vitamins (Continued)

VITAMIN	ADULT RDA AND FOOD PORTION CONTAINING IT*	FUNCTIONS	DEFICIENCY DISEASE	SIGNS AND SYMPTOMS OF DEFICIENCY	SOURCES
Folate (folic acid)	400 mcg 2.8 cups canned pinto beans	Essential to the formation of DNA Participant in formation of heme	No specific term	Bright red tongue Fatigue, weakness Shortness of breath Heart palpitations Megaloblastic anemia	Liver Dried peas, beans, lentils Wheat germ Peanuts Asparagus Endive Lettuce Brussels sprouts Broccoli Spinach Fortified grain products Liver
Cobalamin	2.4 mcg 1.9 oz canned salmon	Synthesis of DNA, RNA, metabolism of amino and fatty acids Synthesis and maintenance of myelin	Pernicious anemia (lack of intrinsic factor, not dietary) Vitamin B_{12} deficiency (avoidance of animal products)	Fatigue Pallor Shortness of breath Heart palpitations Megaloblastic anemia Numbness and tingling of extremities Abnormal gait Possible memory loss Dementia	Meat Fish Poultry Milk Cheese Eggs Vitamin B_{12}-fortified soymilk or tofu
Pantothenic acid	5 mg 1 cup cooked shiitake mushrooms	Coenzyme in fatty acid metabolism Many other metabolic and regulatory processes	No specific term	Burning feet syndrome	Liver Chicken Egg yolk Yogurt Legumes Mushrooms Potatoes Broccoli Whole-grain cereal
Biotin	30 mcg 3 large eggs	Coenzyme is the synthesis of fat, glycogen, and amino acids	No specific term	Alopecia Scaly, red rash around the eyes, nose, and mouth Paresthesias of the extremities Depression, and hallucinations	Liver Eggs Salmon Peanuts Milk Sweet potato Soybeans
Choline	450–550 mg 3.6–4.4 large eggs	Liver and brain function Lipid metabolism Cell membrane structure	No specific term	Liver and muscle damage	Liver Eggs Beef Pork Milk, yogurt Baked beans Broccoli Wheat germ

*Example; not suggested as sole source of the vitamin.

merchant vessels in 1854 happened 101 years after Lind's work.

Most animals manufacture vitamin C in their livers. Humans, along with other primates, guinea pigs, some birds, and fruit-eating bats, cannot synthesize vitamin C. Humans and primates have an inactive form of an encoding gene for the last enzyme in the chain reaction for vitamin C synthesis and therefore must obtain vitamin C from the diet (Padayatty & Levine, 2014).

Absorption, Metabolism, and Excretion

Vitamin C is absorbed from the small intestine. As the amount of vitamin C consumed increases, the proportion of the vitamin absorbed decreases. At usual intakes from food of 30 to 180 milligrams per day, 70% to 90% of vitamin C is absorbed. At intakes greater than 1 gram, typically less than 50% of vitamin C is absorbed (National Institutes of Health, February 11, 2016).

Absorbed vitamin reaches the liver through the hepatic vein and then is accumulated in almost all human tissues. The pituitary and adrenal glands have the highest concentrations of vitamin C, but the greatest total amount is found in the liver. Excretion is via the urine.

Functions

Vitamin C has diverse functions in the body. It contributes to wound, burn, and fracture healing; serves as an antioxidant; enhances the absorption of iron; and assists in the synthesis of hormones and neurotransmitters.

COLLAGEN SYNTHESIS

Vitamin C is necessary in the formation of **collagen**, the strong fibrous protein in connective tissue. Bone, skin, blood vessels, soft dental structures, and scar tissue all contain collagen. Without vitamin C, collagen molecules are inadequately cross-linked, resulting in weak tissue.

ANTIOXIDANT

Vitamin C is a powerful antioxidant. By preventing the uptake of oxygen by other molecules, it deters the destruction of tissue by unstable molecules. It also has been shown to regenerate other antioxidants in the body, including vitamin E (National Institutes of Health, 2016).

IRON ABSORPTION FACILITATOR

Vitamin C facilitates iron absorption by acting with hydrochloric acid to keep iron in the more absorbable **ferrous** form. Four ounces of orange juice, for instance, nearly quadruples the iron absorbed from the plant foods eaten with it.

OTHER FUNCTIONS

High concentrations of vitamin C are found in the **adrenal glands.** These are the organs that secrete adrenaline, the "fight-or-flight" hormone, in times of stress. Vitamin C also aids in the synthesis of norepinephrine and **serotonin.**

Vitamin C has not been shown to prevent common colds in the general population, but prophylactic use has reduced the duration of colds by 8% in adults and 14% in children. In marathon runners, skiers, and soldiers on subarctic exercises, prophylactic vitamin C in doses of 250 to 1,000 milligrams per day reduced the risk of common cold by 50%. When taken after the onset of symptoms, however, vitamin C did not affect cold duration or symptom severity (National Institutes of Health, February 11,2016).

Deficiency

Scurvy is an uncommon disease in developed countries, but can still develop in high-risk populations. Signs of scurvy can appear within 1 month of vitamin C intake of less than 10 milligrams per day (National Institutes of Health, February 11, 2016).

SIGNS AND SYMPTOMS

Early signs of scurvy are tender, sore gums that bleed easily and small skin hemorrhages due to weakened blood vessels. The late manifestations of scurvy relate to the breakdown of collagen. Wound healing is delayed; even healed scars may separate. The ends of long bones soften and become malformed and painful, and fractures appear. Teeth loosen in their sockets and fall out. Hemorrhages occur about the joints, stomach, and heart. Untreated scurvy often progresses to sudden death, probably from internal bleeding.

TREATMENT

An initial intravenous dose may be given. Moderate doses of vitamin C, 100 milligrams orally three times a day, will cure scurvy.

RISK FACTORS

A diagnosis of scurvy may not be considered initially because scurvy today exists primarily within certain populations: the elderly, alcoholics, clients with gastrointestinal disease, and clients with fruit and vegetable allergies (Levavasseur et al, 2015).

Foods that are high in both vitamins A and C are shown in Figure 6-2.

Stability and Preservation

Boiling, cooking, and canning fruits and vegetables lower vitamin C content. During juice processing, temperature and oxygen are the main factors responsible for vitamin C losses.

Easily implemented food preparation procedures can minimize loss of vitamin C:

- Store orange juice in a metal or glass opaque container that holds no more than an amount that can be consumed in a short time.
- Eat vegetables raw when possible or cook them as quickly as possible; crisp-cooked is better than limp-cooked for retaining the vitamin C content.

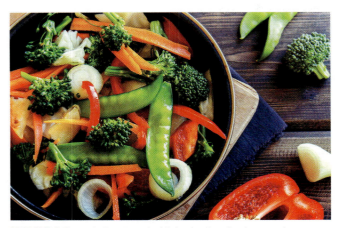

FIGURE 6-2 A salad prepared with broccoli and red pepper is an excellent way to obtain both vitamins A and C.

■ Boil the cooking water for 1 minute before adding the food to eliminate the dissolved oxygen that would otherwise oxidize the vitamin C.

In years past, many food establishments routinely added baking soda to vegetables to enhance their color, but the alkali also destroyed the vitamin C. Fortunately, this practice is now illegal.

Increased Needs

Individuals who smoke require an additional 35 milligrams of vitamin C, and those exposed to secondhand smoke should obtain the RDA daily (National Institutes of Health, February 11, 2016).

Food Processing Use

Vitamin C is used to mitigate undesirable reactions in food. For example, sodium or potassium nitrite is widely used in cured meat products because it inhibits outgrowth and neurotoxin formation by *Clostridium botulinum,* delays the development of oxidative rancidity, develops the characteristic flavor of cured meats, and reacts with myoglobin to stabilize the red meat color. Nitrate reacts with stomach acids to form nitrosamine, a known carcinogen. Because vitamin C blocks the formation of nitrosamines from nitrates, some meat packers add vitamin C to their products to protect against nitrosamine formation.

Toxicity

A dose 10 times the RDA is called a **megadose.** The most common side effects of large amounts (2 grams) of vitamin C are abdominal pain and osmotic diarrhea from bacterial metabolism of the vitamin in the colon.

Because vitamin C increases the amount of nonheme iron absorbed (see Chapter 7), persons with diseases characterized by iron overload such as sickle cell anemia and **hemochromatosis** (see Chapter 7) should avoid large doses of vitamin C but not fruits and vegetables (Levine & Padayatty, 2014).

Individuals prone to kidney stones are sometimes advised not to take megadoses of vitamin C because it is metabolized to oxalate, and kidney stones are often composed of calcium oxalate. In healthy persons without prior kidney stones, vitamin C from food and supplements did not increase stone formation (Levine & Padayatty, 2014).

Excessive vitamin C causes false readings in two common laboratory tests. Some urine glucose tests will read falsely positive. Stool tests for occult blood will read falsely negative.

B-Complex Vitamins

The B-complex group encompasses six traditionally recognized vitamins: thiamin, riboflavin, niacin, vitamin B_6, folate, and vitamin B_{12}. Recently added to the list are the vitamins pantothenic acid and biotin, as well as the essential nutrient choline. Some diseases, including beriberi and pellagra, are associated with deficiencies of a single B vitamin.

Thiamin

For DRIs, see Appendix A. For food and other sources, see Table 6-5. To investigate the vitamin content of a particular item, go to http://ndb.nal.usda.gov or to http://nutritiondata. self.com.

Thiamin is a water-soluble vitamin known as vitamin B1. Thiamin plays a critical role in energy metabolism and the growth, development, and function of cells (National Institutes of Health, February 11, 2016).

ABSORPTION, METABOLISM, AND EXCRETION

The human body contains about 30 milligrams of thiamin, about one-half of it located in the skeletal muscles, but the liver, heart, kidneys, and brain also have relatively high concentrations. Thiamin is absorbed in the small intestine, primarily in the jejunum and ileum. As a person's energy expenditure increases, the need for thiamin increases. Excess thiamin is mainly excreted in the urine.

FUNCTIONS

Thiamin is an essential coenzyme in the metabolism of glucose and energy production, as well as has a role in cellular metabolism.

DEFICIENCY

Beriberi is the deficiency disease caused by a lack of thiamin. The enrichment of food products has almost eliminated this disease, but it is still seen even in developed countries. The need for thiamin increases as kilocaloric consumption increases. Individuals whose thiamin status is marginal may become deficient when an increased need for energy is caused by strenuous activity, pregnancy, a growth spurt, or fever. Parenteral nutrition without thiamin supplementation can cause thiamin deficiency and is entirely preventable (Dabar et al, 2015).

Despite what is known about the functions of thiamin on a cellular level, that knowledge does not explain all the manifestations of the deficiency disease. *Dry beriberi* is seen mostly in adults with chronic low thiamin intake especially if coupled with high carbohydrate intake. It is characterized by muscle weakness and wasting, particularly in the lower extremities and symmetrical sensory and motor conduction problems affecting the distal limbs. Progression to *wet beriberi* involves the cardiovascular system, culminating in right-sided heart failure (Dabar et al, 2015). In *infantile beriberi*, often presenting between 2 and 6 months of age, the child may have a loud, piercing cry and convulsions. Infantile beriberi occurs most commonly in infants who are breastfed from mothers with thiamin deficiencies (Barennes, Sengkhamyong, Rene, & Phimmasane, 2015). Death can occur within several days of symptoms if not treated (Barennes et al, 2015).

In developed countries, thiamin deficiency is often associated with alcoholism because of

1. Inadequate food intake
2. Increased requirements because liver damage impairs the ability to store vitamins

3. Damage to the intestinal mucosa, which reduces the absorption of dietary thiamin by up to 90% (Guerrini & Mundt-Leach, 2012)

The following two neurological disorders are often associated with thiamin deficiency in alcoholism. Clients with **Wernicke encephalopathy,** a neurological disorder caused by thiamin deficiency, display many motor and sensory deficits often involving eye muscles, balance, and memory. Some clients develop **Korsakoff psychosis** characterized by amnesia and impaired conceptual functions. In these conditions, thiamin must be administered parenterally, either intramuscularly or intravenously, to raise plasma levels sufficiently to prevent long-term brain damage (Guerrini & Mundt-Leach, 2012).

STABILITY AND INTERFERING FACTORS

Air and heat destroy thiamin levels, especially in the presence of alkalis. For this reason, adding baking soda to green vegetables to retain their color or to dried beans to soften them inactivates the thiamin in the vegetables. Also, an enzyme in raw fish, raw shellfish, and ferns, **thiaminase,** destroys thiamin, but cooking inactivates the enzyme.

TOXICITY

No adverse effects associated with thiamin from food or supplements have been reported. Neither have side effects reported from oral intakes of 500 milligrams daily.

Riboflavin

For DRIs, see Appendix A. For food and other sources, see Table 6-5. To investigate the vitamin content of a particular item, go to http://ndb.nal.usda.gov or to http://nutritiondata.self.com.

Riboflavin, vitamin B_2, was encountered late in the 19th century, when laboratory workers observed a yellow-green fluorescent pigment that formed crystals. Not until the 1930s was riboflavin isolated and eventually named for a sugar it contains (ribose) and the color yellow (Latin: *flavus*).

ABSORPTION, METABOLISM, AND EXCRETION

Most absorption of riboflavin occurs in the proximal small intestine facilitated by bile. About 95% of the riboflavin from foods is absorbed, up to a maximum of about 27 milligrams per single meal or dose. Normal bacteria in the large intestine synthesize riboflavin, producing larger amounts when a person consumes a vegetable-based diet rather than a meat-based diet.

Small amounts of the vitamin are found in many tissues, with the greatest concentrations in the liver, kidneys, and heart. Body stores are estimated to suffice for 2 to 6 weeks. The kidneys contribute to riboflavin **homeostasis** by excreting the excess.

FUNCTIONS AND PHARMACEUTICAL POTENTIAL

Riboflavin is a coenzyme in the metabolism of protein and of other vitamins. Thyroid and adrenal hormones accelerate the conversion of riboflavin to its active coenzymes, which are involved in many oxidative enzyme systems. Riboflavin needs increase as protein needs increase. Clients undergoing major healing processes, such as those with extensive burns, require more riboflavin than the average person.

DEFICIENCY

Riboflavin deficiency commonly occurs with thiamin and niacin deficiencies. A person who avoids all dairy products, however, may be deficient in riboflavin alone, a condition called **ariboflavinosis.** Other people at risk for riboflavin deficiencies are vegetarian athletes, pregnant and lactating clients, and people with infantile Brown-Vialetto-Van Laere syndrome (National Institutes of Health, February 11, 2016).

STABILITY AND INTERFERING FACTORS

Riboflavin is fairly resistant to heat, oxygen, and acid but is sensitive to UV light. Thus, cardboard milk cartons or opaque plastic bottles are more protective of the vitamin than clear glass bottles. Even phototherapy used to treat hyperbilirubinemia in newborns has demonstrated the ability to cause riboflavin deficiency (Srinivasa, Renukananda, & Srividya, 2015).

TOXICITY

Large oral doses have not yielded reports of toxicity. Doses of 400 milligrams a day for 3 months have demonstrated no adverse effects (National Institutes of Health, February 11, 2016).

Niacin

For DRIs, see Appendix A. Niacin allowances are related to energy intake. For food and other sources, see Table 6-5. To investigate the vitamin content of a particular item, go to http://ndb.nal.usda.gov or to http://nutritiondata.self.com.

Niacin, vitamin B_3, is a generic term for nicotinic acid and nicotinamide.

ABSORPTION, METABOLISM, AND EXCRETION

Preformed niacin can be absorbed in the stomach but is more easily absorbed in the small intestine by carrier-mediated diffusion. Metabolism by the liver and excretion of excess in the urine is the usual pathway. Niacin has a short half-life live and is metabolized from the body within hours of consumption.

Not all of the body's niacin has to come from preformed niacin in food. The liver can convert the essential amino acid tryptophan to niacin.

FUNCTIONS

Requisite for more than 200 enzymes, niacin is a coenzyme required for energy metabolism. Niacin also participates in the synthesis of steroid hormones and fatty acids.

DEFICIENCY

Pellagra is the deficiency disease caused by the lack of niacin. Symptomatic niacin deficiency can present as soon as 60 days after insufficient dietary intake. Currently, pellagra occurs most frequently in people with risk factors for malnutrition such as chronic alcohol intake, homelessness, AIDS, or absorption problems. Symptoms of pellagra include a triad of symptoms: diarrhea, dermatitis, and dementia. See Box 6-2 for the clinical signs and symptoms of pellagra.

To have a deficiency, a person must consume a diet lacking in both niacin and tryptophan. Symptoms can appear after 2 months of niacin-deficient diet and death can result in 4 to 5 years without treatment (Bamanikar & Dhobale, 2014). With treatment, the dermatologic and gastrointestinal symptoms generally resolve within 48 hours, which can confirm the diagnosis.

SOURCES AND STABILITY

Certain assumptions were made in devising the DRIs to allow for niacin from preformed sources and from protein sources providing tryptophan to be converted to niacin. The measurement derived is a **niacin equivalent** (see Clinical Calculation 6-2). Liver function; supplies of riboflavin, vitamin B_6, and iron; and the body's need for protein synthesis would impact the conversion of tryptophan to niacin.

BOX 6-2 ■ Pellagra

The "three D's" are pellagra's major symptoms: dermatitis, diarrhea, and dementia. The fourth D is death. Diarrhea is certainly not unique to niacin deficiency but contributes to worsening nutritional status. The more characteristic symptoms of dermatitis and dementia can vary markedly from person to person, complicating the diagnostic process.

The sun-sensitive dermatitis is a red rash on exposed skin: the face, neck, arms, hands, and feet. The rash is bilaterally symmetrical with a definite border marking its beginning: on the hands and arms, the rash sometimes resembles gloves, on the feet, boots.

Clients may have hallucinations and display paranoid, suicidal, and aggressive behaviors. In epidemics of pellagra, it is likely that inmates in asylums were merely niacin deficient, without the dermatitis, and kept malnourished by the poor food provided. Eleven such residents of the Georgia State Sanitarium were cured of their dementia with a nutrient-rich diet, reported in a 1915 journal. Beginning in 1937, there have been numerous reports of dramatic recoveries from dementia nearly overnight upon receiving nicotinic acid therapy, indicating that niacin deficiency disrupts a short-term process such as neural transmission rather than causing degeneration of brain tissue (Kirkland, 2014).

CLINICAL CALCULATION   6-2

Niacin Equivalents (NEs)

1 NE = 1 milligram preformed niacin = 60 milligrams tryptophan
  1 gram of complete protein is assumed to provide 10 milligrams of tryptophan.

For example, 1% milk fortified with vitamins A and D contains:

0.227 mg preformed niacin
8.22 g protein

Then:

8.22 g protein × 10 mg tryptophan/g protein =
82.2 mg tryptophan
82.2 mg tryptophan ÷ 60 mg per NE =
1.37 NEs from tryptophan
0.227 mg preformed + 1.37 NE *possible* from tryptophan =
1.6 NE per cup of milk

Coffee and tea contain niacin and can prevent pellagra in cultures with low-protein diets but high intakes of these beverages. Niacin has been found to be stable in light, heat, and air and in alkali environments. Despite its water solubility, only small amounts of niacin are lost in cooking water. It is the most environmentally stable vitamin.

TOXICITY

Pharmacological doses of niacin, given to lower blood cholesterol, cause flushing and over the long-term can cause liver damage. Although serious hepatic toxicity from niacin administration has been reported, it is largely confined to the use of slow-release formulations given as unregulated nutritional supplements.

Vitamin B_6

For DRIs, see Appendix A. For food and other sources, see Table 6-5. To investigate the vitamin content of a particular item, go to http://ndb.nal.usda.gov or to http://nutritiondata.self.com.

Vitamin B_6 was first reported in 1934, isolated in 1938, and synthesized in 1939 (da Silva, Mackey, Davis, & Gregory, 2014). Vitamin B_6 has many roles, but no deficiency disease is associated with it. The name for the pharmaceutical preparation of vitamin B_6 is **pyridoxine.**

ABSORPTION, METABOLISM, AND EXCRETION

The body contains from 45 to 185 milligrams of vitamin B_6, 75% to 80% of it in the muscles. The vitamin is absorbed in the small intestine, mainly in the jejunum. The liver is the primary site for vitamin B_6 metabolism, which also requires riboflavin, niacin, and zinc (da Silva et al, 2014). Most excess vitamin B_6 is excreted in the urine, with little eliminated via the feces.

FUNCTIONS

Vitamin B_6 is a coenzyme in the metabolism of amino acids. It is involved in the metabolism of more than 100 enzymes, including those that synthesize niacin from tryptophan and heme for hemoglobin (National Institutes of Health, February 11, 2016). The importance of adequate vitamin B_6 status for proper immune function has been known for many years (da Silva et al, 2014).

DEFICIENCY

A deficiency of B_6 is unlikely in healthy people because large amounts are present in the general diet. Certain subgroups of the population are at risk of suboptimal vitamin B_6 intake and status:

- Alcoholics
- People with renal disease
- People with autoimmune disease
- Women with nausea and vomiting during pregnancy
- People who are obese

Furthermore, factors such as disease, drug interactions, or errors in food processing may cause an actual deficiency. In the 1950s, severe heat treatment of commercial infant formula produced vitamin B_6 deficiency–induced convulsive seizures that were cured by pyridoxine. As a result, fortification of infant formulas with pyridoxine became routine (da Silva et al, 2014).

Vitamin B_6 deficiency may become apparent in 2 to 3 weeks but may take up to $2^1/_2$ months to appear. Clinically, a person with a vitamin B_6 deficiency may present with these signs and symptoms:

- Rash on face, neck, shoulders, and buttocks
- Mouth lesions
- Fatigue and weakness
- Confusion
- Peripheral neuropathy

Interference with heme production may lead to a hypochromic, microcytic anemia (see Chapter 7).

SOURCES AND STABILITY

Vitamin B_6 is widely distributed in foods. Those of animal origin are the best sources, but whole grains, vegetables, some fruits, nuts, and fortified cereals are major contributors of vitamin B_6 to the diet.

TOXICITY

No adverse effects of vitamin B_6 from foods have been reported. Long-term intake of pharmacologic doses of pyridoxine, greater than 500 milligrams per day, is associated with a risk of sensory neuropathies (da Silva et al, 2014).

Folate

For DRIs, see Appendix A. For food and other sources, see Table 6-5. To investigate the vitamin content of a particular item, go to http://ndb.nal.usda.gov or to http://nutritiondata.self.com.

Folate (also known as vitamin B_9) and vitamin B_{12} were discovered during the search for the reason that eating liver cured **megaloblastic anemia.** Folic acid was discovered as a factor in yeast in 1931 and was later isolated from spinach leaves and named from the Italian for "foliage."

The term for this nutrient as it occurs in foods and body tissues is **folate.** The oxidized and more stable form used to fortify foods and in supplements is **folic acid.** Total body folate levels are estimated to range from 11 to 28 milligrams, about half of which is stored in the liver.

ABSORPTION, METABOLISM, AND EXCRETION

Enzymes in the jejunal and pancreatic secretions and bile convert the folate in foods to the absorbable form used in fortified foods and supplements, which is then absorbed in the acid environment of the upper small intestine and transported to the liver. In the liver, some of the folate is processed for storage in the tissues or the liver and some is secreted into bile.

When the gallbladder releases bile into the duodenum, folate may again be split off and absorbed. This recycling process, which may account for 100 micrograms of reabsorbed folate daily, is important in allowing folate stores to be adequate for 2 to 4 months, compared with 1 to 4 weeks for thiamin stores. Excretion of folate occurs via the urine and a minimal amount through the bile into feces.

FUNCTIONS

Folate is involved in protein synthesis, including that of amino acids, **DNA, RNA,** and heme. Thus, folate participates in the reproduction of every cell and is particularly necessary for rapidly growing cells, including those in the gastrointestinal tract, blood, and fetal tissue, where the absence of adequate amounts becomes clinically and often catastrophically apparent. See the Toxicity section for a relationship to cancer.

DEFICIENCY

Poor dietary intake is the most common cause of folate deficiency especially when coupled with abuse of alcohol that causes intestinal malabsorption, decreased hepatic uptake, and increased excretion, mainly via the urine.

Other clients at risk are those with gastrointestinal diseases marked by malabsorption and with increased losses due to hemodialysis.

Folate deficiency results in impaired cell division and protein synthesis, including the faulty synthesis of red blood cells. In addition to laboratory blood changes, a client may have these signs and symptoms of folate deficiency:

- Bright red tongue
- Fatigue and weakness
- Headaches, irritability
- Shortness of breath
- Heart palpitations

DIETARY REFERENCE INTAKES

Folate RDAs and AIs are given in dietary folate equivalents (DFEs).

One DFE equals

- 1 microgram of food folate
- 0.6 microgram of folic acid from fortified food or as a supplement consumed with food
- 0.5 microgram of a supplement taken on an empty stomach (National Institutes of Health, 2016).

Foods that provide at least 40 micrograms of folate per serving are permitted by the FDA to make the health claim: "Healthful diets with adequate folate may reduce a woman's risk of having a child with a neural tube (brain or spinal cord) defect."

SOURCES AND STABILITY

Green, leafy vegetables, for which the nutrient is named, are good sources as are fruits, legumes, and liver that started the search for the vitamin because of its curative powers (see Table 6-5).

In 1998, the United States and Canada began mandatory fortification of flours, grains, and cereals with folic acid (140 micrograms per 100 grams of product) to prevent neural tube defects (see Chapter 10). By 2009, 51 countries had mandatory wheat flour fortification programs that included folic acid. Research has demonstrated that folic acid fortification prevents 1,300 babies annually from developing neural tube defects who otherwise may have been affected (Centers for Disease Control and Prevention, January 15, 2015). It is still recommended that all women of childbearing age consume 400 micrograms of folic acid daily.

Folate is destroyed by heat, oxidation, ultraviolet light, and acids. To minimize losses, folate-rich foods should be eaten raw or cooked quickly in small amounts of water.

INTERFERING FACTORS

Folic acid does not require digestion, but folate does. Zinc deficiency impairs an enzyme that digests folate. Conjugase inhibitors in certain foods prevent the digestion of polyglutamate forms of folate and prevent its absorption.

Methotrexate, an anticancer drug, is a folate antagonist. Its purpose is to interfere with DNA in cancer cells, but it simultaneously affects normal cells. See Chapter 15 for details on the interaction of folic acid and medications.

TOXICITY

No adverse effects of folate from food or folic acid from supplements have been reported.

Folate intakes of 15 times the UL (15,000 micrograms) have been associated with insomnia, irritability, and gastrointestinal distress. High doses of folic acid can mask the effects of vitamin B_{12} deficiency as well as increase the risk of colorectal cancer (National Institutes of Health, 2016).

Vitamin B_{12} (Cobalamin)

For DRIs, see Appendix A. Persons older than 50 years are counseled to obtain vitamin B_{12} from fortified foods or supplements because 10% to 30% of older people have changes in the gastrointestinal tract that limit the absorption of the vitamin from foods. For food and other sources, see Table 6-5. To investigate the vitamin content of a particular item, go to http://ndb.nal.usda.gov or to http://nutritiondata.self.com.

Vitamin B_{12}, also called cobalamin, is an essential coenzyme in the synthesis of DNA, RNA, and **myelin** and is necessary for normal red blood cell formation. Vitamin B_{12} is stored to a greater extent than the other B vitamins, but diverse causes can precipitate vitamin B_{12} deficiency.

ABSORPTION, METABOLISM, AND EXCRETION

Cobalamins in foods must be liberated from the proteins to which they are attached in foods, a digestive process using gastric acid and pepsin in the stomach. Efficient absorption of vitamin B_{12} also requires an explicit protein-binding factor called **intrinsic factor (IF)**, secreted by the gastric mucosal cells in the stomach. Intrinsic factor combines with vitamin B_{12}, also called **extrinsic factor,** in the proximal small intestine to protect vitamin B_{12} from digestive enzymes and intestinal bacteria until the complex reaches the ileum, where the vitamin is absorbed about 4 hours after ingestion. If the intrinsic factor system is working, more than 50% of the cobalamin in a typical meal will be absorbed, but the intrinsic factor system is limited to about 2 micrograms of cobalamin at a time.

Vitamin B_{12} is not freely absorbed. The amount absorbed depends on the body's storage levels and the amount ingested. At low levels of intake, a large amount of the vitamin is absorbed and vice versa. In addition, in healthy persons, the vitamin can be recycled from bile and intestinal secretions before the remainder is excreted in feces.

FUNCTIONS

Vitamin B_{12} is a coenzyme in the synthesis of DNA and RNA and the metabolism of amino acids and fatty acids. Vitamin B_{12} is also essential for the synthesis and maintenance of myelin, the fatty insulation that permits speedy transmission of impulses along the nerves.

SOURCES

Vitamin B_{12} is synonymous with animal products that have derived their cobalamins from microorganisms. Healthy young adults who regularly consume meat, fish, poultry, milk, cheese, or eggs are not at risk of vitamin B_{12} deficiency.

Plant food sources are not available for vitamin B_{12}. For strict vegetarians, nutritional yeast and vitamin B_{12}–fortified products (soymilk or tofu) are required.

The vitamin is fairly stable, resistant to light, heat, and oxidation.

DEFICIENCY

Deficiency of vitamin B_{12} is a common problem affecting up to 20% of the elder population, resulting in hematologic, gastrointestinal, and neurological symptoms (Mavromati & Sentissi, 2013). Persons may be at increased risk of vitamin B_{12} deficiency because of gastrointestinal or dietary causes.

GASTROINTESTINAL CAUSES

AFFECTING ALL COBALAMIN. When a person lacks intrinsic factor, the result is a condition called **pernicious anemia**. The prevalence of this **autoimmune disease** increases with age and is attributed to autoimmune antibodies against both gastric parietal cells and intrinsic factor. Its prevalence is 0.1% in the general population and 1.9% in persons older than 60 years.

Pernicious anemia can also occur after the surgical removal of the stomach or a large portion of the stomach. In those cases, the cause is not autoimmune interference but missing tissue to produce intrinsic factor.

Intestinal diseases can cause severe intrinsic-factor-related malabsorption of vitamin B_{12} in the ileum. Some of those acquired causes are intestinal parasites, surgical alteration of the ileum, radiation therapy, **celiac disease,** and **Crohn disease** (see Chapter 20).

AFFECTING FOOD-BOUND COBALAMIN. Cobalamin release from food is impaired in food cobalamin malabsorption. Because gastric acid facilitates separation of vitamin B_{12} from the foods containing it, vitamin B_{12} deficiency can be caused by conditions that decrease gastric acid such as gastric or bariatric surgery. Similarly, prolonged use of medications that neutralize gastric acid or block its production can impair vitamin B_{12} status.

DIETARY CAUSES

Vitamin B_{12} deficiency can be caused by a diet devoid of animal products. People particularly at risk are the elderly, persons with alcoholism who eat poorly, and vegetarians.

SIGNS AND SYMPTOMS

Symptoms of vitamin B_{12} deficiency can be seen in the circulatory and nervous systems; however, some clients display only one or the other. Circulatory symptoms include megaloblastic anemia and result in the following signs and symptoms:

- Fatigue
- Pallor
- Shortness of breath
- Tachycardia

Neurological manifestations include these signs and symptoms that may be irreparable:

- Numbness and tingling in the extremities
- Difficulty maintaining balance
- Confusion
- Dementia

Diagnosing vitamin B_{12} deficiency by examining red blood cells is difficult in persons consuming ample folate because folate enables the continued manufacturing of red blood cells in the correct size and number. Folic acid cannot maintain myelin, however. As a result of the inability to diagnose the deficiency quickly, the neurological deterioration of pernicious anemia continues unabated.

TREATMENT

In most countries, treatment of vitamin B_{12} deficiency related to pernicious anemia is intramuscular injections of cobalamin. The pharmaceutical names for vitamin B_{12} are **cyanocobalamin** and **hydroxocobalamin.**

Oral cobalamin should be reserved for clients with only hematological manifestations of vitamin B_{12} deficiency.

INTERFERING FACTORS

Excessive intake of alcohol or vitamin C interferes with vitamin B_{12} absorption and utilization. The body's use of vitamin B_{12} is also impaired by a deficiency of vitamin B_6 and by antacids.

TOXICITY

No toxicity from vitamin B_{12} has been recorded from food or supplements or from parenteral doses to clients with pernicious anemia.

Table 6-5 summarizes the information on the ten water-soluble vitamins.

Other Essential Nutrients

Three additional nutrients are so widely distributed in foods that only special circumstances have produced deficiencies. Long-term **parenteral nutrition (PN)** is one such situation. That therapy is detailed in Chapter 14. Two are vitamins and the third technically is not a vitamin, but all three appear in the DRI tables for vitamins.

For DRIs, see Appendix A. To investigate the pantothenic acid or choline content of a particular item, go to http://nutritiondata.self. com/tools.nutrient-search or to www.nal.usda.gov/fnic/foodcomp/ Data/Choline/Choline.html. Partial data on biotin content of foods are available at www.ncbi.nlm.nih.gov/pmc/articles/ PMC1450323.

PANTOTHENIC ACID

This vitamin's name is derived from Greek for "everywhere" because it is widely found in nature. **Pantothenic acid,** B_5, was isolated in 1931, its structure determined in 1939, and it was synthesized in 1940.

Pantothenic acid serves as a coenzyme in fatty acid metabolism and many other metabolic and regulatory processes. Because it is present to some extent in all foods, pantothenic acid deficiency is rare except in severe malnutrition. No cases of deficiency have been documented in people who eat a variety of foods.

Most adults in the United States consume 4 to 7 milligrams per day, of which about 50% is absorbed, principally in the jejunum. The vitamin is excreted intact, primarily in the urine. People with diabetes mellitus (Chapter 17), alcoholism, and inflammatory bowel diseases (Chapter 20) may have an increased need for pantothenic acid. Good food sources include meats, egg yolk, yogurt, and mushrooms. No toxicities have been reported

BIOTIN

In 1931, a substance in liver was recognized as curing a syndrome called *egg white injury*. As a coenzyme in the synthesis of fat, glycogen, and amino acids, **biotin** is an essential nutrient because bacterial synthesis in the large intestine is insufficient to meet a person's needs. Dietary biotin is absorbed primarily in the jejunum, and small amounts are stored in the muscle, liver, and brain. Excretion occurs via the kidney.

Biotin deficiency appears to be common during normal human pregnancy, with fetal concentrations six times higher than the mother's. In animals, biotin deficiency causes birth defects, particularly cleft palates.

Meat, fish, poultry, eggs, and dairy products are rich dietary sources of biotin.

Deficiencies have been caused by parenteral nutrition that omitted biotin but also in children with an autosomal recessive inborn error of biotin metabolism. Biotin deficiency may develop in persons with alcoholism or gastrointestinal diseases and those on long-term anticonvulsant therapy or kidney dialysis. Symptoms include **alopecia;** a scaly, red rash around the eyes, nose, and mouth; **paresthesias** of the extremities; depression; and hallucinations (Serum biotin, 2016).

Toxicity has not been reported.

Avidin, a protein in raw egg white that is thought to serve as a **bacteriostat,** interferes with biotin absorption by irreversibly binding with it. Excessive consumption of raw egg whites has caused biotin deficiency.

CHOLINE

Choline was discovered in 1862, synthesized in 1866, but not recognized as essential for humans until 1998 because investigators thought the body manufactured sufficient amounts of the substance. Although the liver synthesizes choline, the gene for the enzyme catalyzing the synthesis is induced by estrogen.

Choline is essential for liver and brain function, lipid metabolism, and cellular membrane composition and repair. Humans produce choline in insufficient amounts in the liver and require consumption in the diet. Choline is a part of the neurotransmitter **acetylcholine** and of **phospholipids** that are structural components of all human cell membranes. Although not a vitamin by strict definition, choline has been given an AI and is listed in the DRIs with the vitamins. Choline is widely distributed in foods, with the best sources being liver, eggs, beef, and pork.

Effects of excessive intake (10 to 16 grams per day) include sweating, salivation, vomiting, and a fishy body odor.

Table 6-6 lists the sources of vitamins by food groups to clarify the potential for inadequate intake if a person excludes an entire food group.

TABLE 6-6   Good Sources of Vitamins by Food Groups

VITAMIN	SYNTHESIS/ MISCELLANEOUS	MEATS	MILK	FRUITS/ VEGETABLES	GRAINS
A		Liver Egg yolk	Fortified	Deep yellow, dark green leafy	
D	In skin	Saltwater fish	Fortified		Fortified cereals
E				Sunflower, safflower, canola oils Nuts Leafy vegetables	Wheat germ Whole grains Fortified cereals
K	In intestine			Green leafy Canola, soybean oils	
C				Fresh fruit, especially citrus Vegetables	
Thiamin		Pork Beef liver Salmon		Black beans	Wheat germ Fortified cereals
Riboflavin		Meats, esp. liver Eggs	Milk		Fortified cereals
Niacin	Coffee Tea	Meat Fish Poultry			Whole or enriched grains Fortified cereals
B_6		Sirloin steak Salmon Chicken breast		Bananas Nuts Broccoli Carrots	Whole grains Fortified cereals
Folate (folic acid)		Liver		Dried peas, beans, lentils Dark green leafy Peanuts	Fortified grain products Whole grains Wheat germ
B_{12}		Meat Fish Poultry Eggs	Milk Cheese	Fortified soymilk, tofu	
Pantothenic acid	Possibly in intestine	Liver Chicken Egg yolk	Yogurt	Mushrooms Broccoli Potatoes	Whole-grain cereals
Biotin	In intestine	Liver Egg yolk Salmon		Soybeans Peanuts Sweet potato	
Choline	In liver	Liver Eggs Beef Pork	Milk Yogurt	Baked beans Broccoli	Wheat germ

Vitamin Supplements

Vitamin supplements are not intended as substitutes for a healthy diet mainly because foods contain many nutrients and phytochemicals in addition to vitamins. Knowledge of vitamins and the foods containing them is constantly evolving. The single piece of advice given most frequently in the conclusions of researchers, however, is the admonition to eat five servings of fruits and vegetables every day. Fruit eaten out of hand is the original fast food.

No U.S. government health agency, private health group, or health professional organization promotes regular use of a multivitamin/mineral supplement or individual nutrients without first considering the quality of a person's diet (National Institutes of Health, July 8, 2015). For certain groups of people, fortified foods or supplements are recommended. As indicated in this chapter, synthetic vitamins in fortified food or supplements are recommended for women capable of becoming pregnant (folic acid) and individuals older than 50 years (vitamin B_{12}). In addition, vegans should ensure that their intakes of vitamin B_{12} from fortified foods or supplements are adequate (National Institutes of Health, February 11, 2016). The American Academy of Pediatrics recommends infants receive vitamin D supplements until weaned to vitamin D–fortified infant formula, consuming at least 1,000 mL per day, or the infant is 1 year old and weaned to vitamin D–fortified milk (Centers for Disease Control and Prevention, June 17, 2015).

Individuals wishing to take supplements should consider taking a multivitamin instead of a medley of single vitamins and should not exceed 100% of the RDA/AIs. An RDA/AI amount of multivitamins will prevent deficiency in healthy individuals, and toxicity is unlikely. When choosing a vitamin product, people should select one tailored to their age, gender, and situation (e.g., pregnancy). In any event, vitamin taking should be reported to health-care providers along with medication history.

Although not a major expense for individuals, sales of multivitamin/mineral and herb supplements in 2014 in the United States totaled $36.7 billion. Supplement users also tend to have higher micronutrient intakes from their diets than do nonusers. Multivitamins are sold in many formulations. Dollars & Sense 6-1 suggests considerations when shopping for multivitamins.

Dollars & Sense 6-1

Brand Name versus Generic Multivitamins

The Food and Drug Administration (2016) does not have the authority to review dietary supplement products for safety and effectiveness before they are marketed. Reading the label, although a necessary first step, does not automatically indicate the best choice of a supplement. For safety, the FDA (2016) recommends the following:

- Use noncommercial sites if buying supplements online.
- Watch for false claims such as "no side effects" or "totally safe."
- Recognize that "natural" doesn't mean safe.
- Speak with your health-care provider before taking a supplement.

Centrum, recommended for adults under 50 years of age, sold for $12.76 for 200 tablets (6 cents each) on the same day that Walgreens A Thru Z Multivitamin/Multimineral sold for $7.14 for 200 tablets (4 cents each). At these prices, a year's supply of the Walgreen brand would save $7.20 for each person over the Centrum product. Greater savings might be had if larger quantities were purchased, but that is not always the case. Sometimes larger amounts of an item cost more per unit than smaller amounts. It pays to shop carefully.

KEYSTONES

- Vitamins are organic substances required by the body in minute quantities and that do not become part of the structure of the body.

- Vitamins A, D, E, and K are fat soluble and require sufficient dietary fat intake and adequate fat digestion for proper utilization. The water-soluble vitamins, C and the B-complex vitamins, are not stored in the body in appreciable amounts, requiring more frequent intake than fat-soluble ones.

- Deficiency of vitamin A results in xerophthalmia and night blindness, and deficiency of vitamin D causes rickets and osteomalacia.

- Vitamins C, B_{12}, thiamin, and niacin have specific diseases associated with deficiency: scurvy, pernicious anemia, beriberi, and pellagra.

- Vitamin K is present in green leafy vegetables and canola and soybean oils; vitamin C in fresh vegetables and fruit, especially citrus.

- Enrichment is the restoration to a product of nutrients that were lost during processing. Fortification is the addition of nutrients not normally present in a food to increase its nutritional value.

- Pregnant women should avoid excessive intake of preformed vitamin A from foods or supplements because of risk to the fetus. Excessive vitamin D from supplements or multiple fortified foods may be hazardous to children.

■ Good sources of vitamins A and C are broccoli, cantaloupe, and red pepper.

■ People who take vitamins should limit their intake to 100% of the RDA in a multivitamin product, except individuals with special needs.

■ Two large groups of people for whom synthetic vitamins in fortified food or supplements are recommended are women capable of becoming pregnant (folic acid) and individuals older than 50 years (vitamin B_{12}).

CASE STUDY 6-1

Mr. J, a 79-year-old widowed man, prides himself on caring for himself during the past year since his wife died. His typical meal pattern is as follows:

■ Breakfast—egg, toast, jam, coffee
■ Lunch—cheese or lunchmeat sandwich, tea
■ Dinner—canned stew or hash

Although Mr. J has a refrigerator, he avoids buying fresh fruits or vegetables. He says he has difficulty consuming produce before it spoils. He seldom goes out to eat.

For the past few months, Mr. J has noticed that his gums are tender. He stopped wearing his dentures when his gums began to bleed.

The visiting nurse confirmed inflammation of the gums. When the nurse took Mr. J's blood pressure, she noted a red, flat rash on Mr. J's forearm.

CARE PLAN

Subjective Data
Sore gums ■ Diet lacks fresh fruits and vegetables

Objective Data
Inflamed gums ■ Erythematous **petechiae** related to blood pressure measurement

Analysis
Possible vitamin C deficiency related to lack of fresh fruit and vegetables as evidenced by sore bleeding gums and petechiae after sphygmomanometer use.

Plan

DESIRED OUTCOMES EVALUATION CRITERIA	ACTIONS/ INTERVENTIONS	RATIONALE
Will consume foods containing 90 mg of vitamin C every day within 3 days	Teach the importance of daily vitamin C	Little vitamin C is stored in the body; should be consumed nearly every day
	Explore the acceptability of good sources of vitamin C; list amounts necessary to obtain 90 mg; recommend purchasing small quantities	Foods would be better sources than vitamin supplements because food also supplies other nutrients
	If the client selects frozen vegetables, teach to boil water 1 minute before adding vegetables and to cook quickly until crisp-tender	Heat and oxygen destroy vitamin C
	Follow up in 3 days; report to primary care provider if unimproved	

Three days later, the nurse determined that Mr. J had not been grocery shopping, and his bleeding gums and petechiae persisted. After telephone consultation with his physician, she instructed Mr. J to have the vitamin C blood test the physician ordered and to visit the doctor the following week.

TEAMWORK 6-1

PHYSICIAN'S NOTES

The following Physician's Notes are representative of the documentation found in a client's medical record.

When the doctor saw Mr. J, he wrote the following:

Chief complaint: *Referred by home health regarding possible vitamin C deficiency*

Subjective: *Unsure of reason for visit. "Sent by nurse."*

Objective: *Gingival hypertrophy and inflammation, recent bruising on extremities*

Serum ascorbic acid level 0.15 milligrams per 100 milliliters

Analysis: *Scurvy*

Plan: *Replenish vitamin C levels with ascorbic acid: 1 gram per day for 5 days, then 500 milligrams per day until normal levels achieved.*

Follow up in 2 weeks

CRITICAL THINKING QUESTIONS

1. Is this the end of Mr. J's nutritional problems? What additional assessment data would be helpful as you continue to work with Mr. J?

2. Why do you think Mr. J did not follow the nurse's initial advice?

3. Even after the physician prescribes vitamin C, why is it important to improve Mr. J's food intake?

CHAPTER REVIEW

1. Which of the following vitamins are water soluble?
   1. A and C
   2. A, D, E, and K
   3. B and C
   4. B, D, E, and K

2. The vitamin that is essential to the synthesis of several blood clotting factors is:
   1. Vitamin A
   2. Vitamin B_6
   3. Vitamin C
   4. Vitamin K

3. Which of the following groups of foods would be the best sources of carotene?
   1. Apricots, cantaloupe, and squash
   2. Asparagus, beets, and sweet potatoes
   3. Broccoli, lettuce, and lima beans
   4. Lemons, oranges, and strawberries

4. Deficiency of vitamin D causes:
   1. Rickets
   2. Pellagra
   3. Night blindness
   4. Beriberi

5. In general, individuals who elect to take a vitamin supplement should:
   1. Buy the most economical product
   2. Limit the amounts to 100% of RDA levels
   3. Obtain a physician's prescription
   4. Select the most advertised product

CLINICAL ANALYSIS

1. Ms. C is bringing her 3-month-old infant to the well-baby clinic. Ms. C states that the infant is taking 6 ounces of a commercial baby formula every 4 hours. Ms. C has not added solid foods to the infant's diet. She was told to wait until the infant is 4 to 6 months old before adding cereal. Ms. C is giving the baby the multivitamin preparation prescribed. She also has added cod liver oil to the infant's diet. "It's only a teaspoonful," she said. Ms. C's grandmother gave Ms. C cod liver oil as a child. Ms. C credits her grandmother's care during her own childhood for her strong bones and teeth. She admires her grandmother, who at age 75 still stands straight and tall. Which of the following pieces of information should the nurse gather first to focus on the situation presented?

   a. The amount of vitamin C in the multivitamin supplement
   b. The conditions under which the vitamins are stored
   c. Ms. C's technique for measuring the vitamins
   d. The total amount of vitamin D the infant receives each day

2. Mr. S has expressed interest in improving his diet. The nurse assessed Mr. S's usual intake, noting the absence of citrus fruit. He stated that the acids upset his stomach. Which of the following suggestions to maximize vitamin C content in vegetables is appropriate?

   a. Adding baking soda to the cooking water
   b. Cooking thoroughly to kill any bacteria
   c. Eating good sources raw when possible
   d. Keeping food in a mesh bag to allow air to circulate

3. Ms. M is a Seventh-Day Adventist who has elected a vegan lifestyle and who lives an indoor life. For which of the following vitamin deficiencies would she be at greatest risk without professional dietary advice?

   a. Vitamins A, C, and E
   b. Vitamins B_{12}, D, and niacin
   c. Vitamin B_6, folate, and thiamin
   d. Vitamin K, riboflavin, and biotin

Minerals

In a broad sense, minerals are obtained from the Earth's crust. Through the effects of the weather, rocks that contain minerals are ground into smaller particles, which then become part of the soil. Growing plants absorb the minerals from the soil with the water they need. Animals eat the plants, and humans eat both the plants and the animals.

Water is the medium of absorption of nutrients for plants and the basis of the body's nutrient delivery system. In addition, certain forms of minerals are intricately bound to the distribution and movement of water in the body.

Minerals make vital contributions to growth and maintenance of the body's health. This chapter covers minerals important in human nutrition and the role each plays in the body. It describes some general functions of minerals and explains how minerals are classified in nutrition. It details the nutritional implications of the 7 major and 10 trace minerals.

Functions of Minerals

Minerals represent 4% of total body weight. Like vitamins, minerals help to regulate bodily functions without providing energy and are essential to good health. Unlike vitamins, minerals:

1. Are inorganic substances.
2. Become part of the body's composition.

For instance, calcium and phosphorus combine to give bones and teeth their hardness. Iron attaches to the protein globin to form hemoglobin. Iodine becomes part of the thyroid hormones.

Most minerals serve a variety of functions in the body's regulatory and metabolic processes. Sodium is essential for maintaining fluid balance. Sodium, potassium, and calcium have critical functions in nerve and muscle activity. Potassium and phosphorus play significant roles in acid–base balance. A disruption of the body's balance of any one of these minerals, although not necessarily caused by diet, can be life-threatening.

Classification of Minerals

Three groups of minerals are considered in nutrition: major, trace, and ultratrace.

Major minerals (macrominerals) and **trace minerals** (microminerals) are differentiated by:

- Amounts present in the body:
  - Major: more than 5 grams (approximately 1 teaspoonful)
  - Trace: less than 5 grams
- Intake requirements:
  - Major: 100 milligrams (approximately $\frac{1}{50}$ teaspoonful) or more per day
  - Trace: less than 100 milligrams per day
  - Ultratrace: less than 1 milligram per day

Despite their small amounts, trace minerals make vital and often unique contributions to the body's functioning.

Ultratrace minerals appear in the Dietary Reference Intakes (DRI) tables (see Appendix A). The only values that have been set are Tolerable Upper Intake Level (ULs) for three of the five minerals in this category.

Major Minerals

The seven major minerals include calcium, sodium, and potassium, which are familiar to many people in a dietary context. The other four are phosphorus, magnesium, sulfur, and chloride.

Calcium

About 1.5% to 2% of total body weight is calcium, representing 40% of the body's mineral mass. The body of a 150-pound adult contains approximately 3 pounds of calcium, 99% in the bones and teeth. The remaining 1% of the calcium circulates in the body fluids.

Functions

Calcium, with phosphorus, forms the hard substance of bones and teeth. Ample calcium and phosphorus alone will not guarantee strong bones and teeth, however. Vitamin D is necessary for calcium absorption, and protein serves as the matrix that determines the structure of the bone. Exercise, particularly weight-bearing exercise, is also essential for strong bones. Except for slightly demineralized areas, teeth cannot repair themselves and so dental restoration is needed.

Calcium also performs several vital metabolic functions in the nervous, muscular, and cardiovascular systems, for instance:

1. Calcium assists in manufacturing **acetylcholine,** a neurotransmitter (a chemical that enhances transmission of nerve impulses).
2. Calcium acts as a catalyst in initiating and controlling muscle contraction and relaxation. At the beginning of a muscle contraction, calcium is released from its storage area inside the muscle cell. At the end of a contraction, the calcium is gathered into its storage area.
3. Calcium is a catalyst in the clotting process: it aids in the conversion of platelets to thromboplastin and in the conversion of **fibrinogen** to **fibrin.**

Control Mechanisms

Bone remodeling is the process through which bone is renewed to maintain bone strength and mineral homeostasis. In this process, bone cells called **osteoclasts** produce enzymes to destroy the protein matrix that holds the calcium phosphate in place. Other bone cells, called **osteoblasts,** produce new matrix protein, which chemically attracts calcium and other nutrients to rebuild the bone.

Several hormones work together to accomplish these activities. Vitamin D (see Chapter 6) is one of these hormones.

Parathyroid hormone and calcitonin are the other two. Tiny glands behind the thyroid gland in the neck secrete **parathyroid hormone** when the serum calcium level is too low. The thyroid gland secretes **calcitonin** when the serum calcium level is too high.

Figure 7-1 illustrates the complementary actions of parathyroid hormone and calcitonin.

Other hormones also affect the body's use of calcium. One prominent one is estrogen. Decreased estrogen production leads to increased bone resorption and decreased calcium absorption (National Institutes of Health [NIH], November 17, 2016).

Dietary Reference Intakes

For DRIs see Appendix A. In 2010, the values for calcium were upgraded from Adequate Intake (AIs) to Recommended Dietary Allowance (RDAs) for all ages except infants. For food and other sources, see Table 7-1. To investigate the mineral content of a particular item, go to http://ndb.nal.usda.gov or to http://nutritiondata.self.com.

Sources

Calcium can be obtained from animal or vegetable sources, but calcium from animal sources is more readily absorbed.

ANIMAL SOURCES

Milk and milk products are the best animal sources of calcium. In milk, calcium is accompanied by lactose, which increases absorption in infants but not in adults. Another advantageous component of milk is the protein the osteoblasts need to rebuild the bone matrix. In sum, milk is such an important source of calcium that it is virtually impossible to obtain adequate dietary calcium without dairy products. Figure 7-2 shows a child drinking milk with a "fast-food" meal.

See Table 7-2 to evaluate alternate sources of calcium compared to fluid milk. Note the cost in kilocalories.

Milk products supply other nutrients in addition to calcium, such as vitamins A and D, and are also a major source of riboflavin and protein (see Fig. 7-3). Supplements should not substitute for food but sometimes are necessary adjuncts. Clinical Application 7-1 describes the types of calcium supplements available and suggestions for choosing a supplement when necessary.

Calcium supplements should be taken:

- In doses of 500 milligrams or less for optimal absorption
- With meals if calcium carbonate (stomach acid enhances absorption)
- Without regard to meals if calcium citrate

PLANT SOURCES

Good plant sources of calcium include collard greens, broccoli, kale, legumes, and soybeans. Some experts question how much calcium the body is actually able to absorb from plant sources because of multiple interfering factors.

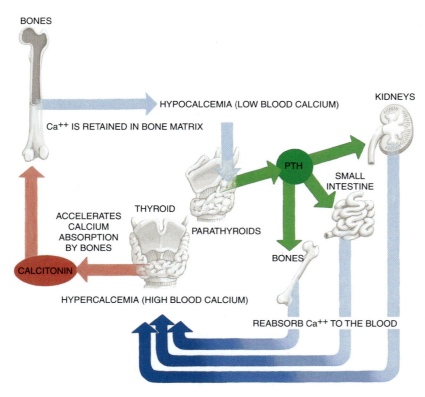

FIGURE 7-1 Parathyroid hormone raises serum calcium levels when they are too low. Calcitonin from the thyroid gland lowers serum calcium levels when they are too high. *(Reprinted from Venes, D [ed]: Taber's Cylcopedic Medical Dictionary, ed 21. FA Davis, Philadelphia, 2010, p. 338, with permission.)*

TABLE 7-1   Major Minerals

MINERAL	ADULT RDA/ AI AND FOOD PORTION*	FUNCTIONS	SIGNS AND SYMPTOMS OF DEFICIENCY	SIGNS AND SYMPTOMS OF EXCESS	GOOD SOURCES IN COMMON FOODS
Calcium	1,000–1,200 mg 3.3–4 cups 1% milk	Structure of bones and teeth Nerve conduction Muscle contraction Blood clotting	Tetany Osteoporosis Rickets (premature infants)	Calcification of soft tissue	Milk products Salmon, sardines with bones Clams Oysters
Phosphorus	700 mg 8.9-oz sockeye salmon	Structure of bones and teeth Component of DNA and RNA Component of buffers and almost all enzymes Component of ADP and ATP	Increased calcium excretion Bone loss Muscle weakness	Tetany Convulsions Renal insufficiency	Lean meat Fish Poultry Milk Nuts Legumes
Sodium	1,200–1,500 mg 0.5–0.65 tsp salt	Fluid balance Transmission of electrochemical impulses along nerve and muscle membranes	Hyponatremia	Hypernatremia	Table salt Processed foods Milk and milk products
Potassium	4.7 g 4 cups canned white beans	Conduction of nerve impulses Muscle contraction	Hypokalemia (not usually dietary)	Hyperkalemia (not usually dietary)	Banana Cantaloupe Winter squash Green leafy vegetables Legumes Salt substitutes
Magnesium	310–420 mg 2.1–2.8 cups spinach	Associated with ADP and ATP Involved in DNA and protein synthesis Influences cardiac and smooth muscle contractility	Impaired CNS function Tetany	Weakness Depressed respirations Cardiac arrest	Green leafy vegetables Seafood Peanut butter Legumes Coffee Cocoa

TABLE 7-1   Major Minerals (Continued)

MINERAL	ADULT RDA/ AI AND FOOD PORTION*	FUNCTIONS	SIGNS AND SYMPTOMS OF DEFICIENCY	SIGNS AND SYMPTOMS OF EXCESS	GOOD SOURCES IN COMMON FOODS
Sulfur	Not established	Component of amino acids methionine and cysteine Gives shape to hair, skin, and nails	None known due solely to sulfur	None known due solely to sulfur	Complete protein foods
Chloride	1,800–2,300 mg 0.5–0.67 tsp salt	Component of hydrochloric acid Helps maintain fluid and acid base balance	In infants: neurological impairments	None known	Table salt Salty snacks Processed foods Eggs Meat Seafood

ADP, adenosine diphosphate; ATP, adenosine triphosphate; CNS, central nervous system.
*Examples only; not suggested for a sole source of a day's intake.

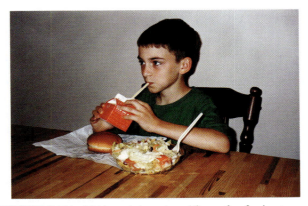

FIGURE 7-2 This child has a balanced meal from a fast-food restaurant: a small hamburger, a salad, and milk. Growing bones and teeth need calcium from milk products.

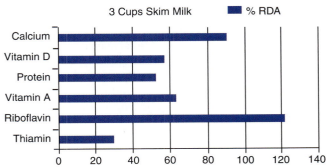

FIGURE 7-3 Milk supplies many nutrients in addition to calcium. Three cups of skim milk provide a woman between 19 and 50 years of age with these percentages of her RDAs: calcium, 90%; vitamin D, 58%; protein, 54%; vitamin A, 64%; riboflavin, 122%; and thiamin, 30%. The kilocaloric cost for all of these nutrients is a minuscule 249 kilocalories.

TABLE 7-2   Food Containing Approximately 300 Milligrams of Calcium, Equal to 1 Cup of Milk

FOOD	AMOUNT	KILOCALORIES
Skim milk	1.0 cup	86
Plain low-fat yogurt	0.7 cup	101
Swiss cheese	1.1 oz	118
Whole milk	1.0 cup	150
Cheddar cheese	1.5 oz	171
Low-fat yogurt with fruit	0.9 cup	199
Cottage cheese, 2% low-fat	2.0 cups	410
Soft ice cream	1.3 cups	479
Cottage cheese, creamed, large curd	2.25 cups	529
Sherbet	2.9 cups	786

CLINICAL APPLICATION   7-1

Calcium Supplements

There are two main types of calcium supplements available: calcium carbonate and calcium citrate. Calcium carbonate contains 40% elemental calcium and is inexpensive, which makes it a popular first choice of supplement. Calcium citrate is more expensive and contains 21% elemental calcium. Calcium carbonate has been shown to cause less gastrointestinal upset than calcium citrate. Calcium citrate is absorbed better in more alkaline environments and is recommended for clients 50 years of age or older because of decreased gastric acids or in clients with absorption problems.

Supplements labeled "USP" or "CL" (see Chapter 15) meet voluntary industry standards for quality, purity, and tablet disintegration or dissolution. To test the dissolvability of a calcium product, place a tablet in one-half cup of vinegar. Stir occasionally over one-half hour, after which no particles should be visible. Dissolvability is only the first step in calcium absorption, however, because of the multiple factors affecting it.

Absorption and Excretion

Calcium is absorbed throughout the small intestine through two distinct processes. In the **duodenum** and proximal **jejunum,** the process is active, through the intestinal cells, and involves vitamin D–dependent calcium-binding transport proteins. In the distal jejunum and ileum, the process is passive, between the intestinal cells.

Net calcium absorption in infants and young children is up to 60%, compared with 15% to 20% absorbed by adults (NIH, November 17, 2016). With decreased estrogen in aging females, calcium absorption may diminish. Excretion takes place in urine and feces, but also through the skin through sweat.

Interfering Factors

Several factors can interfere with the absorption and retention of calcium, as described in Table 7-3.

OXALATES

Some plants contain salts of oxalic acid called **oxalates** that bind with the calcium present in some vegetables to produce calcium oxalate, an insoluble substance excreted in the feces. A few foods high in oxalate are nuts, rhubarb, and Swiss chard. Although it is generally not advised to eliminate all oxalate-containing foods, reducing consumption can help reduce the risk of developing kidney stones.

PHYTATES

Phytic acid, the storage form of phosphorus in seeds, forms an insoluble complex with calcium. Foods that contain high levels of phytic acid, such as legumes, nuts, and cereal, can reduce calcium absorption.

The overall effect of oxalic and phytic acids on calcium availability in most balanced diets usually is not significant. People who avoid dairy products, however, need careful attention to meal planning. Ovovegetarian and vegan clients should seek calcium-fortified products, such as orange juice and calcium-set tofu, to bolster their intake of the mineral.

PROTEIN

The impact of dietary protein on calcium absorption has been a subject of debate. High-protein diets increase urinary calcium excretion and make the urine more acidic. These two effects were suspected to produce a dietary environment favorable for demineralization of the skeleton.

However, increased calcium excretion due to a high-protein diet does not seem to be linked to impaired calcium balance. In contrast, some data indicate that high-protein intakes increase intestinal calcium absorption (NIH, November 17, 2016).

OTHER MINERALS

Because calcium, magnesium, and zinc use the same absorption mechanism, magnesium and zinc can impair the absorption of calcium.

Sodium intake can also have a detrimental effect on calcium balance. When sodium levels are increased, the excess is excreted in urine and calcium is eliminated with it. It is estimated that every 500 milligrams of sodium consumed results in 10 milligrams loss of calcium in the urine. The result of high sodium diets is an increased excretion of calcium through the urine and a decrease in intestinal absorption of calcium. Therefore, dietary sodium has a tremendous potential to influence bone loss at suboptimal calcium intakes in women.

CAFFEINE

Excessive caffeine intake of 300 to 400 mg has demonstrated an increased loss of calcium through both the urine and feces. Several studies have proven that the loss is minimal and can be offset by consuming an ounce, or less, of milk. If a person's calcium intake is low, or he or she has osteoporosis, drinking many caffeinated beverages could adversely affect bone health.

OTHER FACTORS

In certain situations, calcium bioavailability may be reduced by diseases or medications to treat them. In individuals with digestive system diseases producing **steatorrhea,** the excess fat in the bowel combines with calcium, forming insoluble soap, which is then excreted in the feces.

Deficiencies

Calcium deficiency in children can contribute to poor bone and tooth development. Rickets is typically more directly related to vitamin D deficiency than to calcium deficiency except in premature infants, whose skeletons still need increased calcium. Two other conditions related to calcium balance are osteoporosis and tetany.

OSTEOPOROSIS

According to the World Health Organization, **osteopenia** is bone mineral density 1 to 2.5 standard deviations below the mean of healthy young adults, whereas **osteoporosis** is bone mineral density more than 2.5 standard deviations below the mean. Osteoporosis is a progressive systemic disease that leads to bone fragility and fracture with a 30% to 40% lifetime risk for fracture (Begum et al, 2014).

Two major factors in the development of osteoporosis are:

1. The bone mass developed from birth to age 30
2. The rate at which bone mass is lost in later life

TABLE 7-3	Factors Affecting Calcium Absorption and Excretion	
INCREASE ABSORPTION	**DECREASE ABSORPTION**	**INCREASE EXCRETION**
Lactose (infants)	Oxalic acid	Excessive protein
Vitamin D	Phytic acid	Excessive sodium
	Zinc supplements coupled with low calcium intake	Caffeine coupled with low calcium intake

In girls and women, 99% of total bone body mineral content is achieved by age 22, with peak bone mass being achieved by age 30 years. Postmenopausal women will lose 12% to 15% of premenopausal bone mass within 5 years (Casey, 2015). Osteoporosis is most common in postmenopausal, fair-complexioned white women; however, all are not equally affected (see Genomic Gem 7-1). Men and black women lose bone mass also, but because their skeletons are generally heavier, they are at lower risk of osteoporosis.

Figure 7-4 shows normal and osteoporotic cancellous bone. Figure 7-5 displays x-ray films of normal and osteoporotic

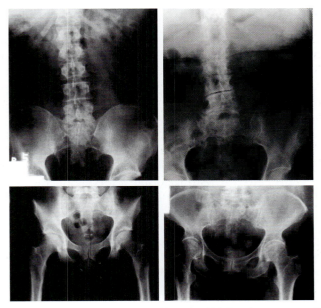

FIGURE 7-5 X-ray films of a normal bone on the left and an osteoporotic bone on the right. *(Courtesy of Dr. Russell Tobe.)*

GENOMIC GEM **7-1**

Osteoporosis Is Familial

Bone Mineral Density

About 80% of the variance in peak bone mass is an inherited trait. A family history of hip fracture may be predictive of a twofold increased risk of hip fracture.

An early marker of genetic influence on bone physiology entails the vitamin D receptor, which has been associated with low bone mineral density in several populations. Women with the low bone mineral density vitamin D receptor genotype not only displayed more rapid bone loss but also failed to increase calcium absorption if calcium intake was low.

Most of the known genes identified with osteoporosis encode components of pathways involved in bone synthesis or resorption. To date, only a small proportion of the total genetic variation implicated in osteoporosis has been ascertained. Progress in this area is expected to accelerate in the future (Tucker & Rosen, 2014).

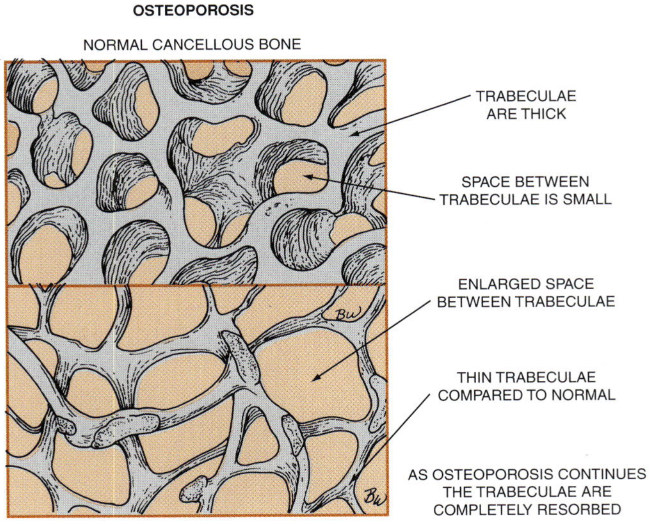

OSTEOPOROSIS

NORMAL CANCELLOUS BONE

TRABECULAE ARE THICK

SPACE BETWEEN TRABECULAE IS SMALL

ENLARGED SPACE BETWEEN TRABECULAE

THIN TRABECULAE COMPARED TO NORMAL

AS OSTEOPOROSIS CONTINUES THE TRABECULAE ARE COMPLETELY RESORBED

OSTEOPOROTIC CANCELLOUS BONE

FIGURE 7-4 Sketch of normal and osteoporotic cancellous bone showing enlarged spaces and thinner bony structure in the latter. *(Reprinted from Venes, D [ed]: Taber's Cyclopedic Medical Dictionary, ed 21. FA Davis, Philadelphia, 2010, p. 1659, with permission.)*

bones. Clinical Application 7-2 details prevalence, major risk factors, diagnostic aids, and treatment approaches for osteoporosis.

Two lifestyle factors impacting bone include:

1. Smoking
2. Alcohol consumption

Relatively minor risk factors for decreased calcium metabolism (alcohol, caffeine, high-protein intake, phytic acid– and oxalic acid–containing foods, sodium, and smoking), when combined, and especially when coupled with low-calcium and vitamin D intake or sunlight aversion, might make a decided difference in an individual's bone health.

TETANY

Despite the hormonal control of serum calcium and the large reservoir in the bones, serum calcium levels sometimes fall below normal. An actual lack of calcium or a lack of ionized calcium may cause tetany. A serum calcium level that is too low is called **hypocalcemia.** If the signs and symptoms described here appear, the condition is called **tetany.** Causes include parathyroid deficiency, **alkalosis,** and (in infants) vitamin D deficiency (see Chapter 6).

Hypocalcemia is a major postoperative complication of total thyroidectomy caused by damage to, or impairment of blood supply to, one or more parathyroid glands during surgery. Hypocalcemia occurs in 10% to 50% of thyroidectomy clients with 0.5% to 2% having permanent hypocalcemia that lasts for up to 1 year (Kim et al, 2017). In **alkalosis,** because of the excessive alkalinity of body fluids, a greater number of calcium ions than usual are bound to serum proteins, effectively inactivating calcium and impairing nerve and muscle function (see

CLINICAL APPLICATION   7-2

Osteoporosis Prevalence, Risk Factors, Diagnosis, and Treatment

PREVALENCE
- An estimated 10 million people in the United States, 80% of them women, have osteoporosis, the major factor in fractures in the elderly (International Osteoporosis Foundation, 2017).
- It is estimated that by 2025 osteoporosis will be responsible for 3 million fractures, resulting in $25.3 billion in health-care costs (National Osteoporosis Foundation, undated).

MAJOR RISK FACTORS IN WHITE POSTMENOPAUSAL WOMEN
- Personal history of fracture as an adult.
- History of fragility fracture in a first-degree relative.
- Low body weight (BMI ≤ 18.5)
- Current smoking
- Use of corticosteroid therapy
- Diseases such as chronic obstructive pulmonary disease (COPD), type 1 and type 2 diabetes, rheumatoid arthritis, and chronic liver or gastrointestinal disease (Casey, 2015).

DIAGNOSIS
- History and physical examination, including assessment for height loss and posture changes
- Measurement of bone mineral density (BMD) if postmenopausal. Until 30% to 40% of bone mass is lost, it is not detectable on x-ray film (see Fig. 7-5), but dual-energy x-ray absorptiometry (DEXA) permits earlier diagnosis.

TREATMENT
- Optimize nutrition, including protein, vitamin D, and calcium. Supplements when indicated. High intakes of calcium reduce bone resorption by reducing parathyroid hormone secretion.
- Exercise to the extent fragility permits.
- Consider medications to affect bone metabolism in conjunction with, not instead of, nutrition and exercise.

Acid–Base Balance in Chapter 8). Alkalosis may be caused by:

- Losing acid (due to vomiting or gastric suction)
- Ingesting alkalis (e.g., sodium bicarbonate)
- Breathing too rapidly, either in response to fear or through mechanical ventilation

The result of rapid breathing is excessive loss of carbon dioxide. In the blood, carbon dioxide is transported as carbonic acid. Thus, when too much carbon dioxide is exhaled, the alkalinity of the blood increases and produces tetany.

Early symptoms of tetany are:

- Nervousness
- Irritability
- Numbness
- Tingling of the extremities and around the mouth
- Muscle cramps

Diagnostic signs of tetany are Trousseau sign and Chvostek sign.

In **Trousseau sign,** inflation of the blood pressure cuff above systolic pressure for 3 minutes causes ischemia of the peripheral nerves, increasing their excitability.

In **Chvostek sign,** a tap over the facial nerve in front of the ear causes a twitch of the facial muscles on that side. Figure 7-6 depicts these diagnostic signs.

Because of the many functions of calcium, tetany is a medical emergency. Untreated, tetany can progress to:

- Blood clotting irregularities
- Heart dilatation
- Respiratory paralysis
- Seizures
- Coma

Toxicity

For basic information on mineral toxicity, see Table 7-4. A serum calcium level that is too high, above 11 milligrams per 100 milliliters of serum in adults, is called **hypercalcemia,** most often caused by cancer or hyperparathyroidism.

Another condition, one that involves ingestion of large amounts of calcium along with absorbable alkali, is

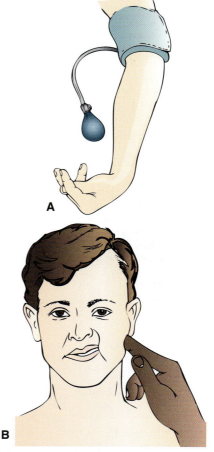

FIGURE 7-6 Indications of hypocalcemia. *A,* Positive Trousseau sign. *B,* Positive Chvostek sign. *(Reprinted from Phillips, L: Manual of I.V. Therapeutics, ed 5. FA Davis, Philadelphia, 2010, pp. 150–151, with permission.)*

TABLE 7-4 Mineral Toxicities

	SIGNS AND SYMPTOMS	NUTRITIONAL CAUSES	ASSOCIATED CONDITIONS
Calcium	Calcium deposits in the soft tissues of the body	Almost never	Hyperparathyroidism Vitamin D poisoning (most frequent in infants) Absorbable antacids Milk-alkali syndrome
Phosphorus	Calcifications in soft tissue	Dietary overload unusual Excessive phospholipids in parenteral nutrition Occurred in infants during the first few weeks of life from diet consisting solely of cow's milk	Kidney disease Overmedication with vitamin D Oral sodium phosphate bowel-cleansing drugs
Sodium	Hypernatremia (Table 7-6)	Healthy people excrete excess sodium without immediate adverse effects except in salt-sensitive individuals	Possible long-range adverse effects due to calcium loss
Potassium	Hyperkalemia (Table 7-6)	Rarely caused by excessive dietary intake Intravenous potassium should be given only to clients excreting urine	Diabetic acidosis Kidney failure Adrenal insufficiency Severe dehydration Transfusion with old blood (see Clinical Application 7-4)
Magnesium	Hypotension Nausea Vomiting Lethargy Confusion Slow pulse Depressed respirations Loss of patellar reflex	Not ordinarily seen	Kidney disease
Sulfur			Environmental causes such as air pollution with sulfur dioxide
Chloride			Environmental release of gas: industry, rail accidents

Iron	Accumulated mineral damages tissues
	Acute:
	    Gastroenteritis
	    Shock
	    Seizures
	    Liver failure
		Most people at little risk of iron toxicity from diet except with homemade beer in Africa
		Accidental overdosing with supplements
			Iron metabolism disorders
			Chronic alcoholism
			Iron poisoning can be fatal.

Iodine	Burning of mouth, throat, and stomach Brassy taste in mouth Increased salivation Nausea, vomiting, diarrhea Acne-like lesions Hypothyroidism Hyperthyroidism Thyroiditis	Chronic increase in consumption	Frequent exposure to x-ray contrast media Prescribed *amiodarone*

Fluoride	Mottled, discolored but sound teeth
	Bone and kidney dysfunction
	Acute toxicity:
	    Nausea, vomiting, diarrhea
	    Acidosis
	    Cardiac arrhythmias
		Drinking water with a fluoride concentration of <2 parts per million rarely problematic
		Overuse, swallowing of fluoridated dental products
		Drinking water with a fluoride concentration of four parts per million (EPA limit)
			Fluorosis possible in children up to 8 years of age
			Increased dental caries
			Rarely, skeletal fluorosis
			Acute toxicity can be fatal

Zinc	Nausea, vomiting Reduced immune response	Supplemental doses three times the Recommended Dietary Allowance	Loss of sense of smell with zinc nasal products

(continued)

TABLE 7-4   Mineral Toxicities (Continued)

	SIGNS AND SYMPTOMS	NUTRITIONAL CAUSES	ASSOCIATED CONDITIONS
Copper	Accumulation of copper in the liver, kidneys, brain, and cornea of the eye	Consuming acidic foods stored in copper vessels Infants fed water high in copper Long-term overdosing with supplements	Wilson disease Clients treated with an artificial kidney that used copper tubing
Selenium	Hair and nail loss Skin lesions Fatigue Gastrointestinal symptoms Nervous system abnormalities (NIH, February 11, 2016).	Overdosing with supplements Manufacturing error with supplements (see Chapter 15)	Miners
Chromium	Disagreeable metallic taste	Contaminated foods or parenteral nutrition solutions Overdosing with supplements	Inhalation of chromium in an industrial setting Possible wear debris from hip prostheses
Manganese	Signs/symptoms similar to Parkinson disease Neurological abnormalities	Parenteral nutrition, especially in neonates Well water high in manganese	Decreased liver function Cholestasis Pica Miners exposed to manganese dust Welders exposed to manganese fumes
Cobalt	Heart, lung signs and symptoms		Occupational exposure in industry Possible wear debris from metal-on-metal hip prostheses
Molybdenum		Eating food from regions with high levels in the soil	Occupational exposure

milk-alkali syndrome. Historically, this syndrome was associated with the milk and cream antacid treatment of peptic ulcers. In the 1970s, the syndrome accounted for just 1% of hypercalcemia cases. Today milk-alkali syndrome is associated with consumption of calcium supplements in the form of calcium carbonate.

Some clients with milk-alkali syndrome present with confusion, which complicates the diagnostic process. These cases emphasize the importance of carefully taking a client's dietary and medication history, as well as teaching a client about over-the-counter and prescription medications. Just because a product is available over the counter does not make it safe regardless of amount or conditions. Early diagnosis of milk-alkali syndrome could limit permanent kidney dysfunction.

Phosphorus

Phosphorus occurs in bones and teeth as calcium phosphate and is second to calcium in amount present in the body, with 85% found in the bones and teeth and the remaining amounts being found in tissues and cells.

Phosphorus is closely associated with calcium in both foods and interrelated metabolic body functions. Their control mechanisms are also entwined.

The storage forms of energy, **adenosine diphosphate (ADP)** and **adenosine triphosphate (ATP)**, contain phosphorus. It is also an essential mineral in **phospholipids,** which are structural components of cells. Lecithin, a part of cell membranes, and myelin, the insulating covering of many nerves, are phospholipids. Phosphorus is contained in almost all enzymes, and phosphorus compounds function as buffers to maintain the blood's pH as slightly alkaline.

Control Mechanisms

Between 50% and 70% of dietary phosphorus is absorbed primarily from the duodenum and jejunum, with greater absorption occurring from animal products and less from phytic acid–containing foods. Vitamin D (calcitriol) is the chief enhancer of absorption. Unabsorbed phosphorus is eliminated in the feces.

Low levels of serum phosphorus stimulate the kidney to produce more active vitamin D (calcitriol). Vitamin D increases the absorption of phosphorus from the intestinal tract and enhances phosphate resorption from the bones. In response to parathyroid hormone, the kidneys, the chief guardians of phosphate balance, excrete excess phosphorus, which can have far-reaching effects, as shown in Clinical Application 7-3.

Dietary Reference Intakes and Sources

For DRIs, see Appendix A. For food and other sources, see Table 7-1. To investigate the mineral content of a particular item, go to http:// ndb.nal.usda.gov or to http://nutritiondata.self.com.

CLINICAL APPLICATION   7-3

Phosphorus Intake and Calcium Balance

In the past, the ratio of calcium to phosphorus was considered crucial to proper calcium balance. Now authorities think that the calcium-to-phosphorus ratio is less important than an adequate calcium intake for adults; however, both premature and term infants require carefully balanced intakes because of immature kidneys (see Chapter 11).

Two related issues attract the attention of researchers:

- Widespread inadequate calcium intake
- Increasing amounts of phosphorus intake

In many countries, phosphorus intake is two to three times the RDA, whereas calcium intake is below the RDA. Phosphate additives are commonly used in frequently consumed foods and beverages in the United States, including chicken and poultry, soft cheeses, and soft drinks, which have contributed to the rise in phosphorus consumption (Chun et al, 2016). A high dietary phosphorus intake may have negative effects on bone through increased parathyroid hormone secretion because a high serum parathyroid hormone concentration increases bone resorption. While data are being gathered and researchers forge it into evidence, a simple solution to the issue of calcium–phosphorus balance is available. Dairy products, which provide large amounts of both nutrients, should be a mainstay of the diet, complemented by moderation in intake of processed foods and cola beverages. Once again, balance, moderation, and variety are keys to a healthy diet.

Deficiency

Although calcium and magnesium impair phosphorus absorption, deficiency is unlikely in healthy persons consuming a normal diet. Deficiency, however, has occurred in clients receiving parenteral nutrition (see Chapter 14) with insufficient phosphorus.

In addition, certain medications or diseases can produce **hypophosphatemia.** For example, persons ingesting a diet low in phosphorus while also taking a phosphate-binding drug, such as the antacid aluminum hydroxide, have experienced hypophosphatemia. Also, the following conditions have precipitated hypophosphatemia:

- Malabsorption disorders
- Severe burns
- Uncontrolled diabetes mellitus

Additionally, **refeeding syndrome,** a condition related to imbalances in phosphorus, occurs when wasted or starved clients are given nutrients in excess of what their bodies can process (see Chapter 22).

Hyperparathyroidism is a disease causing excess excretion of phosphorus. In this disease, parathyroid hormone causes withdrawal of calcium from the bones. Because the two minerals, calcium and phosphorus, are combined in the bones, phosphorus is lost along with calcium. Chronic kidney disease often produces the same result.

Reflecting the wide distribution and functions of phosphorus in the body, deficiency affects many organs and systems. Signs and symptoms of hypophosphatemia include the following:

- Impaired growth
- Osteomalacia
- Proximal muscle atrophy and weakness
- Cardiac arrhythmias
- Respiratory insufficiency
- Nervous system disorders

Toxicity

For basic information on mineral toxicity, see Table 7-4. Decreased renal excretion of phosphorus is the most common cause of **hyperphosphatemia.**

In 2016, the U.S. Food and Drug Administration (FDA) posted a warning regarding over-the-counter sodium phosphate products that are used to treat constipation and can be administered either orally or rectally as an enema. Serious cardiac and renal injury secondary to dehydration and shifts in electrolytes, including calcium, phosphorus, and sodium, have been found in clients who exceeded the daily recommendation. The FDA recognized an increased risk of adverse effects for the following clients:

- Those older than 55 years
- Those with dehydration, kidney disease, acute colitis, or delayed bowel emptying
- Those taking medications that affect kidney function (U.S. Food and Drug Administration [FDA], 2016)

Previous cases of hyperphosphatemia causing serious neurological damage were attributed to sodium phosphate bowel-cleansing products administered rectally to individuals with bowel diseases. Clients with conditions that increase the permeability of the intestine are at special risk when using these products.

Sodium

The body of a 154-pound adult contains about 105 grams (3.5 ounces) of sodium. Approximately 70% of the sodium in the body is in the blood and other extracellular fluids and in nerve and muscle tissue.

Sodium has a major role in maintaining fluid balance in the body and contributes to maintaining acid–base balance as well (see Chapter 8). Sodium is also necessary for the transmission of electrochemical impulses along nerve and muscle membranes.

The intestine readily absorbs sodium. At most, 5% of dietary sodium travels within the intestine to remain in the feces. The remaining 95% of ingested sodium is absorbed into the bloodstream. To maintain a normal level of sodium in the blood, the kidney either reabsorbs sodium and returns it to the bloodstream or allows it to be spilled in the urine. The major hormone controlling sodium excretion, **aldosterone** from the adrenal cortex, stimulates the kidney to return sodium to the bloodstream (see Chapter 8).

Dietary Reference Intakes and Sources

For DRIs, see Appendix A. For food and other sources, see Table 7-1. To investigate the mineral content of a particular item, go to http://ndb.nal.usda.gov or to http://nutritiondata.self.com.

Table salt, the major dietary source of sodium, is 40% sodium and 60% chloride. One teaspoonful (5 grams) of salt contains 2.3 grams of sodium, the UL for adults younger than 50 years. Many foods, such as milk, milk products, and several vegetables, are naturally high in sodium.

The average sodium intake among persons in the United States is greater than 3,400 milligrams per day. The estimated distribution of intake is:

- 77% from packaged and restaurant foods
- 12% from natural sources
- 11% from salt added while cooking or eating a meal (Centers for Disease Control and Prevention [CDC], 2017)

See Figure 7-7, which shows the percentage of U.S. population that exceed the recommended sodium intake.

Despite the fact that salt is not so crucial to maintaining year-round food stocks as it was years ago, when, for instance, meat was salted to preserve it, food processors still find it a useful and inexpensive additive. Manufacturers add sodium for flavor, to alter the texture of the food, or to extend its shelf life. Consequently, food industry participation will be needed to achieve significant reductions in sodium

intake. Table 7-5 compares the sodium content of relatively unprocessed foods with processed versions. Sodium-restricted diets and the legal definitions regarding the sodium content of foods are covered in Chapter 18.

Deficiency

Sodium deficiency is typically caused not by dietary deficiency (because of the abundance of sodium in foods) but by increased sodium loss from:

- Diarrhea
- Vomiting
- Kidney, cardiac, and liver disease
- Heavy sweating

Hyponatremia is the technical name for low serum sodium, less than 135 **milliequivalents** (see Chapter 8) per liter in adults. Low serum sodium because of excess retained water is called **dilutional hyponatremia.** It can result from disordered hormonal control (syndrome of inappropriate antidiuresis, **SIAD**) and from overhydration with plain water by perspiring athletes or military trainees (see Chapter 8).

Because of the rigid confines of the skull, the brain is subject to dysfunction when it fails to control its water content effectively. Hyponatremia can result in cerebral edema and increased intracranial pressure. The impairment of brain function is evident in the signs and symptoms of abnormal sodium and potassium levels listed in Table 7-6.

Toxicity

For basic information on mineral toxicity, see Table 7-4. The reported 4 to 6 grams of sodium in the average American diet is probably an underestimate. Frequently such surveys do not account for all sources of sodium. An excess of sodium in the blood, greater than 145 milliequivalents per liter in adults, is called **hypernatremia.** Its signs and symptoms appear in Table 7-6.

Potassium

The body of a 154-pound adult contains about 245 grams of potassium, approximately 8.6 ounces, and 85% of ingested potassium is absorbed in the ileum and jejunum in the small intestine. From 95% to 98% of the body's potassium is inside the cells, where it helps to control fluid balance.

In addition to fluid balance, potassium is essential for the conduction of nerve impulses and the contraction of muscles, including the heart. Potassium also helps maintain the body's **electrolyte** and acid–base balance (see Chapter 8) and can contribute to cardiovascular health. The FDA has approved this health claim: "Diets containing foods that are good sources of potassium and low in sodium my reduce the risk of high blood pressure and stroke." Qualifying foods must contain at least 350 milligrams of potassium, but no more than:

- 140 milligrams of sodium
- 3 grams of total fat

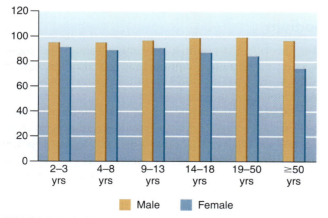

Prevalence of U.S. population aged ≥2 years with usual sodium intake in excess of *2015-2020 Dietary Guidelines for Americans* limits by sex and age group

■ Male ■ Female

FIGURE 7-7 The bars in the graph show the percentage of U.S. population that exceed the recommended sodium intake based on age and gender. Current recommendations are to consume <2,300 mg of sodium per day. (*Data from Centers for Disease Control and Prevention, January 8, 2016. MMWR, Prevalence of Excess Sodium Intake in United States—NHANES, 2009–2012. Available at https://www.cdc.gov/mmwr/preview/mmwrhtml/mm6452a1.htm.*)

TABLE 7-5   Comparison of Sodium Content in Fresh and Processed Foods

FRESH FOOD	SODIUM (MG)	PROCESSED FOOD	SODIUM (MG)
Natural Swiss cheese, 1 oz	74	Pasteurized, processed Swiss cheese, 1 oz	388
Lean roast pork, 3 oz	65	Lean ham, 3 oz	930
Whole raw carrot, 1	25	Canned carrots, 1/2 cup	176
Tomato juice, canned without salt, 1 cup	24	Tomato juice, canned with salt, 1 cup	881

TABLE 7-6   Signs and Symptoms of Abnormal Serum Sodium and Potassium Levels

	LOW	NORMAL	HIGH
Sodium			
Lab value	<135 mEq/L	135–148 mEq/L	>148 mEq/L
Condition	Hyponatremia		Hypernatremia
Symptoms	Weakness Headache Irritability Anxiety		Thirst Fatigue
Signs	Muscle twitching Fingerprinting over the sternum Altered consciousness Seizures Coma Permanent neurological damage Respiratory arrest		Flushed skin Sticky mucous membranes Agitation Coma
Potassium			
Lab value	<3.5 mEq/L	3.5–5.0 mEq/L	>5.0 mEq/L
Condition	Hypokalemia		Hyperkalemia
Symptoms	Nausea Paresthesias, especially lower extremities Disorientation		Irritability Abdominal cramps
Signs	Vomiting Decreased bowel sounds Diminished reflexes Muscle weakness Weak, irregular pulse Coma		Weakness, especially lower extremities Irregular pulse Characteristic electrocardiograph changes Cardiac arrest

- 1 gram of saturated fat
- 20 milligrams of cholesterol
- 15% kilocalories from saturated fat (FDA, April 1, 2015)

Dietary Reference Intakes

For DRIs, see Appendix A. For food and other sources, see Table 7-1. To investigate the mineral content of a particular item, go to http://ndb.nal.usda.gov or to http://nutritiondata.self.com.

Sources of Potassium

Potassium is present in all plant and animal cells, but the best sources are unprocessed foods. Only fats, oils, and white sugar have negligible amounts of potassium (see Table 7-1). Dietary instructions may focus on fruit sources because the client might also need to limit sodium, which frequently occurs in greater amounts in vegetables and dairy products than in fruits. Potassium might also be obtained from salt substitutes that often replace the sodium with potassium. Table 7-7 shows several good sources of potassium that, if prepared without salt, are also very low in sodium.

Deficiency

A potassium deficiency is related to diet only in cases of severe protein-energy malnutrition. **Hypokalemia,** a serum potassium of less than 3.5 milliequivalents per liter, can be fatal if prolonged or severe. Hypokalemia may be caused by:

- Vomiting
- Diarrhea
- Diabetic ketoacidosis
- Potassium-wasting diuretics
- Kidney disease
- Excessive laxative use

For signs and symptoms, see Table 7-6.

TABLE 7-7   Good Sources of Potassium with Very Low Sodium and Moderate Kilocalories

FOOD	PREPARATION	SERVING	MG K+	MG NA+	KILOCALORIES
Acorn squash	Baked Unsalted	1 cup cubes	896	8.2	115
White potato	Baked Unsalted	1 small (5 oz) with skin	738	13.8	128
Banana	Sliced	1 cup	537	1.5	133
Orange juice	Frozen, diluted 1:3	1 cup	473	2.5	112
Cantaloupe	Unsalted	1 cup cubes	427	25.6	54
Prunes	Uncooked, pitted	1/3 cup	425	1.2	139
Apricots	Canned in juice	1 cup	403	9.8	117

Toxicity

For basic information on mineral toxicity, see Table 7-4. A potassium level greater than 5.0 milliequivalents per liter is hyperkalemia. Signs and symptoms of hyperkalemia appear in Table 7-6.

Hyperkalemia is rarely caused by food but rather by impaired kidney function. It may also be caused by excessive destruction of cells in burns, crushing injuries, or severe infections. No symptoms may be apparent until blood levels of potassium are very high and skeletal muscle weakness is seen, followed by cardiac dysfunction that could prove fatal. One adverse effect of blood transfusion with old blood is elevated serum potassium. Clinical Application 7-4 covers that possibility. Other signs, such as results of electrocardiograms, assist in diagnosis of potassium imbalances with peaked T-waves. Dire consequences can result from hyper- or hyponatremia and hyper- or hypokalemia. If the nurse recognizes and reports early signs and symptoms, the need for drastic treatment measures and perhaps permanent damage may be averted.

CLINICAL APPLICATION   7-4

Hyperkalemia After Blood Transfusion

Red blood cells (RBCs) do not survive as long in the blood bank as they do in the human body. Potassium is the major **cation** (see Chapter 8) in red blood cells. When the red blood cells die and their cell walls rupture, potassium is spilled into the surrounding liquid.

Blood that has been stored for a prolonged period may contain up to 30 mEq per liter of potassium due to the destruction of the red blood cells. This may not sound like a large amount, but potassium is usually administered intravenously at a concentration of 40 mEq per liter to a person who is potassium depleted. The person receiving a blood transfusion (or many units of blood) may have a serum potassium level that is nearly normal, and the old blood containing a higher concentration of potassium could precipitate hyperkalemia.

The nurse should be aware of the age of blood products and identify clients at risk of hyperkalemia.

Magnesium

The human body contains about 25 grams (0.9 ounce) of magnesium. About 50% to 60% of the magnesium is in bone, 39% to 49% in soft tissue, and 1% in body fluids (NIH, February 11, 2016).

Absorption, Elimination, and Functions

Magnesium is absorbed throughout the small intestine, mostly in the distal jejunum and ileum and may be absorbed from the colon if disease has impaired small intestine absorption. Of usual intakes, from 30% to 40% is absorbed, with the smaller percentage absorbed at high intakes and the larger percentage at low intakes.

Excess magnesium is eliminated by the kidneys, where it competes with calcium for reabsorption sites. Magnesium is involved in more than 300 different enzymatic reactions. It is associated with ADP and ATP in energy metabolism. Magnesium is involved in DNA synthesis and degradation, in protein synthesis, and insulin action. Magnesium influences the transportation of calcium and potassium across cell membranes, an important process to ensure nerve impulse, muscle contraction, and normal heart rhythm (FDA, February 11, 2016).

Dietary Reference Intakes and Sources

For DRIs see Appendix A. For food and other sources, see Table 7-1. To investigate the mineral content of a particular item, go to http://ndb.nal.usda.gov or to http://nutritiondata.self.com.

Magnesium is widely distributed in foods, especially green, leafy vegetables, in which it is a component of chlorophyll. Removing the germ and outer layers of the wheat kernel can remove more than 75% of its magnesium content. Beverages such as coffee, cocoa, instant tea, and powdered fruit-flavored drinks also contain magnesium.

Interfering Factors and Deficiency

Phosphorus can inhibit magnesium absorption especially when magnesium intake is low and that of phosphorus is high. The two are thought to combine in the intestinal tract, rendering both unavailable for absorption.

Diabetes mellitus is commonly associated with magnesium deficiency, presumably due to renal losses secondary to elevated glucose concentrations in the kidney. Deficiency may also result from the following:

- Malabsorption disorders, such as Crohn and celiac disease
- Excessive alcohol use
- Older adults

Hypomagnesemia is associated with disease processes such as type 2 diabetes, migraine headaches, hypertension and cardiovascular disease, and osteoporosis (FDA, February 11, 2015). Because of its safety, magnesium sulfate has been used for decades as an anticonvulsant for **preeclampsia** and **eclampsia** (see Chapter 10) and contributes to the low mortality rate from these conditions in developed countries. Because magnesium metabolism is intricately linked to calcium metabolism, magnesium-deficient clients display the signs of tetany. Other signs include the following:

- Muscle cramps or twitching
- Insomnia
- Heart irregularity or heart racing
- Seizures
- Drowsiness, fatigue, and confusion

Toxicity

For basic information on mineral toxicity, see Table 7-4. Ordinarily, magnesium levels do not build up in the blood except as a result of kidney disease. In fact, oral magnesium can cause diarrhea—Epsom salt is magnesium sulfate. Because of magnesium's close link to calcium, the effects of magnesium toxicity can be blocked by administering calcium.

Sulfur

The adult body contains approximately 175 grams of sulfur, a component of the cytoplasm of every cell. Sulfur is especially notable in hair, skin, and nails, where it contributes to their shape. Sulfur is a component of thiamin, biotin, insulin, and heparin and of the amino acids methionine and cysteine. A protective function of sulfur is that of combining with toxins to neutralize them.

The major source of sulfate for humans is provided through the amino acid pool (see Fig. 4-1) by catabolism of the sulfur-containing amino acids methionine and cysteine. Dietary intake of foods containing these amino acids helps to replenish the supply (see Table 7-1). Cases of deficiency of sulfur alone are unknown. Only people with a severe protein deficiency lack this mineral. *For basic information on mineral toxicity, see Table 7-4.*

Chloride

Chloride plays a major role in maintaining fluid balance and acid–base balance. The body of a 154-pound adult contains approximately 105 grams of chloride. Of the body's chloride, 88% is found in extracellular fluids such as the hydrochloric acid in the stomach, and 12% is found in intracellular fluids. Chloride also is released by white blood cells as they fight substances foreign to the body. Chloride is almost completely absorbed through the small intestine and is excreted primarily by the kidney.

For DRIs see Appendix A. For food and other sources, see Table 7-1.

The DRI levels were established proportionate to the AI for sodium because nearly all dietary chloride is derived from salt. Table salt, which is 60% chloride, contains about 3 grams of chloride per teaspoon (5 grams). Vegetable sources of chloride include seaweed, tomatoes, olives, and celery. Chlorine toxicity and deficiency are not common in healthy adults. Toxicity is typically the result of renal insufficiency and can lead to fluid retention. Chlorine gas is used to treat drinking water and is regulated by the Safe Drinking Water Act enacted into law in 1974. Deficiency can result from excessive sweating, diarrhea, or vomiting and can lead to metabolic alkalosis. Chloride deficiency has occurred in infants because chloride was omitted from their formulas. A genetic defect in chloride transport regulation causes **cystic fibrosis** (see Chapter 20).

Trace Minerals

Many trace minerals occur in such small amounts that they are difficult to measure and analyze; thus, their physiological functions and possible roles in nutrition are not completely understood.

Ten trace minerals have well-known bodily functions, and nine of them have been assigned RDAs or AIs. Four of them are commonly recognized for their relationship to health:

1. Iron
2. Iodine
3. Fluoride
4. Zinc

The other six are:

1. Selenium
2. Chromium
3. Copper
4. Manganese
5. Cobalt
6. Molybdenum

Five additional trace minerals, arsenic, boron, nickel, silicon, and vanadium, termed ultratrace minerals, appear in the UL tables, but RDAs or AIs are not determinable.

Iron

For a nutrient with functions as vital as those of iron, the amount in the body is slight—males average 4 grams and females average 3.5 grams. The body conserves its supply of iron by recycling the mineral released from the catabolism of worn-out red blood cells.

Functions

Iron is essential to the formation of hemoglobin, the component of the red blood cell that transports approximately 98.5% of the oxygen in the blood. **Hemoglobin** is composed of **heme,** the nonprotein portion that contains iron, and globin, a simple protein.

Iron is also a component of **myoglobin,** a protein located in muscle tissue. Myoglobin stores oxygen within the muscle cells. When the body needs an immediate supply of oxygen, such as during strenuous exercise, myoglobin releases its stored oxygen.

Iron is also present in enzymes that support energy metabolism and the synthesis and catabolism of neurotransmitters. About 80% of the iron in a healthy body is available for carrying oxygen: hemoglobin contains 65%, myoglobin 10%, and iron-containing enzymes 3%. The balance is in the blood or stored in the liver, spleen, and bone marrow for future use. The primary storage form of iron in the body's cells is **ferritin,** a blood protein found primarily in the liver and immune system.

Absorption

The body tightly conserves its supply of iron. Dietary iron is absorbed throughout the small intestine, most efficiently in the duodenum. When red blood cells are destroyed after their usual life span of 120 days, their iron is stored for reuse. Once iron is absorbed, there is no physiological mechanism for excreting the excess. Fortunately, under normal conditions, the body is selective about absorbing iron.

Perhaps the most exciting breakthrough in iron biology is the discovery of **hepcidin,** a peptide hormone that controls the absorption of iron (Zou & Sun, 2017). The liver manufactures hepcidin, a hormone that regulates iron metabolism in the duodenum, liver, spleen, and bone marrow. When the body's iron levels are high, hepcidin is synthesized to inhibit absorption of dietary iron and release of iron from intracellular stores (Mirciov et al, 2017).

FACTORS AFFECTING AMOUNTS

The amount of dietary iron that is absorbed is determined by the amount of ferritin present in the intestinal mucosa. The iron obtained from ingested food is bound to a protein called **apoferritin** in the intestinal mucosa to form ferritin. When the total supply of apoferritin has been bound to iron, any additional iron in the gut is rejected and eliminated in the feces. Absorbed iron combines with a protein in the blood, **transferrin,** which transports iron to the bone marrow for hemoglobin synthesis, to the liver or spleen for storage, or to the body cells for use.

FACTORS AFFECTING ABSORPTION RATES

Two types of iron are found naturally in foods that are absorbed through different mechanisms:

1. Heme iron
2. Nonheme iron

Heme iron is bound to the hemoglobin and myoglobin in meat, fish, and poultry. From 40% to 45% of the total iron in these animal sources is heme iron. Because heme iron is composed of **ferrous iron** (Fe^{2+}), it is rapidly transported and absorbed intact.

Nonheme iron is the other 55% to 60% of the total iron in meat, fish, poultry, and all the iron in plant sources.

The absorption of nonheme iron is slow because it is closely bound to organic molecules in foods as **ferric iron** (Fe^{3+}). In the acidic medium of the stomach, oxygen is removed from ferric iron during a chemical reaction called reduction. The end product is ferrous iron, which is more soluble and bioavailable. See Figure 7-8 for an overview of the steps involved in the process of iron absorption.

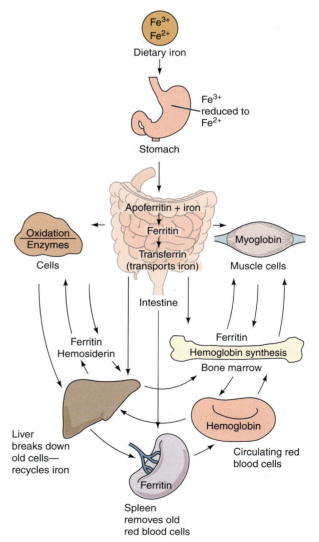

FIGURE 7-8 In the process of dietary iron absorption, iron is absorbed primarily in the small intestine but also is recovered from worn-out cells before being transported or stored to meet the body's needs.

FACTORS ENHANCING ABSORPTION

Several factors increase the absorption of iron through different mechanisms.

- Ascorbic acid, vitamin C, enhances iron absorption.
- Acids, such as ascorbic and citric, increase absorption by combining with the iron in a soluble compound, thus preventing formation of insoluble iron complexes.
- MFP Factor (meat, fish, poultry) increases the absorption of nonheme iron when meat, fish, or poultry is consumed at the same time.

FACTORS INTERFERING WITH ABSORPTION

Other minerals compete with iron for absorption.

- Calcium intake of 300 to 600 mg can inhibit uptake of both heme and nonheme iron.
- Eggs contain a compound that can inhibit absorption.
- Phytate found in soy protein and fiber.
- Oxalic acid from certain berries and vegetables (see the calcium section) combines with iron, reducing its availability.
- Decreased gastric acid, whether because of antacid medications or gastric resection, lessens the iron that is absorbed.
- Polyphenols found in tea and coffee, when consumed with nonheme iron, can reduce iron absorption by more than 50%.

Table 7-8 summarizes the factors that affect iron absorption. People who consume vegetarian diets should be especially careful to construct optimal menus not only because of the elimination of meat but also because of the increased amounts of phytates likely included in the diet.

TABLE 7-8   Factors Affecting Iron Absorption

INCREASE	DECREASE
Large alcohol intake	Phytic or oxalic acids
Meat, fish, or poultry	Coffee or tea (tannins)
Vitamin C	Less gastric acid, antacids Calcium and zinc

Excretion

No known mechanism exists to regulate the excretion of iron. Small amounts of iron are lost daily via the gastrointestinal tract, shed skin cells, and urine even in healthy people. Certain medications and diseases increase the losses.

Dietary Reference Intakes

For DRIs see Appendix A. For food and other sources, see Table 7-9. To investigate the mineral content of a particular item, go to http://ndb.nal.usda.gov or to http://nutritiondata.self.com.

Vegetarian diets are estimated to provide iron at 10% bioavailability, partly because they lack the MPF factor, rather than the 18% from a mixed Western diet. Hence the requirement for iron is 1.8 times higher for vegetarians than for other Americans.

Sources

The Western diet contains an estimated 5 to 7 milligrams of iron per 1,000 kilocalories. In the United States, one-third of dietary iron is supplied by grains, one-third by meats, and one-third by other sources. Absorption also varies among the sources of iron. Ten percent to 30% of iron is absorbed from liver and other meats; less than 10% is absorbed from eggs; less than 5% is absorbed from grains and most vegetables.

Many foods are fortified with iron, but its bioavailability depends on the compounds used. Iron from spinach, iron supplements, and contamination iron are absorbed at a 2% rate.

Deficiency

Perhaps the most significant worldwide nutritional problem, iron deficiency, affects more than 2 billion people, including half the women and children in developing countries (Wessling-Resnick, 2014). Iron-deficiency anemia occurs in 2% to 5% of adult men and postmenopausal women in the developed world often caused by gastrointestinal blood loss. The most important causes of such blood loss are colonic or gastric cancers that need to be ruled out (Goddard, James, McIntyre, & Scott, 2011).

TABLE 7-9   Trace Minerals

MINERAL	ADULT RDA/AI AND FOOD PORTION CONTAINING IT*	FUNCTIONS	SIGNS AND SYMPTOMS OF DEFICIENCY	SIGNS AND SYMPTOMS OF EXCESS	BEST SOURCES
Iron	8–18 mg (female) 8 mg (male) 1 packet fortified, instant oatmeal	Component of hemoglobin	Fatigue, lightheadedness Shortness of breath Hypochromic, microcytic anemia	Hemosiderosis Hemochromatosis	Liver, other red meats Clams Oysters Lima and navy beans Dark green leafy cooked vegetables Dried fruit

(continued)

TABLE 7-9   **Trace Minerals** (Continued)

MINERAL	ADULT RDA/AI AND FOOD PORTION CONTAINING IT*	FUNCTIONS	SIGNS AND SYMPTOMS OF DEFICIENCY	SIGNS AND SYMPTOMS OF EXCESS	BEST SOURCES
Iodine	150 mcg 3/8 tsp iodized salt	Component of thyroid hormones	Goiter Cretinism Myxedema	Acnelike lesions Goiter	Iodized salt Saltwater seafood
Fluoride	3–4 mg 4.3–5.7 L fluoridated water	Hardens teeth	Dental caries	Mottled teeth Increased caries	Fluoridated water Seafood Brewed tea
Zinc	8–11 mg 3.6–5 oz beef chuck roast, lean only	Component of 70 enzymes Involved in DNA and RNA synthesis Necessary for collagen formation Serves role in immunity	Growth failure Hypogonadism Delayed wound healing Impaired night vision Impaired taste Delayed sexual maturation	Copper deficiency Suppressed immune response	Red meat, especially organ meat Seafood, especially oysters Poultry Pork Dairy products Whole grains
Copper	900 mcg 1.8 oz lobster	Cofactor for enzymes involved in hemoglobin synthesis and cell respiration Necessary for melanin formation	Menkes disease Anemia Demineralization of skeleton Depigmentation of skin and hair Impaired immune function	Wilson disease Copper deposits in liver, kidneys, brain, spleen, and cornea	Organ meats Shellfish Nuts Seeds Legumes Dried fruit
Selenium	55 mcg 3.6 large hard-cooked eggs	Part of many enzymes Necessary for iodine metabolism Protects against the toxicity from mercury, cadmium, and silver	Keshan cardiomyopathy	Sour milk or garlic breath odor Fatigue Nail and hair loss	Brazil nuts Meats Seafood Dairy products Eggs
Chromium	20–35 mcg 0.5–0.9 oz American cheese	Thought to potentiate action of insulin	Weight loss Impaired glucose utilization Elevated blood lipids Peripheral neuropathy	Rarely related to food Metallic taste	Meats, especially organ meats Fish Poultry Cheese Peanuts Whole grains
Manganese	1.8–2.3 mg 1.1–1.4 cups cooked spinach	Involved in amino acid and carbohydrate metabolism Required for bone formation	Dermatitis Decreased growth of hair and nails Skeletal defects Changes in hair and beard color	Accumulated mineral in brain In miners: liver damage and Parkinson-like syndrome Central nervous system impairment	Whole grains Dried fruits Nuts Cooked green, leafy vegetables
Cobalt	Not established	Component of vitamin B_{12}	Not reported		Meat Poultry Fish Eggs Milk, cheese
Molybdenum	45 mcg ¼ cup cooked navy beans†	Cofactor for enzymes involved in catabolism of sulfur-containing amino acids and purines	Parenteral nutrition clients only: tachycardia, headache, mental disturbances, coma	Hyperuricemia Gout	Meat Fish Poultry Legumes Whole grains

*Examples only; not suggested for sole source of a day's intake.
†Mineral omitted from many nutrient databases.

Iron deficiency can be determined by laboratory tests such as plasma ferritin, total iron-binding capacity, RBCs, hematocrit, and hemoglobin. When the hemoglobin measures lower than normal, anemia can be diagnosed. A person who is anemic has insufficient hemoglobin to provide oxygen to the cells of the body. The features of the red blood cells are characteristic of various anemias. In iron-deficiency anemia, the red blood cells are microcytic (smaller than normal) and hypochromic (contain less hemoglobin, giving the cell less color than normal).

The anemic client often complains of lightheadedness, shortness of breath on exertion, and possibly soreness of mouth and tongue, and physical examination reveals pallor and probably an increased pulse rate.

RISK OF DEFICIENCY

In the United States, population groups that frequently have inadequate iron intake are as follows:

- Infants and young children
- Pregnant women
- Women with heavy menstrual bleeding
- Clients with cancer
- Frequent blood donors
- Clients with gastrointestinal disease or gastrointestinal surgery
- Clients with heart failure (NIH, February 11, 2015)

More information on iron deficiency in pregnant women is included in Chapter 10. Iron deficiency in children appears in Chapter 11.

ASSESSMENT DATA

Although no single test is diagnostic for iron deficiency, a common test to determine the hemoglobin level of the blood delivers valuable assessment data. The normal level for men is 14 to 18 grams per 100 milliliters of blood; for women, it is 12 to 16 grams. Another common laboratory test is the **hematocrit,** which measures the percentage of red blood cells in a volume of blood. Normal hematocrit levels are 40% to 54% for men and 36% to 46% for women. Persons living above 4,000 feet in altitude will have higher normal values. Low hemoglobin and hematocrit levels are late indicators of iron deficiency.

TREATMENT

Supplemental iron is best absorbed when taken on an empty stomach, but gastrointestinal side effects often provoke noncompliance. Even taking the supplement with food or close to mealtime is better than not taking it at all. Accompanying the supplement with meat or vitamin C–rich foods and avoiding coffee, tea, milk, and cereals with it should increase absorption. Also, beginning at a lower dosage and then increasing it as tolerance develops is sometimes a useful strategy. Enteric-coated preparations are available but may not dissolve until beyond the duodenum, where absorption is most effective.

Hemoglobin levels can be used to monitor the effectiveness of treatment. Iron therapy should be continued for several months after hemoglobin and hematocrit levels return to normal to enable the body to rebuild iron stores.

In developing countries with high levels of infectious diseases, iron administration for anemia has been followed by increased morbidity from infections. Because bacteria also require iron, when the body's supply increases, they thrive. In 2006, the World Health Organization and the United Nations Children's Fund released a joint statement advising that, in regions where the prevalence of malaria and other infectious diseases is high, iron and folic acid supplementation should be limited to those who are identified as iron deficient. When target groups have already been identified as being iron deficient, iron supplementation is the intervention of choice for the treatment of anemia and other manifestations of iron deficiency.

Toxicity

For basic information on mineral toxicity, see Table 7-4. Iron absorption is effectively controlled in healthy people even when meat intake is high and foods are fortified.

Hemochromatosis is a genetic disease that is caused by a mutation of a gene that interferes with normal hepcidin function and causes too much iron to be absorbed from dietary sources (see Genomic Gem 7-2). Surplus iron is stored in the liver as **hemosiderin.** When large amounts of hemosiderin are deposited in the liver and spleen without tissue damage, a condition called **hemosiderosis** results. Clients with alcoholism, although often lacking many other nutrients, sometimes suffer from iron overload. Some alcoholic beverages themselves contain a significant amount of iron. For example, inexpensive red wines contain 10 to 350 milligrams of iron per liter.

Toxicity from supplemental iron tablets is a major threat to children. The body's absorptive controls for dietary iron are circumvented by the large amounts of soluble iron in pharmaceutical preparations. In the United States, iron is the most common cause of accidental pediatric poisoning deaths in children younger than 6 years (see Clinical Application 7-5).

Iron supplements prepared for children contain small amounts of iron; most lethal ingestions among children are from prenatal multivitamins, which contain large amounts of iron.

The Consumer Product Safety Commission requires child-resistant packaging for iron preparations in certain forms and specified strengths, and the FDA requires a warning label on solid dosage forms of iron (FDA, July 1, 2016).

Iodine

In the human body, iodine is usually found and functions in its ionic form, iodide. The body of the average adult can contain 1,500 milligrams of iodine, with the thyroid storing up to 50 milligrams and the rest being stored in other body tissue.

GENOMIC GEM 7-2

Hereditary Hemochromatosis

This **autosomal recessive** disease is associated with mutations in genes with resultant diminished hepcidin synthesis and increased absorption of iron. The disorder has a **homozygous** frequency of 1:200 and a **heterozygous** frequency of 1:8 in people of Northern European ancestry. It is uncommon among blacks and rare among people of Asian ancestry. Of clients with clinical hemochromatosis, 83% are homozygous.

The hemochromatosis gene, abbreviated *HFE*, is located on chromosome 6. It instructs cells in the liver and intestine to produce the HFE protein that

- Interacts with other proteins on the cell surface to detect the amount of iron in the body and
- Regulates the production of hepcidin, the master iron regulatory hormone

More than 20 mutations in the *HFE* gene have been identified as causing the most common type of hemochromatosis. Two particular mutations are responsible for most cases, each substituting one amino acid for another used to make the HFE protein:

- Tyrosine for cysteine at position 282 (C282Y) is the most common cause
- Aspartic acid for histidine at position 63 (H63D)

Signs and symptoms are caused by deposits of iron in various organs and may include fatigue, abdominal pain, hyperpigmentation of the skin, diabetes, joint symptoms, heart and liver disease, and erectile dysfunction. In affected clients, early treatment by phlebotomy can prevent organ damage. Treatment involves regular removal of blood 500 mL per week through **phlebotomy** until a satisfactory serum ferritin level is achieved. Dietary interventions can also be therapeutic:

- Avoid iron and vitamin C supplements, including multivitamin–multimineral preparations.
- Consume red or organ meats in moderation.
- Avoid alcohol.

Untreated, hemochromatosis leads to organ failure and death.

CLINICAL APPLICATION   7-5

Precautions to Prevent Medication Poisoning in Children

Health-care providers should impress upon parents the enormous threat medications and supplements pose for small children. The products should be stored:

- Out of reach
- Out of sight
- With child-resistant caps intact

Adults should ingest medicines out of the child's view to avoid modeling a behavior that could harm the child.

If a child ingests any medication or supplement, a poison control center should be consulted *immediately* without waiting for signs and symptoms to appear.

Function and Control of the Thyroid Gland

The main function of iodine is its participation in the synthesis of thyroid hormones, which are essential for proper maturation of the nervous system, particularly in utero and for the first few years after birth. Devastating consequences result from deficiency of iodine during those years (see Deficiency later in this section).

The thyroid gland secretes **thyroxine (T_4)** and **triiodothyronine (T_3)** in response to **thyroid-stimulating hormone (TSH)** from the anterior pituitary gland. Both T_3 and T_4 increase the rate of oxidation in cells, thereby increasing the rate of metabolism. When serum levels of T_3 and T_4 are adequate, secretion of TSH ceases. This is called a **negative feedback cycle**: TSH stimulates T_4 and T_3 production until a sufficient level of those hormones stops the secretion of TSH; when T_4 and T_3 levels drop, more TSH is secreted.

Absorption and Excretion

Iodine is rapidly absorbed, mostly from the stomach but also from the duodenum, and excreted by the kidneys, which have no mechanism to conserve iodine. After performing their functions, T_4 and T_3 are degraded by the liver, and the iodine content is excreted in bile.

Dietary Reference Intakes and Sources

For DRIs see Appendix A. For food and other sources, see Table 7-9.

Iodine can come from foods, either naturally present or fortified, or from incidental sources.

IN FOODS AND WATER

Foods that are naturally high in iodine include saltwater fish, shellfish, and seaweed. The iodine content in plants varies with the mineral content of the soil in which they are grown. Table salt fortified with iodine (100 micrograms of iodine in ¼ teaspoon of salt) has been available in the United States since 1924.

Iodine has antibacterial properties and is sometimes used to purify drinking water. If the region is also iodine deficient, the mineral in the water can serve both purposes.

INCIDENTAL

Sometimes iodine is present as a side effect of processing. For example, iodine solutions can be used to sterilize milk pasteurization vats; some iodine may remain on the vat and be mixed into the next batch of milk to be processed. Iodine is also used to improve the texture of bread dough.

Deficiency

Since the introduction of iodized salt, overt deficiency has rarely been encountered in North America. Deficiencies have occurred in individuals who avoid iodized salt and seafood and vegans who consume sea salt, which contains virtually no iodine.

LOCAL EFFECTS

When the thyroid gland does not receive sufficient iodine, it increases in size, from a normal adult organ weighing 10 to 25 grams, growing to 500 to 700 grams (1 to 1.5 pounds) in its attempt to increase production of thyroid hormones. This enlargement of the thyroid is called **goiter** (Fig. 7-9). Sometimes the gland may attain sufficient size to impede breathing or swallowing. Unfortunately, in rare cases, replacement of iodine does not reduce the goiter, especially after long-standing deficiency, and so surgery or radiotherapy may be needed.

Because of iodine-poor soil, the Great Lakes States and the Rocky Mountain States once were considered the "goiter belt." Now that food is distributed nationally and internationally and iodized salt is readily available, goiter is less common in the United States. Other countries continue to have significant effects of iodine deficiency (Box 7-1).

SYSTEMIC EFFECTS

Severe **hypothyroidism** during pregnancy results in **cretinism** in the newborn. As a consequence of the mother's thyroid deficiency, the infant exhibits mental and physical retardation. Cretinism is a congenital condition (present at birth). Prevention focuses on diagnosing and treating iodine deficiency in pregnant women.

Hypothyroidism due to iodine deficiency occurring in older children and adults is called **myxedema.**

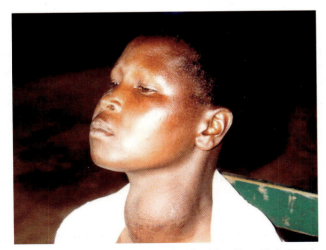

FIGURE 7-9 Woman with a goiter. *(Reprinted from Kenya Medical Mission Web site, with permission.)*

> ### BOX 7-1 ■ Worldwide Iodine Deficiency
>
> Iodine deficiency is uncommon in North America, but remains a public health problem in 54 countries (World Health Organization, 2017). Nearly 2 billion people are at risk for iodine deficiency with total goiter rates at 15.8% globally (Abebe, Gebeye, & Tariku, 2017). Goiter is often the first symptoms of iodine deficiency.
>
> About 45% of households in Europe have access to iodized salt and deficiency is also seen in Africa, Southeast Asia, and the Eastern Mediterranean (NIH, June 24, 2011). In areas with a high prevalence of goiter because of lack of iodine in the food and water, the condition is termed **endemic** goiter.
>
> Progress has been made with the universal iodization of salt since the World Health Organization increased efforts to promote national salt fortification programs. The cost amounts to 2 to 5 U.S. cents per person per year (World Health Organization, 2014).

Interfering Factors

Substances called **goitrogens** may block the body's utilization of iodine. Goitrogens found in vegetables belonging to the cabbage family, including cauliflower, broccoli, Brussels sprouts, rutabaga, and turnips, are unlikely to cause goiter because of the relatively small amounts consumed and because cooking destroys the goitrogens. The only food linked to goiter is cassava, a starchy root eaten in developing countries.

Toxicity

For basic information on mineral toxicity, see Table 7-4. Chronic toxicity may develop with an intake greater than 1.1 milligrams per day. Iodine toxicity produces the same symptoms as deficiency, including goiter (NIH, June 24, 2011).

Fluoride

In body fluids, fluorine exists as fluoride, a salt of hydrofluoric acid, or as an **ion.** About 99% of the body's fluoride accumulates as fluorapatite in bones and teeth. Fluoride seems to make bone mineral less soluble and hence less likely to be reabsorbed.

Nearly 100% of soluble fluoride found in fluoridated water and toothpaste is rapidly absorbed from the stomach and small intestine, but absorption diminishes to 50% to 80% when fluoride is consumed as foods. Calcium and magnesium are thought to form insoluble complexes with fluoride, decreasing its absorption. Excretion of fluoride is through urine.

Functions

Fluoride stimulates osteoblast production and mineral deposition in children's bones.

Fluoride's major contribution to human health relates to its role in preventing dental caries. In **plaque** and saliva, fluoride inhibits demineralization and enhances remineralization of early carious lesions. Whether in water or toothpaste, fluoride works in two main ways:

- By slowing the activity of bacteria that cause decay
- By combining with the enamel on the surface of the teeth to make it stronger and more resistant to decay

Fluoride in drinking water, although at a lower concentration than in toothpaste, maintains a constant low level of fluoride in the dental plaque and saliva all day.

Dietary Reference Intakes and Sources

For DRIs see Appendix A. For food and other sources, see Table 7-9.

Food and beverages prepared with fluoridated water contain increased fluoride. Fluoride is found in many processed foods and drinks such as soda, beer, and sports drinks. Tea is an additional source of fluoride, with black tea averaging 3 to 4 milligrams per liter of fluoride. Previous recommendations for fluoride in drinking water (0.7 to 1.2 milligrams per liter) were based on geographic areas considering variations in water intake in warm climates. Over the past several decades, many factors, including the advent of air-conditioning, have reduced geographic differences in water intake. The new recommendation of 0.7 milligrams of fluoride per liter of water is intended to prevent tooth decay while minimizing the risk for dental **fluorosis.** Besides the environmental changes, the new recommendation acknowledges that more sources of fluoride besides water (over-the-counter dental products, professional dental treatments, and supplements) are available than when water fluoridation was first introduced in the United States (U.S. Department of Health and Human Services Federal Panel on Community Water Fluoridation, 2015).

The U.S. Environmental Protection Agency, which is responsible for the safety and quality of drinking water in the United States, sets a maximum allowable limit for fluoride in community drinking water at 4 milligrams per liter (U.S. Public Health, 2015).

The oral health of Americans over the past 50 years has improved significantly, mostly because of effective prevention and treatment efforts. One major success is community water fluoridation, which now benefits about 70% of Americans who receive water through public water systems. Information on county and community water systems can be obtained at https://www.cdc.gov/fluoridation/index.html. Unfortunately, 42% of children aged 2 to 11 have dental caries (tooth decay) in their primary teeth (National Institute of Dental and Craniofacial Research [NIDCR], 2014).

Concern has been raised that children consuming conditioned water or bottled water instead of fluoridated tap water would receive suboptimal amounts of fluoride. Neither boiling nor charcoal-based water filtration systems remove fluoride from water; however, distillation and reverse osmosis treatments are effective in decreasing fluoride in water (CDC, April 1, 2016).

The FDA does not require bottled water manufacturers participating in interstate commerce to list the fluoride content on the label, but it does require that fluoride additives be listed. Intrastate commerce regulation is left to the individual states. If the label lacks the desired information, consumers should contact the bottled water's manufacturer to ask about the fluoride content of a particular brand (CDC, April 14, 2015).

Toxicity

For basic information on mineral toxicity, see Table 7-4.

Dental fluorosis can result when children regularly consume higher-than-recommended amounts of fluoride during the teeth-forming years, age 8 and younger. Most dental fluorosis in the United States, about 92%, appears as white spots on the tooth surface that often only a dental professional would notice. Moderate and severe forms of dental fluorosis cause more extensive enamel changes. The severe form in which pits may form in the teeth rarely occurs where the level of fluoride in water is less than 2 milligrams per liter (CDC, August 31, 2015).

After the FDA approved a health claim for fluoridated bottled water containing 0.6 to 1.0 milligrams of fluoride per liter to read "Drinking fluoridated water may reduce the risk of dental caries or tooth decay," another concern regarding possible excessive intake arose. Infant formulas as manufactured contain low fluoride levels. To avoid the possibility of excessive fluoride ingestion by infants from preparing powdered or concentrated formulas with fluoridated water, parents can use low-fluoride bottled water to mix infant formula. The infant's health-care provider should be asked about the proportion of the baby's feedings that should be prepared with low-fluoride bottled water products. These waters are labeled as deionized, purified, demineralized, or distilled, unless they specifically list fluoride as an added ingredient (CDC, July 31, 2015).

Acute toxicity has followed accidental ingestion of supplements or of excessive amounts of toothpaste. Package labeling directs caregivers to limit the amount of fluoridated toothpaste for children younger than 6 years to "a pea-sized amount," which should not be swallowed. Parents should consult a dentist or physician before using such toothpaste for a child younger than 2 years.

Zinc

The bodies of adult humans contain 2 to 3 grams of zinc; 90% is found in the muscle and bone and the other 10% in organs and body fluids.

One essential zinc-containing respiratory enzyme, *carbonic anhydrase*, catalyzes carbon dioxide and water into carbonic acid to allow rapid disposal of carbon dioxide. Zinc is essential for the growth and repair of tissues because it is involved in the synthesis of DNA and RNA. Zinc plays a vital role in growth and development during infancy and childhood. Zinc is associated with insulin and is a component of a protein, *gustin*, concerned with taste acuity. The production of active vitamin A for the visual pigment rhodopsin requires zinc. Zinc plays a role in immune function and wound healing. Its effect on the common cold is a matter of debate (see Clinical Application 7-6).

Absorption, Control, and Excretion

Zinc is released from foods in the acid environment of the stomach and absorbed from the small intestine, mainly the duodenum and upper jejunum through some of the same

CLINICAL APPLICATION 7-6

Zinc for the Common Cold?

Whether zinc should be recommended to ward off or minimize symptoms of the common cold has been studied since at least 1993. Two meta-analyses found that zinc shortened the duration of the common cold when started within 24 hours of onset of symptoms. A meta-analysis with 5 trials of low-dose zinc, less than 75 mg, had no effect on the duration of a cold and 3 trials of high-dose zinc, greater than 75 mg, shortened the duration of the cold by 42% (Hemil & Chalker, 2015). A Cochrane review demonstrated that when zinc was taken within 24 hours of symptoms, participants had a decrease in duration and severity of their symptoms (NIH, February 11, 2016). In 2009, the FDA advised consumers not to use zinc-containing nasal gels or sprays marketed as cold remedies after receiving more than 130 reports of users developing **anosmia**, loss of their sense of smell. In some people, the loss was long-lasting or permanent, posing a safety risk if they could not detect noxious odors in the environment such as smoke, a gas leak, or spoiled food (NIH, February 11, 2016).

absorption sites as iron. Control of zinc levels is achieved through limitations on absorption that varies from 10% to 80% but typically amounts to 20% to 30% of the zinc in the U.S. diet.

Up to 80% of zinc excretion occurs via the gastrointestinal tract through feces and biliary and intestinal sections, with smaller amounts being lost in urine and skin.

Dietary Reference Intakes and Sources

For DRIs see Appendix A. For food and other sources, see Table 7-9. To investigate the mineral content of a particular item, go to http://ndb.nal.usda.gov or to http://nutritiondata.self.com.

Zinc is recovered from pancreatic and biliary secretions in the gastrointestinal tract for reuse, which is an important function of the body in the maintenance of zinc balance.

The requirement for dietary zinc may be as much as 50% greater for vegetarians, particularly vegans, as for persons consuming a mixed diet (NIH, February 11, 2016).

Interfering Factors

Less zinc is absorbed from plant foods than from animal foods. Phytates, especially in cereals and legumes, bind with zinc in the intestinal lumen and prevent absorption. Conditions or medications that decrease gastric acidity impede zinc absorption. Iron and zinc compete for the same absorption sites. Zinc and nonheme iron interact when ingested together in solution and when 20 milligrams or more of iron is consumed. The effect is not always apparent when taken with a meal and varies with the form of the nutrients. In a similar reaction, zinc and calcium or copper may interact. In addition, phytates, oxalates, and tannins all reduce the absorption of zinc.

Deficiency

Zinc intake correlates directly with protein consumption. Groups at risk because of limited meat intake include people with low incomes, elderly people, and vegetarians. Zinc deficiency in adults can also occur as a result of diseases that either hinder zinc absorption or cause excessive amounts of zinc to be excreted in urine. Zinc deficiency effects are as follows:

- In children
  - Growth retardation
  - Skeletal abnormalities
  - Delayed sexual maturation
  - Decreased cognition
- In adults
  - Alopecia
  - Loss of taste sensation
  - Poor wound healing
  - Impaired immunity
  - Eye and skin conditions

The World Health Organization and United Nations Children's Fund recommend the routine use of zinc supplementation to help reduce the duration and severity of diarrhea, a leading cause of death in children under the age of 5 globally, and to prevent subsequent episodes (World Health Organization, January 10, 2017). Zinc supplementation in children has been associated with increased immune response with diseases with frequent infections such as HIV, Down syndrome, and sickle cell disease (Goel & Shah, 2014).

Toxicity

For basic information on mineral toxicity, see Table 7-4. Because zinc can be toxic if consumed in excessive amounts, it should be obtained from foods, not from routine or long-term supplementation (see Clinical Application 7-6).

Copper

The healthy adult body contains about 50 to 150 milligrams of copper, found in all body tissues and most secretions. Copper is a cofactor for enzymes involved in hemoglobin synthesis and cell respiration and is required for melanin pigment formation. A mutation in a copper-dependent enzyme causes albinism (Dolinska et al, 2014), the partial or total absence of pigment in the hair, skin, and eyes. It is usually transmitted as an autosomal recessive trait.

Gastric secretions aid in the release of bound copper in foods. Although some absorption is possible in the stomach, most copper is absorbed from the small intestine, chiefly the duodenum. Typically, 50% to 80% of ingested copper is absorbed with higher percentages occurring at low intake levels. The major route of excretion is via bile into the feces, through which the liver maintains copper balance.

Dietary Reference Intakes and Sources

For DRIs, see Appendix A. For food and other sources, see Table 7-9. To investigate the mineral content of a particular item, go to http://ndb.nal.usda.gov or to http://nutritiondata.self.com.

In the United States, adult intake averages 1 to 1.6 milligrams.

Interfering Factors and Deficiency

High intakes of iron and zinc interfere with copper metabolism. Phytates hinder copper absorption, but most people in the United States do not consume enough phytates to affect copper status.

Individuals at increased risk of copper deficiency are those:

- Taking medications that make the stomach less acid
- Consuming zinc supplements, typically 40 milligrams or more per day
- With gastrointestinal diseases permitting malabsorption
- With kidney diseases that increase copper loss

Copper deficiency is a commonly reported long-term complication of **bariatric surgery** (Gletsu-Miller & Wright, 2013). Deficiency has been documented in malnourished and premature infants and as a result of the prolonged administration of parenteral nutrition (see Chapter 14) solutions deficient in copper (Chitambar & Asok, 2014).

Because of copper's link with iron utilization, copper deficiency produces a hypochromic, microcytic anemia that requires treatment with copper, not iron. Other manifestations of copper deficiency are:

- Bone abnormalities
- Impaired immune function
- Depigmentation of the skin and hair (Gropper & Smith, 2013)

A hereditary abnormality causing defective copper elimination from cells is the cause of **Menkes disease**. Most tissues accumulate excess copper but not to toxic levels because the absorption of copper from the gastrointestinal tract is subsequently blocked. The disease is inherited as an **X-linked** recessive trait. Standard treatment involves parenteral administration of *copper-histidine*.

Toxicity

For basic information on mineral toxicity, see Table 7-4.

A genetic mutation causes **Wilson disease,** which is inherited as an autosomal recessive trait affecting copper absorption, leading to toxic copper accumulation in the organs. Clinical manifestations include multisystem damage, such as cirrhosis, neurological symptoms, and muscular skeletal deformity (Yu et al, 2017).

Selenium

The total body selenium is about 20 milligrams. The highest concentrations of this mineral occur in the thyroid gland, kidneys, liver, heart, pancreas, and muscle. An analogue of the amino acid methionine called selenomethionine can be incorporated into body proteins with methionine (NIH Office of Dietary Supplements, 2016).

Selenium is integral to more than 25 enzymes that primarily function as **antioxidants**. Selenium also contributes to thyroid function and a healthy immune system. It also protects against the toxicity of heavy metals mercury, cadmium, and silver.

Selenium does not require digestion, and absorption throughout the small intestine does not appear to be regulated. Homeostasis of the mineral is thought to be maintained by urinary excretion that represents 50% to 60% of selenium losses with the remaining being eliminated through the feces.

Dietary Reference Intakes and Sources

For DRIs, see Appendix A. For food and other sources, see Table 7-9. To investigate the mineral content of a particular item, go to http://ndb.nal.usda.gov or to http://nutritiondata.self.com.

Seafood and organ meats are the richest sourses of selenium (NIH Office of Dietary Supplements, 2016). Other sources include dairy products, eggs, animal meat, and plant sources including nuts, grains, and legumes. The amount of selenium present in plant foods depends on the selenium content of the soil and water where the foods are grown.

Deficiency and Toxicity

Selenium deficiencies have been produced in animals but are unlikely in humans who eat meat on a regular basis. Nevertheless, some exceptions exist, such as clients undergoing hemodialysis, clients with HIV, and clients living in selenium deficient regions (NIH, 2016).

For basic information on mineral toxicity, see Table 7-4. Selenosis, toxicity from selenium, has occurred in miners and people overdosing with supplements. Symptoms of selenium toxicity can include hair and nail loss, skin lesions, fatigue, gastrointestinal symptoms, and nervous system abnormalities (NIH, February 11, 2016).

Chromium

The adult body contains approximately 4 to 6 milligrams of chromium. High concentrations are found in the kidney, liver, muscle, spleen, heart, pancreas, and bone. Only about 0.4% to 2.5% of dietary chromium is absorbed depending on intake, with the greater absorption taking place at lower intake levels. Chromium is absorbed throughout the small intestine, especially the jejunum. Ninety-five percent of excretion is via the urine, the content of which reflects current intake, not chromium status. Small amounts are lost as skin cells are shed.

Chromium is thought to potentiate the action of insulin but the mechanism of action is uncertain. The results of chromium supplementation on insulin sensitivity have been conflicting, and its use for type 2 diabetes is controversial. Chromium plays a role in carbohydrate, fat, and protein metabolism. *For DRIs see Appendix A. For food and other sources, see Table 7-9.*

Vitamin C may enhance absorption, but antacids and phytates decrease absorption of chromium.

Individuals receiving parenteral nutrition (see Chapter 14) without chromium have shown signs of type 2 diabetes and chromium is now routinely added to parenteral therapy.

For basic information on mineral toxicity, see Table 7-4. Chromium toxicity rarely occurs.

Manganese

The body contains only 10 to 20 milligrams of manganese, which is found in highest concentrations in the bones, liver, pancreas, and kidneys. Manganese is involved in the formation of bone and cartilage. Enzymes from nearly every class can be activated by manganese but, with few exceptions, are not manganese specific.

Absorption throughout the small intestine typically is less than 5%, with higher rates of absorption occurring with low intakes and females absorbing greater amounts than males for unknown reasons. Absorption is inhibited by nonheme iron, copper, oxalates, phytates, and fiber. Excretion is accomplished primarily through the liver via bile.

For DRIs, see Appendix A. For food and other sources, see Table 7-9. To investigate the mineral content of a particular item, go to http://ndb.nal.usda.gov or to http://nutritiondata.self.com.

Deficiency is unlikely except when manganese is deliberately eliminated from the diet. Among other signs and symptoms, the client displays:

- Infertility
- Iron-deficiency anemia
- Impaired glucose metabolism

For basic information on mineral toxicity, see Table 7-4. Manganese toxicity most often results from inhalation exposure in occupational settings, characteristically causing Parkinsonian-like symptoms and psychological changes. Toxicity has also been seen in clients receiving parenteral nutrition.

Cobalt

For food and other sources of cobalt, see Table 7-9. DRIs for cobalt have not been established.

As an essential component of the vitamin B_{12} molecule, cobalt is necessary for red blood cell formation. Cobalt deficiency can result in pernicious anemia. Cobalt toxicity can result from environmental exposure through the skin or lungs, and by ingesting too much. There is evidence showing cobalt toxicity resulting from wear on cobalt-containing artificial hip joints.

Molybdenum

The body contains about 2 milligrams of molybdenum, a cofactor for enzymes involved in the metabolism of sulfur-containing amino acids and **purines.** Both in absolute amounts and in concentration, molybdenum is found primarily in the liver, kidneys, and bone. About 50% to 85% of molybdenum in foods is absorbed without digestion from the proximal small intestine. Because it binds to copper in the intestinal tract, *tetrathiomolybdate,* a pharmaceutical preparation of molybdenum, is used in the treatment of copper toxicity, including Wilson disease, and some cancers. Molybdenum is mainly excreted by the kidneys, which are thought to promote homeostasis, but small amounts are lost via bile in feces and in sweat and hair (Gropper & Smith, 2013).

For DRIs, see Appendix A. For food and other sources, see Table 7-9.

An inherited recessive deficiency of sulfite oxidase that requires molybdenum produces severe neurological damage and death in childhood. *For basic information on mineral toxicity, see Table 7-4.*

Ultratrace Minerals

For DRIs for boron, nickel, and vanadium, see ULs in Appendix A. Arsenic, a colorless, odorless mineral, is found mostly in skin, nails, and hair, which can be analyzed to determine long-term exposure. Arsenic occurs naturally in rocks, soil, and water, but agricultural and industrial contamination of those resources is the major contributor to the amount of arsenic in the United States. Residues of arsenic in pesticides remain in the soil for decades to be taken into crops used for foods.

Although some foods contain arsenic in a less toxic organic form, the form in drinking water is the more toxic inorganic form. Inorganic arsenic may be found in foods because it is present in the environment, both as a naturally occurring mineral and because of activity such as past use of arsenic-containing pesticides. Long-term exposure to high levels of arsenic is associated with higher rates of skin, bladder, and lung cancers as well as heart disease (FDA, May 15, 2017). The FDA has set an allowable level for arsenic in bottled drinking water of 10 micrograms per liter (FDA, July 1, 2016), the same value used for public water systems (U.S. Environmental Protection Agency, March 21, 2017) and has proposed the same level for inorganic arsenic in apple juice (FDA, May 17, 2017).

Rice is different from most other grains in that it more readily accumulates arsenic. The FDA has been collecting data on arsenic in foods, including rice, for decades, and in April 2016 established a limit for inorganic arsenic in infant cereal of no more than 100 parts per billion (ppb) or 100 micrograms.

Boron is found mainly in bone, teeth, nails, and hair, the body's content totaling between 3 and 20 milligrams. More than 70% of excretion is in urine as boric acid with smaller amounts of boron lost in feces and sweat. Clear biochemical functions in humans have not been demonstrated, but beneficial effects on bones, cell membranes, and the immune system have been observed. Plant foods are particularly rich in boron, including almonds, red kidney beans, broccoli, bananas, and dried fruit such as raisins, prunes, and apricots.

Nickel is found in highest concentrations in the thyroid and adrenal glands. It is also found in hair, bone, lung, heart, kidney, and liver but the total amount in the body is thought to be about 10 milligrams. No specific biological role in humans has been identified. Nickel is released into the environment with the combustion of nickel-containing products and is found in higher levels in foods of plant rather than animal origin. Most absorbed nickel is excreted in urine, but sweat concentrations can be fairly high and small amounts are lost via bile. *Silicon* is involved in the normal formation, growth, and development of bones, connective tissues, and cartilage. Intake mostly comes from plant foods, with whole cereal grains and root vegetables especially rich sources. The kidney is considered the major organ of excretion; urinary silicon is significantly correlated with intake. Long-term use of silicon-containing antacids appears to contribute to particular types of kidney stones. *Vanadium*, totaling about 100 to 200 micrograms in the body, is found mainly in bone, teeth, lung, and thyroid gland. No specific biological function has been identified. Absorption is less than 10%. Excretion is mainly in urine with small amounts

in bile. Rich food sources include shellfish, black pepper, parsley, and dill seed.

Other Minerals That Have an Impact on Health

Aluminum, lead, and mercury are found in the body not because of nutritional needs but as the result of environmental contamination. Aluminum is stored in various organs, primarily the liver, and it can cross the blood-brain barrier and accumulate over time in the brain (Tian et al, 2017). See Chapter 10 for recommendations regarding mercury avoidance for pregnant women and Clinical Application 7-7 for more information on lead poisoning.

Aluminum, a metal frequently found in the environment, puts clients especially at risk when it contaminates pharmaceutical products used for hemodialysis or parenteral nutrition because such intake bypasses any possible defense by the gastrointestinal system. Aluminum toxicity can cause serious central nervous system and bone effects.

Controversy exists regarding the use of aluminum in the childhood immunizations hepatitis A and pneumococcus. Aluminum is added as an adjuvant that is supposed to increase the immune response. The FDA has established that

CLINICAL APPLICATION   7-7

Lead Poisoning (Plumbism)

Lead is a contaminant in the human body derived from inhalation, ingestion, or skin contact. No age group is immune to the effects of lead poisoning, although children are at the greatest risk. Children can develop profound and permanent adverse health effects to the developing brain and nervous system; pregnant women can suffer miscarriage, premature birth, and low-birth weight infants; and adults can develop hypertension and kidney disease (World Health Organization, September, 2016).

No blood lead level (BLL) has been declared safe. The *level of concern* has been renamed *reference value* (based on the 97.5th percentile of the BLL distribution in U.S. children aged 1–5 years) and lowered from 10 mcg/dL to the current value of 5 mcg/dL (CDC, May 17, 2017). There are no changes in treatment guidelines; chelation is recommended for children who have levels ≥45 mcg/dL (CDC, May 17, 2017). Lead-based paint is the most widespread and dangerous high-dose exposure risk for young children (CDC, December 18, 2015). Children may eat paint chips that have an appealing sweet taste but a principal mode of ingestion is lead dust on hands, toys, and household objects that young children are prone to put into their mouths. Lead paint in homes built before 1977, when residential lead-based paint was discontinued in the United States, pose a particular risk to children and fetuses whose nervous systems are still being developed.

About 90% of total body lead in adults is accumulated in the bones, where it remains for decades and may be released during pregnancy as a side effect of mobilizing calcium for tissue building. Because lead freely crosses the placenta, lead poisoning during

pregnancy harms the woman and invariably produces congenital lead poisoning at BLLs higher than those of the mother.

Other sources of lead have been identified by the CDC including:

- Candy from Mexico. Lead can be found in both the ingredients and packaging.
- Toys not made in the United States or antique toys may have plastic or paint that contains lead.
- Toy jewelry out of vending machines. One 4-year-old child died after swallowing a piece of jewelry made from a lead-based product.
- Artificial turf may contain unhealthy levels of lead-based dust.
- Sindoor, a product found in cosmetics and in religious ceremonies. Hindu women often wear sindoor in the part of their hair to indicate marital status (May 29, 2015).

In addition to lead-based paint, older homes also may have plumbing that could contaminate drinking water. Because boiling increases the concentration of lead in water, the need to boil water for infant formula needs individual evaluation. To decrease the chance of lead leaching into drinking or cooking water:

1. Run water for 2 minutes in the morning before drawing water to drink.
2. Use cold water for cooking and drinking.
3. Use a water filter that has been tested and approved to remove lead.

Local health departments are able to direct people to appropriate laboratories if they wish to have their water tested.

the exposure of aluminum through vaccinations is minimal and poses no long-term risk (February 6, 2015). There has also been controversy regarding the connection of aluminum and the development of neurologic diseases such as Alzheimer. Normal daily exposure to aluminum does not appear to be a factor in the development of the disease.

Mineral Supplementation

Excessive intake of nutrients can be as harmful as insufficient intake. For most healthy people, foods are the preferred source of minerals. For reasons that will be clarified in Chapter 15, mineral supplements produced by a pharmaceutical manufacturer are the best choices.

People who take supplements are advised not to take more than the RDAs or AIs for each mineral without consulting their health-care providers, who should always be informed of supplements their clients take. In the case of some minerals, toxicity is possible at levels slightly above the recommended intake amounts. In addition, an excess of one mineral may cause a deficiency of another. Consideration should also be given to regular intake of fortified foods and beverages when advising use of mineral supplements.

KEYSTONES

- Minerals are inorganic substances that help regulate body functions without providing energy, but unlike vitamins, minerals become part of the body's structure and enzymes.

- Major minerals are present in the body in amounts of 5 grams (1 teaspoonful) or more; the daily recommended intake is 100 milligrams or more. Trace minerals are those with lesser amounts. Calcium, sodium, and potassium are major minerals. Iron, iodine, and zinc are trace minerals.

- Calcium is essential to the structure of bones and teeth and to nerve conduction, muscle contraction, and blood clotting. Milk, seafood with bones, and fortified orange juice are good sources of calcium.

- Iron is an essential component of hemoglobin that transports oxygen throughout the body. Red meat; cooked dark green, leafy vegetables; and fortified cereals are good sources of iron.

- Calcium, sodium, and potassium are essential to normal nerve and muscle function.

- Deficiency of iodine can result in goiter; of selenium, in cardiomyopathy; and of fluoride, in dental caries.

- Iron deficiency is one type of anemia; cretinism and goiter are caused by iodine deficiency. Menkes and Wilson diseases are inherited inabilities to metabolize copper producing deficiency and toxicity, respectively.

- Assuming no related diseases, individuals who should be assessed for potential mineral imbalances are those who shun whole categories of foods, vegetarians, dairy avoiders, and consumers of supplemental minerals in excess of the RDA/AIs.

- Persons fed artificially in which normal gastrointestinal absorptive processes are bypassed or whose intake consists of compounded formulas or of foods particularly rich in single nutrients should be carefully monitored. Additionally, storage vessels made of copper or containing lead have caused toxicities, as have medical devices that released aluminum into treatment solutions.

- Teaching clients to safeguard iron-containing supplements from children and to seek immediate medical attention should ingestion occur is of prime importance in preventing those poisoning deaths. Careful assessment of the swallowing or overuse of nonfood items could identify potentially hazardous practices that have led to zinc- and fluoride-poisoning deaths.

CASE STUDY 7-1

Mrs. B is a 34-year-old woman who has related her fear of osteoporosis to the nurse. A recent visit to a 75-year-old aunt crystallized this fear. The aunt has become stooped and recently broke her hip. Mrs. B is especially concerned because she has often been told that she resembles this aunt. Mrs. B asks, "Is there anything I can do to prevent this from happening to me?"

A 24-hour recall of dietary intake revealed a total of 1 cup of milk and no other dairy products. Mrs. B did consume two 3-oz servings of meat. Mrs. B has three small children and stated that they are exercise enough for her. She sits outside and watches them play on every nice day.

Mrs. B is 5 feet 3 inches tall and weighs 110 lb. She is white with fair skin.

CARE PLAN

Subjective Data

Fear of osteoporosis ■ Family history positive for osteoporosis ■ Less than RDA for calcium previous 24 hours ■ Met MyPlate guideline for protein group previous 24 hours ■ No planned exercise program

Objective Data

Height: 5 ft 3 in. ■ Weight: 110 lb (BMI 19.5) ■ White, fair, slight build

Analysis

Self-identified need regarding prevention of osteoporosis related to aunt's history of disease.

Plan

DESIRED OUTCOMES EVALUATION CRITERIA	ACTIONS/ INTERVENTIONS	RATIONALE
Client will list appropriate actions to maintain a strong skeleton after teaching session	Teach client how to consume 1,000 mg of calcium daily: 3 cups of milk or equivalent	One cup of milk contains approximately 300 mg of calcium + 100 mg from other sources
	Teach client factors favoring calcium absorption: vitamin D	If client chooses unfortified dairy products for calcium content, vitamin D may become insufficient depending on available sun exposure
	Teach client role of exercise in strengthening bones	Weight-bearing exercise stimulates the osteoblasts to build bone

At a follow-up visit, Mrs. B indicated that she had increased her consumption of dairy products but had not begun a planned exercise program. The nurse referred Mrs. B to a local Women's Health Center.

TEAMWORK 7-1

DIRECTOR OF WOMEN'S HEALTH CENTER'S NOTES

The following Director of Women's Health Center's Notes are representative of teamwork documentation.

Subjective: *Interested in strengthening bones due to fear of familial osteoporosis*

States no activity impediments

Objective: *BMI = 19.5*

Passed intake activity screen

Analysis: *Increased risk of osteoporosis based on family history and physical characteristics*

Plan: *Suggest ultrasound heel bone mineral density for baseline value*

Beginning-level walking program with group 3 times weekly, solo 3 times weekly.

CRITICAL THINKING QUESTIONS

1. What additional dietary information would you need before recommending good sources of calcium for Mrs. B?

2. What other assessment data would be helpful to broaden the scope of preventing osteoporosis?

3. Is the problem described in the Case Study a significant one for a 34-year-old woman? Why or why not?

CHAPTER REVIEW

1. Like vitamins, minerals give no energy to the body. Unlike vitamins, which of the following is true regarding minerals:
   1. Are completely absorbed from the intestinal tract
   2. Become part of the structure of the body
   3. Cause few clinical problems because of their widespread abundance in foods
   4. Cannot accumulate to the extent that they cause problems

2. Which of the following foods are the best sources of iron? Select all that apply.
   1. Eggs
   2. Baked beans
   3. Beef
   4. Spinach
   5. Low-fat milk

3. Which of the following individuals would be at greatest risk for a mineral deficiency?
   1. Someone who consumes no dairy products
   2. Someone who consumes no shellfish
   3. Someone who consumes no red meat
   4. Someone who drinks tea or coffee with every meal

4. Cretinism and goiter are caused by deficiency of _____.
   1. Copper
   2. Selenium
   3. Iodine
   4. Zinc

5. Calcium is necessary for strong bones and teeth. It is also necessary for:
   1. Assisting with the production of insulin
   2. Maintaining stomach acidity
   3. Preventing blood clots
   4. Enabling muscle contraction

CLINICAL ANALYSIS

1. Mrs. H is a 30-year-old mother of three children, all younger than 5 years. On her 6-week postpartum visit, her hemoglobin level was 10 grams per 100 milliliters of blood. She is given a prescription for ferrous sulfate and referred to the office nurse for nutrition counseling regarding her iron intake.

   Mrs. H tells the nurse that she eats what the children eat: cold cereal and milk for breakfast, peanut butter and jelly sandwiches, and maybe a banana for lunch and casseroles of tuna or hamburger for dinner. Mrs. H is a heavy coffee drinker, consuming 10 cups per day, 2 with each meal and a total of 4 others during "coffee breaks." The H family is lower-middle class. Mr. H is a long-distance truck driver and is away from home for long intervals.

   Mrs. H has some knowledge of iron needs and sources because of her three pregnancies. She is reluctant to continue the ferrous sulfate she has been taking throughout her pregnancy. "It binds me up," she tells the nurse. Also, Mrs. H maintains she cannot eat liver: "It gags me."

   Which of the following statements by Mrs. H would indicate that she understood the nurse's instructions correctly?
   a. "I should eat a little meat, fish, or poultry with every meal containing grain, fruit, and vegetable sources of iron."
   b. "I should increase the fiber in my diet because it will increase the absorption of iron."
   c. "If I want an alcoholic beverage, beer contains the most iron in a readily absorbable form."
   d. "Since I am taking an iron supplement, it is not important how I eat."

2. To meet the safety needs of the H children, the nurse instructs Mrs. H to keep her ferrous sulfate in a locked cupboard. The reason for this is:
   a. Interactions of iron tablets with vitamin supplements intended for children can cause deficiencies of water-soluble vitamins.
   b. The human body has no effective means of excreting an overload of iron.
   c. Iron poisoning, although rare, can occur if a child ingests more than 30 tablets of ferrous sulfate.
   d. Because iron binds with calcium, an overdose of iron would cause rickets.

3. Based on her current habits, which of the following changes to her lifestyle would be likely to increase Mrs. H's iron absorption from food?
   a. Changing her meal times to allow 5 hours to elapse between them.
   b. Avoiding citrus fruits and juices with meals.
   c. Trying alternate forms of liver such as in sausage.
   d. Delaying coffee and tea drinking to 2 hours after a meal.

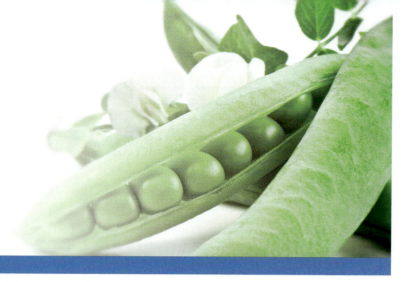

CHAPTER 8

Water

After completing this chapter, the student should be able to:

- List the functions of water in the body.
- Relate locations of the water by age and gender to the potential for harm caused by imbalances.
- Describe the initial stimulus and the end results of the hormonal control mechanism of water balance in the body.
- Connect the concept of osmolality to choices for providing the body's nutrient needs.
- Recognize the roles of the two major organs that maintain acid–base balance.

- Categorize average gains and losses of fluid in a healthy adult over a 24-hour period.
- Contrast the regulation, costs, and benefits of tap versus bottled water.
- Identify methods of assessing water balance in the body.
- Distinguish between the signs and symptoms of heat exhaustion and heatstroke and first-aid treatment.
- Outline situations in which water deficit or excess may become lethal.

Water in Human Nutrition

Water is the largest single constituent of the human body, and the need for water is more urgent than the need for any other nutrient. Humans can live a month without food but only 6 days without water.

More than half of body weight is water, which is found in and around the cells, within the blood and lymph vessels, and in various body cavities. Some tissues have significantly more water than others:

- Muscle and kidneys are 79% water.
- Brain and heart are 73% water.
- Skin contains 64% water.
- Bone tissue is 31% water.

Babies are born comprised of about 78% water, which drops to 65% at 1 year of age. Adult men are about 60% water and women 55% because women have a higher percentage of body fat. Lean muscle mass contains more water than fat (U.S. Geological Survey, 2016).

Fluid Compartments

Body fluids are contained in intracellular and extracellular compartments (Fig. 8-1). These compartments are separated by semipermeable membranes, which allow some substances to pass through and prevent the passage of other substances. Water passes freely through the membranes.

Thirteen water transport proteins, called aquaporins (AQP), have been identified in humans (Tamma, Goswami,

Reichmuth, De Santo, & Valenti, 2015). Aquaporins are membrane proteins that function as water-selective channels in the plasma membranes of many cells and help to explain the speed at which water moves across cell membranes, including the selective absorption found in different areas of the kidney (National Institutes of Health [NIH], 2016; NIH, 2017).

Intracellular Fluid

The fluid inside the cells is called intracellular. In adults, intracellular water constitutes about 65% of body water. In infants, approximately 46% of the body water is intracellular.

Extracellular Fluid

All fluid outside cells is extracellular. In adults, about 35% of the body's water is extracellular, whereas in infants, the approximate proportion is 54%. Figure 8-2 illustrates those relationships. The difference is important because extracellular fluid is more easily and rapidly excreted than is intracellular fluid. **Extracellular fluid** includes interstitial, intravascular, lymph, and transcellular fluids.

INTERSTITIAL FLUID

Located between the cells or surrounding the cells, interstitial fluid assists in transporting substances between the cells and the blood and lymph vessels.

INTRAVASCULAR FLUID

Intravascular fluid is found within the blood vessels, arteries, arterioles, capillaries, venules, and veins. The liquid part of the blood is called **plasma;** the liquid part of the blood

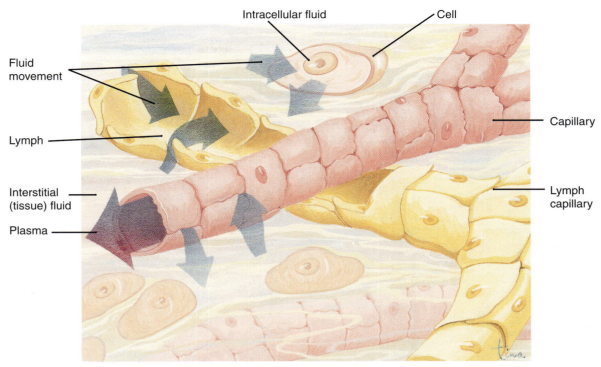

FIGURE 8-1 Water compartments, showing the names water is given in its different locations and the ways in which water moves between compartments. *(Reprinted from Scanlon, VC, and Sanders, T: Essentials of Anatomy and Physiology, 6th ed. FA Davis, Philadelphia, 2011, p. 30, with permission.)*

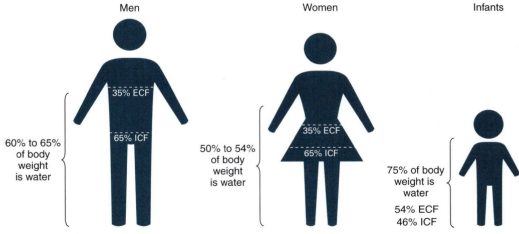

FIGURE 8-2 The relative amounts of body weight that are intracellular and extracellular water in men, women, and infants.

without the clotting elements is called **serum.** As is illustrated in Figure 8-3, 91.5% of plasma is water.

LYMPHATIC FLUID

The venous system cannot collect and return all the fluid from the tissues to the heart. **Lymph,** via the lymphatic vessels, assists in returning the fluid part of blood to the heart.

TRANSCELLULAR FLUID

Transcellular fluids include cerebrospinal fluid, pericardial fluid, pleural fluid, synovial fluid, intraocular fluids, and gastrointestinal secretions. Transcellular fluids are constantly being secreted into their spaces and reabsorbed into

the vascular system. Figure 8-4 shows the approximate distribution of water in the four compartments.

Usage

No storage tanks for water exist in the body; water continually moves from one body compartment to another and is often reused by the body to perform different tasks.

Functions

As a component of cells, water helps give the body shape and form, and as the major constituent of blood, it helps to maintain blood volume and blood pressure. It is part of

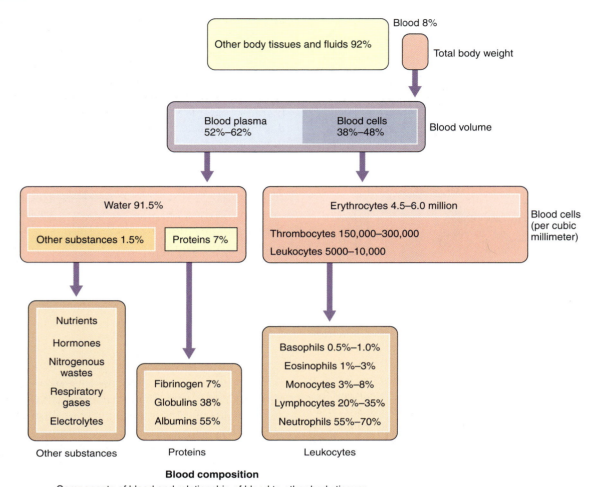

Blood 8%

Other body tissues and fluids 92%

Total body weight

Blood plasma 52%–62% | Blood cells 38%–48%   Blood volume

Water 91.5%

Other substances 1.5%   Proteins 7%

Erythrocytes 4.5–6.0 million

Thrombocytes 150,000–300,000

Leukocytes 5000–10,000

Blood cells (per cubic millimeter)

Nutrients

Hormones

Nitrogenous wastes

Respiratory gases

Electrolytes

Fibrinogen 7%

Globulins 38%

Albumins 55%

Basophils 0.5%–1.0%

Eosinophils 1%–3%

Monocytes 3%–8%

Lymphocytes 20%–35%

Neutrophils 55%–70%

Other substances   Proteins   Leukocytes

Blood composition

Components of blood and relationship of blood to other body tissues

FIGURE 8-3 Blood constitutes 8% of body weight. The largest single component of the blood is water. *(Reprinted from Venes, D [ed]: Taber's Cyclopedic Medical Dictionary, 21st ed. FA Davis, Philadelphia, 2009, p. 283, with permission.)*

☐ Intracellular

☐ Intravascular

☐ Interstitial

☐ Transcellular

FIGURE 8-4 Proportionate amounts of water in the four fluid compartments in the body. *(Reprinted from Williams, L, and Hopper, P: Understanding Medical Surgical Nursing, 4th ed. FA Davis, Philadelphia, 2011, p. 70, with permission.)*

the structure of many of the body's large molecules, such as protein and glycogen. Some body water also serves as a lubricant, as in mucus secretions and joint fluid.

Water helps to regulate body temperature by absorbing the heat produced by fever and the heat resulting from metabolic processes. On average, tissue metabolism generates 100 kilocalories per hour. The blood carries excess heat to the skin, where it is dissipated by perspiration or radiation.

Water is a **solvent** for minerals, vitamins, glucose, and other small molecules. (The substance that is dissolved in a solvent is called a **solute**.) See Box 8-1 for a list of the functions of water in the body.

BOX 8-1 ■ Functions of Water

- Gives shape and form to cells
- Maintains blood volume and blood pressure
- Helps form the structure of large molecules
- Serves as a lubricant and a solvent
- Helps regulate body temperature
- Transports nutrients to and waste away from cells
- Is a medium for and participant in chemical reactions

Absorption

A small amount of water can be absorbed into the bloodstream from the stomach, but a liter of water can be absorbed from the small intestine in an hour. The daily absorption of water by the small intestine is up to 15 liters per day and by the colon 5 liters per day (Popkin, D'Anci, & Rosenberg, 2010).

Under conditions that disrupt an individual's automatic adaptive mechanisms, water may be retained. The accumulation of excessive amounts of fluid between the cells (in the interstitial spaces) is called **edema.** Conditions that may cause such water retention include:

- Venous or lymphatic blockage
- Heart failure
- Severe protein deficiency (see Chapter 4)
- Sodium retention
- Some kidney conditions

When finger pressure displaces excess fluid over a bony area the sign is termed **pitting edema.** Although the fluid remains inside the body, it is lost to circulation (Fig. 8-5).

As a result of injury or trauma, the capillaries become more permeable so that more fluid and cells can travel to the site of the injury to begin repairs, or healing. This process also causes swelling, or edema, at the site of an injury—blisters at the site of burns, for example, where fluid leaves the vessels and accumulates in the skin. As is noted in Chapter 22, correct fluid replacement is a high priority for severely burned clients.

In most cases, localized edema is not deadly; however, accumulation of fluid in the brain (cerebral edema) or in lung tissue (pulmonary edema) is life-threatening. Cerebral edema may result from tumors, toxic chemicals, or infection. Pulmonary edema can be a consequence of a failing

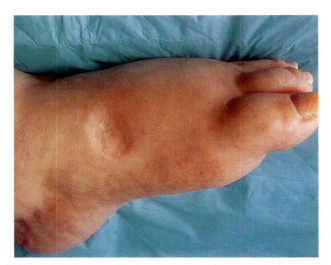

FIGURE 8-5 Finger or thumb pressure over a bony area displaces edematous fluid; shown here as pitting edema of the foot. *(Reprinted from Williams, L, and Hopper, P: Understanding Medical Surgical Nursing, 4th ed. FA Davis, Philadelphia, 2011, p. 397, with permission.)*

heart or irritation of the lung, as seen in a client who inhales toxic gases.

Excessive water also can be dispersed throughout the body. This condition is called **water intoxication,** which can be caused by excessive water intake (either by the intravenous or gastrointestinal route), cerebral concussion, or hormonal disorders. Many of the symptoms are caused by diluting the concentration of the minerals in the body's fluid compartments.

Dietary Reference Intakes

Dietary Reference Intakes (DRIs) have been established for total water from food and beverages; see Appendix A. For all ages and physiological conditions, the level of certainty is an Adequate Intake (AI), not a Recommended Dietary Allowance (RDA).

Approximately 80% of water needs are expected to come from fluids and 20% from foods. Larger intakes are required by physically active people or those in hot environments.

The previously publicized negative effects of caffeine and alcohol on water balance have been refuted by evidence showing the diuretic effects of those substances to be transient. Appropriately responding to thirst sensation and mealtime beverages are usually adequate to maintain hydration. Acute water toxicity is a hazard in individuals rapidly consuming much more than the kidneys' maximal excretion rate of 0.7 to 1.0 liter per hour (Institute of Medicine, 2005).

Ordinarily, breast milk alone can supply an infant's needed water even in a desert. At the opposite end of the age spectrum, older adults often have a blunted sense of thirst, and their water needs may be affected by disease and medication.

Physiology of Body Fluids
The Effect of Electrolytes on Water Balance

Each fluid compartment has an electrolyte composition that serves its needs and has automatic mechanisms designed to keep it electrically neutral, or balanced. The positive ions within a compartment must equal the negative ones. When shifts and losses occur, compensating shifts and gains reestablish electroneutrality.

Important Body Electrolytes

Mineral ions strongly influence not only water balance but also osmotic pressure, blood pressure, and acid–base balance. See Table 8-1 for a summary of the major body electrolytes, and Clinical Application 8-1 for the diagnostic uses and hazards of electrolytes.

Because electrical activity is determined by the concentration of electrolytes in a given solution, electrolytes are measured by the total number of particles in solution rather than their total weight. The unit of measure in the United States is the **milliequivalent (mEq),** expressed as mEq/liter.

TABLE 8-1   Major Body Electrolytes

ELECTROLYTE	FLUID COMPARTMENT*	FUNCTIONS
Cations		
Sodium (Na^+)	Extracellular	Major cation in extracellular fluid. Na^+ concentration in fluids determines the distribution of H_2O by osmosis. The kidney uses Na^+ with H^+ and HCO_3^- to regulate acid–base balance.
Potassium (K^+)	Intracellular	Major cation in intracellular fluid. K^+ with Na^+ maintains water balance. The kidney uses K^+ with Na^+ and HCO_3^-, to regulate acid–base balance.
Calcium (Ca^{2+})	Extracellular†	Participates in permeability of cell membranes, transmission of nerve impulses, muscle action.
Magnesium (Mg^{2+})	Intracellular	Regulates nerve stimulation and normal muscle action.
Anions		
Chloride (Cl^-)	Extracellular	Major anion in extracellular fluid. With Na^+, helps maintain water balance and acid–base balance.
Bicarbonate (HCO_3^-)	Extracellular	Most important extracellular fluid buffer.
Phosphate (HPO_4^{2-})	Intracellular	Within the intracellular fluid, phosphates and proteins buffer 95% of the body's carbonic acid and 50% of other acids.

*Extracellular fluid and intracellular fluid both contain all the cations and anions listed in this table but are labeled as either extracellular fluid or intracellular fluid according to the concentration. For example, sodium ions make up 142 of the total 155 milliequivalents per liter (of the cations) in the extracellular fluid.
†Of the cations, 3% in extracellular fluid and 1% in intracellular fluid.

CLINICAL APPLICATION   8-1

Diagnostic Uses and Potential Hazards of Electrolytes

Skin sensors attached to an electrocardiograph can trace the electrical activity of the heart. The resulting graphic record is called an **electrocardiogram (ECG).** The machine's sensors on the skin can detect the electric current because blood is an electrolyte solution and thus capable of conducting electricity. The same principle applies to the use of an electroencephalograph, a device that traces brainwave activity. The record obtained from this machine is called an **electroencephalogram (EEG).**

The characteristics of electrolyte solutions that allow these machines to sense electrical activity can also be hazardous. A fluid-filled tube, such as a nasogastric tube or catheter, can conduct stray electricity from faulty electrical devices to the client's heart and could result in dysrhythmias. The electricity in the shock may be minuscule but enough to be fatal if it happens at the wrong time in the cardiac cycle. The health-care worker should be vigilant for defective electrical equipment, tagging it for repair and replacing it immediately.

The concentration of a pharmaceutical solution is also measured in milliequivalents. Clinical Calculation 8-1 shows the conversion of milligrams of sodium chloride to milliequivalents.

Osmotic Pressure

Osmosis is the movement of water (or another solvent) across a semipermeable membrane from an area with fewer particles to one with more particles. The result, as long as the difference is reasonable, is an equalization of concentration on either side of the membrane. Clinical Application 8-2 describes an experiment to demonstrate osmosis.

CLINICAL CALCULATION   8-1

Converting Milligrams to Milliequivalents

Milligram is a measure of weight. Milliequivalent is a measure of the concentration of electrolytes (number of particles) per volume of solution. The concentration of electrolytes in any given solution determines its chemical activity.

Electrolytes are expressed as milliequivalents per liter of solution whether referring to blood values or intravenous solutions.

To convert milligrams to milliequivalents, it is necessary to know

- the number of milligrams per liter,
- the molecular weight of the substance, and
- its valence, a number indicating the combining power of an atom, found in many dictionaries.

A teaspoonful of table salt in 1 liter of water will produce a 0.5% solution. A teaspoonful is roughly 5 grams. Because table salt is 40% sodium and 60% chloride, the liter of 0.5% salt water would contain 2 grams (2,000 mg) of sodium and 3 grams (3,000 mg) of chloride.

Two other values are needed: atomic or molecular weights and valences. The atomic weight for sodium is 22.9898. Sodium has a valence of 1. The formula for converting milligrams to milliequivalents is:

$$mEq/L = \frac{(mg/L) \times valence}{molecular\ weight} = \frac{2,000 \times 1}{22.9898} = 87\ mEq/L\ of\ sodium$$

Continuing, we can use the same formula with different values to calculate the milliequivalents of chloride. The atomic weight for chlorine is 35.453. Chlorine has a valence of 1.

Filling in the values for chloride, we have:

$$mEq/L = \frac{(mg/L) \times valence}{molecular\ weight} = \frac{3,000 \times 1}{35.453} = 85\ mEq/L\ of\ chloride$$

Then, adding the sodium and chloride, we have:

$$87 + 85 = 172\ mEq/L\ in\ the\ 0.5\%\ solution.$$

CLINICAL APPLICATION 8-2

Osmosis in the Kitchen

To make sauerkraut, cabbage is sliced finely and placed in the bottom of a crock. Salt is added to the dry cabbage in layers that are tamped down until the crock is full. At this point, liquid will have gathered, pulled from the cabbage pieces by the concentrated salt. A heavy plate topped with bags of water is placed atop the cabbage to continue squeezing the water from the cabbage as it ferments. The crock is covered with a cloth. After 5 or 6 weeks, the crock is full of juice, and the cabbage has become sauerkraut.

To make a small batch of sauerkraut, use 2 teaspoons of canning salt per pound of cabbage.

The size of the molecule and its ability to ionize determines the number of particles in a given concentration. Electrolytes readily ionize in solution. Disaccharides and monosaccharides do not ionize.

Osmosis is a passive process. The movement of some substances, however, is active. Some substances require active transport mechanisms to push them through a membrane. Two such transport mechanisms are the sodium pump and the potassium pump. Located in cell membranes, these pumps are actually proteins that move ions.

Sodium pumps move sodium ions out of cells (and water follows).

Potassium pumps move potassium ions into cells.

In this manner, the body maintains electrolyte concentrations of the intracellular and extracellular fluid compartments. Active transport requires energy to operate.

DETERMINATION OF OSMOTIC PRESSURE

When two solutions on either side of a semipermeable membrane have different concentrations, pressure develops. This pressure, which is exerted on the semipermeable membrane, is called **osmotic pressure.** Osmotic pressure causes a solvent such as water to cross the membrane, but the solutes (particles) that are outside the membrane cannot go through.

OSMOLALITY AND NUTRITION

The measure of the osmotic pressure exerted by the number of particles per volume of liquid is referred to as its **osmolarity.** The unit of measure for osmotic activity is the **milliosmole.** Clinically, osmolarity is usually reported in milliosmoles per *liter.* **Osmolality,** in contrast, is the measure of the osmotic pressure exerted by the number of particles per weight of solvent, usually reported in milliosmoles per *kilogram.* The normal value for osmolality of human blood serum is about 275 to 290 milliosmoles per kilogram. The primary determinant of osmolality in the extracellular fluid is sodium (Lewis, 2016a).

Fluids are designated **isotonic** if they approximate the osmolality of blood plasma. Two commonly administered isotonic intravenous fluids are 5% glucose in water and 0.9% sodium chloride. Fluids exerting less osmotic pressure than plasma are labeled **hypotonic.** Those exerting greater osmotic pressure than plasma are called **hypertonic.**

Achieving the correct osmolality of fluids administered intravenously (by needle or tube into the vein) is crucial. A solution that is too concentrated pulls water out of the red blood cells, and the cells shrivel and die. A solution that is too weak allows water to be pulled into the red blood cells until the cells burst. For these reasons, isotonic solutions are given with red blood cell products.

Intravenous solutions containing sufficient nutrients to provide all a person's known needs are so hypertonic that they must be infused into a very large vein so that they are diluted quickly by the substantial volume of blood flowing past the infusion port or catheter. This procedure is called parenteral nutrition and is described in Chapter 14.

Oral fluids also can be categorized by osmotic pressure. Plain water is hypotonic. Whole milk at 275 milliosmoles per liter is close to isotonic but is not recommended for infants for another reason related to its metabolism (see Chapter 11). Ginger ale, with 510 milliosmoles per liter, and 7-Up®, with 640, are both hypertonic. The significance of these differences will become apparent in the section on treatment of fluid volume abnormalities.

SERUM ELECTROLYTES

The electrolyte content of blood can also be reported in milliequivalents per liter. The normal serum sodium level is 135 to 145 milliequivalents per liter. In most cases, because sodium is the most influential extracellular ion, osmolarity of the extracellular fluid can be estimated clinically by doubling the serum sodium value. Normal serum sodium doubled would be 270 to 296 milliosmoles per liter. Normal osmolality of the serum is about 300 milliosmoles per kilogram. This simple method gives a close approximation.

The other ion that health-care providers monitor carefully in clients with potential fluid and electrolyte imbalances is potassium. Most of the potassium in the body is inside the cells, at a concentration of 150 milliequivalents per liter. By contrast, potassium concentration in the blood is only 3.5 to 5.0 milliequivalents per liter. Even slight variations above or below these values can produce severe consequences. The heart muscle is particularly sensitive to high or low levels of potassium; abnormal levels can produce cardiac arrest.

Although proteins play a role in fluid balance (discussed subsequently), they normally remain in the cell or extracellular fluid. Therefore, sodium, potassium, and chloride ions provide the most movement across cell membranes to maintain osmotic pressure and fluid balance (Lewis, 2016a).

The Effect of Plasma Proteins on Water Balance

The body has highly developed mechanisms that maintain a constant flow of water and:

- Nutrients to cells
- Waste materials from cells

Adequate blood pressure is necessary for this transport system to function. Blood pressure is the force exerted against the walls of the arteries by the beating heart. It is reported in two numbers, for example, 120/80 (measured in millimeters of mercury, mm Hg). The top number is the pressure when the heart beats, called **systolic pressure.** The bottom number is the pressure between beats, called the **diastolic pressure.** One of the factors necessary to maintain blood pressure is a sufficient volume of blood in the arteries and veins.

Water and nutrients in the blood are pushed out through the thin walls of the capillaries into the interstitial fluid by **hydrostatic pressure** (blood pressure) supplied by the heart. From the interstitial compartment, the water and nutrients cross cell membranes to bathe and nourish the cell. Plasma proteins, including **albumin,** remain in the capillaries because they are too large to squeeze through the capillary wall.

Inside the capillaries, the remaining plasma proteins exert **colloidal osmotic pressure (COP).** At this point, the COP is greater than the hydrostatic pressure, thereby pulling water and waste materials from the interstitial fluid into the capillaries to maintain blood volume. Low serum protein is the cause of water imbalance in the body, resulting in an accumulation of water in the interstitial spaces. This edema develops because there are not enough plasma proteins in the capillaries to hold the water within the circulatory system.

Regulation of Water Intake and Excretion

The body has mechanisms regulating both the intake and the excretion of water. To achieve homeostasis, the body's automatic monitoring and regulating mechanisms are activated by deficits or excesses of water amounting to only a few hundred milliliters (Popkin et al, 2010).

Normally, thirst governs water intake. Excretion is controlled mainly by two hormones:

1. Antidiuretic hormone causes the body to reabsorb (retain) water.
2. Aldosterone causes the body to retain sodium.

Thirst Mechanism

Thirst is the desire for fluids, especially water. Thirst normally occurs when 10% of the intravascular volume is lost or when cellular volume is reduced by 1% to 2%. When blood contains too little water, its osmotic pressure increases. Special sensors in the **hypothalamus** monitor the osmotic pressure as the blood circulates in the brain. When the hypothalamus detects an increase in osmotic pressure, the gland triggers a desire to drink.

Antidiuretic Hormone

If thirst is not alleviated, the hypothalamus increases production of **antidiuretic hormone (ADH),** which is then secreted from the posterior pituitary gland. ADH, also named **vasopressin,** causes the kidneys to return more water to the bloodstream rather than spill it into the urine. A rise in osmolality by 2% to 3% stimulates enough ADH to maximally concentrate the urine. The opposite is also true: a decline in osmolality by 2% to 3% produces maximally dilute urine (Bailey, Sands, & Franch, 2014; Wisse, Zieve, & Black, 2015).

ADH also constricts arteries to increase blood pressure. A similar situation occurs by putting a finger over the end of a garden hose, narrowing its diameter, thereby increasing pressure of the flowing water.

In **diabetes insipidus,** the hypothalamus does not secrete ADH or the kidneys do not respond appropriately. If the hypothalamus is not secreting ADH, a pharmaceutical preparation can be given. Clinical Application 8-3 provides information about a condition called syndrome of inappropriate antidiuretic hormone secretion (SIADH) also known as syndrome of inappropriate antidiuresis (SIAD).

CLINICAL APPLICATION   8-3

Syndrome of Inappropriate Antidiuretic Hormone Secretion (SIADH)

The syndrome of inappropriate secretion of antidiuretic hormone (SIADH), also called the syndrome of inappropriate antidiuresis (SIAD), is the most frequent cause of hyponatremia (Sahay & Sahay, 2014; Wisse et al, 2015). Normally, increased blood osmolality stimulates the posterior pituitary gland to release ADH. When enough water is returned to the bloodstream by the kidney, ADH secretion stops. Common causes of SIADH include the following:

- Lung disease (pneumonia, tuberculosis, cystic fibrosis, asthma)
- Some tumors (oat cell of lung, carcinoma of pancreas, lymphoma, leukemia)
- Certain drugs (selective serotonin reuptake inhibitors [SSRIs], chemotherapeutic agents, antidepressants, type 2 diabetes drugs)
- Surgery, brain and bone

The signs and symptoms of SIAD are those of hyponatremia (see Table 7-6). Familiarity with the client's usual behavior is crucial because there may be changes in mental status, such as confusion and memory problems.

Hyponatremic clients without serious signs or symptoms of cerebral edema do not require urgent therapy to raise the serum sodium, but the underlying causes should be treated. Chronic or mild hyponatremia has been linked to falls, impaired gait and attention, and fractures. Depending on their extracellular fluid volume status, management of their fluid intakes may be part of the therapeutic plan (Wisse et al, 2015).

In stark contrast, hyponatremia with cerebral symptoms is a medical emergency in which treatment delay may prove fatal. The emerging consensus calls for prompt bolus treatment of symptomatic hyponatremia with hypertonic saline or saline infusions (Lewis, 2017).

Aldosterone

The release of **aldosterone,** a hormone secreted by the adrenal glands, is another water-balancing mechanism in the body. Aldosterone causes sodium ions to be returned to the bloodstream by the kidneys rather than to be spilled into urine. Sodium, the most influential extracellular ion, pulls water along with it.

The stimulus for the release of aldosterone is decreased pressure of the blood-supplying kidney tissue. In response, the kidneys produce **renin** that acts with secretions from the liver and the lungs to produce **angiotensin II.** The cascade continues as shown in Figure 8-6.

The other side of sodium retention is potassium loss. Within fluid compartments, positively charged particles must equal negatively charged ones. When sodium is retained, to maintain electroneutrality, the kidney excretes more potassium under the influence of aldosterone.

Acid–Base Balance

The body is well equipped to digest and metabolize acidic and basic foods without jeopardizing its acid–base balance, assuming normal amounts are ingested. The use of substances such as baking soda to treat an upset stomach should be discouraged, however, because the baking soda can be absorbed into the blood, thereby affecting the whole body. Nonabsorbable antacids designed to treat stomach upsets and used according to directions are a better choice than baking soda.

Acids are compounds that yield hydrogen ions when dissociated in solution. The more hydrogen ions a solution contains, the more concentrated the acid. Bases, or alkalis, are substances that accept hydrogen ions. Acidity or alkalinity is measured by a scale called **pH** for *potential of hydrogen.*

The pH scale ranges from 0 to 14: acids are rated 0 to 6.999; 7.0 is neutral; bases (alkalis) are greater than 7. On the scale, 1 would indicate a strong acid, and 14 a strong base. Figure 8-7 illustrates the pH scale, showing placement of acid, neutral, and alkaline fluids. The difference between units is 10-fold. Thus, lemon juice at a pH of 2 is 10 times as acidic as orange juice with a pH of 3.

Physiologically, a substance is an acid or base depending on whether it will donate or accept a hydrogen ion after metabolism in the body. For example, both citric acid in fruit sodas and phosphoric acid in colas are classified as acids chemically, but citric acid becomes a base after metabolism in the liver, whereas phosphoric acid is unchanged (Bailey et al, 2014). See Chapter 7 for the effects of phosphorus on calcium intake.

The action of the lungs, kidneys, and buffer systems of the body maintains the balance between too much and too little acid in body fluids. These buffer systems minimize significant changes in the pH of body fluids by controlling the hydrogen ion (H^+) concentration.

Buffers are substances that can neutralize both acids and bases. Proteins (hemoglobin) and the **bicarbonate** (HCO_3^-)–carbonic acid (H_2CO_3) system are the most

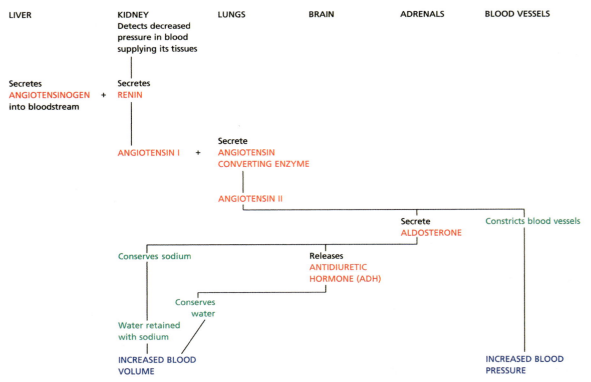

FIGURE 8-6 Hormonal control of water balance. Although the kidneys do most of the work, the complex process also involves the liver, lungs, brain, adrenal glands, and blood vessels.

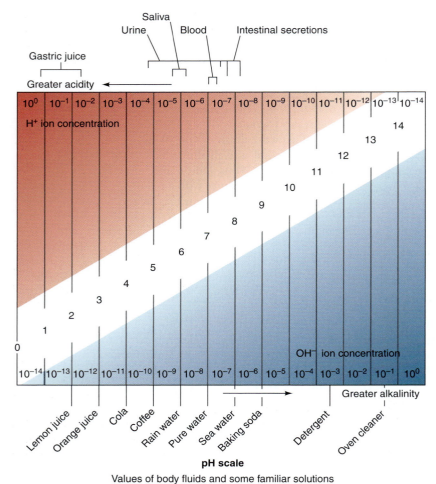

FIGURE 8-7 Representation of the pH scale with usual readings for body fluids, beverages, and household products. *(Reprinted from Venes, D [ed]: Taber's Cyclopedic Medical Dictionary, 21st ed. FA Davis, Philadelphia, 2009, p. 1764, with permission.)*

important buffers in the extracellular fluid. Phosphate (HPO_4^{2-}) and proteins are two important buffers in the intracellular fluid.

Extracellular Fluid

The normal pH of the extracellular fluid is 7.35 to 7.45. The body is continually working to maintain the pH within this narrow range, which is slightly alkaline despite the acidity of the waste products of metabolism. A blood pH below 6.8 or above 7.8 is usually fatal (Fournier, 2009). A pH of 6.8 produces shock, coma, and respiratory failure. The symptoms of severe alkalemia are those of hypocalcemia because at a pH greater than 7.75, not enough ionized calcium is available for cardiac contractility, leading to death if uncorrected (Bailey et al, 2014).

Extracellular fluid contains both positive sodium ions (Na^+) and negative bicarbonate ions (HCO_3^-). When a strong acid is introduced into the fluid, a chemical reaction takes place, yielding sodium chloride (a salt), which is neutral, and carbonic acid (a weak acid). **Carbonic acid** breaks down to carbon dioxide and water, which are excreted by the lungs (exhaled) and kidneys, respectively.

When a strong base (alkali) enters the system, carbon dioxide and water (the two main waste products of cellular

metabolism) react to form carbonic acid to counteract the alkaline effect of the base. The end products of this reaction are water and a weak base that does not drastically affect the pH.

RESPIRATORY SYSTEM

The lungs help maintain pH by varying the amount of carbon dioxide (CO_2) exhaled. Retained carbon dioxide makes the body fluids more acidic because it reacts to form carbonic acid, a source of hydrogen ions. Too much carbonic acid, or too much of any acid, results in **acidosis,** a condition that causes the lungs to automatically increase the rate and depth of breathing, eliminating more carbon dioxide and water.

This respiratory response to acidosis begins within minutes of an increase in acidity. Respiratory compensation for acidosis is 50% to 75% effective and is an extremely important component in the regulation of pH. The respiratory system acts quickly but can eliminate only carbonic acid.

The homeostatic system can be subverted by rapid breathing caused by anxiety, which triggers paresthesias (peripheral and perioral), peripheral tetany (e.g., stiffness of fingers or arms), fainting, and sometimes all of these findings. Tetany occurs because respiratory **alkalosis** causes both hypophosphatemia and hypocalcemia (Tabers.com). See hypocalcemia in Chapter 7.

The first aid recommended for hyperventilation resulting from anxiety is breathing through only one nostril with the mouth closed. The previous technique, breathing into a paper bag, can lead to hypoxia (Tabers.com).

RENAL SYSTEM

Metabolic acids, usually derived from the diet, as well as excess carbonic acid, must be eliminated in urine. The main metabolic acid is sulfuric acid obtained from the metabolism of the sulfur-containing amino acids methionine and cysteine. Inorganic phosphates used as food additives (e.g., colas) may also increase the acid content of the diet (Bailey et al, 2014).

The kidney spills or retains hydrogen, sodium, and bicarbonate ions as necessary to maintain an acceptable pH in blood. For example, in response to acidosis, the kidneys excrete hydrogen ions and reabsorb sodium and bicarbonate ions. Conversely, in response to **alkalosis,** the kidneys conserve hydrogen ions and excrete sodium and bicarbonate ions. The kidneys initiate these actions within 24 hours but require 3 to 4 days to compensate for changes in blood pH.

Intracellular Fluid

The normal pH of the intracellular fluid is 6.8 to 7.0, slightly acid to neutral. Within the intracellular fluid, organic phosphates and proteins are the most important buffers. These substances buffer 95% of the body's carbonic acid and 50% of other acids. Protein is the most powerful and plentiful buffer system in the body.

Of the body's proteins, hemoglobin has the largest buffering capacity. Thus, red blood cells have 70% of the buffering power of the blood. This buffering capacity allows large quantities of carbon dioxide to be transported from the tissues to the lungs, with only a small change in venous pH compared with arterial pH.

When blood contains excessive hydrogen ions, the ions move into the cells to be buffered. Then, to maintain electroneutrality, potassium moves from the intracellular to the intravascular compartment, raising serum potassium levels.

Water Balance and Imbalances

Getting enough water to maintain hydration each day, through water, beverages, and foods is important to good health (Centers for Disease Control and Prevention [CDC], 2016). The exact amount of water intake required each day is difficult to determine. This is due, in part, because accurately studying water intake has utilized differing data collection methodologies (Gandy, 2015). Additionally, individual needs vary based upon individual's health, living environment, and activity level. The Institute of Medicine set Dietary Reference Intakes across the different age groups (Appendix A). The Mayo Clinic generally advises drinking enough fluid so that one is rarely thirsty, though advanced age may decrease the trigger for thirst (Lewis, 2016a), and urine is light yellow to colorless (Mayo Clinic, 2014). Additional research is required before more definitive recommendations can be made regarding recommendations for water requirements (Gandy, 2015).

Sources of Water

Plain water from the tap and bottled water are obvious sources, but much of our water is consumed in other beverages. Skim milk is 91% water, and whole milk is 88% water. Water itself may contain other nutrients in varying amounts. Hard water has calcium, magnesium, and often iron. Water conditioners used to soften water replace those minerals with sodium or potassium. Drinking softened water increases some people's sodium intake, though not significantly for most healthy individuals. The Mayo Clinic recommends that for individuals utilizing a water softener and are concerned by sodium intake switch to potassium chloride for their water-purification system (Sheps, 2016).

We obtain about four cups of water per day in foods. Some foods that are solids also have high water content: head lettuce is 96% water, celery is 95% water, and raw carrots are 88% water. *To investigate the water content of a particular item, click on "Foods by Nutrient" at http://nutritiondata. self.com. If you select a 100-gram portion, the grams of water listed is also the percentage.*

Water is also a product of metabolism, which yields about 1 cup of water per day in the average person. Each energy nutrient produces a different amount of metabolic water:

- 1 gram of carbohydrate produces 0.60 gram of water.
- 1 gram of fat produces 1.07 grams of water.
- 1 gram of protein produces 0.41 gram of water.
- *But* 1 ounce of pure alcohol *requires* 8 ounces of water for its metabolism.

The Centers for Disease Control and Prevention (CDC) estimates that Americans spend billions of dollars each year on bottled water. Bottled water is not automatically safer than tap water in the United States (CDC, 2014). It is estimated that 25% of all bottled water is tap water. The CDC recommends that immunocompromised individuals should consume water that has been through reverse osmosis, distillation, or filtration with an absolute 1-micron filter (CDC, 2014). It takes 1.63 liters of water to make every liter of bottled water (Postman, 2016).

See Table 8-2 for a brief comparison of these two main sources of drinking water, and Figure 8-8 for a serving suggestion.

Losses of Water

We lose water in obvious ways, called **sensible water losses,** as in perspiration and urine. We also lose water in less obvious ways, called **insensible water losses,** as through breathing.

TABLE 8-2   Comparison of Bottled Water and Municipal Water Regulations

	BOTTLED WATER	PUBLIC WATER
Regulatory agency	Food and Drug Administration (FDA)	Environmental Protection Agency (EPA)
Subject to regulation	Only that sold state-to-state, = 30%–40% of bottled water	All systems with >14 service connections or serving >24 people
Number of states regulating intrastate bottlers	40	
Testing for bacteria	Once a week	20 times/month for small systems 100 + times/month for large systems
Chemical testing	Annually	Quarterly
Allowable lead level	5 parts per billion	15 parts per billion*
Allowable arsenic level	10 parts per billion	10 parts per billion
Certified labs to test	No	Yes
Required reporting to state or federal governments	No	Yes

Requires treatment to reduce level. Level set considering aging pipes.
Source: U.S. Environmental Protection Agency, 2017.

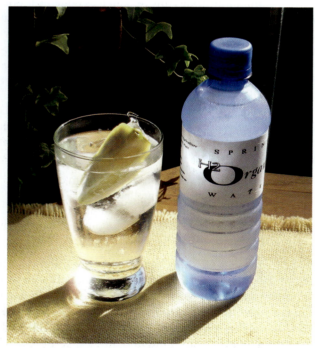

FIGURE 8-8 Either choice will hydrate a person. Although cost is not the only factor to consider, it is significantly less for a glass of tap water (even with ice and a lemon wedge) than a bottle of water.

Sensible Water Losses

Sensible water losses include losses of the major extracellular ions, sodium and chloride. Three important routes commonly account for sensible water losses:

1. Through the skin as perspiration
2. Through the kidney as urine
3. Through the gastrointestinal tract in the feces

PERSPIRATION

Evaporation of sweat is the main means of dissipating the body's heat produced by exercise. In extreme cases, a person may perspire at the rate of 2 liters per hour. For example, during a marathon race, runners may lose 6% to 8% of their body weight, primarily as perspiration. A 150-pound person could then lose 9 to 10½ pounds, or 4.3 to 5 liters, of fluid.

Sweat is not pure water. It is salty to the taste and hypotonic, and its composition varies from person to person. On average, 1 liter of perspiration contains, with wide ranges for each, approximately:

- 40 to 45 milliequivalents of sodium
- 3.9 milliequivalents of potassium
- 3.3 milliequivalents of magnesium
- 39 milliequivalents of chloride

Consequently, even a sweat loss of 5 or 6 liters entails small amounts of electrolytes so that rehydration with water should be adequate (Gropper & Smith, 2013; Lissoway & Weiss, 2014). An unconditioned person's sweat may contain 100 milliequivalents of sodium per liter, whereas the sweat of a well-conditioned individual may contain just 30 mEq/L (Bailey et al, 2014).

See Clinical Application 8-4 for information on heat-related illnesses.

URINE

In the normal, healthy person with average exertion throughout the day, urine output is roughly equal to liquid intake. A well-hydrated individual produces light yellow or straw-colored urine. A minimum amount of urine must be excreted each day to carry away the waste products resulting from metabolic processes. This function, called obligatory excretion, eliminates 400 to 600 milliliters per day. The kidneys function more efficiently when they receive an abundant water supply because economizing on water while

CLINICAL APPLICATION   8-4

Heat-Related Illnesses

Heat-related deaths in the United States occur an average of 618 per year. Causes can be high ambient temperatures over a period of days (classic heatstroke) or vigorous exercising in warm or hot environments that affects the person quickly (exertional heatstroke). Delayed access to cooling is the leading cause of morbidity and mortality in persons with heatstroke. Moving the affected person to a cool place, placing cool, wet clothes on the person, and cool water immersion are the treatments of choice when available (CDC, 2017).

See Table 8-3 for a summary comparison of heat exhaustion and heatstroke.

Persons at greatest risk of classic heat-related illness are:

- Young children
- Older adults
- Individuals with chronic medical (especially heart and lung or mental) disorders
- Clients taking medications that interfere with salt and water balance (CDC 2017; Lissoway & Weiss, 2014)

To help prevent heat-related incidents, acclimatization to heat should occur over 8–11 days while increasing the level and amount of activity. Thirst is a poor indicator of hydration and adequate fluids should be consumed every few hours. Maximum fluid absorption occurs up to 30% faster than plain water with a beverage containing 6%–7% carbohydrate (Lissoway & Weiss, 2014). During exertion, 1/2 to 1 cup of fluid every 15–20 minutes is recommended depending on heat and exertion level (Johnston, 2016).

CLINICAL CALCULATION   8-2

Hourly Urine Output in Children

Children should excrete 1 milliliter of urine per kilogram of body weight per hour. What would be a normal hourly urine output for a child who weighs 50 pounds?

First, convert pounds to kilograms. There are 2.2 pounds per kilogram.

$$\frac{50 \text{ lb}}{2.2 \text{ lb/kg}} = 22.7 \text{ kg}$$

Then multiply weight in kg × 1 mL/hour

$$22.7 \times 1 = 22.7 \text{ mL/h}$$

Thus, a 50-lb child normally should excrete 22.7 mL of urine per hour.

---

producing more concentrated urine takes more energy and increases wear on the kidney tissues. Strong evidence supports reduced risk of kidney stones in individuals with good hydration (National Kidney Foundation, 2016).

The hourly urine output of seriously ill clients is monitored but the amounts must be interpreted in relation to the client's situation. Even if a person is losing massive amounts of fluid through the gastrointestinal tract, such losses do not rid the body of metabolic wastes as efficiently as the kidney does. Adults should excrete 40 to 80 milliliters of urine per hour, although the amount varies throughout the day and night. Children's urine output should be at least 1 mL/kg body weight/hour (see Clinical Calculation 8-2).

GASTROINTESTINAL SECRETIONS

Regarding water balance, normally the gastrointestinal tract's net activity down to the level of the jejunum is secretion of water and electrolytes. Beyond that point, the net activity is resorption of water and electrolytes (Bailey et al, 2014).

Abnormal gastrointestinal function can cause extensive fluid loss. Location of the loss determines signs and symptoms. Gastric juice is acid, whereas intestinal juices are alkaline. Therefore, conceptually, gastrointestinal losses are divided into those lost above the outlet of the stomach, the **pyloric sphincter,** and those lost below it.

ABOVE THE PYLORUS. The common causes of losses above the pylorus are vomiting or stomach suctioning. Two organs secrete digestive juices above the pylorus: the salivary glands in the mouth and the gastric glands in the stomach. The ions lost in secretions above the pylorus are:

- Sodium
- Potassium
- Chloride
- Hydrogen

About 1 liter of saliva per day is mixed with food or just swallowed. The stomach secretes about 1.5 to 2.5 liters of gastric juice per day. If gastric juices are lost, hydrogen ions in the hydrochloric acid are also lost, putting the person at risk for alkalosis.

BELOW THE PYLORUS. The usual causes of losses below the pylorus are diarrhea and intestinal suctioning. Gastrointestinal secretions below the pylorus contain:

- Sodium
- Potassium
- Bicarbonate

Two to three liters of intestinal secretions per day flow into the bowel to digest food. Normally, bile is released from the gallbladder into the small intestine at the rate of 1 liter per day. The total gastrointestinal secretions amount to 6.5 to 8.5 liters per day. Yet because water is absorbed back into the blood from the large intestine, normal feces from an adult contain only 100 to 200 milliliters of water.

Insensible Water Losses

An invisible amount of water is lost through the lungs and the skin. These are insensible losses amounting to between 800 and 1,000 milliliters of water daily. Breath is visible only in cold weather. Even in warmer weather and indoors, people lose 400 milliliters of water per day in exhaled air. Deep respirations or a dry climate increase the amount of water lost.

The insensible loss of water through the skin is evaporative. It is almost pure water and nearly electrolyte-free. This insensible water loss amounts to 6 milliliters per kilogram of body weight in 24 hours, which is a baseline amount.

Environmental conditions influence the amount of water lost. Greater losses occur:

- At high temperatures
- At high altitudes
- In low humidity

Clinical Calculation 8-3 shows how to estimate insensible water loss. Burns, phototherapy, radiant warmers, or fever will increase the amount of insensible water loss. Fever increases evaporative losses by about 12% per degree Celsius of temperature elevation.

Clinical Calculation 8-4 shows how fever affects **evaporative water losses**. Table 8-4 lists average fluid gains and losses for 24 hours.

Assessment of Water Balance

Gathering data on water losses is straightforward: daily weight or documenting intake and output.

Weight

Daily weight is the single most important indicator of fluid status. One liter is 1 kilogram or 2.2 pounds.

Acute weight loss in adults is rated as follows:

Mild volume deficit, 2% to 5% loss
Moderate volume deficit, 5% to 10% loss
Severe volume deficit, >10% loss

Fluid balance in an infant is much more precarious than in an adult. Because a greater proportion of the infant's body water is in the extracellular space, infants can lose water more rapidly than adults. Therefore, a loss of 5% of body weight (or other findings in Table 8-5) in an infant merits medical attention. Proportionate concern is justified for children up to the age of 3 years when adult proportions

---

CLINICAL CALCULATION 8-3

Insensible Water Loss Through the Skin

The rule of thumb for insensible water loss through the skin is 6 mL/kg per 24 hours. How much insensible water loss would be expected for a 154-lb client?

First, convert pounds to kilograms:

$$\frac{154\ lb}{2.2\ lb/kg} = 70\ kg$$

Then multiply the client's weight in kilograms by the estimated standard:

$$70\ kg \times 6\ mL/kg = 420\ mL$$

Thus, this client's insensible water loss in a 24-hour period is expected to be 420 mL.

CLINICAL CALCULATION 8-4

Evaporative Water Loss in Fever

Fever increases the amount of evaporative loss by 12% for every degree Celsius of fever. If the 154-lb client in Clinical Calculation 8-3 had a fever of 102.2°F, how much additional evaporative loss would he or she sustain?

Temperatures can be reported in Fahrenheit or Celsius degrees, and the conversion formulas account for the fact that the Celsius scale sets freezing at zero and the Fahrenheit sets it at 32°

To convert Fahrenheit to Celsius, subtract 32 and multiply by 5/9.

$$102.2 - 32 = 70.2 \times 5/9 = 39°C$$

This client's temperature would be 39°C.

Likewise, a normal temperature of 98.6°F would be converted as

$$98.6 - 32 = 66.6 \times 5/9 = 37°C.$$

The client had insensible losses of 420 mL.

The client has an elevation of 2°C, which would increase evaporative loss by 24%.

$$420\ mL \times 0.24 = 100.8\ mL\ \text{additional evaporative water loss}$$
$$420\ mL + 100.8\ mL = 520.8\ \text{total insensible water loss through the skin}$$

To convert from Celsius to Fahrenheit, the formula is: $(°C \times 9/5) + 32$.

---

of fluid distribution normally occurs and the child usually can verbalize thirst.

Weight changes can be caused by metabolic events as well as by fluid shifts. If a client receives no oral, enteral, or parenteral nutrition, the loss of body tissue may amount to 0.3 to 0.5 kilogram per day.

Similarly, the loss of effective circulatory volume is not always an external loss. Weight gain may accompany circulatory loss. See Clinical Application 8-5 for insight into internal fluid losses.

Intake and Output

In a healthy person, liquid intake and output should be approximately equal. Measuring intake is easier than measuring output, but it still is frequently inaccurate. Most institutions post the amounts that food and beverage containers hold. Amounts remaining should be measured and subtracted from the total liquid served.

Rather than assuming that clients have consumed everything missing from the pitcher or tray, the nurse should ask if they drank the fluid (as opposed to, for instance, giving it to a visitor). Updating the intake form throughout the day rather than at the end of a shift is likely to produce a more complete record. Record the amount of water from ice chips as one-half of their volume. One cup of ice chips yields only ¹/₂ cup of water.

Fluid lost into a dressing or a diaper can be estimated by weighing it. Subtract the dry material's weight from

TABLE 8-3 Serious Heat-Related Illnesses

	HEAT EXHAUSTION	HEATSTROKE—MEDICAL EMERGENCY
Pathophysiology	Loss of water and salt in sweat	Loss of body temperature regulation Progresses to multiple organ dysfunctions
Symptoms	Headache Weakness, fatigue Dizziness, fainting Muscle cramps	Lethargy Throbbing headache Disorientation
Signs	Coherent	Delirium Convulsions Coma
Temperature	Usually <102.2°F (39°C)	>104°F (40°C)
Pulse	Weak, thready, rapid	Full, bounding, rapid
Respirations	Shallow, rapid, quiet	Difficult, loud
Skin	Cool, clammy, sweaty	Flushed, hot, dry (unless from exertion or just progressed from heat exhaustion)
First-aid treatment	Move to cool location Lie down Elevate feet Loosen clothing Monitor temperature If able to drink: ½ tsp salt in ½ glass of water orally every 15 min until medical help arrives	Move to cool location Lie down Elevate head Remove clothing Ice bags to neck, axillae, groin Spray with water while fanning Monitor airway, breathing, circulation until medical help arrives

TABLE 8-4 Average Fluid Gains and Losses in Adults in 24 Hours

FLUID GAINS		FLUID LOSSES*	
Energy metabolism	300 mL	Kidneys	1,200–1,500 mL
		Skin	500–600 mL
Oral fluids	1,100–1,400 mL	Lungs	400 mL
Solid foods	800–1,000 mL	Intestines	100–200 mL
Total gains	2,200–2,700 mL	Total losses	2,200–2,700 mL

*Includes sensible and insensible losses.

CLINICAL APPLICATION 8-5

Identifying Third-Space Losses

Large amounts of fluid can accumulate in several places in the body outside the circulatory system. These losses are called **third-space losses.** Certain diseases cause **ascites,** the accumulation of fluid (often amounting to several liters), not within the bowel but around it in the abdominal cavity. Other third-space losses involve internal bleeding or the collection of fluid in the chest cavity. An alert nurse can spot an early clue to third-space losses: decreasing urine output despite seemingly adequate fluid intake.

the total. One gram of weight equals 1 milliliter of water. **Specific gravity** is the weight of a substance compared with that of distilled water. Normal specific gravity of urine is 1.010 to 1.025, but a lower value is common in newborns. So although the weight of a diaper wet with

urine is not exactly the same as if it were wet with water, this method of recording incontinent urine is adequate in most situations.

In a sick person, intake and output totals may not balance every day. The client's intake and output should be assessed over a period of several days because a single-day evaluation can lead to missing the big picture. See Clinical Application 8-6 for teaching and documentation tips regarding fluid intake and Box 8-2 for a practical assessment tip regarding output.

CLINICAL APPLICATION 8-6

Avoiding Misinterpretation

One client was told to "drink a lot of fluid" when he was discharged from the hospital. He interpreted this to be 3 to 4 gallons per day! His kidneys did their best, but kidneys cannot excrete plain water. In a few days, the client was back in the hospital for correction of electrolyte imbalance.

- Be specific when teaching clients.
- Document both the teaching content and the client's response to the information.

BOX 8-2 ■ Visual Assessment of Fluid Balance

In persons with normal organ function, a good day-to-day measure of hydration status is the color of urine. Urine of light yellow color usually reflects normal fluid balance, whereas concentrated urine of a deeper color may indicate dehydration.

Water Imbalances

Fluid volume is unbalanced if it is insufficient or excessive. Signs and symptoms of both are shown in Table 8-5. To assess fluid volume through observation of hand veins, raise the client's hand above the heart. Normally, the veins will collapse in 3 to 5 seconds. Then lower the hand below the heart. The veins should refill in 3 to 5 seconds. The veins of a person with insufficient fluid volume require more than 5 seconds to refill. Reverse the procedure to assess excessive fluid volume in which the veins will take more than 5 seconds to empty.

Fluid compartments do not operate in isolation: if one is out of balance, the other compartments eventually will be affected as the body attempts to equalize osmotic pressure across the compartments.

Insufficient Fluid Volume

Treating insufficient fluid volume with appropriate fluids is essential, as is correcting the cause. Hypotonic fluids are given to replace fluid volume and correct electrolyte imbalances orally if possible but by nasogastric tube or intravenously if necessary (Clinical Application 8-7). Although hypotonic, plain water orally is not advised for treating insufficient fluid volume because it is likely to inhibit thirst and to increase urine output.

Parents should be informed of the desired treatment outcomes for a child with diarrhea. Oral electrolyte solutions, although clearly life-saving and effective in maintaining hydration, do not necessarily reduce stool volume or

CLINICAL APPLICATION 8-7

Oral Electrolyte Solutions

Originally, oral electrolyte solutions were designed to combat diarrheal diseases in developing countries. They proved so useful that they have since been modified for use in industrialized nations. One commonly used oral electrolyte solution is Pedialyte®, available over-the-counter without a prescription. One liter of Pedialyte contains sodium chloride and potassium citrate yielding the following electrolytes:

45 mEq sodium (Na^+)	35 mEq chloride (Cl^-)
20 mEq potassium (K^+)	30 mEq citrate, a base ($^-$)
65 mEq cations	65 mEq anions

Pedialyte is mildly hypotonic, about 250 milliosmoles per liter. It also contains a concentration of glucose that promotes sodium and water absorption, 25 g/L, which also contributes 100 kilocalories per liter.

Pedialyte is designed for hydration maintenance of an infant or child experiencing vomiting or diarrhea. If the client becomes dehydrated, as evidenced by loss of 5% of body weight, medical attention is needed. Intravenous fluids or an oral rehydration solution of different composition from Pedialyte may be prescribed for the dehydrated child.

the duration of diarrhea. Rapid oral rehydration with the appropriate solution has been shown to be as effective as intravenous fluid therapy in the treatment of dehydrated clients. Sodium and glucose in the correct proportions can be passively cotransported with fluid from the gut lumen

---

TABLE 8-5   Signs and Symptoms of Abnormal Fluid Volume

	INSUFFICIENT FLUID VOLUME	EXCESSIVE FLUID VOLUME
Symptoms		
Gastrointestinal	Thirst Loss of appetite (decreased blood to intestines)	Nausea Loss of appetite (edema of the bowel)
Signs		
General	Weight loss Depressed fontanel (infant) Sunken eyes (infant) Lack of tears when crying (infant)	Weight gain Edema
Skin and mucous membranes	Dry mucous membranes Decreased skin **turgor** (not reliable in elderly)	Skin stretched and shiny
Cardiovascular system	**Orthostatic hypotension** (pressure decrease of 15 mm Hg in systolic or diastolic) Increased pulse rate upon standing Increased hematocrit values (unless red blood cells also lost) Narrowing **pulse pressure** Filling of dependent hand veins takes longer than 5 seconds	Decreased hematocrit values Increasing **pulse pressure** Emptying of elevated hand veins takes longer than 5 seconds
Urinary	Decreased urine output Concentrated, dark urine	**Polyuria** Dilute, light urine
Gastrointestinal	Vomiting (decreased blood to intestines) Longitudinal furrows on tongue	Vomiting (edema of intestines)
Central nervous system	Confusion, disorientation	Deteriorating consciousness

into the circulation to restore intravascular volume. All of the commercial rehydration fluids are acceptable for oral rehydration therapy (ORT). They contain the following:

- 2 to 3 g/dL of glucose
- 45 to 90 mEq/L of sodium
- 30 mEq/L of base
- 20 to 25 mEq/L of potassium
- Osmolality of 200 to 310 mOsm/L (Huang, Anchala, Ellsbury, & George, 2012)

If hypertonic solutions are given orally to correct fluid loss, the concentrated solution would remain in the stomach longer than water, providing satiety and restraining water intake. In addition, hypertonic solutions draw fluid from the bowel wall into the lumen, resulting in osmotic diarrhea. Some commercial laxatives and enemas are hypertonic solutions.

In addition to causing osmotic diarrhea, hypertonic solutions allow less sodium and water to be absorbed than from the ORT solutions. Ginger ale (565 milliosmoles per liter [mOsm/L]) and apple juice (700 mOsm/L) are poor choices for rehydration in prolonged diarrhea, owing to their high glucose and low electrolyte concentrations. Another popular choice, chicken broth, is also not advised. It contains no carbohydrate, just 2 mEq of sodium, with an osmolality of 330 mOsm/L (Huang et al, 2012).

Thickened hydration solutions are also available for clients who have difficulty swallowing thin liquids. A dietitian should be consulted before using food thickeners, inasmuch as some of them bind with water, making water less available for absorption.

An alternative to intravenous rehydration in selected clients is the use of hypodermoclysis. In this technique, fluid is introduced into the subcutaneous tissue, in the thighs or abdomen, for instance, usually by means of a pair of long needles. A drug may be used to aid in dispersal of the solution.

Excessive Fluid Volume

Overhydration normally does not occur in healthy individuals who consume excessive fluids if the kidneys, liver, and heart are functioning normally. To exceed the body's ability to excrete excessive fluid, a young adult would have to regularly drink more than 6 gallons of water daily (Lewis, 2016b). When a person becomes ill and the control mechanisms stop working, the individual can retain fluid intracellularly or extracellularly.

As with insufficient fluid volume, the remedy for excessive fluid volume is to treat the cause. Osmotic diuretic drugs such as *mannitol* remain in the extracellular space. By increasing the osmotic pressure there, these drugs pull excess fluid from the cells to be excreted by the kidney.

Nutritionally, the client may be on a restricted fluid regimen. The physician may prescribe an intake of no more than 1,000 milliliters in 24 hours. This amount compensates for insensible losses through the skin and lungs. It is essential to supply fluid as prescribed and to teach the client the reason for the restriction. Over a period of several days, the obligatory urine output and any diuretic therapy will help the client's body excrete the excess fluid.

KEYSTONES

- Water transports nutrients to cells and heat and waste from cells; provides the volume needed to maintain blood pressure; becomes a structural component of cells and large molecules; and serves as a lubricant, solvent, and medium for chemical reactions.

- Of an adult's body weight, 55% to 60% is water, 35% of it extracellular. Of an infant's body weight, 78% is water, 54% of this extracellular, which can be lost quickly under adverse conditions.

- When the kidneys detect decreased blood pressure supplying its tissues, it begins a complex sequence of hormonal release involving the lungs, the adrenals, and the brain. The result is constricted blood vessels that increase blood pressure and conservation of sodium and water by the kidney that increases blood volume.

- Osmolality measures the osmotic pressure of fluids in the body or administered to it. Fluids are isotonic, hypotonic, or hypertonic compared with the osmolality of human serum. Hypertonic intravenous solutions require large vessels to quickly dilute the solution, and hypertonic oral solutions may counteract efforts to rehydrate an individual with diarrhea.

- Within minutes of detected acidosis, the lungs help to maintain acid–base balance by varying the amount of carbon dioxide exhaled; however, these organs are limited to eliminating carbonic acid. The kidneys eliminate excess carbonic acid and other acids but react slowly, within 24 hours, and may take 4 days to correct acid–base imbalances.

- The average adult gains fluids from oral fluids (1,250 mL), solid foods (900 mL), and metabolism (300 mL), which total 2,450 mL in 24 hours. During the same time, fluid would be lost through the kidneys (1,350 mL), skin (550 mL), lungs (400 mL), and intestines (150 mL) to again total 2,450 mL.

■ The Environmental Protection Agency requires that all but the smallest public water systems be tested by certified laboratories more frequently than bottled water manufacturers, with results reported to governmental bodies. The Food and Drug Administration regulates bottled water as a food, exempting intrastate sales and labeling for naturally occurring fluoride but mandating a lower allowable lead level than in tap water, although at a cost of up to 10,000 times the cost of tap water.

■ Daily weight is the single most important indicator of fluid status, but consideration must be given to the complete clinical situation when interpreting results. The second major technique to assess water balance in the body is an accurate intake and output record, including visual inspection of urine color.

■ Heat exhaustion, resulting from loss of water and salt in sweat, is differentiated from heatstroke by mental clarity; a temperature below 102.2°F (39°C); weak, thready pulse; shallow, quiet respirations; and a cool, clammy skin. Heatstroke presents with the opposite signs, results from a loss of body temperature regulation, and can progress to multiple organ failure. First aid while awaiting emergency medical technicians involves salt water orally for heat exhaustion if possible and rapid cooling of the body with water, ice packs, and fanning for heatstroke.

■ Dehydration from fluid losses can be lethal, with infants at high risk. Hyponatremia from dysregulation of hormonal water balance or from voluntary overhydration has proved fatal.

CASE STUDY 8-1

Mr. N, a 75-year-old retired office worker, recently arrived from his summer home in the north to his winter home in Florida. After leaving temperatures in the 40s, he had looked forward to enjoying the 85°F (29.4°C) weather. Although Mr. N had hired someone to care for his small yard while he was away from Florida, he still had to do a number of chores, which he tackled with a vengeance.

After 1½ hours, Mr. N began to get a headache. He felt a bit weak and dizzy but continued his work. He was nearly finished with the outside tasks.

Half an hour later, Ms. N found her husband lying on the ground and called to their neighbor, a retired nurse.

The nurse noted that Mr. N's skin was pale and cool but that he was perspiring profusely. He was conscious and coherent but said that he felt weak. The nurse took Mr. N's pulse. It was 90 beats per minute, regular but weak. His respirations were 12 per minute and shallow.

The nurse provided the emergency care described in the following care plan. (Of course, she did not write it all out before helping Mr. N.)

CARE PLAN

Subjective Data

Had worked outside in 85°F (29.4°C) heat for 2 hours ■ Headache, weakness, dizziness ■ Recently arrived from colder climate

Objective Data

Conscious, coherent ■ Skin pale, cool, wet with perspiration ■ Pulse 90, regular and weak ■ Respirations 24 and shallow

Analysis

Heat stress related to excessive loss of hypotonic fluid (sweat) as evidenced by wet, pale skin and weak, rapid pulse.

Plan

DESIRED OUTCOMES EVALUATION CRITERIA	ACTIONS/ INTERVENTIONS	RATIONALE
Client will remain conscious and oriented, with a pulse rate no greater than 90 beats/min, until the emergency team arrives.	Instruct Ms. N to call emergency medical services and return to help.	In an emergency situation, the nurse stays with the client. Potential electrolyte imbalance requires medical care.
	Loosen Mr. N's clothing.	Loosening the clothing will allow maximum air exchange and permit relaxation.
	With Ms. N, move client to shade or provide shade where he lies.	Mr. N must get out of the sun. Depending on the situation, he might be moved indoors, but perhaps the two women could not manage to move him.

DESIRED OUTCOMES EVALUATION CRITERIA	ACTIONS/ INTERVENTIONS	RATIONALE
	Keep client lying down with legs elevated slightly.	Lying down permits maximum blood circulation to the brain. Raising the legs increases the return of blood to the heart. The head should not be lowered because this causes venous congestion in the brain.
	Ask Ms. N to provide water, a diluted sport drink (to obtain 7–8 grams of carbohydrate per serving) to Mr. N.	Water and dilute carbohydrate drinks are readily absorbed by the intestine.

TEAMWORK 8-1

EMERGENCY MEDICAL TECHNICIAN'S NOTES

The following emergency medical technician's notes are representative of teamwork documentation.

Chief complaint: *Collapsed while performing yard work*

Subjective: *Oriented to person, place, time*

Hesitant in answers

Wife reports 75 years old, no chronic illnesses, baby aspirin daily for cardiovascular prevention

Objective: *Temperature 101.0°F (38.3°C) axillary*

Pulse 108, weak, thready

Respirations 22, shallow

B/P 105/70

Skin cool, clammy

Analysis: *Heat exhaustion*

Plan: *Rehydrate with 0.9% sodium chloride at 250 mL/hour*

Monitor vital signs every 5 minutes

Transport to emergency department

CRITICAL THINKING QUESTIONS

1. Reread the narrative. At what points in the narrative or in your expansion of the story could you envision Mr. N avoiding this incident?

2. The case study narrative does not discuss Mr. N's usual dietary intake. What dietary modifications can you think of that would make Mr. N's situation of overworking in the heat more critical?

3. What would you include in a presentation on preventing heat-related illnesses for an audience of elderly residents such as Mr. N, who follow the sun for the winter?

CHAPTER REVIEW

1. Which of the following people has the greatest percentage of body weight as water?
   1. A 154-pound man
   2. A 120-pound woman
   3. An 18-pound boy, 14 months old
   4. An 8-pound girl, 4 days old

2. Which of the following areas of regulation is stricter for bottled water than for tap water?
   1. Allowable lead level
   2. Frequency of testing for bacteria and chemicals
   3. Number of customers affected
   4. Requirements to report to authorities

3. Which of the following amounts is correct for average gains from oral fluids in adults for 24 hours?
   1. 500 to 600 mL
   2. 800 to 1,000 mL
   3. 1,100 to 1,400 mL
   4. 2,200 to 2,700 mL

4. The single most important indicator of fluid status in the body is:
   1. Collapsing of hand veins
   2. Daily weight
   3. Intake and output records
   4. Pulse pressure changes

5. Heat exhaustion is caused by:
   1. Insufficient secretion of antidiuretic hormone (ADH)
   2. Loss of water and salt in sweat
   3. Inability to perspire
   4. Retention of excessive water

CLINICAL ANALYSIS

1. Baby I, a 4-month-old boy, is being seen at a neighborhood clinic because he has developed diarrheal stools within the past 2 days. At birth, he weighed 7 pounds, 8 ounces. Since then he has gained steadily. Three days ago, he weighed 12 pounds, 8 ounces. Baby I's present weight is 12 pounds, 2 ounces. Mrs. I has been feeding the baby his usual formula. He drinks eagerly but then has an explosive bowel movement with loud crying. Baby I has had six bowel movements per day instead of his usual two. With this history, what physical assessment measures would the nurse include initially?
   a. Condition of hair, strength of grasp, presence of sucking reflex
   b. Heart sounds, lung sounds, blood pressure
   c. Skin turgor, fontanel fullness, moisture of mucous membranes
   d. Urine specific gravity, observation of diaper rash

2. Which of the following recommendations by the nurse would show understanding of supportive care of this client?
   a. Give Baby I whole milk to maintain nutrition.
   b. Continue, as Mrs. I has been doing, to allow the bowel to empty itself.
   c. Substitute orange juice for the formula for 3 days.
   d. Start Baby I on an oral electrolyte solution.

3. The nurse instructs Mrs. I to return for additional care for Baby I if one of the following events occurs. Which one would indicate the need to reassess Baby I?
   a. The baby sleeps soundly and has to be awakened for a night feeding.
   b. The baby has three loose bowel movements the day after beginning treatment.
   c. The baby continues to lose weight or passes blood in the stool.
   d. The baby gains more than two ounces per day.

CHAPTER 9

Digestion, Absorption, Metabolism, and Excretion

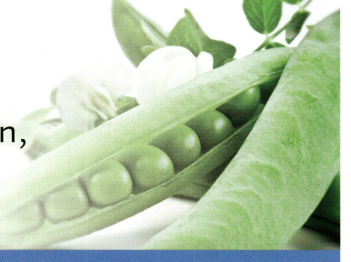

Every part of the human body requires nutrients from food for energy, maintenance, and growth. Food is composed of complex substances that must be broken down to simpler forms for cell use.

The **cell** is the ultimate destination for food's nutrients. Digestion, absorption, and metabolism are the three interrelated processes that act on food to prepare it for use. A fourth process, excretion, is the elimination of indigestible or unusable substances. This chapter discusses all the bodily activities, organs, and systems involved in these major processes.

Overview of the Major Processes

The first step in preparing food for use is digestion. During **digestion,** food is broken down mechanically and chemically in the gastrointestinal tract into forms small enough for **absorption** into the blood or lymphatic system.

After absorption, the nutrients usually are transported to the liver, where they may be adjusted to suit the body's needs. **Metabolism,** the sum of all physical and chemical changes that take place in the body, determines the final use of individual nutrients as well as medications. What the cells cannot use becomes waste that is eliminated through **excretion.**

Digestion

Digestion takes place in the alimentary canal with the aid of its accessory organs.

Alimentary Canal

The **alimentary canal** is a long, muscular tube that extends through the body from the mouth to the anus. It includes:

- The oral cavity
- Pharynx
- Esophagus
- Stomach
- Small intestine
- Large intestine

Muscle rings, called **sphincters,** separate segments of the alimentary canal. The sphincters act as valves to control the passage of food. When the muscles contract, the passageway closes; when the muscles relax, the passageway opens.

The **mucosa** lines the alimentary canal and secretes **mucus,** which lubricates the canal and helps facilitate the smooth passage of food. The mucosa secretes the digestive enzymes of the stomach and small intestine.

Accessory Organs

Three **organs** located outside of the alimentary canal are considered part of the digestive system—the liver, gallbladder, and pancreas. They make important contributions to the digestive process.

Liver

The **liver** is the second largest single organ in the body (skin is the largest). The liver performs many functions, but its primary digestive function is the production of **bile,** which breaks down dietary fats. Bile exits the liver via the hepatic **duct** (a narrow tube that permits the movement of fluid from one organ to another).

Gallbladder

The **gallbladder** is a 3- to 4-inch sac that concentrates and stores bile until it is needed in the small intestine. Bile is delivered to the small intestine through the common bile duct. About 2 to 3 cups of bile are secreted each day into the alimentary canal.

Pancreas

The **pancreas** secretes enzymes that are involved in the digestion of all the energy nutrients. These secretions are collectively known as pancreatic juice. Pancreatic juice is carried to the small intestine via the pancreatic and common bile ducts.

Digestive Action

Mechanical and chemical digestion occur simultaneously throughout the alimentary canal. **Mechanical digestion** is the physical breaking down of food into smaller pieces. **Chemical digestion** involves the splitting of complex molecules into simpler forms.

Mechanical Digestion

Examples of mechanical digestion include chewing, or **mastication,** and swallowing, peristalsis, and emulsification. **Peristalsis** is a wavelike movement that propels food through the entire length of the alimentary canal. This one-way movement is caused by the alternate contraction and relaxation of the circular and longitudinal muscles that make up the external muscle layer of the alimentary canal. Other muscular activity churns the food, reducing it to successively smaller particles and mixing it with digestive secretions. All of these muscular actions are regulated by a network of nerves within the wall of the alimentary canal.

Chemical Digestion

Many **chemical reactions** are involved in digestion. **Hydrolysis** is a chemical reaction in which a substance is split into two smaller and simpler substances by the addition or the taking up of the elements of water. When the substance is split, one hydrogen (H) attaches to one of the products and the hydroxyl (OH) attaches to the other product. For example, the conversion of starch to maltose, of fat to glycerol and fatty acids, and of protein to amino acids all involve hydrolysis. The hydrolysis of nutrients is achieved mostly through the action of digestive enzymes, which are present in:

- Saliva
- Gastric juice
- Pancreatic juice
- Intestinal juice

Each enzyme is specific in its action, and it acts only on a particular substance. Enzymes sometimes require the presence of additional substances, such as activators, coenzymes, or hormones, for activation. More than 500 enzymes are involved in the digestive process; this chapter discusses a few of the major ones.

In addition to enzymes, other secretions and chemicals are used in digestion. For example, mucus lubricates passages and facilitates the movement of food. It also protects the inside walls of the alimentary canal from acidic solutions. Another example is **electrolytes,** which are substances that conduct an electric current in solution. **Hydrochloric acid (HCl)** is an electrolyte and performs many functions necessary to the digestive process. A third example is bicarbonate, which is a basic solution that enters the small intestine and assists in digestion. Bicarbonate is defined in Chapter 8.

SECRETIONS

The quantity of mucus, electrolytes, water, and enzymes released during the digestive process depends on several factors.

Hormones frequently initiate a given secretion. For example, the presence of food in the stomach stimulates the cells to release a hormone called gastrin. Gastrin stimulates the release of hydrochloric acid. When the stomach's content is sufficiently acidic, it turns off further release of gastrin. When gastrin is no longer being released, hydrochloric acid is no longer released.

Emotions and conditioned responses can affect the amount of a secretion released. For example, the smell of a roasting turkey on Thanksgiving causes the release of hydrochloric acid in the stomach. Stress and tension can also produce this effect, sometimes with deleterious results.

The food in the gastrointestinal tract can influence the release of alimentary canal secretions. Drinking coffee, for instance, causes a hormone to be released into the stomach that in turn causes the secretion of hydrochloric acid. Another trigger for the release of bile from the gallbladder is the presence of fat in the small intestine. A chain of reactions in which one event causes another, and then another, is common in all biological **systems.**

END PRODUCTS

Four to 6 hours after a meal, the body has broken down the food into some trillion molecules. Each of the energy nutrients is broken down into simpler molecules.

- Carbohydrates are digested into monosaccharides.
- Fats are broken down into molecules of glycerol, fatty acids, and monoglycerides.
- The end products of protein digestion are amino acids and small peptides.

Researchers think that as much as one-third of dietary protein is absorbed into mucosal cells as dipeptides and tripeptides. Vitamins, minerals, and water are also released during digestion.

The Food Pathway

Food passes through the mouth into the oral cavity, where it is chewed and exposed to chemicals in the saliva. The tongue voluntarily forces the mass of food, called a **bolus,** into the pharynx, which is responsible for the reflex action of swallowing. The bolus then enters the esophagus, a muscular, mucus-lined tube, and is propelled downward by peristalsis to the stomach.

Both mechanical and chemical digestion occur in the stomach, reducing the food to a semifluid mass that is released into the small intestine. Further digestion takes place in the small intestine, and most of the absorption of nutrients occurs there as well. Any food remaining after digestion and absorption passes into the large intestine and is excreted as fecal matter.

Oral Cavity

The **oral cavity,** the hollow space in the skull directly behind the mouth, includes the roof of the mouth, the cheeks, and the floor of the mouth. Within the oral cavity are the teeth, tongue, and openings of the ducts of the salivary glands.

DIGESTIVE ACTION

Food entering the oral cavity is chewed and broken down into smaller particles. This mechanical action increases the surface area of the food for exposure to saliva, a digestive secretion produced by the **salivary glands.** Saliva moistens and softens the food for swallowing and contains the digestive enzyme known as **salivary amylase,** which converts starch to maltose (a disaccharide) or to the shorter chains of glucose. Because simple sugars (monosaccharides) require no digestion, some absorption may occur in the mouth. The chemical digestion of more complex carbohydrates (starch) continues until the hydrochloric acid in the stomach halts the action of the salivary amylase.

Pharynx

The **pharynx** is a muscular passage between the oral cavity and the esophagus. No digestive action occurs there. The pharynx continues the movement of the bolus by the reflexive action of swallowing. The bolus then enters the esophagus. Box 9-1 discusses the dietary treatment of dysphagia, and Figure 9-1 outlines the standardized international dysphagia diet definition framework.

BOX 9-1 ■ Dietary Treatment for Dysphagia

The American Speech-Language-Hearing Association estimates that annually, 1 in 15 adults will experience a swallowing disorder called dysphagia, literally meaning difficulty swallowing (http://www.asha.org). There are two types of dysphagia:

- Oropharyngeal—difficulty in safe transfer of a liquid or food bolus from the mouth to the esophagus
- Esophageal—difficulty in passing food down the esophagus

A swallowing disorder may cause coughing, but not always. As a result, food particles may pass into the lungs (aspiration), allowing bacteria to multiply, which may cause aspiration pneumonia. Dysphagia may be seen after some surgeries and radiation treatment to the head, neck, and/or esophagus, especially for cancer treatment. Premature infants may have difficulty with their suck, swallow and breathing coordination. Individuals with cognitive decline or **traumatic brain injury (TBI)** may also have difficulty swallowing. Dysphagia is commonly seen in clients with neurologic disorders such as stroke, Parkinson disease, multiple sclerosis, and amyotrophic lateral sclerosis.

Diets for dysphagia that safely meet nutrient needs range from nothing by mouth (NPO) to total oral feedings. Candidates for oral feedings should demonstrate the ability to perform a safe swallow by a bedside evaluation or a modified **barium swallow,** be alert and able to follow directions, and be oriented to self and the task of eating.

Dysphagia diets provide graduated steps from the most easily managed food to the ones most difficult to manage:

- Liquids range from extremely thick to thin.
- Solids range from liquidized to regular.
- Liquids and solids may be progressed independently.

Precise diet orders specify both the texture of solid foods and the consistency of liquids as well as other therapeutic modifications. To address the multiplicity of dysphagia diet terminology and practices, a multidisciplinary task force developed the International Dysphagia Diet Standardisation Initiative (IDDSI) based on existing scientific evidence (Marcason, 2017). The IDDSI has eight levels:

Level 0: Thin
- Flows like water

Level 1: Slightly Thick
- Thicker than water, flows through a straw, syringe, nipple

Level 2: Mildly Thick
- Flows off a spoon, sippable, effort required to drink through standard straw

Level 3: Moderately Thick/Liquidized
- Can be drunk from a cup, can be eaten with a spoon, no oral processing or chewing required, smooth texture, some effort required to suck through a straw

Level 4: Extremely Thick/Pureed
- Eaten with a spoon, cannot be poured, cannot be sucked through a straw, no biting or chewing, smooth texture

Level 5: Extremely Minced and Moist
- Eaten with a fork or spoon, can be scooped and shaped. Soft and moist with no separate thin liquid, minimal chewing required, easily mashed with a fork

Level 6: Soft and Bite-Sized
- Eaten with a fork or spoon, soft, tender and moist throughout without separation of thin liquids, biting is not required, chewing is required

Level 7: Regular
- Normal foods of various textures that require the ability to bite and chew

Hydration is also a challenge for clients with dysphagia; as a result, thickening agents are commonly used to increase a client's fluid intake. Using thickening agents to modify beverages, soups, and pureed foods is both an art and a science. Commercial thickening agents, or prethickened liquids should be used when a speech pathologist orders thickened liquids for a client. Only someone who has had training on the use of thickeners should mix them into food products because thickeners may:

- Become thicker with time.
- Add significant carbohydrate kilocalories to clients' diets.
- React differently in various foods; precise measurements are essential.
- Affect palatability of the thickened item.

In addition, being aware that some foods, such as ice cream and gelatin, change their consistency at body temperature is important, and so is following recipes and mixing complementary flavors. Each client needs his or her diet highly individualized. A preprinted sheet of dos and don'ts is of limited usefulness for many clients. A nurse, speech therapist, occupational therapist, and registered dietitian may collectively devote many sessions to the developing individualized diet plans and determining the best positions for clients during feeding times.

(continued)

BOX 9-1 ■ Dietary Treatment for Dysphagia—cont'd

The nurse is an essential part of the team because he or she is in constant contact with the client. The nurse can monitor the diet's implementation and identify any issues or problems that may occur.

Signs and symptoms of dysphagia include the following:
- "Gurgly" voice
- Coughing or choking with food and fluid intake
- Nasal regurgitation
- Pocketing of food in cheeks
- Drooling
- Difficulty in initiating a swallow
- Excessive chewing
- Poor tongue control
- Poor lip closure
- Lack of body position control
- Slurred speech
- Refusal to eat
- Absence of gag reflux
- Excessive time spent eating
- Multiple swallows required to clear a single bolus of food

- Pain on swallowing
- Verbal complaints of food stuck in the throat
- Lack of attention to eating

On observation, these clients may have a documented weight loss, edema, poor skin turgor, and open wounds. These are all signs of poor nutrition.

For the client, safe swallowing includes the following tips:
- Eat slowly.
- Avoid distractions while eating.
- Do not talk while eating.
- Remove loose dentures.
- Sit up while eating.
- Position head correctly.
- Use a teaspoon and take only one-half teaspoon of food or liquids at a time.
- Swallow completely between bites or sips.
- Select foods and fluids of appropriate consistency.

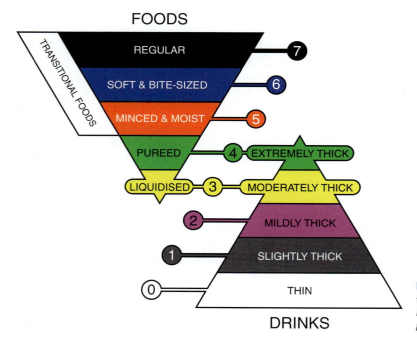

FIGURE 9-1 International Dysphagia Diet definitions for texture-modified foods and liquids. (© *The International Dysphagia Diet Standardisation Initiative 2016 @ http://iddsi.org/framework/.)*

Esophagus

The **esophagus** is a muscular tube about 10 inches long that takes food from the pharynx to the stomach. No digestive action occurs there. Peristalsis forces the bolus into the stomach with the help of mucous secretions. Between the esophagus and the stomach is the **cardiac sphincter** (the first portion of the stomach is called the cardia), which opens to permit passage of food. The sphincter then closes to prevent the backup of stomach contents.

Stomach

The **stomach** is a J-shaped sac that extends from the esophagus to the small intestine. Folds in the mucous membrane, called **rugae,** allow the stomach to expand and to smooth out when full. There is no need to eat constantly, partly because the stomach serves as a reservoir for food—it takes 4 to 6 hours for food to pass completely through to the small intestine. The presence of food in the stomach stimulates the production of the hormone gastrin, which in turn stimulates the production of gastric juice (Tabers, 2017).

Gastric juice, the collective secretions of the stomach, consists of hydrochloric acid, mucus, and the enzymes pepsin, **rennin,** and **gastric lipase.** Many factors influence the rate of gastric emptying, including the amount of gastric juice, meal composition (percent of fat, carbohydrate, or protein), meal particle size, and some hormones. Liquids empty in less time than solids do.

DIGESTIVE ACTION

In the stomach, the chemical digestion of protein begins, and further mechanical digestion takes place. Some water and minerals, certain drugs, and alcohol are absorbed in the stomach. Even before food enters the mouth, the sight or smell of it can cause the gastric mucosa to excrete the hormone **gastrin.** This hormone stimulates the secretion of gastric juice so that there is some present in the stomach when the food arrives. Mucus partially protects the stomach's lining from the corrosive effects of gastric juice.

The hydrolysis of protein begins when hydrochloric acid activates and then converts **pepsinogen** to its active form, **pepsin.** A protein molecule consists of hundreds of amino acids joined by **peptide bonds.** Such chains of amino acids linked by peptide bonds are called **polypeptides.** Pepsin breaks down large polypeptides into smaller ones. In infants, the milk protein casein is broken down by the enzyme rennin, which coagulates (curdles) the milk. In addition to activating pepsin, hydrochloric acid destroys harmful bacteria, makes certain minerals such as iron and calcium more absorbable, and maintains the pH (1 to 2) of the gastric juice.

Another enzyme, gastric lipase, breaks down some milk butterfat molecules into smaller ones. This enzyme is most active in infants; the more alkaline environment of an infant's stomach enables gastric lipase to work more effectively than it does in adults.

The mechanical digestion occurring in the stomach comes from the churning action of the stomach's muscular walls. This activity agitates the contents of the stomach, thoroughly mixing the food with gastric juice. In this way, the food is reduced to a semifluid mass of partially digested material called **chyme.** Peristaltic waves push the chyme toward the **pyloric sphincter,** the valve separating the stomach from the small intestine. With each peristaltic wave, a small amount of **chyme** is forced through the pyloric sphincter into the small intestine.

Gastroparesis, delayed gastric emptying, can be caused by a variety of pathologies, including diabetes mellitus, neuropathic disorders, connective tissue diseases, infiltrating diseases, and postsurgical complications. Symptoms of gastroparesis include:

- Nausea
- Vomiting
- Early satiety
- Bloating or fullness
- Abdominal discomfort

Many clients are asymptomatic (no symptoms). Complications of gastroparesis include:

- Fluid and electrolyte abnormalities
- Inadequate nutritional intake
- Weight loss
- Difficult blood glucose control

Dietary treatment includes small feedings, low-fat foods, low-residue foods, and frequent feedings. Gastric motor and sensory function is complex, and the care of clients with gastroparesis is a challenge.

Ileus, a temporary loss of peristalsis, is another common pathology of gastrointestinal motility. Dietary treatment for ileus is nothing by mouth, or NPO, until the problem is resolved medically.

Small Intestine

The **small intestine** is the longest portion of the alimentary canal, approximately 20 feet (610 cm) in length. It extends from the pyloric sphincter of the stomach to the large intestine. The small intestine is looped and coiled in the central part of the abdominal cavity, surrounded by the large intestine. It consists of three parts: the **duodenum** is the first 10 inches, the **jejunum** is the middle 8 feet, and the **ileum** is the last 11 feet. Ninety percent of the digestive action in the alimentary canal and nearly all end-product absorption of digestion occur in the small intestine.

The entry of chyme into the duodenum stimulates the secretion of two hormones, secretin and **cholecystokinin (CCK).** Collectively, these hormones are responsible for the secretion and release of bile and the secretion of pancreatic juice.

Secretin stimulates the production of bile by the liver and the secretion of sodium bicarbonate juice by the pancreas. The bile salts in bile emulsify fats, and sodium bicarbonate juice (which is alkaline) neutralizes the gastric juice that enters the duodenum. This neutralization is necessary to prevent damage to the lining of the duodenum. Mucus secreted by intestinal glands also provides some measure of protection against such damage.

CCK stimulates the contraction of the gallbladder, an action that forces stored bile into the duodenum. It also stimulates the secretion of pancreatic enzymes, which are essential for the breakdown of carbohydrates, fats, and proteins.

Intestinal juice is also secreted in response to the presence of chyme in the duodenum. The peristaltic action of the small intestine mixes the bile, the pancreatic juice, and the intestinal juice with the chyme as it moves toward the colon. The collective action of these juices yields the final products of digestion.

DIGESTION OF CARBOHYDRATES

The action of pancreatic and intestinal enzymes completes carbohydrate digestion. Pancreatic **amylase** breaks down any remaining starch into maltose. And the action of three enzymes (maltase, sucrose, and lactase) located in the walls of the small intestine reduces the disaccharides maltose, sucrose, and lactose to monosaccharides. Each of these enzymes is specific for a given disaccharide:

Maltase breaks down maltose to glucose and glucose.
Sucrase breaks down sucrose to glucose and fructose.
Lactase breaks down lactose to glucose and galactose.

Often, low levels of these intestinal enzymes lead to intolerances for the respective disaccharides.

In fact, approximately 65% of the world's population has some degree of lactose intolerance from a lack of the intestinal enzyme lactase (National Institutes of Health, 2017). Clinical Application 9-1 discusses carbohydrate intolerances, including lactose intolerance. Table 9-1 lists food items that are lactose-free, low in lactose, and high in lactose. Table 9-2 contains a lactose-restricted diet with a sample menu.

LACTOSE IN MISCELLANEOUS PRODUCTS. Clients on a lactose-free diet should read all labels carefully to see if milk or milk solids, lactose, or whey have been added to the products. Many toothpastes and over-the-counter medications contain a small amount of lactose. Generally, the amount is very small and is tolerated well.

Lactaid is an over-the-counter product specially designed for individuals with lactose intolerance. Lactaid is a natural enzyme that is available in a tablet form. Some grocery stores also sell milk that has been pretreated with the lactase enzyme. This product will digest 70% of the lactose in milk into glucose and galactose. As a result, most lactose-intolerant persons can drink Lactaid-treated milk or, after consuming the tablets, eat foods that contain lactose and digest the lactose comfortably. Milk treated with Lactaid is slightly sweeter than regular milk. The sweeter

TABLE 9-1   Lactose in Foods

Lactose-Free Foods

Broth-based soups unless made with added whey

Plain meat, fish, poultry, peanut butter

Breads that do not contain milk, dry milk solids, or whey

Cereal, crackers

Fruit, plain vegetables

Desserts made without milk, dry milk solids, or whey

Tofu and tofu products, such as tofu-based ice cream substitute

Nondairy creamers

Low-Lactose Foods (0–2 grams/serving)

Milk treated with lactase enzyme, $1/2$ cup

Sherbet, $1/2$ cup

Aged cheese, 1–2 oz

Processed cheese, 1 oz

Butter or margarine

Commercially prepared foods containing dry milk solids or whey

Some medications and vitamin preparations may contain a small amount of lactose. Generally, the amount is minimal and is tolerated well.

High-Lactose Foods (5–8 grams/serving)

Milk (whole, skim, 1%, 2%, buttermilk, sweet acidophilus), $1/2$ cup

Powdered dry milk (whole, nonfat, buttermilk—before reconstituting), $1/8$ cup

Evaporated milk, $1/4$ cup

Sweetened condensed milk, 3 tbsp

Party chip dip or potato topping, $1/2$ cup

White sauce, $1/2$ cup

Creamed or low-fat cottage cheese, $3/4$ cup

Dry cottage cheese, 1 cup

Ricotta cheese, $3/4$ cup

Cheese food or cheese spread, 2 oz*

Sour cream, $1/2$ cup

Heavy cream, $3/4$ cup

Ice cream or ice milk, $3/4$ cup

Half and half, $1/2$ cup

Yogurt, $1/2$ cup†

*Lactose content is higher than that of aged cheese and of processed cheese because of the addition of whey powder and dry milk solids.
†Yogurt may be tolerated better than foods with similar lactose content because of hydrolysis of lactose by bacterial lactase found in the culture. Tolerance may vary with the brand and processing method.

CLINICAL APPLICATION   9-1

Intolerances

Some individuals are deficient in the enzyme lactase and are unable to digest lactose into glucose and galactose. The resulting condition is called lactose intolerance.

Lactose intolerance, the most common of these conditions, can be hereditary or secondary to other disease processes involving the small intestine. After eating or drinking milk products, the client commonly experiences these symptoms of lactose intolerance:

- Abdominal cramping and pain
- Loose stools
- Flatulence (gas)

Dietary treatment of lactose intolerance involves three steps:

1. Identifying food items that contain lactose.
2. Eliminating all sources of lactose from the diet.
3. Establishing an individual tolerance level on a trial-and-error basis. The tolerance levels for lactose vary widely.

taste results naturally when lactose is broken into glucose and galactose.

A lactose-restricted diet may be low in calcium, riboflavin, and vitamin D. Clients should be instructed in alternative sources of these nutrients or may need evaluation for supplements.

DIGESTION OF FATS

Fats are emulsified by bile salts in the small intestine before they are digested further. **Emulsification** is the physical

TABLE 9-2   Lactose-Restricted Diet

Description

This diet restricts foods that contain lactose. Soy-milk substitutes are used as a milk replacement. Individual tolerances should be taken into consideration because some clients may tolerate foods low in lactose (see Table 9-1).

Note: All labels should be read carefully for the addition of milk, lactose, or whey.

Indications

This diet is used for the management of clients exhibiting the signs and symptoms of lactose intolerance, Crohn disease, short bowel syndrome, or colitis. Persistent diarrhea and excessive amounts of gas may be lessened by decreasing lactose intake.

Nutritional Adequacy

This diet is low in calcium, riboflavin, and vitamin D. Supplementation may be recommended.

FOOD GROUP	ALLOWED	AVOIDED
Milk	Hard, ripened cheese Ensure® Boost® Ensure Plus® Soy milk Lactaid-treated milk Coffee Rich®	Unripened cheese Fluid milk Powdered milk Milk chocolate Cream Most chocolate drink mixes Most coffee creamers

Breads and cereals	Most water-based bread (French, Italian,
	  Jewish, Graham crackers)
	Ritz crackers without cheese
		Bread to which milk or lactose has been
		  added (check label)

Fruits	Any	None
Vegetables	Fresh, frozen, or canned without milk	Creamed, buttered, or breaded vegetables
Meat	Those not listed under "Avoided" Kosher prepared meat and/or milk products	Breaded or creamed meats, fish, or poultry Most luncheon meats Sausage Frankfurters
Desserts and miscellaneous items	Angel food cake Gelatin desserts Milk-free cookies Popcorn made with milk-free margarine Pretzels Mustard, catsup, pickles	Most commercially made desserts Sherbet Ice cream Toffee Cream candies Most chewing gums

SAMPLE MENU

Breakfast	Lunch/Dinner	
1/2 cup orange juice	3 oz baked chicken	1 slice milk-free bread
1/2 cup cream of wheat	Baked potato	2 tsp milk-free margarine
2 slices whole-grain milk-free bread	1/2 cup carrots	Angel food cake with fresh fruit topping
2 tsp milk-free margarine	Sliced tomato	Coffee
Jelly		
Coffee		
1/2 cup nondairy "creamer"		

breaking up of fats into tiny droplets. In this way, more surface area of the fat is exposed to the chemical action of the enzyme pancreatic lipase. Pancreatic lipase completes the digestion of fats by reducing triglycerides to diglycerides and monoglycerides, fatty acids, and glycerol.

DIGESTION OF PROTEIN

Although hundreds of enzymes are involved in protein digestion, this text reviews only a few of the major ones. The shorter polypeptides, resulting from the stomach's digestive action, are broken down further by pancreatic and intestinal enzymes. Two of the major pancreatic enzymes are **trypsin** and **chymotrypsin,** which have inactive precursors that are activated by other enzymes.

The intestinal wall also secretes a group of enzymes known as **peptidases,** which act on the smaller molecules produced by the pancreatic enzymes, reducing them to single amino acids and small peptides, the final products of protein digestion.

Table 9-3 summarizes the digestion of carbohydrates, fats, and proteins by body organ (mouth, stomach, and small intestine) and identifies action as mechanical or chemical.

TABLE 9-3   Summary of Digestion

NUTRIENT	MOUTH AND ESOPHAGUS	STOMACH	SMALL INTESTINE
Carbohydrates yield	Mechanical Mastication Swallowing Peristalsis Mucus Chemical Salivary amylase	Mechanical Peristalsis Mucus Chemical None	Mechanical Peristalsis Mucus Chemical Pancreatic enzymes: pancreatic amylase Intestine enzymes Maltase Sucrase Lactase
Monosaccharides			
Fats yield	Mechanical Mastication Swallowing Peristalsis Mucus Chemical None Lingual lipase in infants	Mechanical Peristalsis Mucus Chemical Gastric lipase†	Mechanical Peristalsis Mucus Gallbladder: bile* Chemical Pancreatic enzymes: pancreatic lipase
Glycerol, fatty acids, and monoglycerides			
Proteins yield	Mechanical Mastication Swallowing Peristalsis Mucus Chemical None	Mechanical Peristalsis Mucus Chemical Rennin Pepsin Hydrochloric acid	Mechanical Peristalsis Mucus Chemical Pancreatic enzymes: trypsin, chymotrypsin Intestinal enzymes: peptidases Mechanical
Amino acids and small peptides			

*Emulsifies fat.
†Digests butterfat only.

Absorption

The end products of digestion move from the gastrointestinal tract into the blood or lymphatic system in a process called **absorption.** The **lymphatic system** transports **lymph** from the tissues to the bloodstream, which is technically part of the circulatory or cardiovascular system. All fluid in the lymphatic system enters the blood after it collects in the thoracic duct, which opens into the subclavian vein. Lymph enters the bloodstream through the subclavian vein. Only after nutrients have been absorbed into either the blood or lymphatic system can the body's cells use them.

The end products of digestion include monosaccharides from carbohydrate digestion, fatty acids and glycerol (and often monoglycerides) from fats, and small peptides and amino acids from protein digestion. Absorption occurs primarily in the small intestine.

Small Intestine

The inner surface of the small intestine has mucosal folds, villi, and microvilli to increase the surface area for maximum absorption (Fig. 9-2). The mucosal folds are like pleats in fabric. On each fold (pleat) are millions of finger-like projections, called **villi.** Each villus has hundreds of microscopic, hair-like projections (resembling bristles on a brush), called **microvilli,** on its surface. The large surface area resulting from this arrangement fosters the movement of nutrients into the blood or lymphatic system. The structure of the mucosa serves as a unit that accomplishes the absorption of nutrients.

Within each villus is a network of blood capillaries and a central lymph vessel called a **lacteal.** The villi absorb nutrients from the chyme by way of these blood and lymph vessels. Monosaccharides, amino acids, glycerol (which is water soluble), minerals, and water-soluble vitamins are absorbed into the blood in the **capillary** network. Because short- and medium-chain fatty acids have fewer carbons in their chain length, they are more water soluble than long-chain fatty acids. Thus, they are absorbed directly into the blood as well.

These water-soluble nutrients, including short- and medium-chain fatty acids, eventually enter into hepatic portal circulation (via the portal vein) and travel to the liver. **Hepatic portal circulation** is a subdivision of the vascular system by which blood from the digestive organs and spleen circulates through the liver before returning to the heart. In the liver, the nutrients are modified according to the body's needs.

Because long-chain fats are not soluble in water and blood is chiefly water, fat-soluble nutrients cannot be absorbed directly into the blood. Instead, fat-soluble nutrients—including

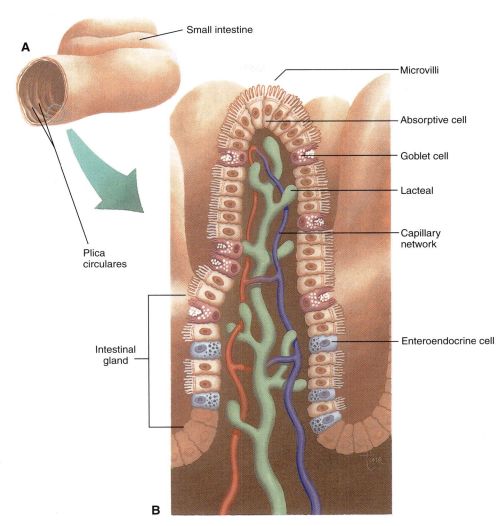

A — Small intestine

Microvilli

Absorptive cell

Goblet cell

Lacteal

Capillary network

Enteroendocrine cell

Plica circulares

Intestinal gland

B

FIGURE 9-2 Cross section of the small intestine. The multiple folds greatly increase the surface area of the small intestine. *(Reprinted from Scanlon, VC, and Sanders, T: Essentials of Anatomy and Physiology. FA Davis, Philadelphia, 2003, with permission.)*

long-chain fatty acids, any monoglycerides remaining from fat digestion, and fat-soluble vitamins—are first combined with bile salts as a carrier. This complex of fat-soluble materials is then absorbed into the cells lining the intestinal wall.

After the fat is absorbed, the bile separates from it and returns to recirculate. Within the intestinal cells, an enzyme reduces any remaining monoglycerides to fatty acids and glycerol. In a process called triglyceride synthesis, the fatty acids, glycerol, and absorbed long-chain fatty acids recombine (within the intestinal cells) to form human triglycerides.

Next, special proteins cover the newly formed triglycerides and any other fat present (such as cholesterol) to form lipoproteins called **chylomicrons,** which are released into the lymphatic system via the lacteals. Remember that the lymphatic system is connected to the blood system. The protein wrapping these packages of fat enables the chylomicrons to move into the blood via the **thoracic** lymphatic duct (and hence into portal blood). In the liver, lipids are also modified to suit the needs of the body before distribution to body cells. Table 9-4 describes some of the nutrient modifications made in the liver.

TABLE 9-4	Metabolic Modifications in the Liver
ENERGY NUTRIENT	MODIFICATION
Carbohydrates	Fructose and galactose changed to glucose, excess glucose converted to glycogen
Lipids	Lipoproteins formed, cholesterol synthesized, triglycerides broken down and built
Amino acids	Nonessential amino acids manufactured, excess amino acids deaminated and then changed to carbohydrates or fats, ammonia removed from the blood, plasma proteins made
Other	Alcohol, drugs, and poisons detoxified

The **ileocecal valve,** which relaxes and closes with each peristaltic wave controls further passage of undigested food. This valve prevents backflow and ensures that chyme remains in the small intestine long enough for sufficient digestion and absorption.

The small intestine's structure decreases in size, or wastes away, during starvation, stress, medically indicated bowel rest, and whenever the small bowel is not used. After 1 week of a protein-deficient diet, the microvilli shorten (Colaizzo-Anas, 2007). Even an individual who is ill with a flulike virus and does not eat for several days may need several additional days to regain his appetite after recovery from the illness. Eating six small low-fat meals daily assists in appetite recovery. See Dollars & Sense 9-1.

Large Intestine

The **large intestine,** also called the **colon,** extends from the ileum (last part of the small intestine) to the anus. When chyme leaves the small intestine, it enters the first portion of the large intestine, the **cecum** (the appendix, an organ with no known function, is attached to the cecum). It then travels slowly through the remaining parts of the large intestine: the ascending colon, the transverse colon, the descending colon, the sigmoid colon, the **rectum,** and the anal canal.

Water is the main substance absorbed by the large intestine. However, the absorption of some minerals and vitamins also occurs in the colon. Up to 80% of the water is extracted in the cecum and the ascending colon and returned to the bloodstream. Vitamins synthesized by intestinal bacteria, including vitamin K and some of the B complexes, are absorbed from the colon. After absorption and digestion have taken place, the remaining waste products are eliminated in the feces through the rectum.

Elimination

Absorption of water into the bloodstream slowly reduces the water content of the material left inside the large intestine, and the waste product (feces) has a solid consistency. Mucus, the only secretion of the large intestine, provides lubrication for the smooth passage of the feces. By the time feces reach the rectum, it consists of 75% water and 25% solids. The solids include cellular wastes, undigested dietary fiber, undigested food, bile salts, cholesterol, mucus, and bacteria.

Indigestible Carbohydrates

The body cannot digest some forms of carbohydrates because it lacks the necessary enzyme to split the appropriate molecule. Some vegetables and legumes contain these indigestible sugars and fibers. Intestinal gas is formed partly in the colon by the decomposition of undigested materials. Foods that may cause intestinal gas in one person may not in another because each person has slightly different bacterial colonies in the colon.

Factors Interfering With Absorption

Malabsorption is the inadequate movement of digested food from the small intestine into the blood or lymphatic system. Malabsorption can cause malnutrition. Table 9-5 lists factors that interfere with the absorption of nutrients. Note in the table that many diseases, medications, and some medical treatments have a negative impact on the absorption of nutrients. Clinical Application 9-2 discusses surgical removal of all or part of the alimentary canal and the effect on absorption. Clinical Application 9-3 discusses inadequate absorption.

The cells lining the inside layer of the small intestine have a very short life. The smallest structures are replaced every 2 to 3 days. Although this rapid cell turnover helps to promote healing after injury, it also allows vulnerability to any nutritional deficiency or process that might interfere with cell reproduction. Genomic Gem 9-1 describes celiac

---

Dollars & Sense 9-1

Reintroducing Food After an Illness

Dehydration can be costly if it involves a trip to the emergency department. The cells of the gastrointestinal tract turn over every few days; therefore, if one cannot or will not eat for just a few days, gastrointestinal cell replacement ceases. Among the reasons for not eating are the stomach flu, common cold, a major dental procedure, or childhood illnesses such as measles.

In all these situations, the client will experience some discomfort when food is reintroduced. Symptoms may include abdominal cramping and diarrhea. To prevent a costly trip to the emergency department because of dehydration, everyone should consume liquids if at all possible when ill. If emeses (vomiting) prevent intake, introduce liquids first during recovery, not spicy or solid foods. Good liquid choices include the following:

- Popsicles
- Apple juice
- Grape juice
- Cranberry juice
- Broth
- Tea
- Gelatin

TABLE 9-5   Factors Decreasing Absorption

Medications	Antacids
	Laxatives
	Birth control pills
	Anticonvulsants
	Antibiotics
Parasites	Tapeworm
	Hookworm
Surgical procedures	Gastric resections
	Any surgery on the small intestine
	Some surgical procedures on the large intestine
	Infection
Disease states	Tropical sprue
	Gluten-sensitive enteropathy
	Hepatic disease
	Pancreatic insufficiency
	Lactase deficiency
	Sucrase deficiency
	Maltase deficiency
	Circulatory disorders
	Cancers involving the alimentary canal
Medical complications	Effects of radiation therapy
	Chemotherapy

Note: Most of these conditions are discussed in later chapters.

CLINICAL APPLICATION 9-2

Surgical Removal of All or Part of the Alimentary Canal

Clients may need to have a portion of the small intestine surgically removed for a variety of reasons. These clients are frequently at a nutritional risk because they are either permanently or temporarily unable to absorb essential nutrients. In such cases, a nutritional assessment is indicated. In the past, some clients elected to have a portion of the alimentary canal removed to lose weight. This procedure is discussed in Chapter 16.

CLINICAL APPLICATION 9-3

Inadequate Absorption

Visually inspecting a client's feces can confirm a suspicion of poor digestion or absorption. Large chunks of food indicate a problem with digestion. A large amount of liquid or near-liquid stools suggests poor absorption. A simple question directed to the client, such as "Are your stools formed?" can provide some information. Sometimes, however, a client's concept of normal may be different from the health-care provider's.

GENOMIC GEM 9-1

Celiac Disease

Celiac disease is also known as celiac sprue, nontropical sprue, and **gluten-sensitive enteropathy.** It is an immune response to gluten, a protein found in wheat, rye, and barley. Oats may also be problematic if they were grown in soil previously planted with wheat, rye, or barley. In the United States, crop rotation is a common practice. Individuals with celiac disease suffer from a wide variety of nutritional problems.

Gluten is mainly found in foods but may also be found in medicines, vitamins, and lip balms. It is a digestive disease, affecting 1 in 133 people in the United States or 1% of the population. It damages the small intestine and interferes with absorption of nutrients from food. Celiac disease is a genetically determined condition. Some grain proteins cause an autoimmune response that damages the lining of the small intestine, causing damage to, or destroying of, the villi and malabsorption of nutrients (National Institutes of Health, 2012a, 2012b; Beyond Celiac, 2017). This effect may be related to an allergic reaction and can be either severe or mild. In the severe form, the loss of intestinal mucosa causes malnutrition by impairing the intestine's ability to absorb nutrients, including carbohydrates, proteins, fats, and fat-soluble vitamins.

Lactose intolerance is common in clients with celiac disease. Because the mucosa of the small intestine is damaged, there is a resulting decrease in lactase, an intestinal enzyme that helps digest lactose from milk.

Treatment of celiac combined with lactose intolerance involves using a lactose-free, gluten-free diet. This is a complex diet for a dietitian to plan and for the client to follow. Clients benefit from being kept on the lactose-free restriction only until intestinal cell regeneration occurs, often between 6 months to a year but can take up to 2 years (Ojetti et al, 2007).

Because untreated celiac disease results in intestinal villous damage and malabsorption, nutritional assessment to prevent and treat malnutrition and iron deficiency anemia is imperative (Academy of Nutrition and Dietetics, 2013). See Table 9-6 for lists of foods containing gluten, including several prepared foods containing thickened sauces. For a positive outcome, the client on a gluten-restricted diet must have extensive teaching. Table 9-7 lists products that can be substituted for flour in many recipes.

TABLE 9-6 Gluten-Restricted Diet

Description
This diet is free of cereals that contain gluten: wheat, oats, rye, and barley. Oats may be included in the diet if the oats are guaranteed to be gluten-free.

Indications
This diet is used to treat the primary intestinal malabsorption found in celiac disease.

Adequacy
Kilocalorie (energy) intake may be inadequate to replace previous weight loss. This diet may not meet the recommended dietary allowances for B-complex vitamins, especially thiamin. Iron intake may be inadequate for the premenopausal woman.

FOOD GROUPS	FOODS THAT CONTAIN GLUTEN	FOODS THAT MAY CONTAIN GLUTEN	FOODS THAT DO NOT CONTAIN GLUTEN
Beverage	Cereal beverages (e.g., Postum®), malt, Ovaltine®, beer, and ale	Commercial* chocolate milk, cocoa mixes, other beverage mixes, dietary supplements	Coffee, tea, decaffeinated coffee, carbonated beverages, chocolate drinks made with pure cocoa powder, wine, distilled liquor

(continued)

TABLE 9-6   Gluten-Restricted Diet (Continued)

FOOD GROUPS	FOODS THAT CONTAIN GLUTEN	FOODS THAT MAY CONTAIN GLUTEN	FOODS THAT DO NOT CONTAIN GLUTEN
Meat and meat substitutes		Meat loaf and patties, cold cuts and prepared meats, stuffing, breaded meats, cheese foods and spreads; commercial soufflés, omelets, and fondue; soy protein meat substitutes	Pure meat, fish, fowl, egg, cottage cheese, peanut butter
Fat and oils		Commercial salad dressing and mayo, gravy, white and cream sauces, nondairy creamer	Butter, margarine, vegetable oil
Milk	Milk beverages that contain malt	Commercial chocolate milk	Whole, low-fat, and skim milk; buttermilk
Grains and grain products	Bread, crackers, cereal, and pasta that contain wheat, oats (if not gluten free), rye, malt, malt flavoring, graham flour, Durham flour, pastry flour, bran, or wheat germ; barley; millet; pretzels; communion wafers	Commercial seasoned rice and potato mixes	Specially prepared breads made with wheat starch,† rice, potato, or soybean flour or cornmeal; pure corn or rice cereals; hominy grits; white, brown, and wild rice; popcorn; low-protein pasta made from wheat starch
Vegetables		Commercially seasoned vegetable mixes; commercial vegetables with cream or cheese sauce; canned baked beans	All fresh vegetables; plain commercially frozen or canned vegetables
Fruits		Commercial pie fillings	All plain or sweetened fruits; fruit thickened with tapioca or cornstarch
Soup	Soup that contains wheat pasta; soup thickened with wheat flour or other gluten-containing grains	Commercial soup, broth, and soup mixes	Soup thickened with cornstarch, potato rice or soybean flour; pure broth
Desserts	Commercial cakes, cookies, and pastries	Commercial ice cream and sherbet	Gelatin; custard; fruit ice; specially prepared cakes, cookies, and pastries made with gluten-free flour or starch; pudding and fruit filling thickened with tapioca, cornstarch, or arrowroot flour
Sweets		Commercial candies, especially chocolates	
Miscellaneous		Ketchup, prepared mustard, soy sauce, commercially prepared meat sauces and pickles, vinegar, flavoring syrups (syrups for pancakes or ice cream)	Monosodium glutamate, salt, pepper, pure spices and herbs, yeast, pure baking chocolate or cocoa powder, carob, flavoring extracts, artificial flavoring

SAMPLE MENU

Breakfast	Lunch/Dinner
½ cup orange juice	Chicken breast
Cocoa Puffs®, Sugar Pops®, Puffed Rice®	Baked potato
2 slices gluten-free bread	½ cup broccoli
1 poached egg	Lettuce/tomato salad
1 cup milk	French dressing
2 tsp margarine	Sour cream
Jelly	½ cup milk
	Cornstarch pudding

*The terms *commercially prepared* and *commercial* are used to refer to partially prepared foods purchased from a grocery or food market and to prepared foods purchased from a restaurant.

†*Wheat starch may contain trace amounts of gluten. Avoid if not tolerated.*

Note: Medications may contain trace amounts of gluten. A pharmacist may be able to provide information on the gluten content of medications.

TABLE 9-7	Gluten-Free Substitutions for 2 Tablespoons of Wheat Flour
3 tsp cornstarch	
3 tsp potato starch	
3 tsp arrowroot starch	
3 tsp quick-cooking tapioca	
3 tbsp white or brown rice flour	

disease, in which ingestion of gluten causes an autoimmune response that damages the lining of the small intestine.

Gut failure describes a situation in which the small intestine fails to absorb nutrients properly. Symptoms of gut failure include:

- Diarrhea
- Malabsorption
- Poor response to oral feedings

A vicious cycle starts when the cells lining the small intestine fail to reproduce because they do not have the necessary nutrients for cell replacement. The result is chronic diarrhea caused by malabsorption. In turn, the malabsorption leads to malnutrition, which prevents cell reproduction (see Fig. 9-3).

Steatorrhea

Some diseases and medications result in the malabsorption of fat. In these conditions, clients have **steatorrhea**, or fat in the stools. In many cases, the inhibition of pancreatic lipase, an enzyme necessary for the digestion of fats, causes the condition. Treatment typically involves using medications and decreasing dietary fat.

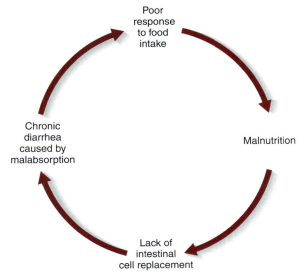

FIGURE 9-3 "Gut failure." Gut failure is a self-perpetuating cycle. Poor response to food intake leads to poor intestinal cell regeneration, which leads to chronic diarrhea caused by malabsorption.

Food Allergies

A food **allergy** is sensitivity to a food that does not cause a negative reaction in most people. Clients commonly use the term **food allergy** as a generic term that encompasses a broad range of symptoms triggered by certain foods. The medical community reserves the term to immunologically mediated abnormal reactions to foods that are life-threatening.

A true allergy requires meticulous avoidance of the implicated food to minimize the risk of potentially life-threatening reactions. Avoidance includes:

- No eating
- No touching
- No smelling

Individuals may be genetically predisposed to a food allergy.

Some food allergies may be due to an alteration in absorption. The susceptible person absorbs a part of a food before it has been completely digested. The incomplete digestion of protein in particular is responsible for many allergic reactions. Box 9-2 provides a list of food allergy triggers.

Metabolism

After digestion and absorption, nutrients are carried by the blood (usually after being modified in the liver cells) to all cells of the body. After entry into the cells, the nutrients from food undergo many chemical changes, which result in either the release of energy or the use of energy.

Metabolism is the sum of all chemical and physical processes continuously going on in living organisms, comprising both anabolism and catabolism. Catabolic reactions usually result in the release of energy. Anabolic reactions require energy.

Catabolic Reactions

In the cells, glucose, glycerol, fatty acids, and amino acids can be broken down even further. These nutrients are held together by bonds that require energy to form and that,

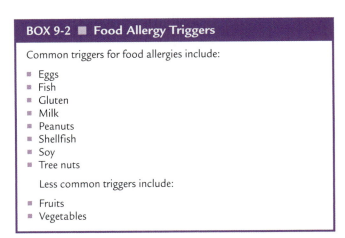

BOX 9-2 ■ Food Allergy Triggers

Common triggers for food allergies include:

- Eggs
- Fish
- Gluten
- Milk
- Peanuts
- Shellfish
- Soy
- Tree nuts

Less common triggers include:

- Fruits
- Vegetables

when broken, release energy. The breakdown of the fuel-producing nutrients yields carbon dioxide, water, heat, and other forms of energy. Eventually, the carbon dioxide is exhaled, and the water becomes part of the body fluids or is eliminated in urine. Fifty percent or more of the total potential energy usually is lost as heat. The remaining available energy is temporarily stored in the cells as adenosine triphosphate (ATP).

ATP, a high-energy compound that has three phosphate groups in its structure, is available in all cells. Practically speaking, ATP is the storage form of energy for the cells because each cell has enzymes that can initiate the hydrolysis (breakdown through the addition of water) of ATP. In this reaction, one or more phosphate groups split off and subsequently release energy. If one phosphate group is removed, the result is ADP (adenosine diphosphate) plus phosphate.

Many steps are involved in the catabolic process responsible for the release of this energy. These steps require one or more of the following agents: enzymes, coenzymes, or hormones. Some vitamins and minerals act as coenzymes. Oxygen is also necessary for the full release of any potential energy. The addition of oxygen to the reaction is called **oxidation.** During the many steps that occur, energy is released little by little and stored as ATP.

The breakdown process includes the formation of intermediate chemical compounds such as **pyruvate** (pyruvic acid) and **acetyl CoA.** Acetyl CoA can be broken down further by entering a series of chemical reactions known as the **Krebs cycle** or the TCA (tricarboxylic acid) cycle. Figure 9-4 is a simplified schematic of the steps involved in the release of energy by the cells.

Storage of Excess Nutrients

If the cells do not have immediate energy needs, the excess nutrients are stored. Glucose is stored as glycogen in liver and muscle tissue; surplus amounts are converted to fat. Glycerol and fatty acids are reassembled into triglycerides and stored in adipose tissue. Amino acids are used to make body proteins; any excess is deaminated (stripped of nitrogen) and ultimately used for glucose formation or stored as fat. If energy is not available from food, the cells will seek energy in those body stores. Fat cannot be used to meet the body's need for glucose; however, protein can be converted into glucose. If carbohydrate intake is inadequate, the body will break down lean body mass (protein stores) to meet its glucose need.

Anabolic Reactions

Once immediate energy needs have been met, cells utilize nutrients as needed for growth and repair of body tissue. The cellular supply of ATP is used first. When this instant energy source is exhausted, glycogen and fat stores are used. In addition to building up body protein, other anabolic

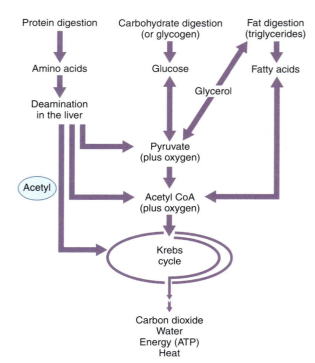

FIGURE 9-4 Energy production in the cells. Energy is released bit by bit during the further breakdown of amino acids, glucose, glycerol, and fatty acids.

reactions include the recombination of glycerol and fatty acids to form triglycerides and the formation of glycogen from glucose.

Excretion of Waste

Materials of no use to the cells become waste that is eliminated through excretion. Solid waste and some liquid is disposed of in the feces. The digestive system needs assistance from other body systems in the disposal of nonsolid waste. The lungs dispose of gaseous waste. Most liquid waste is sent first to the kidneys and then to the **bladder** to be eliminated in the urine. Some liquid waste is disposed of by the skin through perspiration.

Carbon dioxide (CO_2) is a gas that is eliminated through the lungs each time one exhales. The amount of carbon dioxide exhaled depends on the type of fuel (lipid, protein, or carbohydrate) or the source of fuel that the body is currently burning for energy. For example, more CO_2 is produced when carbohydrates are utilized than when protein or fat are used.

The skin removes some of the liquid waste in the form of perspiration or water, and some is excreted in the feces. The kidneys eliminate most of the excess water, sodium, hydrogen, and urea. **Urea** is synthesized in the liver from the nitrogen resulting from the breakdown of amino acids. Some water is also removed from the body each time one exhales.

KEYSTONES

- The cell is the ultimate destination for the nutrients in food.
- Digestion is the process through which food is broken down for use by cells: carbohydrates are broken down to monosaccharides, fats are reduced to glycerol and fatty acids, and proteins are split to yield amino acids.
- Secretions from the salivary glands, stomach, small intestine, liver, and pancreas assist in chemical digestion.
- Absorption refers to the movement of food from the gastrointestinal tract into the blood and lymphatic systems.
- Metabolism involves anabolism and catabolism. The liver plays a major role in metabolism.
- Energy is released little by little from the end products of digestion in a series of chemical reactions.

- Energy nutrients not needed immediately by the cells are stored as glycogen and adipose tissue.
- The human body cannot convert fat into glucose, but it can convert protein into glucose.
- The metabolism of food produces waste. Waste products are released from the body in feces, urine, perspiration, and exhaled air.
- Many ailments and diseases, including malabsorption, disaccharide intolerances, allergies, and gluten-sensitive enteropathy, are related to the structure and function of the gastrointestinal system.

CASE STUDY 9-1

Mr. H is 25 years old, 6 feet tall, and weighs 170 lb (dressed without shoes). He has a medium frame, as determined by measuring his wrist circumference. Mr. H has been admitted to the hospital for an elective arthroscopic (surgical procedure) on his right knee. During the nursing admission process, Mr. H complained of gas pains and frequent loose stools. He stated that he does not avoid any particular foods and has a healthy appetite. He claims to drink about 3 cups of milk each day. The client complains of losing 5 lb during the previous month. Mr. H uses the restroom twice during the interview to "move his bowels." The second time you inspect the stool. The client's stool is loose and unformed.

The next day you note that a diagnosis of lactose intolerance has been made. A lactose-restricted diet is ordered.

The following nursing care plan originates on the day the client is admitted. The physician uses the information collected from the nurse in making his or her diagnosis. Please note that the client has already met the first desired outcome and part of the second; the outcomes have been charted. The client has not met the third desired outcome.

CARE PLAN

Subjective Data
Client complains of gas pains and loose stools. Client states that he does not avoid any particular foods. He drinks milk.

Objective Data
Client observed to use the restroom twice in 9 minutes to defecate. Visual inspection shows loose and unformed stool.

Analysis
Diarrhea related to client's complaints of loose unformed stools as evidenced by the client's need to use the restroom twice in a 9-minute period and by direct observation of one loose and unformed stool.

Plan

DESIRED OUTCOMES EVALUATION CRITERIA	ACTIONS/ INTERVENTIONS	RATIONALE
The client will assist in ruling out causes for his loose stools and report his signs and symptoms to the nurse.	Teach the client to observe and record the pattern, onset, frequency, characteristics, amount, time of day, and precipitating events related to occurrence of diarrhea.	Observation and documentation of the client's response to these factors will assist in determining the cause of his loose stools.

(Continued on the following page)

DESIRED OUTCOMES EVALUATION CRITERIA	ACTIONS/ INTERVENTIONS	RATIONALE
	Refer client to the dietitian to determine usual food intake and nutritional status.	
	Determine exposure to recent environmental contaminants, such as drinking water, food-handling practices, and proximity to others who are ill.	
	Review drug intake for medications affecting absorption (see Table 9-5).	
The client will eliminate causative factors at once after these factors have been determined.	Follow through with the elimination of causative factors, restrict intake if necessary, and note change in drug therapy, if any.	Elimination of the causative factors should decrease the frequency of loose, unformed stools. The client needs to be instructed on the relationship of his or her diarrhea to causative factors.
The client will have formed stools within 24 hours after the causative factors have been eliminated.	Document stool consistency.	Whenever possible, an objective measure should be used to evaluate the success of any client intervention. Stool consistency is an objective measure for treatment response to diarrhea and malabsorption.
If he or she is willing, refer the client to the registered dietitian.		

TEAMWORK 9-1

DIETITIAN'S NOTE

The following Dietitian's Notes are representative of the documentation found in a client's medical record. The SOAP acronym refers to subjective and objective information, assessment, and plan. Subjective is what the client reports. Objective is what has been previously documented, such as doctor's diagnosis, laboratory information, results of diagnostic procedures, and measurements. Assessment is the interviewer's interpretation of the subjective and objective information combined. Dietitians may chart the nutrition diagnosis here. Plan is action or actions the provider intends to do as a result of the assessment.

Subjective: *Client states that he has no previous knowledge of food- and nutrition-related recommendations. States that he feels much better after milk restriction. Client expressed interest in learning more about diet. Formerly client drank three glasses of milk per day. He is concerned about calcium and vitamin D deficiencies. He misses eating soft and fresh cheese. Client claims a recent 5-pound weight loss that he attributes to frequent loose stools.*

Objective: *Prescribed diet (Rx) = lactose-restricted diet; medical diagnosis (Dx) = lactose intolerance*

Assessment: *Food- and nutrition-related knowledge deficit related to weight loss and loose stools as evidenced by client statements that he has no prior exposure to lactose-restricted diet and cessation of loose stools 24 hours after the diet was started. Oral and written instructions were provided. Special emphasis was placed on food sources of calcium and vitamin D that are low in lactose. Client demonstrated an understanding of the diet by verbally planning a lactose-free menu for one diet without error.*

Plan: *Recommend a calcium and vitamin D supplement. Client instructed to call the outpatient dietitian with questions. The phone number was provided. Follow-up visit in 1 week.*

CRITICAL THINKING QUESTIONS

1. The client asks you how long he will need to follow this diet and whether he will ever be able to reintroduce milk to his diet. What do you tell him?

2. What would you tell the client if the diet were only partially effective in controlling the diarrhea?

CHAPTER REVIEW

1. An appropriate snack for a child on a gluten-free diet would be:
   1. Crackers and peanut butter
   2. Half of a cheese sandwich
   3. Potato chips and an oatmeal cookie
   4. Rice cakes and a banana

2. Solid body waste is stored in the:
   1. Large intestine
   2. Gallbladder
   3. Small intestine
   4. Stomach

3. Gaseous waste is expelled:
   1. In the urine
   2. In the feces
   3. Through the lungs
   4. Through the skin

4. The end products of protein digestion are:
   1. Glycerol and fatty acids
   2. Amino acids
   3. Fatty acids
   4. Monosaccharides

5. A food commonly responsible for an allergic reaction is:
   1. Chicken
   2. Peanuts
   3. Rice
   4. Carrots

CLINICAL ANALYSIS

1. The nurse is visiting Mr. D, who is receiving home health care. His caregiver is concerned that Mr. D chokes on liquids but swallows semisolid food well. Which of the following actions by the nurse would be the most appropriate?
   a. Recommend a soft diet.
   b. Recommend a fluid restriction.
   c. Refer Mr. D to a speech pathologist.
   d. First, advise client to drink thickened liquids and then refer to both a speech therapist and then a registered dietitian.

2. Brenda, a 3-year-old, has been admitted to the pediatric unit with a diagnosis of celiac disease. The doctor ordered a gluten-free diet. Which of the following meals would be compatible with the diet order?
   a. Goulash, green beans, and milk
   b. Hamburger on bun, French fries, and a chocolate shake
   c. Tomato soup, grilled cheese, applesauce, and a cookie
   d. Baked chicken, baked potato, sour cream, green beans, peaches, and milk

3. Mr. P is on a low-fat diet (20 grams) to control his steatorrhea. An appropriate snack would be:
   a. Fruit
   b. Nuts
   c. Cheese
   d. Cookies

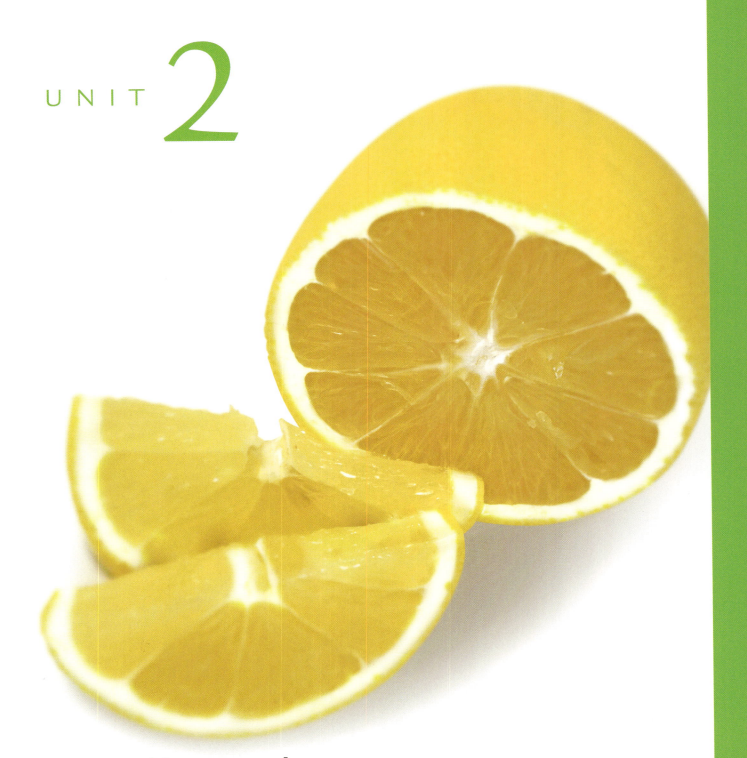

UNIT 2

Family and Community Nutrition

CHAPTER 10

Life Cycle Nutrition: Pregnancy and Lactation

LEARNING OBJECTIVES

After completing this chapter, the student should be able to:

- Compare the nutritional needs of a pregnant woman with those of a nonpregnant woman of the same age.
- Contrast the nutritional needs of a pregnant adolescent with those of a pregnant adult.
- Explain why folic acid intake is critical for women of childbearing age.
- Identify substances to be avoided by pregnant and breastfeeding women.
- Discuss the dietary treatment of common problems of pregnancy.
- List three advantages that breastfeeding confers on the mother.

The needs for many nutrients change at different stages of life. Human beings are most vulnerable to the impact of poor nutrition during periods of rapid growth. This chapter focuses on the period of most rapid growth, that of the unborn child. If the essential nutrients are not present to support growth during that critical time, permanent damage to tissues and organs can occur.

Nutrition During Pregnancy

An expectant mother's nutritional status can affect the outcome of pregnancy. For example, during the first month of **gestation,** the mother must be well nourished so that the **placenta** that forms will be healthy. Because the entire **embryo** and **fetus's** major body organs form within 2 to 3 months of conception, nutrition during this time is critical to the health of the child. Required nutrients come from the mother's diet or body stores.

The placenta is not just a passive conduit for nutrients, however. The placenta performs multiple functions that are essential for fetal survival, growth, and development. These functions include transport of gases, nutrients, and waste products. The placenta also provides a barrier to the transfer of some substances such as maternal red blood cells and bacteria.

After the birth and weaning of a child, the mother needs time to rebuild her nutrient stores. Research has demonstrated that pregnancies that are less than 18 months apart are associated with higher risks of infants being born premature, of **low birth weight (LBW).** Whether related to birth spacing or not, these complications are not evenly distributed throughout the population. A significant association has been demonstrated for black women to be at a higher risk for having an infant who is delivered of LBW,

with 13% of black infants being born with LBW annually (March of Dimes, 2014). The best action an expectant mother can take for her unborn child is to enter the pregnancy with good nutrient stores and to consume a well-balanced diet while pregnant. She must also avoid harmful substances, such as alcohol and contraindicated drugs, including over-the-counter and prescription preparations.

From **implantation** to birth, the fertilized **ovum** (which weighs less than 100 mcg) develops into an infant who weighs about 3.4 kilograms (7.5 pounds) on average. During this period of rapid growth and development, the mother needs additional nutrients, including kilocalories, protein, and certain vitamins and minerals.

Energy Needs

For dietary reference intakes (DRIs) for macronutrients, see Appendix A. For digestible carbohydrate and protein DRIs, see Table 10-1.

Increased energy is needed to sustain the mother and for the development of the fetus and the placenta. From the fourth through the sixth month, the second trimester, much of this energy supports the growth of the uterus (womb) and other maternal tissues. During the seventh through ninth months, the third trimester, much of the energy supports the fetus and the placenta. To meet this increased metabolic workload and to spare protein for tissue building, a pregnant woman needs an extra:

- 340 kilocalories per day in the second trimester
- 452 kilocalories per day in the third trimester

On average the pregnant woman will need to increase daily caloric intake by approximately 300 kilocalories per day.

TABLE 10-1 RDAs and AIs for Selected Minerals and Energy Nutrients

LIFE STAGE GROUP	CALCIUM (MG/DAY)	FLUORIDE* (MG/DAY)	IODINE (MCG/DAY)	IRON (MG/DAY)	ZINC (MG/DAY)	CARBOHYDRATE (G/DAY)†	PROTEIN (G/DAY)
Pregnancy							
<19 years	**1,300**	3	220	27	12	175	71
19–50 years	**1,000**	3	220	27	11	175	71
Lactation							
<19 years	**1,300**	3	290	10	13	210	71
19–50 years	**1,000**	3	290	9	12	210	71

AI, adequate intake; RDA, recommended dietary allowance.
*AI.
†Based on its role as primary energy source for the brain.
Values in boldface indicate RDA; AIs are in light face.
Source: https://www.ncbi.nlm.nih.gov/books/NBK56068/table/summarytables.t4/?report=objectonly
https://www.ncbi.nlm.nih.gov/books/NBK56068/table/summarytables.t3/?report=objectonly

The increase in calories should be from high-nutrient-density foods such as fruits, vegetables, lean protein, and whole grains.

Fat Needs

For DRIs for fat, see Appendix A.

Long-chain polyunsaturated fatty acids (LC-PUFAs) have demonstrated crucial importance in fetal growth and the development of the fetal retina and brain (Christian et al, 2016). Fatty acids accumulate in the fetal brain rapidly during the third trimester of gestation and during the first postpartum month (Giuseppe, Roggi, & Cena, 2014). These essential fatty acids can be supplied directly from the diet or synthesized from the omega-6 fatty acids and omega-3 fatty acid families. Because of the importance of DHA to fetal brain development, it is recommended that pregnant women consume 200 mg each day (March of Dimes, 2016). See Chapter 18 for more information on omega-3 fatty acids.

The adequate intakes (AIs) for omega-6 fatty acids (linoleic acid) and omega-3 fatty acids (alpha-linolenic acid) are increased during pregnancy and lactation compared to amounts designated for other women.

Food sources of linoleic acid are the following oils:

- Corn
- Safflower
- Sunflower

Alpha-linolenic acid is found in these oils:

- Canola
- Flaxseed
- Soybean
- Walnut (see Chapter 18)

Important sources of DHA are fish and shellfish, because conversion by the body is not required. Consequently, a pregnant woman's diet should contain oils as well as seafood within the limits described in the section Certain Species and Amounts of Fish.

Protein Needs

For DRIs for protein, see Appendix A and Table 10-1.

Protein is required to build fetal **tissue.** The mother also needs adequate protein for growth of her tissues. Her blood volume increases in anticipation of blood loss at delivery. Her breasts develop in preparation for lactation. Her uterus enlarges and contains a sac filled with **amniotic fluid.** For those reasons, the recommended dietary allowance (RDA) for protein for pregnant women is 54% more than for nonpregnant women or 71 grams.

Protein intake becomes a hazard to the fetus when the mother has phenylketonuria and is eating inappropriately. The goal of treatment with phenylketonuria is to maintain phenylalanine levels within safe limits. The limit in pregnant women is 120 to 360 µmol/L to ensure normal growth and prevent mental retardation in the fetus. All women should be asked directly if they have ever had a special diet prescription. The health-care provider should investigate further when a woman cites a history of troubled pregnancies, congenital abnormalities, an infant with intellectual disabilities, spontaneous abortion, or stillbirth.

Vitamin Needs

Pregnant women have an increased need for some vitamins. They must avoid taking excessive amounts of others because of potential hazard to the fetus.

Water-Soluble Vitamins

For DRIs for vitamins during pregnancy and lactation, see Appendix A. For selected vitamins during pregnancy and lactation, see Table 10-2.

A pregnant woman's RDA for vitamin C is 13% higher than that of a nonpregnant woman. Vitamin C is necessary for collagen formation and tissue building.

The RDAs for all the B vitamins except biotin are modestly increased for pregnancy. The increased requirements are understandable—particularly for thiamin, niacin, and

TABLE 10-2   RDAs for Selected Vitamins for Pregnancy and Lactation

LIFE STAGE GROUP	VITAMIN A (MCG/DAY)	VITAMIN C* (MG/DAY)	VITAMIN D (MCG/DAY)	VITAMIN E (MG/DAY)	THIAMIN (MG/DAY)	NIACIN (MG/DAY)[†]	VITAMIN B$_6$ (MG/DAY)	FOLATE[†] (MCG/DAY)	VITAMIN B$_{12}$ (MCG/DAY)
Pregnancy									
<19 years	750	80	15	15	1.4	18	1.9	600	2.6
19–50 years	770	85	15	15	1.4	18	1.9	600	2.6
Lactation									
<19 years	1,200	115	15	19	1.4	17	2.0	500	2.8
19–50 years	1,300	120	15	19	1.4	17	2.0	500	2.8

RDA, recommended dietary allowance.
*Smokers require an additional 35 mg/day of vitamin C.
†Women able to become pregnant should consume 400 micrograms of synthetic folic acid from fortified foods/supplements besides food folate.
Source: https://www.ncbi.nlm.nih.gov/books/NBK56068/table/summarytables.t2/?report=objectonly

vitamin B$_6$, which are coenzymes involved in energy metabolism. See the section on hyperemesis gravidarum for information specific to thiamin deficiency. Two other B vitamins are of special concern in pregnancy: vitamin B$_{12}$ and folic acid.

VITAMIN B$_{12}$

For DRIs for vitamins during pregnancy and lactation, see Appendix A. For selected vitamins during pregnancy and lactation, see Table 10-2.

The vitamin B$_{12}$ RDA is only slightly increased for pregnant and lactating women. The placenta appears to concentrate vitamin B$_{12}$ because serum levels in the newborn are about twice the maternal levels. Vitamin B$_{12}$ is concentrated and stored in the fetal liver during pregnancy and provides the infant with stores to sustain them for the first several months of life.

Strict vegetarians and vegans are at a higher risk of vitamin B$_{12}$ deficiency (see Chapter 6). Vegetarians need to ensure adequate intake of vitamin B$_{12}$ from fortified foods or supplements. Fortified food and supplements made from cobalamin provide a physiologically active form of the vitamin, whereas products that list only vitamin B$_{12}$ might include nonbioavailable sources. Vitamin B$_{12}$ deficiencies have shown to result in neurological insult to the infant.

FOLIC ACID

For DRIs for vitamins during pregnancy and lactation, see Appendix A. For selected vitamins during pregnancy and lactation, see Table 10-2.

The RDA for folic acid for all women of childbearing potential specifies synthetic folic acid from fortified foods or supplements. In addition, food folate from a varied diet is expected to be consumed.

These recommendations are based on clinical studies that showed that 4 mg of folic acid daily prevented 72% of **neural tube defects (NTDs)** in infants of women who have already delivered a child afflicted with the defect (Demilew & Asres Nigussie, 2017) (see Box 10-1). The Centers for Disease Control and Prevention (CDC) quickly recommended the treatment for such high-risk women beginning folic acid

---

BOX 10-1 ■ Neural Tube Defects: Occurrence, Pathophysiology, and Side Effects of Supplementation

Neural tube defects (NTDs) are the most common preventable type of birth defect in the world, and affect approximately 300,000 children worldwide (CDC, January 11, 2017).

The neural tube is embryonic tissue that develops into the brain and spinal cord. A critical time in the development of this structure is from conception through the fourth week of pregnancy. Interference with normal development at that time produces major congenital defects, including **anencephaly, meningoencephalocele, spina bifida,** and **meningocele.** Unfortunately, the neural tube develops before many women are aware they are pregnant.

As a multifactorial condition, the exact connection of NTDs to folic acid is unclear, but folate is directly or indirectly essential for cell function, division, and differentiation.

---

1 month before conception and continuing until 3 months of pregnancy. Studies have demonstrated that periconceptional consumption of adequate folic acid, of 4 mg daily, can prevent 50% to 70% of NTDs (Centers for Disease Control and Prevention [CDC], 2016).

Despite recommendations for women of childbearing age to increase folic acid intake, most women have not done so. Consequently, folic acid has been added to the enrichment protocol for cereal-grain products in the United States since January 1998; 140 mcg of folic acid has been incorporated into each 100 grams of grain. Studies have demonstrated notable declines in neural tube defects, including spinal bifida, anencephaly, and encephalocele, in countries that have implemented mandatory fortification of grains with folic acid (Atta et al, 2016). Data demonstrate that Hispanic women continue to be at a significantly greater risk for having a baby affected with NTD than non-Hispanic white women and black women, who also have the lowest risk (CDC, 2016). See Genomic Gem 10-1 for more information on risk factors for NTDs.

Although there are strong data that conclusively confirm a decreased incidence in NTD when women consume adequate folic acid before and during pregnancy, data suggest

GENOMIC GEM 10-1

The Genesis of Neural Tube Defects

Most cases of neural tube defects (NTD) occur in women without a history of the disorder, but there is evidence of a genetic component to this multifactorial condition. There is a higher recurrence risk to siblings in families with an NTD child. Because folic acid is so clearly protective, much research has focused on its metabolic pathways. Variants of several folate-related genes have been significantly associated with risk for NTDs.

Among other findings suggesting a genetic component are the following:

- There is a 4-out-of-100 chance of having a baby with NTD if there is a family history and a 1-out-of-10 chance if there are two siblings with NTD (March of Dimes, 2017).
- Ethnic and racial differences in NTD prevalence—Hispanic women continue to have higher rates of NTD than non-Hispanic white women (National Center on Birth Defects and Developmental Disabilities, 2017).
- Other risks that are being studied are maternal diabetes, maternal obesity, maternal hyperthermia, and antiepileptic medications (Mayo Clinic, 2014). While awaiting clear understanding of causality, the ability to prevent approximately 70% of NTDs through the administration of folic acid is a remarkable advance.

that less than 40% of women of childbearing age are actually taking folic acid daily (CDC, 2016). A woman's knowledge of folic acid and its role in preventing NTDs is essential for reducing the risk of NTD. Health-care providers need to increase their efforts to promote adequate folic acid intake among fertile women. Specific target populations include the following:

- Young women
- Hispanic women
- Women with low incomes

Fat-Soluble Vitamins

For DRIs for vitamins during pregnancy and lactation, see Appendix A. For selected vitamins during pregnancy and lactation, see Table 10-2.

The RDA for vitamin E and the AI for vitamin K are the same for pregnant women as for mature, nonpregnant women. Interfering with normal physiology can create problems, however. During normal pregnancy, the placenta transfers limited amounts of vitamin K to the fetus. Significant bleeding problems are rare, but infants are treated with vitamin K at birth (see Chapter 11). Vitamins D and A merit special mention even for normal pregnancies.

VITAMIN D

The same controversy about the adequacy of the AI for vitamin D (see Chapter 7) spills into discussions regarding the needs of pregnant women.

Vitamin D has multiple functions in the growth and development of the fetus, and maternal deficiency can result in impaired fetal skeletal formation and low bone mass, LBW, small-for-gestational-age, and intrauterine growth retardation (Amegah, Klevor, & Wagner, 2017). Attention is being brought to the effects of maternal vitamin D deficiency in relationship to the development and outcomes of the infant. Research is also showing that vitamin D deficiency can result in adverse effects for the mother, including gestational diabetes, bacterial vaginosis, and preeclampsia (Weinert & Silveiro, 2015).

Further research is being done to investigate the current vitamin D recommendations for pregnant women.

VITAMIN A

Vitamin A excess in pregnant women has been related to birth defects. Vitamin A as retinol or retinoic acid in excess of 10,000 IU per day or treatment with **isotretinoin** during the first trimester increases the risk of **retinoic acid syndrome.** The characteristic fetal deformities include the following:

- Small or no ears
- Abnormal or missing ear canals
- Brain malformation
- Heart defects

Three ounces of beef liver may contain 27,000 IU, and 3 oz of chicken liver, 12,000 IU. A pregnant woman who eats liver regularly may consume enough vitamin A to pose a risk to her baby. A well-balanced diet should supply the RDA for pregnant women.

Some prenatal vitamins substitute beta-carotene, which is not associated with birth defects, for preformed vitamin A or omit vitamin A entirely. Table 10-3 lists the RDAs and ULs in micrograms and International Units for vitamin A for pregnancy and lactation. Remember that the conversion to IUs depends on the source (see Clinical Calculation 6-1).

Isotretinoin, a vitamin A metabolite used to treat severe acne, is hazardous to the fetus, with almost a 335% risk of malformations if a woman is exposed to isotretinoin beyond the first 15 days of conception (Wilson, 2016). Despite a pregnancy prevention program started by the manufacturer of isotretinoin in 1988 and subsequent upgrades (one called iPLEDGE), women are still becoming pregnant while taking the drug. Requiring client registration and negative pregnancy tests before each prescription is dispensed have not eliminated the danger to fetuses.

Women of childbearing age taking isotretinoin should adhere to strict contraceptive protocols, including simultaneous use of two reliable methods.

In contrast, vitamin A deficiency (VAD) is a greater problem than toxicity in developing countries. VAD affects both the pregnant woman and the infant. Adverse health consequences are not likely to develop during periods of rapid growth, such as pregnancy, lactation, and infancy (National Institutes of Health, 2016).

TABLE 10-3   **DRIs for Vitamin A During Pregnancy and Lactation**

	RDA		UL	
	Micrograms as RAEs	IUs	Micrograms as Preformed Only	IUs
Pregnancy				
<19 years	750	2,475	2,800	9,240
19–50 years	770	2,541	3,000	9,900
Lactation				
<19 years	1,200	3,960	2,800	9,240
19–50 years	1,300	4,290	3,000	9,900

DRI, dietary reference intakes; IUs, international units; RAEs, retinol activity equivalents; RDA, recommended dietary allowance.

Mineral Needs

For DRIs for minerals during pregnancy and lactation, see Appendix A. For selected minerals during pregnancy and lactation, see Table 10-1.

The trace mineral iron plays a major role in the health of the mother and fetus and therefore appears first in the discussion. Other minerals of special concern in pregnancy are calcium, iodine, fluoride, and zinc.

Iron

For DRIs for minerals during pregnancy and lactation, see Appendix A. For selected minerals during pregnancy and lactation, see Table 10-1.

During pregnancy, the mother's plasma volume increases by about 45% to 50% by the 34th week of gestation, and her red cell mass increases by about 33%. Besides supporting the mother's increased blood volume, iron supports the red blood cells in the fetus, placenta, and umbilical cord. As a result, the net iron cost of a singleton (one fetus) pregnancy is estimated at 1 gram. Even moderate iron-deficiency anemia (IDA) is associated with twice the risk of maternal death.

IDA in pregnancy can result in adverse effects such as preterm delivery and LBW, and severe deficiency can lead to irreversible damage to the central nervous system (Kumar, Dubey, & Khare, 2017).

Fortunately, the body adjusts to limited or abundant iron sources, and iron absorption is enhanced in the second and third trimesters of pregnancy. Rates of iron absorption vary so that women who begin pregnancy:

■ With adequate iron stores, absorb about 10% of ingested iron
■ With low iron stores, absorb about 20%
■ Anemic, absorb about 40%

The RDA for iron for pregnancy assumes an absorption rate of 20%. Prophylactic iron 30 to 60 mg per day is recommended by the World Health Organization for all pregnant women to reduce the risks of maternal anemia and LBW, and preterm birth (World Health Organization, 2017). Even when she takes supplements, a woman's hemoglobin and hematocrit should be monitored regularly.

Lower values are expected during the first and second trimesters because expanding blood volume dilutes the concentration of red blood cells.

Prescribed iron supplements may not be taken. Economic factors or side effects, such as nausea, cramps, gas, and constipation, may influence intake. Although oral iron preparations are best absorbed if taken 1 hour before or 2 hours after meals, individualizing the schedule is better than the client choosing to eliminate the supplement altogether. Iron supplements should be taken as directed. Clinical Application 10-1 illustrates the principle of knowing the client as well as the subject matter.

CLINICAL APPLICATION   10-1

Effective Teaching

Health-care providers must identify the client's learning needs and assess how the client learns best. Examples would be

1. The client will understand the function of iron and why it is important in pregnancy.
   a. Prevention of anemia and complications associated with pregnancy.
   b. Discuss signs and symptoms of anemia.
2. The client will identify foods that are high in iron.
   a. Animal food products such as beef, chicken fish, and eggs, and plant sources such as green leafy vegetables and dried beans.
3. If an iron supplement is required, the client will understand how and when to take.
   a. Take supplement with a vitamin C–containing drink, such as orange juice, for absorption.
   b. Take the supplement 1 hour before or 2 hours after a meal.
   c. A stool softener may be required if constipation develops.
   d. Do not stop taking the iron if symptoms of anemia improve.

Teaching is more than presenting facts, especially when the goal is changed behavior. Local knowledge and cultural perspective are essential to the health-care provider promoting a new health practice.

Calcium

For DRIs for minerals during pregnancy and lactation, see Appendix A. For selected minerals during pregnancy and lactation, see Table 10-1.

Calcium plays an important role in the development of the fetus and in maintaining good health of the mother. Calcium absorption increases during pregnancy and additional calcium is not required, but the RDA for calcium should be obtained during pregnancy and lactation. Throughout pregnancy, approximately 30 grams of calcium is transferred to the fetus, most of it in the third trimester. It is estimated that approximately 5% of maternal bone mass is mobilized during pregnancy and lactation, with the loss reversing after cessation of lactation (Ettinger et al, 2014).

Studies have demonstrated that the use of calcium supplements of at least 1,000 milligrams reduces the risk of hypertension, preeclampsia, maternal death, and LBW infants (Hart, 2014). Deficiency in calcium may result in skeletal and neurologic disorders in the infant and an increased risk of maternal osteoporosis (Ezzell & Castelow, 2014). Chapters 6 and 7 describe the effects and interactions of calcium and vitamin D.

Transient osteoporosis is a rare, self-limiting syndrome typically characterized by hip pain in the third trimester of pregnancy accompanied by radiologic osteopenia; other joints may be affected as well. Etiology is unclear, with the left hip more often involved than the right and bilateral hips affected in 25% to 30% of pregnant women. Usual treatment is supportive during the mean duration of 6 to 8 months.

Iodine, Fluoride, and Zinc

For DRIs for minerals during pregnancy and lactation, see Appendix A. For selected minerals during pregnancy and lactation, see Table 10-1.

As part of thyroid hormones, iodine is essential to the control of metabolism. During the second half of pregnancy, resting energy expenditure increases by as much as 23%. The RDAs for iodine are increased by 46% and 93% for pregnant and lactating women over those of other women. In the United States, a pregnant woman's usual need for iodine is met by the use of iodized salt. Severe maternal deficiency can cause cretinism in the newborn (see Chapter 7).

The fetus begins to develop teeth at the 10th to 12th week of pregnancy. Fluoride crosses the placenta so that the concentration in fetal circulation is one-fourth that of the mother; fluoride is found in fetal bones and teeth. The American Academy of Pediatric Dentistry (2012) does not support the use of prenatal fluoride supplements. The AI for pregnancy and lactation is the same as for nonpregnant women.

Zinc is not mobilized from the mother's tissues. To provide for the fetus, the mother needs regular intake. Sixty percent of the fetal zinc store is acquired during the third trimester and deficiency can have negative effects on the endocrine system, leading to growth failure (Mashad, Sayed, & Elghorab, 2016). The RDAs for pregnant and lactating women are about 50% higher than those for other women. Lean meat from beef chuck roast, 3.5 to 4 ounces, would provide these RDAs.

Water and Weight Gain

Plasma volume during pregnancy expands by about 50%, necessitating a fluid intake of about 9 cups daily.

The recommended weight gain during pregnancy has varied over the years. Clinical Calculation 10-1 shows how to determine a goal for weight gain in pregnancy based on prepregnancy weight. On average, a woman of normal weight should gain 2 to 4 pounds during the first trimester, followed by 1 pound per week for the remainder of the pregnancy. There are charts that can be used to plot weight gain based on prepregnancy BMI. Informational charts and a BMI calculator can be found at: https://www.cdc.gov/reproductivehealth/maternalinfanthealth/pregnancy-weight-gain.htm. Table 10-4 shows the typical distribution of pounds between the baby and the mother's tissues.

Gaining more than recommended is associated with hypertension, preeclampsia, gestational diabetes, and cesarean delivery. Gaining less than recommended is associated with fetal growth retardation, LBW, and increased **perinatal mortality.**

CLINICAL CALCULATION 10-1

Determining Recommended Weight Gain During Pregnancy

Body mass index (BMI) = Weight in kilograms/Height in meters^2
Suppose a woman is 5 ft 4 in. tall and weighs 125 lb.

$$5 \text{ ft } 4 \text{ in.} = 64 \text{ in.}$$
$$1 \text{ m} = 39.371 \text{ in.}$$
$$\frac{64}{39.371} = 1.6 \text{ m}$$
$$\frac{125 \text{ lb}}{2.2 \text{ lb/kg}} = 56.8 \text{ kg}$$
$$\text{BMI} = \frac{56.8}{(1.6)^2} = \frac{56.8}{2.56} = 22.2$$

Looking at the following table, we see that 22.2 is in the normal category. Recommended weight gain for this woman is 25–35 lb.

RECOMMENDED WEIGHT GAIN FOR PREGNANCY

BMI CATEGORY	KILOGRAMS	POUNDS
<18.5 = underweight	12.5–18	28–40
18.5–24.9 = normal	11.5–16	25–35
25–29.9 = overweight	7–11.5	15–25
>30 = obese	5–9	11–20

Short women and women of various racial or ethnic groups should follow the same recommendations. Teenagers who are pregnant should also use BMI as a guide to weight gain.

TABLE 10-4 Here's How It All Adds Up

Baby	7–8 pounds
Amniotic fluid	2 pounds
Placenta	1½ pounds
Increased blood volume	3–4 pounds
Increase fluid volume	3–4 pounds
Increased weight of uterus	2 pounds
Breasts	2 pounds
Mother's fat stores	6–8 pounds
Total	25–35 pounds

Source: Adapted from Mayo Clinic Pregnancy Week by Week (2017).

Studies have demonstrated that overweight or obese women are twice as likely to experience excessive weight gain in pregnancy as normal-weight women (Liu, Wilcox, Whitaker, Blake, & Addy, 2015). It is also noted that African American and lower-income women are at an increased risk of excessive gestational weight gain (Liu et al, 2015).

Meal Pattern

Mature women who become pregnant require relatively few modifications in MyPlate recommendations for adults.

Except for iron, MyPlate recommendations should suffice for healthy women. Healthy People 2020 recommends that women who are capable of becoming pregnant choose food high in heme iron and take an iron supplement as needed. Pregnant women should eat a diet that is varied in fruits, vegetables, lean proteins, and whole grains to ensure adequate nutrient consumption.

Pregnant teenagers need nutrients to provide for their own growth as well as that of the fetus. A client, 16 years old, weighing 120 pounds who is physically active 30 to 60 minutes per day would require additional grains, vegetables, and meat/beans in the second and third trimesters. Clinical Application 10-2 relates the particular hazards of teenage pregnancy.

Women of dissimilar ages, sizes, and lifestyles would require different intakes. Individualized meal planning based on age, height, prepregnancy weight, and activity level is available at https://www.choosemyplate.gov/MyPlate-Daily-Checklist-input.

Careful food selection is critical for all pregnant women but especially for pregnant teens who may have unbalanced diets and for women who restrict or eliminate whole categories of food such as vegetarians. Thorough nutritional assessment, ideally before pregnancy or at least very early in pregnancy, could yield huge dividends by decreasing complications and improving newborns' health. Dollars & Sense 10-1 describes some food assistance programs available to improve nutrition.

Substances to Avoid

While pregnant or nursing, women are urged to limit caffeine intake and to eliminate these items from their diets:

- Alcohol
- Soft cheeses and ready-to-eat meats
- Certain species and amounts of fish
- Undercooked meat and unwashed produce

Serious allergies to nuts and seeds affect less than 1% of the population. See Chapter 11 for information on food allergies. There is no evidence supporting the restriction of foods during pregnancy or lactation to reduce the risk of food allergy development.

Alcohol

A pregnant woman who drinks alcoholic beverages is endangering her baby because alcohol readily crosses the placenta, and the fetus has inadequate enzymes to detoxify it. The amniotic fluid accumulates alcohol and its metabolities, which prolongs fetal exposure (Van Heertum & Rossi, 2017). Moderate alcohol intake increases the risk of miscarriage, preterm birth, stillbirth, and behavioral or cognitive deficits (Dunney, Muldoon, & Murphy, 2015). The fetus is most vulnerable during the first trimester when basic structural development occurs.

First recognized in 1973, **fetal alcohol syndrome (FAS)** is most easily diagnosed between 4 and 14 years of age. FAS has specific diagnostic criteria:

- Three characteristic facial features: smooth philtrum, thin upper lip, and short palpebral fissures (Fig. 10-1)

CLINICAL APPLICATION 10-2

Teenage Pregnancy

The average girl does not reach her full height or attain gynecologic maturity until age 17. When pregnant before that age, she is still growing but has a fetus to nourish as well. Infants born to still-growing adolescents weigh an average of 155 grams (0.3 lb) less than those born to adult women. Rates of spontaneous abortion, preterm delivery, and LBW are higher in growing than in nongrowing adolescents.

Because many pregnant adolescents have low incomes, referral to appropriate sources of assistance is a crucial part of their nutritional care.

Dollars & Sense 10-1

Food Assistance

Supplemental food assistance is available for families in the Supplemental Nutrition Assistance Program **(SNAP)** and for women and children in the **Supplemental Feeding Program for Women, Infants, and Children (WIC).** It provides supplemental foods monthly to low-income pregnant or postpartum women, infants, and children up to age 5. WIC is available in all 50 states plus 40 other territories and jurisdictions. Fifty-three percent of infants born in the United States receive benefits from WIC (U.S. Department of Agriculture [USDA], 2015).

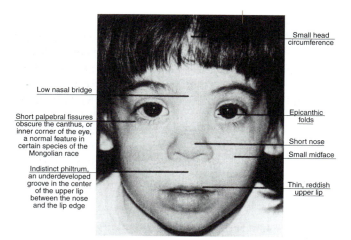

Small head circumference

Low nasal bridge

Short palpebral fissures obscure the canthus, or inner corner of the eye, a normal feature in certain species of the Mongolian race

Epicanthic folds

Short nose

Small midface

Indistinct philtrum, an underdeveloped groove in the center of the upper lip between the nose and the lip edge

Thin, reddish upper lip

FIGURE 10-1 Specific facial signs of fetal alcohol syndrome include microcephaly, or small head size; small eyes and/or short eye openings; and an underdeveloped upper lip with flat upper lip ridges. *(Reprinted from Feldmen, EB: Essentials of Clinical Nutrition. FA Davis, Philadelphia, 1988, p. 164, with permission.)*

- Prenatal and postnatal growth deficits
- Central nervous system abnormalities, such as head circumference at or below the 10th percentile, neurological problems, or functional deficits

In 1996, the term *fetal alcohol spectrum disorder* was introduced to encompass several diagnostic categories covering the wider range of alcohol effects in infants and children that do not meet the criteria for FAS.

Because researchers have not been able to determine safe levels of alcohol during pregnancy, women should be encouraged to abstain. The task of protecting the unborn is formidable. One of the goals of Healthy People 2020 is to increase the percentage of pregnant women abstaining from alcohol use to 98% (Office of Disease Prevention and Health Promotion [ODPHP], 2017). Despite warnings on the effects alcohol can have on fetal development and outcomes, one out of two women of childbearing age drink alcohol and 18% of this group report binge drinking and 10% of pregnant women drink alcohol (CDC, March 7, 2016).

Approximately 50% of pregnancies in the United States are unplanned; for women engaging in risky drinking behaviors and not using effective contraceptive methods, the risk of FAS is increased. Brief interventions by health-care providers have succeeded in reducing such risks (CDC, February 2, 2016). Information on prenatal alcohol screening and intervention program is available at: https://www.samhsa.gov/treatment. In addition, curricular materials for parents, educators, and juvenile justice workers are available at: www.cdc.gov/NCBDDD/fasd/freematerials.html.

Soft Cheeses and Ready-to-Eat Meats

Listeriosis is a bacterial foodborne illness caused by *Listeria monocytogenes*. For the mother, the symptoms of listeriosis tend to be mild and flulike, but the bacteria can be passed via the placenta to the fetus, resulting in spontaneous

abortion, premature delivery, stillbirth, neonatal meningitis, and septicemia (Imanishi et al, 2015).

The organism can withstand freezing, heat, and exposure to alcohol. Outbreaks of listeriosis have been associated with raw or contaminated milk, soft cheeses, smoked seafood, sprouts, and ready-to-eat meats. The CDC estimates that 1,600 people get sick from listeria each year with 260 deaths (December 12, 2016).

The **incubation period** may be 3 to 70 days after a person has eaten the contaminated food. In addition to the general rules for safe food handling, pregnant women should:

- Avoid soft cheeses (feta, Brie, Camembert, blue-veined, and Mexican-style cheese like queso fresco). However, hard cheeses, processed cheeses, cream cheese, cottage cheese, and yogurt may be eaten safely. Eat only cheeses that are labeled as made with pasteurized milk.
- Cook leftover foods or ready-to-eat foods (hot dogs, sausage, deli meats) until steaming hot ($165°$F [$73.9°$C]).
- Not eat refrigerated meat spreads at all or refrigerated smoked seafood without cooking it.
- Not consume unpasteurized milk or foods made from it.
- Refrigerate foods within 2 hours and use leftovers within 3 to 4 days.
- Use a thermometer and keep the refrigerator at $40°$F ($4.4°$C) or lower and the freezer at $0°$F ($-17.8°$C) or lower.

Certain Species and Amounts of Fish

Fish and shellfish can be a major source of **methylmercury**, a widespread environmental neurotoxin that can be harmful to fetal brain development. Because of high levels of mercury in some species of fish (those that grow larger and live longer), the Food and Drug Administration (FDA) and the Environmental Protection Agency have advised pregnant women and women who may become pregnant, nursing mothers, and young children to avoid eating:

- Shark
- Swordfish
- King mackerel
- Tilefish

If chosen as the week's seafood meals, albacore tuna or tuna steak should be limited to 6 ounces per week, whereas up to 12 ounces per week may be consumed of species of seafood with lower amounts of mercury:

- Shrimp
- Canned light tuna
- Salmon
- Pollock
- Catfish

Fish sticks and fish sandwiches at fast food restaurants generally contain species with lower amounts of mercury. Local advisories should be sought to determine the safety of recreationally caught fish. Women can find fish consumption advisories at: http://water.epa.gov/scitech/swguidance/fishshellfish/fishadvisories.

Developing nervous tissue is at particular risk, hence the warning regarding pregnant women and young children. Effects of methylmercury can include:

- Fetal abnormalities
- Microcephaly
- Severe mental and physical retardation

Over time, the body eliminates mercury, but it can accumulate in the body faster than it can be removed.

Undercooked Meat, Unwashed Produce, and Cat Litter

Health-care providers should reinforce the principles of food hygiene to pregnant women. An infection with *Toxoplasma gondii*, a harmful parasite, causes an estimated 400 to 4,000 cases of congenital **toxoplasmosis** annually, producing:

- Mental retardation
- Blindness
- Epilepsy

The wide range of the estimate occurs because the disease is not nationally reportable or widely recognized as a threat by pregnant women. Only 48% of mothers of affected infants recognized risk factors of the disease, a situation that could possibly have been prevented by education.

The diagnosis is made through serological testing for *Toxoplasma* immunoglobulin (Ig)G and IgM. Mothers who contract the disease are often asymptomatic, but the risk of transmitting to the fetus remains. Currently in the United States, there is not universal screening of pregnant women. The protozoan is spread via undercooked meat, unwashed fruits and vegetables, contaminated soil, and cat feces. To prevent the infection, pregnant women should:

- Cook meat, poultry, and seafood thoroughly.
- Clean items that those raw foods have contacted with hot soapy water.
- Peel or meticulously wash raw fruits and vegetables before eating.
- Keep cats indoors and feed them only cooked food or prepared cat food.
- Avoid changing cat litter or, if not possible, use mask and gloves and wash hands carefully afterward.
- Use a thermometer and keep the refrigerator at 40°F (4.4°C) or lower and the freezer at 0°F (−17.8°C) or lower.

The FDA has compiled an extensive free educational kit on food safety for pregnant women and medical professionals. Available in English and Spanish, topics include methylmercury, *Listeria*, and *Toxoplasma*. Health educators can learn how to obtain the materials at www.fda.gov/downloads/Food/ResourcesForYou/HealthEducators/UCM094856.pdf.

Caffeine

Pregnant women have slower caffeine metabolism rates than nonpregnant women. Studies have shown that caffeine has been detected in amniotic fluid, umbilical cord, urine, and plasma of the fetus, which indicates that caffeine does transmit through the placenta (Rhee et al, 2015). There have been numerous studies regarding the ingestion of caffeine and the effects on pregnancy with inconsistent results.

Overall, caffeine intake of less than 300 mg per day is unlikely to delay conception or to increase the risk of spontaneous abortion or birth defects.

Problems and Complications of Pregnancy Affecting Nutrition

The physiological changes that take place in a woman's body during pregnancy may cause a variety of conditions. Some of the common problems, such as morning sickness and leg cramps, are usually annoying but only occasionally require medical intervention. Other conditions, such as hypertensive disorders of pregnancy and gestational diabetes, can be hazardous and demand medical intervention.

Common Problems

Four of the most common problems of pregnancy are:

1. Nausea and vomiting
2. Leg cramps
3. Constipation
4. Heartburn
5. Pica

NAUSEA AND VOMITING

Hormonal changes, some which produce relaxed gastrointestinal muscle tone, cause the nausea and vomiting of pregnancy. It is estimated that approximately 80% of pregnant women will develop nausea and vomiting during pregnancy (Argenbright, 2017). The occurrence and duration of these events vary widely, and they are not confined to mornings. Women who experience nausea and vomiting consume significantly less meat and more carbohydrates in the first trimester when compared to women who did not experience nausea and vomiting. These differences were maintained throughout the pregnancies.

Control of the problem without medication is the goal. Suggestions are as follows:

- Avoid fatty and/or spicy foods.
- Eat small, frequent meals.
- Consume dry carbohydrates between meals and before getting out of bed.
- Drink liquids between rather than with meals.
- Eat a high-protein snack at bedtime.
- Stop smoking.

In most cases, nausea and vomiting subsides after the first trimester. With the usual caution regarding herbal products (see Chapter 15), ginger, lemon oil, or chamomile can be used as a treatment for nausea and vomiting. Vitamin B_6 and thiamine can be used to reduce the severity of nausea.

LEG CRAMPS

Pregnant women often complain of leg cramps. One cause may be neuromuscular irritability due to low serum calcium, but the evidence that supplemental calcium reduces cramping is weak. Because of its close link to calcium metabolism, magnesium deficiency has been postulated to cause leg cramps.

Staying well hydrated is of primary importance, followed by maintaining adequate intakes of potassium, sodium, calcium, and magnesium. A noninvasive procedure to prevent muscle cramps is to stretch the muscles before exercise and, for nighttime cramps, before bedtime.

CONSTIPATION

Decreased gastrointestinal muscle tone, increased water absorption from the intestines, and the growing uterus pressing on the intestines cause constipation, which can affect up to 38% of pregnant women (Lamb & Sanders, 2015). Adequate fluid intake, regular exercise, and a high-fiber diet should relieve this condition. Ideally, the suggested amount of fiber intake, 30 grams per day, should be achieved with food rather than pharmaceutical preparations. Foods high in fiber but relatively low in kilocalories are listed in Table 10-5. Women experiencing constipation during pregnancy are also encouraged to increase daily water intake and participate in moderate amounts of activity daily.

HEARTBURN

A burning sensation beneath the breastbone is called heartburn. Hormonal changes cause relaxation of the cardiac sphincter, located between the esophagus and the stomach. That and the upward pressure on the diaphragm from the enlarging uterus can cause reflux of gastric contents into the esophagus and the burning sensation.

Avoiding spicy or acidic foods and taking small, frequent meals can control heartburn. Other helpful measures include sitting up for an hour after a meal as well as elevating the head while sleeping. Pregnant women should not self-medicate with sodium bicarbonate or antacids. The bicarbonate can be absorbed, producing alkalosis. Antacids decrease iron absorption by decreasing gastric acids, thus increasing the risk of anemia.

PICA

Pica is the compulsive ingestion of nonfood items, usually dirt, clay, laundry starch, baking soda, or ice. Physiologic causes of pica can include deficiency in zinc, iron, calcium, thiamine, or vitamin C (Johnson, 2017). Many women with pica have it only during pregnancy, believing that it cures the annoyances of pregnancy or ensures a beautiful baby. Others contend that the substances they ingest taste good to them.

Health concerns about pica include:

- Inadequate nutrition due to substitution of nonfood items for nutritious foods
- Iron-deficiency anemia

TABLE 10-5   Nutrient-Dense Foods High in Fiber

FOOD	QUANTITY	GRAMS OF DIETARY FIBER	KILOCALORIES
Grains			
All bran	½ cup	9	81
Bran buds	⅓ cup	13	75
100% bran	⅓ cup	8	83
Fruits			
Apple, raw with skin, chopped	1 cup	3	65
Orange sections, raw	1 cup	4	85
Pear, raw with skin	One small	5	86
Prunes, cooked, unsweetened	½ cup	4	133
Vegetables/ legumes			
Baked beans, in tomato sauce with pork	½ cup	5	116
Brussels sprouts, cooked from frozen	1 cup	6	65
Kidney beans, canned	½ cup	7	108
Navy beans, cooked from dry	½ cup	10	128
Green peas, cooked from frozen	½ cup	4	62

- Constipation
- Lead poisoning

Women who have migrated to an area where pica is uncommon may continue the custom. A caring, nonjudgmental interviewer may encourage a woman to reveal that she has a craving for and is eating nonfood items. The interview could lead to preventive therapy and a teaching opportunity.

Complications of Pregnancy

Two complications of pregnancy with nutritional ramifications are:

- Hyperemesis gravidarum
- Gestational diabetes

HYPEREMESIS GRAVIDARUM

Severe nausea and vomiting persisting after the 14th week of pregnancy is called **hyperemesis gravidarum.** Its incidence is reported to be higher in multiple pregnancies and other conditions associated with increased pregnancy hormone levels. The etiology and pathogenesis are unknown. It develops most often in Western countries and in first pregnancies.

Hospitalization will occur in approximately 1% to 1.5% of women with hyperemesis for the treatment of:

- Severe dehydration
- Electrolyte imbalance
- Weight loss greater than 5%
- Ketonuria and/or <500 mL of urine in 24 hours (Dean, 2014)

Major vitamin deficiencies have resulted from hyperemesis gravidarum:

- Hyponatremia can cause symptoms of headache, nausea, and vomiting.
- Deficiencies of vitamins B_6 and B_{12} can result in peripheral neuropathy.
- Deficiency of thiamine has caused Wernicke encephalopathy in pregnant clients.

See Chapters 6 and 20 for information on Wernicke encephalopathy. This disease has resulted in fatal outcomes in the mother or the fetus (Ashraf, Prijesh, Praveenkumar, & Saifudheen, 2016). Prophylactic thiamine supplementation should be considered in the care of hyperemesis.

Hyperemesis gravidarum requires treatment for the health of the woman and the fetus. There are conflicting studies regarding hyperemesis gravidarum's relationship to shorter gestational duration and infants born with LBW (Koudijs et al, 2016). Many approaches have been used to treat hyperemesis gravidarum:

- Pyridoxine
- Ginger
- Rehydration
- Enteral and parenteral nutritional support
- Antiemetics (without teratogenic effects)
- Corticosteroid therapy

GESTATIONAL DIABETES

The emergence of diabetes in pregnancy, **gestational diabetes**, is defined as hyperglycemia in the second or third trimester in a woman who has not had diabetes (Feng et al, 2017). It affects 5% to 9% of pregnancies in the United States and that number is on the rise (Wilson-Reece, Parihar, & LoBello, 2014).

Among the changes of pregnancy that contribute to gestational diabetes is the production of hormones by the placenta that decrease insulin sensitivity and increase insulin resistance in the mother to ensure a constant, optimum level of glucose for the fetus. When the mother's insulin supply is inadequate or ineffective, her high blood glucose is transferred to the fetus, who secretes his own insulin to lower the glucose content of his blood by converting it to fat, hence the hallmark result of diabetes in pregnant women: large newborns.

Risk factors for gestational diabetes are:

- Occurrence of gestational diabetes in a previous pregnancy
- Previous delivery of an infant weighing more than 9 pounds
- Family history of diabetes
- Maternal obesity (greater than 120% of ideal body weight)

Most women return to normal glucose levels after delivery; however, these same women are at a greater risk of developing type 2 diabetes in 15 to 20 years. Lifestyle modifications aiming for a 5% to 7% reduction in body weight and participating in exercise regimes are two interventions that can be effective in the prevention of developing type 2 diabetes (Guo, Chen, Whittemore, & Whitaker, 2016).

Treatment of gestational diabetes, requiring an aggressive team approach, is included in Chapter 17. The cornerstone of treatment is diet therapy and women should be referred for dietary therapy. Because insulin does not cross the placenta in measurable amounts, insulin is the recommended medication used to controlling blood glucose during pregnancy when dietary approaches alone have failed (American Diabetes Association, 2017).

The Breastfeeding Mother

The goal of Healthy People 2020 is to increase breastfeeding rates to:

- 82% of mothers who ever breastfeed
- 61% of those who breastfeed until the infant is 6 months old
- 34% of those who breastfeed until the infant is 1 year old

Initiation of breastfeeding rates in the United States continues to rise, from 74.6% in 2008 to 76.9% in 2009, exceeding the Healthy People 2010 goal. Mexican American and non-Hispanic whites exceeded the goal, but just 65% of non-Hispanic black infants were ever breastfed, still a significant increase from 36% in 1993 to 1994.

Figure 10-2 shows the percentage of 6-month-old infants by race/ethnicity being exclusively breastfed in the United States between 2011 and 2015. Chapter 11 covers the advantages of breast milk for the infant.

Nutritional Needs

For DRIs during pregnancy and lactation, see Appendix A. For selected energy nutrients and minerals, see Table 10-1.

MyPlate recommendations are for the mother to enter a "Daily Food Plan for Moms" to individualize an eating plan while following the general MyPlate recommendations. The site can be found at: https://www.choosemyplate.gov/moms-pregnancy-breastfeeding.

A common recommendation for the breastfeeding woman is to drink a glass of fluid with meals and to limit caffeinated beverages to two to three cups per day.

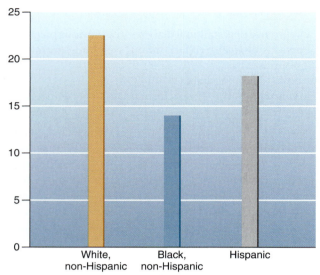

FIGURE 10-2 U.S. breastfeeding rates, 2011–2015: percentage of infants who were exclusively breastfed at 6 months of age by race/ethnicity group. *(Data from Centers for Disease Control and Prevention, July 12, 2017. MMWR, Racial and Geographic Differences in Breastfeeding— United States, 2011–2015. Available at https://www.cdc.gov/mmwr/volumes/66/wr/mm6627a3.htm?s_cid=mm6627a3_w.)*

Calcium

The primary source of calcium in human milk is calcium resorbed from the mother's bones, a process that is not prevented by increased calcium intake from foods or supplements. Moreover, the lost skeletal calcium is rapidly replaced after weaning with complete recovery occurring in most women even with closely spaced pregnancies and long periods of lactation.

Mobilization of calcium from the mother's bones also frees sequestered lead. Lead can be transferred through breast milk, but is not a concern for women who have lead blood levels of less than 5 micrograms/dL.

Energy

The average lactating woman produces 26 ounces of milk daily, but the amount varies greatly. Emptying the breast stimulates more milk production. Breast milk contains about 20 kilocalories per ounce, now the standard for term infant formulas (see Chapter 11). Some of the energy for the milk comes from the mother's dietary intake, some from fat stores accumulated during pregnancy.

Effect of Maternal Deficiencies

The mammary gland can extract most nutrients from the circulation so that breast milk may contain adequate levels of nutrients even when the mother's intake is inadequate. Levels of water-soluble vitamins in human milk depend on maternal intake, and evidence suggests that the mammary gland may take priority in folate use over the mother's own blood-forming needs. Persistent maternal vitamin deficiencies, however, may result in inadequate concentrations in the milk. For instance, vitamin B_{12} deficiency in strict vegetarian women can cause severe and permanent neurologic damage in infancy before diagnosis (CDC, February 11, 2016).

Iodine is a trace mineral that must be consumed through the mother's diet. As recounted in Chapter 7, iodine is critical for normal neurological development and is the one mineral, along with vitamins thiamin, riboflavin, vitamins B_6 and B_{12}, and vitamin A, categorized as priority nutrients. Because low maternal intake or stores of these nutrients are reflected in human milk, supplementing the lactating mother can restore her milk to adequate levels, thus providing a healthier intake for the nursing infant.

Benefits to the Mother

Several advantages to the mother are associated with breastfeeding. Breast milk is less expensive than formula (Dollars & Sense 10-2) and is always ready at the correct temperature. Contamination during formula making is usually not a concern. Nursing the infant encourages the new mother to sit down several times a day. On the other hand, without pumping her breasts and storing the milk (see Chapter 11), the task of feeding the infant is hers alone.

Breastfeeding has unique advantages:

1. Helps the uterus return to its nonpregnant state more quickly.
2. Assists in birth spacing under certain conditions.
3. May be protective against later breast cancer.

Aids Uterine Involution

During breastfeeding, the sucking of the infant stimulates the release of **oxytocin** from the posterior pituitary gland in the brain. Oxytocin causes the uterine muscles to contract and helps return the uterus to its nonpregnant size while reducing postpartum blood loss.

Assists in Birth Spacing

Lactational amenorrhea (LAM) has been found to be an effective form of birth control when the following strict criteria are followed:

- Amenorrhea
- Fully or nearly fully breastfeeding (no interval greater than 4 to 6 hours between breastfeeding)
- Less than 6 months postpartum (CDC, February 1, 2017)

Dollars & Sense 10-2

Savings With Breastfeeding

Breastfeeding is less costly than bottle-feeding. The additional foods the mother consumes are less expensive than infant formula, which may cost a family $1,200 the first year. In addition to individual benefits, breastfeeding can help the environment by reducing costs and waste associated with formula production, marketing, and distribution.

LAM was found to be less effective if expressed milk was used routinely. Consequently, breastfeeding is not suggested as the sole means of birth spacing if other methods are available and acceptable to the client. Because estrogen inhibits lactation, means of contraception other than those containing estrogen are advised if the woman continues to breastfeed.

Lessens Risk of Cancer

Over the long-term, breastfeeding has been associated with a decreased risk of breast cancer and ovarian cancer later in life, especially among premenopausal women. Some of the factors in cancer's complex etiology are described in Chapter 21.

Techniques of Breastfeeding

The medical and nursing staff will assist the mother to start breastfeeding her infant. Even mothers of twins and premature babies can successfully breastfeed with additional education and support. Some general principles to aid in breastfeeding have been established.

The mother and infant should be permitted to spend as much time together as possible during the first 24 hours after birth. This practice permits bonding of infant and mother. Some areas encourage fathers to "room in" also to bond with the baby.

One correct position for breastfeeding is shown in Figure 10-3. It is "tummy-to-tummy." The infant should face the breast squarely. If the breast is very large, the mother must take care to prevent it from blocking the infant's nose lest it impede infant's breathing. When nursing, the infant should grasp the entire areola (the colored portion around the nipple) to prevent the nipples from becoming sore.

Most infants will take 80% to 90% of the milk from each breast in the first 4 minutes of nursing. Because nursing stimulates further milk production, the mother should alternate which breast she offers first to start the feeding. This technique will stimulate further milk production because a breast that baby has completely drained will produce milk at a faster rate than one that has only been partially emptied. Allowing the baby to nurse on one breast at each feeding allows the baby to receive both foremilk and hindmilk.

Encouraging Breastfeeding

Pediatricians are encouraged to provide information on the benefits and methods of breastfeeding so that the mother can make an informed choice. Prenatal encouragement increases breastfeeding rates and identifies potential problem areas.

Hospital and birthing center practices should focus on rooming in, early and frequent breastfeeding, skilled support, and avoidance of artificial nipples, pacifiers, and formula. Box 10-2 summarizes a program to increase breastfeeding worldwide.

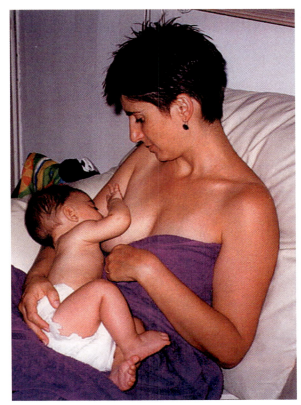

FIGURE 10-3 One correct breastfeeding position, "tummy-to-tummy." The infant takes the entire areola in its mouth. Notice how focused the mother is on the baby.

Adoptive mothers have successfully breastfed their infants by using physical stimulation and breast pumps to establish a milk supply. Breastfeeding supplementary systems, the Lact-Aid or Medla SNS Nursing Trainer System, are available to provide additional milk while the infant is nursing at the breast.

On the other hand, overselling of the benefits and ease of breastfeeding has resulted in starvation deaths of infants (see Chapter 11). Not only should the mother's choice be respected and supported, but also the infant's condition should be monitored appropriately regardless of the feeding method chosen.

Maternal Contraindications to Breastfeeding

Most women can feed their infants at breast. A few contraindications to breastfeeding include the mother's use of illegal drugs and certain medications, particular illnesses in the mother, and the mother's exposure to toxic chemicals. **Galactosemia,** an absolute contraindication due to a metabolic defect in the infant, is covered in Chapter 11.

Medication Use

Breastfeeding mothers are sometimes counseled to interrupt breastfeeding or to wean the infant due to lack of provider knowledge regarding medication safety in relationship to

BOX 10-2 ■ The Baby-Friendly Hospital Initiative

The Baby-Friendly Hospital Initiative (BFHI) is a global UNICEF/World Health Organization (WHO)–sponsored effort to promote breastfeeding. As of 2017, 449 U.S. hospitals and birthing centers in 50 states are designated Baby-Friendly (Baby-Friendly, August 25, 2017). This is currently 5.8%, which is below the Healthy People 2020 goal of 8%.

WHO and UNICEF recommend implementing the following practices in every facility providing maternity services and care for newborn infants:

Ten Steps to Successful Breastfeeding

1. Have a written breastfeeding policy routinely communicated to all health-care staff.
2. Train all health-care staff in skills necessary to implement this policy.
3. Inform all pregnant women about the benefits and management of breastfeeding.
4. Help mothers initiate breastfeeding within a half hour (United States, 1 hour) of birth.
5. Show mothers how to breastfeed and how to maintain lactation even if they are separated from their infants.
6. Give infants no food or drink other than breast milk unless medically indicated.
7. Practice rooming-in: allow mothers and infants to remain together 24 hours a day.
8. Encourage breastfeeding on demand.
9. Give no pacifiers or artificial nipples to breastfeeding infants.
10. Foster the establishment of breastfeeding support groups and refer mothers to them on discharge from the hospital or clinic.

In addition, Baby-Friendly institutions are expected to abide by the WHO International Code of Marketing of Breast Milk Substitutes (Baby Friendly, 2016) that forbids accepting free formula or other gifts and grants from formula producers. Distributing sample packs of formula or literature bearing the name of a formula product to breastfeeding mothers is also not permitted.

GENOMIC GEM 10-2

Ultrarapid Metabolizers of Codeine

In 2007, the FDA issued a warning to health-care providers about a rare but potentially lethal side effect that can affect the infants of nursing mothers who are taking codeine-containing analgesics. Some people are ultrarapid metabolizers of codeine with a specific **cytochrome P450 enzyme** (CYP2D6 genotype). See Chapter 15 for a discussion of these isoenzymes.

People with a certain variation in a liver enzyme allow them to convert codeine to its active metabolite, morphine, more rapidly and completely than other people. A breastfeeding mother with this genotype can accumulate unusually high morphine levels in her serum and breast milk, putting her nursing infant at risk for morphine overdose. One healthy, 13-day-old breastfeeding baby died of such a morphine overdose even though his mother was taking codeine at a reduced dose because she too had suffered side effects (U.S. Food and Drug Administration, August 14, 2013).

The prevalence of the ultrarapid metabolizers of codeine varies among different populations and is less than 10% for most groups. The FDA has cleared a genetic test that can determine a person's CYP2D6 genotype, thus identifying individuals who can rapidly metabolize codeine, although the test is not routinely used.

Because codeine has been used for postpartum pain for decades and is generally considered the safest narcotic pain reliever for breastfeeding mothers, absent genotyping of every new mother, careful, informed observation of mothers and infants is critical. Health-care providers should teach nursing mothers who may be taking codeine about the signs of morphine overdose in themselves (extreme sleepiness and constipation) and in infants (increased sleepiness, trouble breastfeeding, breathing difficulties, and limpness). The mother should report any of those signs to her health-care provider or seek medical attention immediately.

Newborn breastfed babies usually nurse every 2 to 3 hours and should not sleep more than 4 hours at a time. Mothers should also be aware that morphine may remain in the infant's body for up to several days after the last codeine dose.

lactation. Although many medications the mother takes are secreted in breast milk, most do not affect the milk supply or the infant when taken in recommended doses. The great majority of antidepressants are safe during breastfeeding.

Particularly if the medication can be administered directly to infants, the amount received in breast milk is unlikely to be harmful, but the capabilities of the livers and kidneys of premature and young infants as well as the characteristics of the medication should be considered. In rare cases, a mother's metabolism of a drug endangers a breastfeeding infant. See Genomic Gem 10-2.

Diagnostic radioactive compounds require temporary cessation of breastfeeding until the drug has left the mother's system; therapeutic doses are a contraindication. Cytotoxic drugs, illegal drugs, psychotropic drugs, heavy alcohol use, and women who are opioid dependent should be discouraged from breastfeeding because of the potential risk to the infant (The Academy of Breastfeeding Medicine, 2015). The physician should be consulted about both prescription and nonprescription drugs the mother takes.

Substances that are commonly not thought of as drugs may also affect the breastfed infant. These include alcohol and caffeine. The American Academy of Pediatrics (AAP; November 21, 2015) recommends against the habitual use of alcohol by breastfeeding mothers except for an occasional small drink and then only if a 2-hour delay occurs until the next feeding. Alcohol is water soluble and passes effortlessly into breast milk.

Caffeine in breast milk usually contains less than 1% of the caffeine ingested by the mother. The AAP recommends no more than three cups of caffeine-containing drinks a day.

Altered Physiology or Pathology

The AAP states that contraindications to breastfeeding are limited and include galactosemia and mothers who are positive for human T-cell lymphotrophic virus type I or II or untreated brucellosis. Mothers with untreated tuberculosis, who have active herpes simplex lesions on their breasts or who have developed varicella 5 days before or 2 days after delivery, and those infected with H1N1 influenza should not breastfeed but may express their milk for feedings.

Exposure to Toxic Chemicals

Certain chemicals, such as dichlorodiphenyltrichloroethane (DDT) and polychlorinated biphenyls (PCBs), have been shown to be **teratogenic,** causing congenital defects. Concern has been raised about the transmission of toxic chemicals to the infant through breast milk. Once ingested, if the body has no means of excreting the chemicals, the contaminants are stored in adipose tissue. When the lactating mother's fat stores are mobilized to produce milk, it too contains the chemicals.

Some experts think that the risk to the infant is minimal unless the mobilization of the mother's fat is due to inadequate intake. Others say that there is no hazard unless the woman has had occupational exposure to the chemicals or has consumed a large amount of fish from contaminated waters. Women with concerns about the issue should discuss them with their health-care providers.

KEYSTONES

- To support her own and the fetus's growth, a pregnant woman requires increased intake of many nutrients, especially kilocalories, protein, folic acid, and iron. Vitamin B_{12} status should be assessed in vegetarians and vegans.

- All women capable of becoming pregnant should consume 400 mcg of folic acid from fortified foods or supplements to decrease risk of neural tube defects in the embryo.

- The pregnant woman should avoid ingesting alcohol, soft cheeses, ready-to-eat meats, certain species and amounts of fish, undercooked meats, unwashed produce, and immoderate amounts of preformed vitamin A.

- Nutritional interventions are sometimes helpful for common complaints of pregnancy: nausea and vomiting, leg cramps, constipation, and heartburn. Tact and diplomacy may be required to counsel women who have pica.

- Medical intervention and nutritional support are indicated for clients with hyperemesis gravidarum, hypertensive disorders of pregnancy, or gestational diabetes.

- Some maternal contraindications to breastfeeding are ingestion of certain medications and drugs; some illnesses, including HIV and untreated tuberculosis; and exposure to toxic chemicals.

CASE STUDY 10-1

Ms. T is a 21-year-old sexually active woman who has been followed in a family planning clinic for 3 years. She has been faithful about keeping appointments and taking her oral contraceptives. She also takes the multivitamin/multimineral supplement containing 400 mcg of folic acid about four times a week "when she remembers and eats breakfast." She is taking no other medications. She and her immediate family have no known allergies. Now she relates that she is seriously considering becoming pregnant and wonders if they can afford to start a family. Her boyfriend proposed at her 21st birthday celebration. The couple has no pets but they do enjoy outdoor sports. Ms. T denies knowledge of means to minimize fetal risk and states that she drinks a beer or a glass of wine on Saturdays and Sundays. She does not smoke. She received the standard measles, mumps, and rubella (MMR) vaccination as a child.

Ms. T is 5 ft 3 in. and weighs 104 lb. She has a small frame. Her hemoglobin was 14 g/dL, and hematocrit was 42% last month.

CARE PLAN

Subjective Data

Expressed interest in becoming pregnant ■ Concerned about the costs of parenthood ■ Regular moderate alcohol intake ■ History of compliance with medical regimen ■ Immunized against MMR

(Continued on the following page)

Objective Data

BMI 18.4 (underweight) ■ Hemoglobin 14 g/dL, within normal limits (WNL) ■ Hematocrit 42%, within normal limits (WNL)

Analysis

Increased risk to potential fetus related to current lifestyle and underweight

Plan

DESIRED OUTCOMES EVALUATION CRITERIA	ACTIONS/ INTERVENTIONS	RATIONALE
Will affirm today her intention to abstain from alcohol when attempting to achieve a pregnancy and throughout gestation.	Teach Ms. T about fetal alcohol syndrome.	No amount of alcohol is presumed to be safe in pregnancy.
	Use photographs of affected children.	"A picture is worth 1,000 words." Photographs introduce visual learning and have an impact on feelings.
Will take multivitamin, multimineral supplement every day beginning tomorrow.	Reiterate that vitamin preparation should contain 400 micrograms of folic acid.	This is the RDA for all women capable of becoming pregnant.
	Review the value of a varied diet and good sources of food folate.	The RDA also emphasizes the importance of food folate.
Will eat breakfast or equivalent morning nourishment every day beginning tomorrow.	Review dietary guidelines with Ms. T. Explore means to take nourishment in morning.	This is a good habit to acquire. Once Ms. T achieves pregnancy, supplying the embryo/fetus with a steady supply of nutrients is critical.
Will recount the limits to vitamin A intake during pregnancy by next visit.	Inform Ms. T of RDA for vitamin A in pregnancy. Alert Ms. T to the large amounts of preformed vitamin A in liver and liver products. Caution against supplements of vitamin A in addition to the multivitamin, multimineral tablet.	Teratogenic effects usually occur during the first trimester.
	Discuss the safety of beta-carotene (provitamin A) in pregnancy.	Beta-carotene has not been associated with birth defects. Supplements containing provitamin A are considered safe for pregnant women at the RDA level.
Will list actions to take to minimize exposure to *Listeria* infection by 10 weeks before attempted conception.	Provide Ms. T with a list of cheeses to avoid and those that are considered safe. Review rules for safe handling of ready-to-eat meats.	Because the incubation period of *Listeria* is up to 10 weeks, avoidance of possibly contaminated food should begin well before conception.
	Alert her to report flulike symptoms promptly to her primary health-care provider.	Antimicrobial therapy may prevent fetal infection and the associated high mortality.
Will monitor own intake of fish to remain within recommended limits by conception.	Emphasize complete abstinence from shark, swordfish, king mackerel, and tilefish. If available, use food models showing the weekly limits of 12 ounces or 6 ounces of fish.	These advisories from the FDA and the EPA to minimize the exposure of the fetus to methylmercury show the seriousness of the threat.
Will discuss discontinuing oral contraceptive therapy and attempting conception with the primary health-care provider before changing her regimen.	Advise Ms. T about the possibility of birth defects with some oral contraceptives.	Progestins may cause birth defects if taken early in pregnancy.
Will continue planning optimal nutrition for herself and her prospective child.	Refer Ms. T to local Supplemental Feeding Program for Women, Infants, and Children.	If eligible, she could begin receiving food assistance when she becomes pregnant.

TEAMWORK 10-1

WIC PROGRAM DIRECTOR'S NOTES

The following Supplemental Feeding Program for Women, Infants, and Children (WIC) Program Director's Notes are representative of the documentation found in a client's medical record.

Subjective: *Interested in possible food assistance when she achieves pregnancy*

Objective: *Completed WIC application*

Analysis: *Meets eligibility requirements for*

- *Residency in state*
- *Household income*
- *Nutrition risk due to underweight—documented by family planning nurse*

Does not currently meet categorical eligibility requirement:

- *Is not pregnant*
- *Has no dependent children*

Plan: *Place application in pending file*

Encourage client to activate application when she becomes pregnant.

CRITICAL THINKING QUESTIONS

1. If Ms. T were to achieve a pregnancy, what would her month-by-month recommended weight gain be? If she expresses concern about "gaining too much weight" when within the recommended amounts, how would you counsel her?

2. Are there other issues you believe ought to be raised with Ms. T before she attempts to become pregnant? Are they more or less important than the ones addressed in the Care Plan? Why?

3. Assuming Ms. T becomes pregnant, how would you approach anticipatory guidance regarding complications of pregnancy affected by nutrition?

CHAPTER REVIEW

1. Throughout pregnancy and lactation, how many whole grains should a woman consume?
   1. All grains should be whole grains
   2. Half of grains consumed should be whole
   3. One serving of whole grains per day
   4. Whole grains should be avoided

2. Which of the following substances are contraindicated during pregnancy? Select all that apply.
   1. Alcohol
   2. Swordfish
   3. Coffee
   4. Cheddar cheese
   5. Well-done beef

3. Which of the following principles is not recommended by the Baby-Friendly Hospital Initiative?
   1. Feeding on demand
   2. Keeping mother and infant together 24 hours a day
   3. Hydrating the infant with sterile water until the mother's milk supply is established
   4. Putting the infant to breast within 1 hour of birth

4. The RDA for folic acid specifies 400 mcg of synthetic folic acid from fortified foods or supplements for:
   1. All women capable of becoming pregnant
   2. Women taking oral contraceptive medications
   3. Women of Northern European descent
   4. Breastfeeding mothers

5. If a pregnant woman complains of heartburn, she should be instructed to:
   1. Increase her intake of milk products
   2. Decrease her overall food intake
   3. Rest in bed after eating
   4. Avoid spicy or acidic foods

CLINICAL ANALYSIS

1. Ms. S is a 15-year-old girl who thinks that she is 2 months pregnant. She has not told anyone else of the pregnancy. She is unsure if she wants to keep the baby or not. Her purpose in disclosing the information to the school nurse is to obtain assistance with weight control so she has more time to make up her mind.

   On the basis of the above information, which one of the following interventions would be of highest priority at this time?
   a. Designing a weight-control program that is high in calcium
   b. Giving information on the desirability of breastfeeding the infant
   c. Instructing the girl regarding substances that are likely to harm the fetus
   d. Scheduling a visit with a social worker to help the girl decide on a course of action

2. Knowing that adolescents are often lacking in certain nutrients, the nurse would want to assess the girl's intake of:
   a. Cola, coffee, and tea
   b. Fruits, vegetables, milk, and red meat
   c. Fried foods and pastries
   d. Poultry, seafood, and white bread

3. Ms. S complains of morning sickness. The nurse instructs her to:
   a. Eat breakfast later in the morning
   b. Drink at least two glasses of liquid with every meal
   c. Increase her intake of whole-grain breads and cereals to 2 ounces per meal
   d. Drink a large glass of skim milk at bedtime

CHAPTER 11

Life Cycle Nutrition: Infancy, Childhood, and Adolescence

After completing this chapter, the student should be able to:

- Describe normal growth patterns and corresponding nutritional needs for a full-term infant, a toddler, a school-age child, and an adolescent.
- Explain why breast milk is uniquely suited to the human infant's capabilities.
- Discuss the rationale for the sequence in which semisolid foods are introduced into an infant's diet.
- List causes and treatments of five common nutritional problems of infancy.

- Summarize common nutritional problems of the preschool child.
- Relate ways in which a child can be encouraged to establish good nutritional habits.
- Identify areas of concern regarding the typical adolescent's diet.
- Devise a comprehensive plan to prevent obesity in a target population of children or adolescents.

Good nutrition is essential for infants and children. Because of public health efforts, U.S. infant mortality rates have decreased significantly, but still almost 7 out of every 1,000 infants born in the United States die annually (Centers for Disease Control and Prevention [CDC], September 27, 2016).

The goal of Healthy People 2020 is to reduce the infant mortality rate (IMR) to 6.0 per 1,000 live births or less for all racial/ethnic groups (Office of Disease Prevention and Health Promotion, May, 20, 2017). The Centers for Disease Control and Prevention (CDC) reports that over 23,000 infants died in 2014, within the first year of life, with black infants' mortality rate being twice that of white infants (September 28, 2017). Low birth weight (LBW) and short gestational age are leading causes of IMR in the United States. In 2015, the LBW rate for non-Hispanic black women was 13.35%, 6.93% for non-Hispanic white women, and 7.21% for Hispanic women (Martin et al, 2017). Nutritional management with adequate nutrition supply has a major function in survival and subsequent growth and development of LBW infants (Nakstad et al, 2016).

This chapter focuses on periods of rapid **growth** during infancy, childhood, and adolescence. In addition to nutritional needs for all periods of growth, the chapter considers the stages of physical and **psychosocial development** for these ages, noting ways in which food relates to psychosocial development. Toward the end of the chapter is a discussion of overweight and obesity, major public health issues for children and adolescents that, unless checked, do not bode well for the health of Americans.

Psychosocial Development

American psychoanalyst **Erik Erikson** divided life into eight stages, each of which involves a psychosocial developmental task to be mastered and an opposite negative trait that emerges if the task is not mastered. Even if a developmental task is successfully mastered, a new situation may arise, challenging the person to reaffirm his or her mastery. Erikson's developmental tasks through adolescence appear in Table 11-1.

Nutrition in Infancy

Infancy, the first year of life, is a critical period for growth and development.

Growth

Growth is the progressive maturation and increase in size of a living thing. The only time humans grow faster than in infancy is the 40 weeks before they are born. An infant's birth weight should:

- Double by 4 to 6 months of age
- Triple by 1 year

From a birth length of about 20 inches, an infant grows to about 30 inches by age 1.

An infant's *rate of growth* is more significant than absolute values. The growth charts at www.cdc.gov/growthcharts reflect growth patterns of all children in the United States.

TABLE 11-1	Erikson's Theory of Psychosocial Development	
STAGE OF LIFE	DEVELOPMENTAL TASK	OPPOSING NEGATIVE TRAIT
Infancy	Trust	Distrust
Toddler	Autonomy	Doubt
Preschooler	Initiative	Guilt
School-age child	Industry	Inferiority
Adolescent	Identity	Role confusion

In 2006, the World Health Organization (WHO) released new standards for growth and development. The infants measured for these standards are based on established growth of breastfed infant as the norm (WHO, September 9, 2010). The standards are applicable to all children regardless of ethnicity, socioeconomic status, or type of feeding. During the first few days after birth, an infant loses weight as he or she adjusts to his or her new environment and food supply. Among his or her adaptations is learning to feed compared with receiving a continuous supply of nutrients in utero. The amount of weight lost in these first few days should not exceed 10% of the birth weight (Tawia & McGuire, 2014). The newborn (or *neonate*, as an infant is called during the first 28 days after birth) usually returns to its birth weight within 14 days.

The period most critical to brain development extends from conception into the second year of life. Brain cells increase most rapidly before birth and during the first 5 or 6 months after birth. To attain maximum brain growth, the infant needs optimal nutrition.

Development

The gradual process of changing from a simple to a more complex organism is **development.** Becoming a mature individual involves psychosocial and physical changes, not only an increase in size.

Psychosocial Development of the Infant

The psychosocial developmental task of the infant is to learn to **trust** (see Table 11-1). The parent who responds promptly and lovingly to the infant's cries is teaching the infant to trust. If the caregiver handles the infant inconsistently—gently one time and roughly the next—however, the infant learns to mistrust.

Failure to thrive (FTT) is a descriptive term used to describe inadequate growth or the inability to maintain growth. A child may receive a diagnosis of FTT when his or her arc of growth slips by two major percentiles or when growth falls below the third or fifth percentile on a growth chart or when weight falls below the fifth percentile on multiple occasions.

Inadequate caloric intake is the most common etiology associated with FTT and can be related to problems with feeding, including poor sucking and swallowing, breastfeeding difficulties or difficulty transitioning to solid foods, insufficient breast milk or formula, excessive juice consumption, or caloric absorption problems that can be associated with cardiac and gastrointestinal conditions. It can be helpful to assess caregiver–infant interactions related to feeding practices. In situations in which physical care is provided but a tender relationship does not develop, infants may actually suffer stunted physical growth. Caregiver education regarding feeding techniques, child cues, and developmental stages can be helpful in addressing nonorganic causes of FTT.

Physical Development

Development proceeds at a different pace in various tissues and organs. Proper feeding practices are based on the maturation rate of body organs (see Table 11-2).

Nutritional Needs of the Term Infant

For DRIs, see Appendix A. In general, infants' values are based on the contents of breast milk. In 2008, the American Academy of Pediatrics recommended that all infants receive a daily intake of 400 IU of vitamin D beginning in the first few days of life (CDC, June 17, 2015).

A normal pregnancy is 38 to 42 weeks. An infant born after a normal pregnancy is a **term infant.** Breast milk is the species-specific food for human infants. Its characteristics are the standard for infant formulas, which replicate many of the components of breast milk but cannot supply all of its desirable qualities.

Energy and Macronutrients

Resting metabolic rates of infants are high as evidenced by:

- Normal pulse rate of 120 to 150 beats/min
- Normal respiratory rate of 30 to 50 breaths/min
- Large proportion of skin surface to body size requiring energy for temperature regulation

An activity such as crying may double the infant's energy expenditure.

Energy needs for the first 6 months of life are 108 kilocalories per kilogram of body weight per day. From 6 to 12 months of age, the energy need is 98 kilocalories per kilogram per day.

Table 11-3 lists the macronutrients of special importance for infants with comparisons of the relevant components of breast milk and cow's milk. Clinical Application 11-1 discusses a carbohydrate source that should not be given to infants. Box 11-1 identifies some research linking cognitive development to breastfeeding.

Micronutrients

The general recommendations for vitamin and mineral supplementation in infants are listed in Table 11-4.

TABLE 11-2 Physical Characteristics of Infant That Affect Nutrition

SYSTEM	INFANT'S LIMITED CAPACITY	ADAPTATIONS AND MATURATIONS	ADJUSTMENT IN FEEDING	BY 1 YEAR OF AGE
Gastrointestinal	Salivary and pancreatic amylases are inadequate to digest complex carbohydrates for several months.	Has lingual lipase to digest fat, an enzyme lacking in adults.	Delay offering complex carbohydrates.	
	Intestine permits absorption of whole proteins.		Delay offering foods likely to be allergenic until 1 year old.	
	Stomach holds about 1 oz.		Frequent feedings	Stomach holds about 8 oz.
Nervous	Suckles with up-and-down motion of the tongue for 3–4 months.	Rooting reflex well developed. When the infant's cheek is stroked, the head turns toward that side to nurse.	Feed breast milk or infant formula. If semisolid food is offered at this time, the natural motion of the tongue tends to spit it out.	
		After 4 months, the infant can suck using orofacial muscles. The tongue moves back and forth instead of up and down.	Semisolid food is more likely to be swallowed than spit out.	
		At 6 months has hand-to-eye coordination to put food into mouth.	Offer appropriate finger foods.	
		At 7 months can chew appropriate foods.	Increase variety of food offered.	
Urinary	Young infant's kidneys have limited capacity to filter solutes.	By end of the second month of life, kidneys can excrete the waste of semisolid foods.	Delay semisolid foods at least until 2 months of age, preferably 4–6 months.	Kidneys at full functional capacity.

TABLE 11-3 Macronutrient Needs of Term Infant

	NUTRIENT NEEDED	BREAST MILK	COW'S MILK	CONTRAINDICATIONS
Carbohydrate	Galactose is necessary for brain cell formation.	Breast milk is 40% lactose.	12 grams of carbohydrate in 1 cup of whole milk	Honey (see Clinical Application 11-1)
Fat	Fat and cholesterol are necessary for rapidly growing brain and nervous system, bile, and hormones.	Provides 50% of kilocalories from fat as concentrated energy source. Contains lipase to begin digestion for the infant so about 95%–98% of the fat in human milk is absorbed.	8 grams of fat in 1 cup of whole milk	Reduced-fat milks before age 2
	The developing nervous system needs arachidonic and docosahexaenoic (DHA) fatty acids, the main omega-6 and omega-3 fatty acids of the central nervous system.	These two fatty acids, essential for retinal and neural development, are found in human milk.	Not present	
Protein		Human milk contains 60% whey (easily digested) and 40% casein. The major whey protein in breast milk is lactoferrin, which provides antimicrobial, antioxidant, and anti-inflammatory actions.	18% whey, 82% casein	

Adapted from USDA (2009, March); Rollo, Radmacher, Turcu, Myers, & Adamkin (2014); Prell & Koletzko (2016).

CLINICAL APPLICATION   11-1

Honey Is a Danger to Infants

Infants should not be given honey until after their first birthday because honey frequently contains botulism spores acquired from plants or the soil. Up to 25% of honey products have been found to contain spores. Processing the honey does not destroy these spores.

There were 199 confirmed cases of botulism in the United States in 2015. Of the 199 cases, 141, or 71%, of cases were infant botulism (CDC, 2017).

If the spores are ingested by an infant, they become active in his or her intestinal tract and produce a neurotoxin. Symptoms include:

- Constipation
- Lethargy
- Weak cry
- Poor feeding
- Poor muscle tone (CDC, May 8, 2017)

The spectrum of symptoms can range from the mild end of the spectrum, in which the infant does not require hospitalization but may develop feeding difficulties and FTT, to the severe end, characterized by paralysis that causes respiratory difficulties resulting in death.

Physicians are required to report all cases of infant botulism promptly to state and local health departments.

VITAMINS

The routine administration of vitamin K to all infants is mandatory. Infants are at a higher risk for hemorrhagic disease due to lack of vitamin K transfer across the placenta and low levels in breast milk. Vitamin K deficiency bleeding (VKDB) can occur from birth through 12 weeks of life, with highest mortality resulting from intracranial hemorrhage.

BOX 11-1 ■ Research Linking Cognitive Abilities to Breastfeeding

Early research associated breastfeeding with slightly enhanced performance on tests of cognitive development but this remains an issue of debate. Breast milk contains arachidonic (ARA) and docosahexaenoic (DHA) fatty acids, which accumulate during brain growth during the third trimester of pregnancy until age 18 months.

- One study identified that the duration of breast feeding is associated with higher white matter in the brains of 8-year-old children (Stadler et al, 2016).
- Another study indicated that breastfed infants had IQ scores that are two to three points higher as adolescents and adults related to higher DHA and ARA levels (Prell & Koletzko, 2016). Factors such as higher socioeconomic status and level of education are also demonstrating an effect on cognition. This issue is still under investigation. Adding ARA and DHA to infant formulas corresponds to other efforts to mimic breast milk. Neither supplemented formula nor breastfeeding should be viewed as a magic elixir to boost intelligence.

MINERALS

Compared with cow's milk, breast milk contains:

- One-third the sodium, potassium, and chloride
- One-eighth the phosphorus of cow's milk, an amount that accommodates the limited function of the infant's kidneys

Water

The infant's body is about 75% water. The daily turnover of water in the infant is approximately 15% of body weight.

The Breastfed Infant

Breast milk is designed for human infants and is the standard against which substitute milks are measured. Breastfeeding rates in the United States are at an all-time high (see Fig. 10-2), but compared with other countries, they are still low.

Benefits of breastfeeding include decreased rates of:

- Otitis media
- Lower respiratory tract infections
- Asthma
- Childhood obesity
- Eczema
- Diarrhea and vomiting
- Necrotizing enterocolitis
- Sudden infant death syndrome
- Type 2 diabetes (Office on Women's Health, May 3, 2017)

The goals of Healthy People 2020 are to increase breastfeeding rates to:

- 81.9% of mothers who ever breastfeed
- 25.5% who exclusively breastfeed until infants are 6 months old
- 34.1% who breastfeed until infants are 1 year old

The American Academy of Pediatrics recommends exclusive breastfeeding (nothing but breast milk and vitamins, minerals, and medications) for the first 6 months of life.

Practices conducive to breastfeeding and lactation are covered in Chapter 10. Clinical Application 11-2 explains the procedures for storing human milk.

Composition of Breast Milk

Breast milk accommodates the infant's needs during the weeks an infant is nursing, even during the course of a single feeding. Breast milk varies from mother to mother and even in one mother with the time of day. It also varies with the lactation cycle. The variation in content also offers the infant a variety of taste experiences (see Table 11-5).

Unique Advantages of Breastfeeding

One well-documented advantage to breastfeeding that has not been duplicated by formulas is protection against infectious disease. Other advantages are limited improvement in the presentation of allergic disease and a possible negative association with obesity.

TABLE 11-4   Vitamin and Mineral Supplementation for Infants

SUPPLEMENT	PRESCRIBED FOR	SITUATION	RATIONALE
Vitamin			
D	Breastfed infants Partially breastfed infants Formula-fed infants ingesting <1 L of fortified formula	Beginning in the first few days of life	Most breastfed infants are unable to synthesize vitamin D from sunlight sources.
K	All infants	Single intramuscular dose of vitamin K after the first breastfeeding and within 6 hours of birth	Until the infant's intestine becomes colonized with *Escherichia coli* from the environment, he or she is at risk for bleeding problems
C	Breast milk and formula contain adequate amounts.		
B_{12} as cobalamin	Breastfed infant, if mother is strict vegetarian	See Chapter 10	Growth failure and neurological impairment due to cobalamin deficiency occurred in breastfeeding infants of vegetarian mothers
Mineral			
Calcium	Premature infants	See Clinical Application 11-5	Breast milk contains about one-sixth to one-quarter the calcium in cow's milk 67% of breast milk calcium is absorbed vs. 25% of cow's milk calcium
Phosphorus	Premature infants	See Clinical Application 11-5	
Iron	Term infant, when birth weight has doubled Formula-fed premature, from onset Fortified human milk-fed premature, when full enteral feeding established	Iron-fortified formula is recommended	Breast milk contains about 0.5 mg iron/L but 50% is absorbed Only 10% is absorbed from cow's milk or fortified formulas
Fluoride	All children >6 months of age Children >3 years of age	If drinking water contains <0.3 ppm If drinking water contains <0.6 ppm	

Sources: CDC (June 17, 2015); NIH (February 11, 2016a); NIH (February 11, 2016b); WHO (2011); Clark & Slayton (2014).

CLINICAL APPLICATION   11-2

Storage of Human Milk

Careful collection and storage are necessary to preserve the sterility and quality of expressed human milk. The Centers for Disease Control and Prevention has specific guidelines for the collection and storage of human breast milk, including storage at room temperature for no longer than 6 to 8 hours, in an insulated cooler for 24 hours, in the refrigerator for 5 days, and in the freezer of the refrigerator for 3 to 6 months. Breast milk can be frozen for longer periods of time, up to 6 to 12 months, if stored in a chest or upright freezer.

Human breast milk banks make milk available for infants whose mothers do not produce enough milk or have a contraindication to breastfeeding. The Human Milk Banking Association of North America follows strict guidelines in screening for infectious disease, criteria of pasteurization, storage, and distributions of donated milk (2015–2016). The majority of donated milk is provided to premature, hospitalized infants.

PROTECTION AGAINST DISEASE

Breast milk contains bioactive components that protect the infant from disease by the transfer of passive immunity from mother to infant. Among the infection-fighting agents in breast milk are immunoglobulin (Ig)A and leukocytes or white blood cells (WBCs).

PREVENTION OF ALLERGIES

The young infant's gastrointestinal tract can permit the passage of whole proteins into the bloodstream. These proteins can stimulate an allergic response in susceptible infants.

Breastfeeding is protective against allergies for infants with at least one first-degree relative with allergic disease. If breast milk is unavailable or insufficient, infants at high risk of **atopy** may be fed special formulas. **Hydrolysis** splits whole proteins into smaller particles that are less likely to cause allergic reactions. One study demonstrated that infants with a family history of allergies were 18% less likely to develop atopic dermatitis if fed a hydrolyzed protein

TABLE 11-5   Breast Milk Components

	SECRETED	APPEARANCE	COMPONENTS
Colostrum	1–7 days after delivery	Thin, yellow, cloudy fluid	High kilocalorie High protein Antibodies White blood cells Fat-soluble vitamins Minerals
Mature	20 days after delivery As long as breastfeeding continues	Milky	High lactose High vitamin E Calcium:phosphorus ratio of 2:1 (prevents calcium deficient tetany) Antibodies (decreased at 3 months) Antioxidants Foremilk (beginning of feeding): less fat Hindmilk (end of feeding): more fat to increase satiety At 3 months, fewer immunoglobulins

Sources: Infant Nutrition Council, undated. Available at http://www.infantnutritioncouncil.com/resources/breastmilk-information/.

formula in the first months of life (Prell & Koletzko, 2016). Current evidence does not support a major role for maternal dietary restrictions during pregnancy or lactation as protective against allergies. In addition, little evidence backs the delayed introduction of complementary foods beyond 4 to 6 months of age as a strategy to prevent atopic disease.

NEGATIVE ASSOCIATION WITH OBESITY

There is strong evidence that suggests that breastfed infants have a lower risk of later obesity than formula-fed infants. There is a 15% reduction in adolescent and adult obesity rates if any breastfeeding occurs in infancy and a 30% to 50% reduced risk of overweight or obesity if exclusively breastfed for 6 months (Gunnell, Neher, & Safranek, 2016).

The mechanisms involved, although poorly understood, include aspects of the feeding process as well as the components of breast milk. Breastfed infants gain weight more slowly and are leaner than formula-fed infants. In the United States, whereas rates of breastfeeding have risen slowly, childhood obesity rates have increased dramatically. In the United States, between the years 2011 and 2014, the prevalence of obesity was 8.9% in children aged between 2 and 5 (CDC, April 10, 2017). Breastfeeding is just one intervention that can be used to help prevent childhood obesity.

Genetic Abnormalities Affecting Breastfeeding

Among the conditions commonly included in newborn screening tests are two that have profound implications for the infant's nutritional intake. One affects carbohydrate metabolism and the other protein metabolism.

In **galactosemia,** the infant's lack of an enzyme to metabolize galactose is an absolute contraindication to breastfeeding. Galactosemia is inherited as an autosomal recessive trait. If untreated, the child will suffer growth failure, mental retardation, or death. Treatment involves a soy formula

containing no lactose or galactose and lifelong avoidance of milk products.

The mother of an infant with phenylketonuria (see Clinical Application 11-3) often chooses to feed the child only the special formula. Breastfeeding the infant requires both limited amounts of breast milk and the special formula. To determine the amount of breast milk the infant may consume to keep his or her blood levels within the therapeutic limits requires constant monitoring and consultations, but it has been done successfully. Every state has at least one medical center for treating metabolic defects. The maternal and child health division of the state health department can assist with locating such a facility.

The Formula-Fed Infant

As good as it is, exclusive breastfeeding is not possible for all mothers and infants. Infant formula is the only food that is regulated by its own law, the Infant Formula Act of 1980, which sets minimum levels of 29 nutrients and maximal levels of 9 nutrients. Formulas for full-term infants must contain 20 kilocalories per ounce. As much as possible, commercial formulas are designed to match the qualities of human breast milk.

Formulas contain more protein than breast milk. The cow's milk proteins do not contain the optimal amino acids for human infants. Enough protein is included in the formula to provide a sufficient distribution of amino acids.

The saturated fats of cow's milk are poorly digested by the infant. In formulas, vegetable oils replace the saturated fats.

Formula Preparations

Commercial formulas come in three forms: powder (to mix with water), liquid concentrate, and ready-to-feed (see Table 11-6).

CLINICAL APPLICATION   11-3

Phenylketonuria Essentials

Persons with phenylketonuria (PKU) are unable to convert the essential amino acid phenylalanine to tyrosine because the enzyme phenylalanine hydroxylase (PAH) is lacking or defective. In the United States PKU occurs in 1 in 10,000 to 15,000 newborns (National Institutes of Health, August 22, 2017). Phenylalanine occurs in all protein foods, including milk. Once feeding starts, affected infants are at risk of accumulating high blood levels of phenylalanine and consequent intellectual disabilities. All infants in the United States are screened for PKU disease within the first days of life.

DIETARY TREATMENT

Immediate and lifelong avoidance of excess phenylalanine is the principal treatment. Because phenylalanine is an essential amino acid, small amounts of breast milk or infant formula are given to provide just the amounts of phenylalanine the infant needs and can use for growth and metabolism without excessive accumulation. Special phenylalanine-free formulas provide the remaining amino acids. These formulas tend to be high in cost and tend to have an unpalatable taste, which can result in failure to adhere to the strict diet (Durrer, Allen, & Hunt von Herbing, 2017). Diets will consist of special foods that are low in protein, fruits, vegetables, and limited amounts of grains. When solids are introduced it is important to weigh food and calculate the amount of protein and phenylalanine that is consumed each day. Resources are available at websites such as https://howmuchphe.org/ which provide tools to track daily protein intake.

The artificial sweetener aspartame (Equal®, NutraSweet®), which is composed of aspartic acid and phenylalanine, bears a warning label regarding PKU. This disease requires frequent monitoring of growth and blood levels of phenylalanine and tyrosine that should be provided by specialists in the field.

TABLE 11-6   Forms of Formulas

	ADVANTAGES	DISADVANTAGES
Liquid concentrate	Relatively easy to prepare	Opened cans require refrigeration Must be used within 48 hours
Powder	Less waste Possible to prepare a small amount	Unsterile powder may be unsafe for premature infants
Ready-to-feed	Most convenient No calculating or measuring	Most expensive (see Dollars & Sense 11-1)

Dollars & Sense 11-1

Cost of Different Preparations of One Brand of Infant Formula

	Package Size	Price	Cost per Prepared Ounce
Powder	12.5 oz	$16.99	$0.19
Liquid concentrate	13 fl oz	$4.99	$0.19
Ready-to-feed	32 fl oz	$6.99	$0.22

Directions for preparing the formula will be given by the health-care provider. Commonly discussed issues include:

- Cleanliness/sterility of equipment
- Water to use for dilution:
  - Sterility
  - Fluoride content
  - Possible lead contamination (see Clinical Application 7-7)
- Safe storage

- Use of correct strength formula (Formula too concentrated or too diluted can cause severe electrolyte imbalances. Some cases have been fatal.)
- Safe heating of the formula before feeding the infant
- Discarding prepared bottles of formula unrefrigerated for 1 hour or partially consumed

Using a microwave oven for infant foods is not recommended. Heat may be unevenly distributed and continues to build even after the food has been removed from the oven.

Feeding Techniques

Approximately every 4 hours, the infant awakens for feedings. By the age of 2 to 3 months, the baby probably will have eliminated one feeding, so the schedule is five times a day. By 6 months, most infants are feeding four times a day.

The baby is positioned in the crook of the arm semi-upright. The parent's or caregiver's touch is important to the infant's development. Correct techniques include the following:

- The nipple holes should be large enough for milk to drip out on its own without shaking the bottle.
- The nipple should always be filled with milk to prevent the infant from swallowing air while feeding.
- Daily formula intake for an infant should be 1.5 to 2 ounces per pound of body weight, but growth is a better measure of health than the amount of formula swallowed.
- A single feeding should not exceed 8 ounces.

Propping an infant with a bottle is never acceptable because choking is a real hazard.

Special Formulas

Special formulas are available for infants who are allergic to cow's milk, those with galactosemia or lactose intolerance, and those with fat-absorption problems. See Clinical Application 11-4 for a brief description of such formulas, which are commonly soy based.

CLINICAL APPLICATION   11-4

Soy Protein Formulas

The isolated soy protein formulas marketed today are all free of cow's milk protein and lactose and are iron-fortified.

The American Academy of Pediatrics recommends using soy protein–based formulas in term infants for:

- Galactosemia and hereditary lactase deficiency
- Those whose parents desire a vegetarian diet
- Infants with a documented IgE allergy to cow milk who are not allergic to soy protein.
- Those with a transient lactose intolerance

In contrast, the Academy *does not* recommend soy protein–based formula under the following circumstances:

- Preterm infants
- Cow milk protein–induced enterocolitis
- Routine treatment of colic
- Healthy or high-risk infants to prevent atopic disease

Adapted from healthychildren.org: Where We Stand: Soy Formula (November 21, 2015).

For a formula to be considered hypoallergenic, it should be well tolerated by at least 90% of individuals who are allergic to the parent protein from which that formula has been derived.

Palatability becomes an issue as the infant develops more discerning tastes. Hydrolysis produces bitter-tasting peptides. Soy formulas and rice formula were judged to have the best tastes, followed by the whey hydrolysates. The full-term infant's digestive, nervous, and urinary systems are immature—an even greater issue for premature infants. Clinical Application 11-5 summarizes some of the nutritional problems and appropriate interventions used for premature infants.

Hazards of Formula Feeding

On a few occasions, improperly manufactured formulas have been responsible for vitamin and mineral deficiencies in infants. This is an unacceptable, but fortunately rare, occurrence. A more common hazard, and one an individual nurse can monitor, is the improper preparation and use of formulas by the parent. Formulas can be:

- The wrong strength
- Prepared with contaminated water, equipment, or hands
- Kept at feeding temperature too long. Body temperature is "just right" for bacteria to multiply, whether in the body or in a formula bottle.

Choice of Breast or Bottle

In the United States, infants can be well nourished whether breastfed or bottle-fed. To raise a child successfully takes more than simply supplying the correct ratio of nutrients. The mother's informed decision should be supported and appropriate teaching provided.

An estimated 5% of women may be unable to produce a full milk supply for anatomic or medical reasons. Moreover, because infants' sucking stimulates milk production, difficulty with the process may result in diminished milk supply.

It is not uncommon for infants to lose weight in the first days of breastfeeding, which can lead to loss of maternal confidence in breastfeeding and then to discontinuation or formula supplementation. Most infants will regain weight that is lost and not require supplementation with formula. Infants should:

- Be observed while suckling at 2 to 4 days of age by a knowledgeable health-care provider
- Have its weight monitored by the same health-care provider

All parents should be taught to expect the infant to have at least:

- Four good-sized bowel movements
- Six saturated diapers per day

Most important, enthusiastic support for breastfeeding should never delay provision of formula when medically indicated.

Advancing the Diet

Teaching the infant to consume the foods he or she will receive throughout life is a gradual process. First, semisolid foods are given to complement breast milk or formula. Eventually drinking from a cup will replace suckling.

Semisolid Foods

No proof exists of the folk wisdom that the early feeding of solid food to infants promotes their sleeping through the night. At 3 months, 75% of infants sleep all night, regardless of diet. If solid foods are introduced too early, the infant may develop allergies because of the permeability of the intestine.

The American Academy of Pediatrics supports exclusive breastfeeding (nothing but breast milk and vitamins, minerals, and medications) for 6 months while recognizing that infants are often developmentally ready for complementary foods between 4 and 6 months of age.

The infant should achieve voluntary control of swallowing at 3 to 4 months. Before being offered solid food, the infant should be able to control his or her head and trunk. With this ability, the baby can turn away when satisfied. By this time, the infant is drinking 8 ounces of formula or a similar estimated amount of breast milk and yet becomes hungry in less than 4 hours.

In introducing solid food, it is best to follow the infant's lead. To avoid later feeding problems, solid foods should be started when the baby is interested. Babies ready for solid food are hungry and not fussy about tastes (Fig. 11-2). Children learn from adults; parents should avoid showing distaste for particular foods.

CLINICAL APPLICATION

11-5

Premature Infants

Premature infants are born before 37 weeks' gestation. By birth weight, premature infants are categorized as:

- Low birth weight (LBW)—less than 2,500 g (5.5 lb) at birth
- Very low birth weight (VLBW)—less than 1,500 g (3.3 lb)
- Extremely low birth weight (ELBW)—less than 1,000 g (2.2 lb).

An infant can be both premature and LBW or VLBW. Not all premature infants weigh less than 2,500 grams. Nor are all LBW infants premature, but birth weight is the most powerful single predictor of an infant's future health status. LBW infants are approximately 13 times more likely to die within the first 28 days of life than heavier babies (Namiiro, Mugalu, McAdams, & Ndeezi, 2012).

Maternal factors associated with prematurity include smoking, alcohol, or drugs use; previous premature delivery; history of chronic disease; infection; teen mothers; women over age 35; and either very low or high BMI (CDC, November 17, 2016). A genetic variant has also been implicated.

PROVIDING NOURISHMENT

The World Health Organization (2011) recommends the following interventions to improve immediate and long-term health of LBW and VLBW infants.

- Human milk from the infant's mother is the gold standard to nourish VLBW infants. Compared with term mothers' milk, preterm milk has more protein, sodium, and host defense factors but less calcium, phosphorus, and magnesium. Human milk fortifiers add protein, carbohydrate, vitamins, and minerals to the breast milk (see Fig. 11-1). Moreover, the mother's

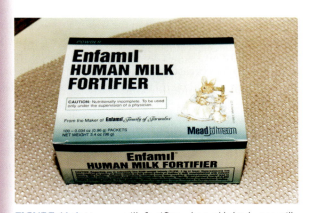

FIGURE 11-1 Human milk fortifier, when *added to human milk*, increases the amount of protein, carbohydrates, and selected vitamins and minerals available to meet the needs of rapidly growing low-birth-weight infants. These are not nutritionally complete supplements. *(With permission from Mead Johnson & Company.)*

enzymes and antibodies are still available to the baby. If the infant cannot be fed mother's own milk, donor milk should be provided.

- If mother's own milk or donor milk cannot be used, the infant should be fed a standard infant formula until age 6 months. VLBW infants should be given preterm infant formula if they fail to gain weight despite adequate feeding with standard infant formula.
- VLBW infants should be given vitamin D supplements ranging from 400–1,000 IU per day until 6 months of age.
- VLBW infants who are fed mother's own milk or donor milk should be given calcium and phosphorus supplementation.
- VLBW infants who are fed mother's own milk or donor milk should be given 2–4 milligrams per kilogram of body weight per day iron supplementation from age 2 weeks to 6 months.

TRACKING PROGRESS

Premature infants should not be evaluated against standards set for term infants.

- Premature infants should have their chronological age corrected by gestational age.
- Special growth grids for premature infants to 38-month gestational age are available.
- Premature infants will have periods of catch-up growth that will initially be seen in head circumference followed by weight and length.

NECROTIZING ENTEROCOLITIS

The most serious gastrointestinal disorder of neonates is **necrotizing enterocolitis (NEC)**, an acquired injury to the bowel. This inflammatory bowel disease of neonates results in inflammation and bacterial colonization of the bowel wall (Claud, 2009). NEC occurs in 5% to 10% of VLBW infants, with mortality rates between 15% and 30% (Sanuels, van de Graaf, de Jonge, Reiss, & Vermeulen, 2017).

Established risk factors include:

- Preterm birth
- Low-birth weight
- Enteral feeding
- Presence of bacteria (Chowdhury et al, 2016)

The precise etiology of this multifactorial disease process remains elusive. Consequently, treatments are symptomatic and surgical. The single most important predictor of outcome, besides gestational age, is whether the disease has progressed to a point requiring surgical intervention. Breastfeeding is the most effective preventative measure for NEC. Breast milk helps to provide immunity to the infant and promote healthy normal flora in the gastrointestinal tract of the infant.

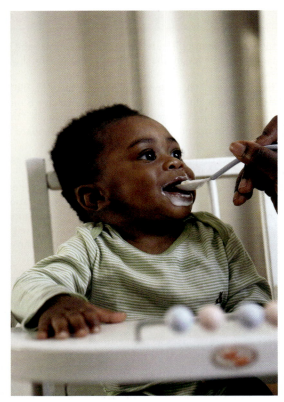

FIGURE 11-2 This baby is experiencing semisolid food for the first time and is clearly eager and ready to eat from the spoon.

A commonly used schedule for introducing new foods appears in Table 11-7. The baby's physician may modify it to meet individual needs. No evidence supports the superiority of a particular sequence of food introduction. In particular, infants might benefit from early introduction of iron-rich foods such as iron-fortified cereals and pureed meats, especially if being breastfed, to prevent the development of iron-deficiency anemia. Single-ingredient food and food that the infant can chew and swallow safely should be offered (Clinical Application 11-6).

The parent should heat a small amount to serve the infant. Food that has been heated and not consumed should be discarded because of possible contamination with salivary enzymes and bacteria. Food that has been opened but not heated should be stored in the covered jar in the refrigerator and used within 3 days.

LEARNING ABOUT FLAVORS

Eating adult foods is a skill that babies must learn, but their culture affects the food choices they will be offered. The fetus will experience flavors from the mother's diet in swallowed amniotic fluid. One study found that infants whose mother drank carrot juice in the third trimester enjoyed carrot-flavored cereals more than infants whose mother did not drink carrot juice or eat carrots. Infants will later experience some of these flavors in breast milk that reflects the foods, spices, and beverages consumed by the mother.

Weaning the Infant

Teaching the infant to use a cup is a gradual process. In most cases, the baby will show interest in the cup at 4 to 6 months. For these early attempts, and if the infant is not exclusively breastfed, water can be offered. If the mother decides to wean the child from breast or bottle before its first birthday, the replacement should be infant formula, not unmodified cow's milk.

The bottle-fed infant may not be ready to give up the bottle until 12 to 14 months of age. If bedtime bottles have not been used, weaning will proceed more rapidly. It is best to substitute the cup for the bottle for one

Waiting too long to introduce solid foods may delay the infant's acquiring the skill to manipulate the tongue and mouth appropriately. Early in the transition to semisolid foods, the amount consumed is likely to be small, so the main source of nutrients continues to be milk.

FEEDING

New foods should be introduced one at a time and a week apart so that if a problem develops, the responsible food can be readily identified. A food should be tried for 3 to 5 days before the infant is permitted to reject it. Only a taste or two is sufficient for the first try.

TABLE 11-7	Suggested Progression for Offering Foods to Infant at Low Risk of Allergies	
AGE OF INFANT	FOOD	RATIONALE/PRECAUTIONS
4 months	Infant cereal mixed with formula	Because of risk of allergies, rice offered first; wheat after age 12 months. Read labels: some mixed infant cereals contain wheat.
5–6 months	Strained vegetables	Less sweet than fruits; thought less likely to be rejected if offered before fruit.
6–7 months	Strained fruits	Will be well accepted; humans have strong preference for sweets.
6–8 months	Finger foods (bananas, crackers)	Encourages self-feeding. Different textures may aid speech development.
7–8 months	Strained meats	May be introduced earlier to add iron and zinc to the diet. Offer variety.
10 months	Strained or mashed egg yolk	Start with ½ tsp. Due to possible allergy, delay egg white until 1 year old.
10 months	Bite-sized cooked foods	Select appropriate foods. See Clinical Application 11-6.
12 months	Foods from adult table	Select suitable foods, prepared according to baby's abilities.

CLINICAL APPLICATION   **11-6**

Avoiding Choking Accidents

Each year, several hundred infants, as well as older children, choke on food. On average, one death every 5 days is reported in children from infancy to 9 years of age.

- Hot dogs, or frankfurters, are involved most often in infant choking. Apples, cookies, and biscuits are also frequent causes of choking in infants. Peanuts and grapes are the most dangerous for 2-year-old children, whereas 3-year-olds still face a risk from hot dogs.
- Other foods typically implicated in choking accidents appear in the following table by category. Because the child can safely eat many other foods, the prudent course is to avoid the listed foods when possible. If a choking incident occurs, any caregiver should be able to perform cardiopulmonary resuscitation (CPR) should it become necessary.
- Small children should always be supervised while they are eating, and they should be seated at a table to eat. Likewise, eating in a moving vehicle is discouraged.

HARD FOODS	STRINGY FOODS	STICKY FOODS	PLUG-SHAPED FOODS
Apples	Beans	Bread	Whole grapes
Carrots	Celery	Chewing gum	Hot dogs
Cookies	String beans	Peanut butter	Grape tomatoes
Corn		Marshmallows	
Hard candy			
Nuts			
Peanuts			
Popcorn			
Raisins			
Other raw vegetables			
Seedy items (e.g., watermelon)			

feeding period at a time. After using the new schedule for 5 days or so, the new method is substituted for a second feeding.

Nutritional Problems in Infancy

Common problems of nutrition in infancy are summarized in Table 11-8. The table includes some home remedies, but if an infant does not improve rapidly from a nutrition-related problem, parents should seek medical attention.

Allergies

Food allergies affect approximately 4% to 6% of children in the United States (CDC, May 9, 2017). Food allergies can be IgE mediated, non-IgE mediated, or a combination of both.

IGE-MEDIATED ALLERGIES

Because true food allergies can have fatal consequences, identifying children with allergies is critical. An **allergen** is a substance that provokes an abnormal individual hypersensitivity

or **allergy.** The steps in allergy production are illustrated in Figure 11-3.

The number of people with allergies is increasing rapidly both in developed and developing countries but not in underdeveloped areas. The fewer the germs in the environment, the more time the immune system has to process and react to allergens.

COMMON FOOD ALLERGENS

The following eight protein families account for the majority of food allergies:

1. Milk
2. Egg
3. Peanut
4. Tree nuts
5. Fish
6. Crustacean shellfish
7. Soy
8. Wheat

TABLE 11-8 Common Nutritional Problems in Infancy

PROBLEM	INTERVENTION	COMMENTS
Regurgitation of milk	Handle baby gently. Burp well; sit up after feeding.	Very common for first 6 months; not serious unless vomiting is projectile or bile-tinged or baby has persistent respiratory symptoms or poor weight gain.
Constipation	Apple or pear juice after the first month of life. 1 oz per day for each month of life up to 4 oz.	Rare in breastfed infants.
Burns to mouth	Swirl formula after heating; test well	Use water bath to heat. Formula warmed in a microwave oven continues to increase in temperature after removal.
Nursing-bottle syndrome	Do not use milk or juice as bedtime bottle; do not put sweetener on pacifier	See Chapter 3.

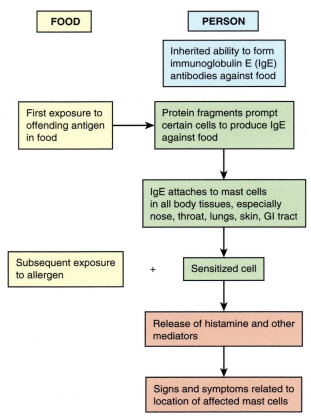

FIGURE 11-3 Development of an allergic reaction to food. *(Adapted from Formanek, 2001; Taylor & Hefle, 2006.)*

In children, the most common allergenic foods are:

- Eggs
- Milk
- Peanuts
- Soybeans
- Wheat

Children typically outgrow allergies to:

- Eggs
- Milk
- Soy
- Wheat

but not to:

- Peanuts
- Tree nuts
- Fish
- Shellfish

Clinical Application 11-7 describes symptoms of **anaphylaxis** after ingestion of a food allergen. The seriousness of food allergies should never be underestimated.

NONFOOD TRANSFERS OF ALLERGENS

Allergens can be transferred by modes other than ingestion:

- Inhalation:
  - An 11-year-old boy had anaphylaxis while his mother was cooking rice.

CLINICAL APPLICATION   11-7

Anaphylactic Reactions to Food

Allergy to food can be fatal. About 30,000 cases of food allergy–related anaphylaxis are seen annually in emergency departments.

Symptoms can develop within seconds of ingestion but typically will begin within 15 minutes of exposure, and respiratory arrest can occur within 30 minutes of exposure. Symptoms include:

- Difficulty swallowing/breathing
- Cough and wheezing, shortness of breath
- Hoarse voice and/or stridor
- Edema of face and hands
- Paleness and clamminess
- Tachycardia
- Loss of consciousness

Treatment and education of clients, families, health professionals, and the community need focus on the following:

- Accidental peanut ingestion should be avoided and early signs and symptoms of allergic reaction recognized. Food label awareness should be taught.
- Epinephrine should be prescribed, kept available, and used for clients with IgE-mediated food allergies.
- Children and adolescents who have an allergic reaction to food should be observed for 3 to 4 hours after the reaction at a center capable of dealing with anaphylaxis.
- Parents of such children should be taught to ensure that an emergency plan is developed and is provided to schools and other relevant institutions.
- Schools need to have training related to identification and emergency treatment of anaphylaxis, have written emergency plans, and have labeled emergency kits.

Of clients who have experienced life-threatening symptoms on initial reaction, 71% will have similarly severe reactions in subsequent episodes. When allergy seems possible, a thorough history and a food diary may yield a list of suspected foods to test further. Skin tests and blood tests can confirm the diagnosis.

Sources: Proudfoot & Saul, 2016; Skolnik, 2015.

- An 8-year-old girl developed anaphylaxis while white potatoes were being boiled at home.
- An 8-year-old boy who had a severe milk allergy had repeated anaphylaxis after intake of dry powder inhaler, which contained trace amounts of lactose (Ramirez & Bahna, 2009).
- Blood transfusion: An 8-year-old boy who underwent multiple blood product transfusion developed allergic reaction to food (Phillips, 2015).

Allergens from dissimilar sources also can evoke an allergic response. Cautions pertaining to cross-sensitivity to latex among persons allergic to various foods are listed in Clinical Application 11-8.

DIAGNOSIS

Self-diagnosis or parental diagnosis is a common practice but prone to error. Misdiagnosis leads to elimination of the wrong food or too many foods.

CLINICAL APPLICATION   11-8

Latex Allergies and Food Hypersensitivity

Individuals allergic to latex have demonstrated hypersensitivity to foods botanically unrelated to latex but that may share allergenic components. Allergies to certain fruits are described in 30% to 70% of latex-allergic clients, which is referred to as latex-fruit syndrome. The fruits most commonly involved are the following:

- Avocado
- Banana
- Chestnut
- Kiwi
- Tomato

Latex allergy should be ruled out in individuals allergic to any of those foods before performing clinical procedures using latex gloves.

For infants, the timing of new foods is well advised. The signs and symptoms of food allergies may appear as long as 5 days after exposure to an allergen. Thus, allowing at least 5 days to elapse between new foods will increase chances of identifying allergens.

TREATMENT OF ALLERGIES

The key to treatment is avoidance of the allergen. Reading labels is likely to take over the lives of the family.

Since the beginning of 2006, when the Food Allergen Labeling and Consumer Protection Act took effect, food labels are required to state clearly whether the food contains a major food allergen. The law identifies a major food allergen as any of the eight listed earlier and any ingredient that contains protein derived from them. So if a product contains casein or whey, for example, the label must include the word *milk*. The plain language declaration requirement also applies to flavorings, colorings, and incidental additives that are or contain a major food allergen (Food Allergy Research & Education [FARE], 2017).

FARE provides educational materials to assist in analyzing labels for ingredients with allergenic potential. Its Web site has notifications of products with ingredients not included on labels. For teachers and caregivers, the organization also has a model emergency plan in English and Spanish (FARE, 2017).

Pharmacologic management of allergy signs and symptoms includes the following:

- Antihistamines that block histamine receptors in the tissues for mild to moderate symptoms
- Epinephrine (adrenalin) with bronchodilator and vasopressor actions for severe reactions; self-administered epinephrine can be lifesaving.

Anaphylaxis guidelines suggest:

- Treatment with epinephrine
- Teaching about self-injectable epinephrine
- Referral to an allergist

- Sending the client home with an anaphylaxis emergency plan
- Teaching about anaphylaxis and its treatment

RELATED FOOD TECHNOLOGY

In any single day, our immune systems are exposed to thousands of proteins from the environment and the food we eat. All foods we consume are potential allergens. The discrepancy between the vast numbers of proteins we encounter and the limited number that actually become allergens led to an allergy assessment strategy for genetically modified foods. This technology enables adding or changing the genes that contribute to food allergies. Biotechnology products are extensively tested for allergic effects before commercialization, which contributes to increased safety.

Cow's Milk Protein–Sensitive Enteropathy

Cow's milk allergy is thought to affect 2% to 3% of children younger than 3 years (FARE, 2017). In an IgE-mediated allergy, an immune system response to a specific protein leads to inflammatory changes in the gastrointestinal tract.

Symptoms resolve within 48 to 72 hours after eliminating cow's milk protein from the diet. Children will often develop a tolerance of cow's milk with age. The physician should be reminded of dietary limitations so that an appropriate time can be chosen to reintroduce the offending foods.

Colic

Infantile colic occurs in 10% to 25% of infants. Although the cause of colic is unknown, the condition is named for the presumed manifestation, spasms of the muscles of the colon. The abdomen is tense, and the infant flexes his or her legs up to the belly and may appear flushed. The infant may cry for hours, starting late in the afternoon, just when caregivers are also tired and cranky. The classic definition of colic is the "Rule of Threes," crying for more than:

- 3 hours a day
- 3 days per week
- 3 weeks (Goldman & Beaumont, 2017)

POSSIBLE CAUSES

Although conclusive evidence on the cause of colic has not been found, suggested causes fall into two main groups:

- Gastrointestinal (food protein hypersensitivity or allergy)
- Nongastrointestinal (parental–child or maternal–child interaction problems)

The various factors act together, gastrointestinal, psychosocial, and neurodevelopmental disorders, have been suggested as causes for colic (Goldman & Beaumont, 2017). Physiological causes have been proposed:

- Some infants with colic have demonstrated low amounts of lactobacilli and increased amounts of coliform bacteria, which can contribute to increased gas production and gut dysmotility (Savino, Ceratto, De Marco, & Cordero di Montezemolo, 2014).

- Food allergy or sensitivity to milk or soy
- Gastroesophageal reflux

TREATMENT

The following interventions have sometimes helped:

- Holding the baby upright
- Burping
- Providing warm water to drink
- Diluting the formula
- Offering dairy-free formulas
- Swaddling
- Carrying the infant
- Rocking
- Making soft repetitive sounds

Newer research is emerging on the use of probiotics in the treatment of colic but more evidence is required. Even though their baby's condition is stressful for them, the parents should try not to be overly concerned. Most infants grow and gain weight despite colic.

The one proven treatment is time: 80% to 90% of infants with colic have diminished symptoms by age 3 months.

Diarrhea

WHO defines diarrhea as the passage of more than three loose, watery stools a day (WHO, 2017). In developing countries, diarrhea is the second leading cause of mortality among children younger than 5 years, with an estimated half million deaths annually (CDC, December 17, 2015).

Seventy-five percent of an infant's body weight is water, 54% of it extracellular. For this reason, an infant is at high risk of rapid dehydration from diarrhea. The degree of dehydration can be estimated from the infant's weight loss with severe dehydration being classified as a weight loss of more than 10%.

CAUSES

Infants are subject to osmotic diarrhea. Overfeeding and food intolerances are common causes of diarrhea.

The most common cause of infectious **enteritis** in human infants is **rotavirus.** Before the introduction of the rotavirus vaccination, rotavirus in children younger than 5 years accounted for 55,000 to 70,000 hospitalizations per year and 20 to 60 deaths annually in the United States (CDC, May 12, 2014). Those who remain at risk in the United States are children who are unvaccinated. Severe vomiting may accompany the diarrhea.

Children between 3 months and 3 years of age are most susceptible. By age 3, most children have antibodies against the virus. The fecal–oral route is its mode of transmission, but the virus survives for long periods on hard surfaces, in contaminated water, and on hands.

The only single prevention and control measure is vaccines against rotavirus gastroenteritis.

PATHOPHYSIOLOGY

As a result of diarrhea, the wall of the intestine may become inflamed. The inflammation diminishes the amount of lactase produced, so the infant may exhibit temporary lactose intolerance. Distension, cramps, and osmotic diarrhea ensue.

TREATMENT

Treatment should begin at home at the onset of the diarrhea. Caregivers should be instructed regarding signs and symptoms of dehydration and other parameters of treatment failure. The usual protocol is as follows:

- **Oral rehydration solutions (ORS)** should be used for rehydration, which should be accomplished in 3 to 4 hours.
- An age-appropriate, unrestricted diet should be given as soon as dehydration is corrected.
- For breastfed infants, nursing should be continued.
- For formula-fed infants, diluted formula is not recommended, and special formula is not necessary.
- Additional ORS should be administered for ongoing losses through diarrhea.
- No unnecessary laboratory tests or medications should be administered.

ORSs (see Chapter 8) are lifesaving not only in developing countries but also in North America. Most infants who are vomiting can be rehydrated with oral fluids. Provide sips of ORS by teaspoon to provide 50 milliliters per kilogram over 4 hours. A child weighing 40 pounds would require 900 milliliters over 4 hours or 225 milliliters, 45 teaspoons, per hour. Parents can administer one teaspoon of ORS every 1 to 2 minutes as tolerated. Ceralyte®, Oralyte®, and Pedialyte®, as well as store brands, are available at nearly all drug stores and grocery stores.

Sports drinks are not adequate substitutes for these solutions. Large amounts of fluids containing simple sugars, such as carbonated soft drinks, juice, and gelatin desserts, should be avoided because they might increase osmotic diarrhea. Liquids at room temperature are often better tolerated than warm or cold beverages.

WHEN TO CALL THE HEALTH-CARE PROVIDER

Parents should be instructed to call the primary health-care provider regarding an infant's diarrhea under the following conditions:

- Young or small infant
  - <6 months of age
  - <17.6 pounds in weight
- History of premature birth, chronic medical conditions, or concurrent illness
- Fever
  - 38°C (100.4°F) for infants aged <3 months
  - >39°C (102.2°F) for children aged 3 to 36 months
- Visible blood in stool
- High output, including frequent and substantial volumes of diarrhea
- Persistent vomiting
- Signs of dehydration
  - Sunken eyes
  - Decreased tears

- Dry mucous membranes
- Decreased urine output
- Change in mental status (e.g., irritability, apathy, or lethargy)
- Suboptimal response to oral rehydration therapy (ORT) already administered or inability of the caregiver to administer ORT.

ORS has been shown to have several benefits compared with intravenous fluid therapy (IVT), which include:

- Convenient to administer
- No associated pain or phlebitis
- ORS has been shown to have similar effectiveness in treating acute gastroenteritis in children

Risk factors for increased mortality from acute diarrhea in the United States are:

- Prematurity
- Young maternal age
- Black race
- Rural residence

The decision to hospitalize an infant should consider these factors along with degree of dehydration.

Nutrition of the Toddler (Age 1 to 3 Years)

The child's nutritional needs become more like those of adults after the first birthday. During the toddler years, growth is slower than during infancy, and although activity increases, the proportional need for kilocalories decreases compared with infancy. Thus, the child's appetite slackens.

How and what the family eats will influence the child's habits and tastes for many years. Being forced to eat a distasteful food because "it's good for you" has imprinted permanent avoidance behaviors on some individuals. Conversely, some parents expand their repertory of menu choices to set good examples for their children.

Psychosocial Development

Autonomy, or independence, is the psychosocial developmental task of the toddler. Every 2-year-old knows the word *no*. One way parents can assist a toddler achieve autonomy is to encourage choices from acceptable food alternatives (Fig. 11-4). If parents insist that a child eat certain items or amounts, the child may learn to use food rejection as a means of gaining attention. Later, more serious eating problems may result from such interactions. The parent can, however, create structure in the child's day by insisting the child remain at the table during mealtime whether or not items are consumed.

Physical Growth and Development

During the toddler years, growth slows. The expected weight gain in the second year may be just 4 to 6 pounds. Height may increase by about 4 inches. By age 2, however, head

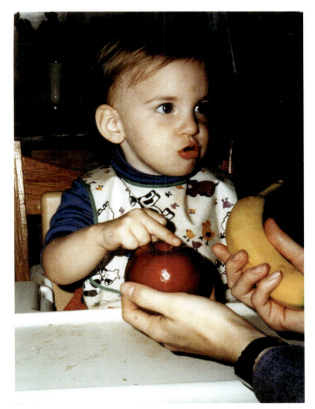

FIGURE 11-4 Autonomy is achieved in small steps. This 19-month-old girl is choosing her dessert.

circumference reaches two-thirds of its adult size. *See "Growth Charts" at www.cdc.gov/growthcharts.*

The toddler is aptly named. One of the skills acquired during this time is walking upright. As this skill is being perfected, the child's muscles of the back, buttocks, and thighs are enlarging. The bones are becoming more mineralized, and "baby fat" is disappearing.

Along with the gross motor skill of walking, the toddler's fine motor control improves. He or she is able to use eating utensils with more finesse. The spoon is likely to reach the mouth still filled with food. The toddler's mouth is more sensitive than an adult's mouth. Foods are eaten better at lukewarm temperatures rather than hot. Thus, dawdling at the table may have a physiological basis.

Nutrient Needs and Intake

For DRIs, see Appendix A. In 2008, the American Academy of Pediatrics recommended that all children receive a daily intake of 400 IU of vitamin D.

The need for many nutrients increases proportionately with body size throughout the growth years. These needs, coupled with the toddler's poorer appetite, stretch parents' ingenuity and patience. See Table 11-9 for MyPlate recommendations for 2- to 3-year-olds.

According to the American Academy of Pediatrics, despite the toddler's poorer appetite, vitamin supplements are

TABLE 11-9   MyPlate Guidelines for 2- to 3-Year-Olds Based on 1,000 Calories/Day

FOOD GROUP	SERVING SIZE	SERVING SUGGESTIONS
Grains	3 ounces	Make half your grains whole. Aim for minimum of 1½ ounces of whole grains a day.
Fruit	1 cup	Eat a variety of fruit. Choose whole or cut-up fruits more often than fruit juice.
Vegetable	1 cup	Vary your veggies. Each week aim for the following: Dark green = ½ cup Red and orange = 2½ cups Beans and peas = ½ cup Starchy veggies = 2 cups Other veggies = 1½ cups
Protein foods	2 ounces	Vary proteins to include seafood, eggs, lean meats, poultry, beans, peas, nuts, and seeds. Keep meat and poultry portions small and lean.
Dairy	2 cups	Drink fat-free or low-fat (1%) milk. Serve fat-free or low-fat yogurt and cheese. If serving soy products make sure that they are calcium-fortified and low fat or fat-free.
Fats, sugar, sodium	3 teaspoons oil Limit saturated fat to less than 11 grams and added sugar to less than 25 grams Sodium less than 1,500 mg	Serve low-fat dairy. Serve lean proteins. Avoid sugary snacks and beverages. Serve fruits in natural form instead of canned fruits packed in water. Avoid processed foods.

probably unnecessary for healthy children older than 1 year (see Dollars & Sense 11-2). Special circumstances may indicate a need for supplementation.

Food Likes

Toddlers like finger foods and can learn about texture by eating them. Toddlers prefer plain foods to most mixtures such as casseroles. Familiar combinations, such as macaroni and cheese, spaghetti, and pizza, however, may be relished. Unfamiliar foods that are rejected the first time should be offered again at a later time.

Dollars & Sense 11-2

Children's Vitamins

Although the American Academy of Pediatrics does not recommend vitamin and mineral supplements for healthy children, many families provide them as insurance. If parents choose to give vitamin and mineral supplements to a child, they should be aware of the cost per year. For example:

Age	Brand Name Product	Price/ Daily Dose	Total Cost
1–12 years	Children's chewable	$0.12	$43.80
12–18 years	Adult tablet	$0.08	$29.20
Total per family with 2 children			$73.00

Mealtimes

Toddlers are learning social skills as well as good nutritional habits. Eating is a social experience for adults most of the time; toddlers also appreciate company. Parents should be encouraged to sit down and eat with the toddler. Visiting other homes might introduce food items and experiences not encountered at home.

Keeping to a regular schedule will help maintain the child's food intake. A 1-year-old's stomach holds just 1 cup, necessitating small servings. A serving is one-fourth to one-fifth the size of an adult's recommended serving. A good rule of thumb is to serve 1 tablespoonful for each year of age.

Eating regular meals and nutritious snacks helps to prevent fatigue and control the appetite. If high-sugar snacks are used to assuage hunger before a meal, however, the more nutritious foods at the meal may be taken poorly.

New Foods

After the pureed foods of infancy, parents will be pleased to offer more attractive plates of food to the toddler. Brightly colored foods are appealing. Nevertheless, chewing may not be well developed. Tough meat or very fibrous vegetables are not for the toddler.

Foods not recommended until after the first birthday can be gradually introduced if family history of allergies is not a concern. These foods include unmodified cow's milk, egg white, wheat, citrus fruits, seafood, chocolate, and nut butters. Parents should continue to introduce foods one at a time at weekly intervals and to watch for reactions.

Even very young children make their wishes known through body movements, pushing food away, closing their mouths, and turning away from the feeder. The astute parent will respond to these cues before the child resorts to crying to communicate distress. Parents should be advised to avoid the use of external cues such as prompts, rewards, or forcing a child to clean their plate.

Daily intake should include:

- One serving of a vitamin C–rich fruit or vegetable
- One serving of a green leafy or yellow vegetable
- Limited sugar
- 19 grams of fiber

Parents should continue to avoid giving the toddler hazardous foods (Clinical Application 11-6). Sometimes chopping the food into tiny pieces eliminates a choking hazard. Nevertheless, a toddler should not be left alone while eating.

Because the kidneys become mature at about age 1, the toddler can tolerate salt in moderation. Preference for salty foods is an acquired taste. Because of the association between salt and high blood pressure later in life, the prudent parent will discourage the consumption of heavily salted foods.

Nutritional Concerns

Toddlers are at risk for iron-deficiency anemia. Misguided food choices may lead to inadequate intakes of nutrients and interfere with growth and development.

Iron-Deficiency Anemia

Iron deficiency affects 2.4 million children in the United States. Childhood iron-deficiency **anemia** is associated with behavioral and cognitive delays. The National Institutes of Health (February 11, 2016) reports that in the United States, 6% of toddlers aged 1 to 3 years are anemic and 12% of these toddlers are Hispanic. Globally, iron-deficiency anemia affects 43% of children under age 5 years (Evaluation of Injectable, 2016).

Overindulging in milk is thought to decrease the appetite for iron-rich foods, enriched cereals, meats, and some fruits and vegetables. Therefore, milk intake should be limited to 24 ounces per day for children aged 1 to 5 years. The term *milk anemia* refers to iron-deficiency anemia caused by overconsumption of milk and underconsumption of iron-rich foods. Juice for toddlers should not exceed 6 ounces per day (Box 11-2).

Treatment of iron-deficiency anemia may include medication and ingestion of iron-fortified foods or foods naturally high in iron. The recommendation for iron supplements is 3 milligrams per kilogram per day with normal hemoglobin resulting within 1 to 2 months. Vegetarian diets may pose a risk for iron deficiency in toddlers. The position of the Academy of Nutrition and Dietetics is that a *well-planned* vegetarian diet can provide all the nutrients needed by children at varying stages of growth. Extremely restrictive diets such as fruitarian and raw foods diets, however, have been associated

---

BOX 11-2 ■ Recommendations for Juice Consumption

For Infants
- No juice before 1 year of age unless clinically indicated for the treatment of constipation
- No juice from bottles or covered cups that permit consumption throughout the day
- No juice at bedtime
- No unpasteurized juice

For Children and Adolescents
- Age 1 to 3: Limit juice to 4 ounces per day
- Age 4 to 6: Limit juice to 4 to 6 ounces per day
- Age 7 and older: Limit juice to 8 ounces per day
- Encourage consumption of whole fruits
- No unpasteurized juice

Assessment and Interventions
- Determine amount of juice intake for children with overnutrition or undernutrition and those with chronic diarrhea or abdominal symptoms.
- Determine the amount and means of juice intake for children with dental caries.
- Teach parents the difference between juice and juice drinks.

Source: Summarized from American Academy of Pediatrics. Abrams, S.A. (2017, May 22). Weighing in on Fruit Juice: AAP Now Says No Juice Before Age 1. *AAP News*. Available at http://www.aappublications.org/news/2017/05/22/FruitJuice052217.

---

with impaired growth and are not recommended for infants and children.

Milk Intake

To support brain growth and development, 1- to 2-year-old children should continue to drink whole milk. At age 2, fat intake should gradually be reduced to 30% to 40% of a child's intake and transitioning to low-fat or fat-free milk is recommended.

Nutrition of the Preschool Child (Age 3 to 6 Years)

This is a delightful time of enthusiastic learning, including food preferences.

Psychosocial Development

Initiative is the psychosocial task to be mastered by the preschool child. Within their capabilities, children should be encouraged to set and achieve some goals of their own. Children can participate in planning and preparation of meals, and they should help in the kitchen, not just with cleanup. Preschool children can help make gelatin desserts, roll cookie dough and use cookie cutters, crack eggs, and stir ingredients to foster a sense of accomplishment.

By making the meal a social time and eating slowly themselves, parents can encourage the same behavior in a child. Exemplifying good manners will be more productive than criticizing the child's manners.

Having company their own age is helpful. Children stay at the table longer and eat more in the company of their peers. Exchanging visits with a friend's child will begin to broaden the child's horizons.

Physical Growth and Development

From the third to the sixth year, a child continues to gain 4 to 5 pounds per year. A gain in height of about 2 inches per year is average so that by age 5, birth length will have doubled. Half the adult height is attained by approximately age 2 years.

Adequacy of growth should be assessed every 6 to 12 months. Growth charts remain the standard against which a given assessment is judged. *See "Growth Charts" at www.cdc.gov/growthcharts.*

Nutrient Needs and Intake

For DRIs, see Appendix A. In 2008, the American Academy of Pediatrics recommended that all children receive a daily intake of 400 IU of vitamin D.

Preschool children are very active. A 3-year-old may need 1,300 to 1,500 kilocalories per day. Serving sizes for 4- to 6-year-old children are the same as those *recommended* for adults.

Developing Good Habits

The preschool child responds best to regular mealtimes. When the adult meal will be served late, the parents have to decide if it would be better to allow the child to socialize with adults at a late meal or to feed the child early.

Preschoolers cannot eat enough in only three meals to meet their needs. By age 3, a child is able to verbalize hunger. Some nutrient-dense, low-fat choices are:

- Cottage cheese
- Low-fat yogurt
- Fresh fruit
- Raw vegetables
- Low-fat milk
- Fruit juices
- Graham crackers
- Fig bars

Concentrated sweets such as candy and soda pop should be limited.

However, too much control is undesirable. Young children naturally obey inner cues of hunger and satiety. Parents who override those cues by insisting the child eat a given amount are teaching the child to overeat. It is better to acknowledge that the child cannot consume enough at mealtime and to provide healthy snacks.

Tableware should be appropriate for the preschool child. Unbreakable dishes that are designed for stability, with deep sides to permit scooping the food onto a spoon or fork, are practical choices. Small glasses and cups, also unbreakable, with a squat design and low center of gravity, will minimize accidents and mealtime tension.

It is not too early to emphasize the importance of cleanliness. Regularly washing hands before meals and brushing teeth after meals will cultivate good health habits.

New Foods

Parents should offer new foods one at a time in small amounts. Trying something new is most acceptable at the beginning of the meal when the child is hungriest. A taste or two is sufficient if new foods are offered at regular intervals. Often 8 to 10 tries are necessary before the child develops a taste for a new food.

Parents have the advantage of being able to select the food offered. Items the parents dislike will not grace the family table regularly, if at all. Children too should be permitted their preferences. If an argument over food develops into a power struggle, as sometimes happens, the child will not admit to liking the food, even when it turns out to be quite tasty.

Nutritional Concerns

Preschool children should be monitored for problems. See Box 11-3 for data that can be included in pediatric nutritional screening.

In addition, dental caries and the nutritional quality in day-care programs may be of concern.

Dental Health

The destruction of tooth enamel by dental caries (see Chapter 2) is a problem for children in all economic groups. The "baby" teeth, as well as the permanent teeth, deserve care and professional attention. For teeth to be

---

BOX 11-3 ■ Nutrition Screening for Young Children

Nutritional screening in young children is important to ensure proper growth and development and for early detection of nutritional-related problems such as obesity and failure to thrive. Nutritional screening also allows time for anticipatory guidance. Various screening tools can be used that provide both subjective and objective data.

Objective data should include:

- Height/length of child and parents
- Weight
- Objective data should be plotted on growth charts at each assessment

Subjective data can include data such as:

- How many ounces of milk and juice does the child consume each day?
- How many servings of fruits and vegetables does the child eat per day?
- How many servings of whole grains does the child eat per day?
- What are main protein sources?
- How many hours of television or video watching per day?
- How many times per week does the child eat fast food meals?
- How many minutes of physical activity does the child participate in each day?

correctly brushed, the parent may have to do it. Fluorosis (see Chapter 7) has occurred as a result of the overuse of supplements and the ingestion of fluoridated toothpaste. Children younger than 6 years are likely to swallow rather than to expectorate toothpaste. A pea-sized portion of toothpaste is sufficient. Regular dental checkups should be a part of the preschool child's routine.

There is an economic disparity associated with early childhood carries (ECC) with children living in lower socioeconomic environments having higher rates of decay (Anil & Anand, 2017). Adequate dentition and good nutrition are mutually supportive. Nutritional counseling for parents is an important intervention for the prevention of dental carries in children.

Childcare Programs

It is estimated that approximately three-quarters of children aged 3 to 6 years in the United States spend time in organized child care. Childcare centers offering meals through the Child and Adult Care Food Program have guidelines that they must follow. Some pertinent recommendations are:

- Fruit juice must be 100% fruit juice and can only be offered once daily.
- Breakfast cereal must contain no more than 6 grams of sugar per ounce.
- Yogurt can contain no more than 23 grams of sugar per 6 ounces.
- Flavored milk should not be offered to children under age 5 years, and when offered to children older than 5 years it should contain no more than 22 grams of sugar per 8 ounces.

Nutrition of the School-Age Child (Age 6 to 12 Years)

A balanced diet suitable for healthy adults will also be good for a school-age child.

Diets should not be restricted because of the energy (kilocalorie), fat, or sugar content of any one food, nor should foods be labeled *good* or *bad*. In the first case, food may be regarded as medicine, and in the second, as "forbidden fruit." Neither viewpoint fosters positive attitudes.

Psychosocial Development

According to Erikson, the developmental task of the school-age child is **industry.** The school years are the years to build competence in many different skills. Making and keeping commitments is part of developing industry.

School-age children can participate in planning menus, shopping for food, preparing the meals, as well as cleaning up afterward (Fig. 11-5). Limiting the child's role to washing the dishes or taking out the garbage will be more likely to foster a sense of inferiority than habits of industry.

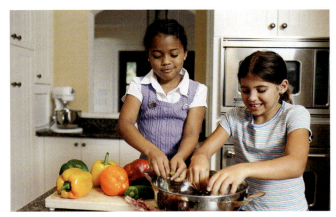

FIGURE 11-5 Preparing dinner with a friend can involve culinary practice.

Physical Growth and Development

The average yearly growth during the school years is 7 pounds and 2.5 inches. The growth is not evenly distributed throughout the year, reflected in an inconsistent appetite. A child's progress should be tracked on the CDC growth charts to determine if growth is within the normal range. *See "Growth Charts" at www.cdc.gov/growthcharts.*

Exercise can help the school-age child's growth and development by stimulating osteoblasts and expending energy to control weight. Activities that are likely to become lifetime interests should be especially encouraged. Unlike sports such as football that are played by few adults, tennis or similar skill sports may provide an outlet for a lifetime.

By school age, the effects of good or poor nutrition will begin to be apparent. The well-nourished child will display most of the qualities listed in Table 11-10.

Nutritional Needs and Concerns

For DRIs, see Appendix A. In 2008, the American Academy of Pediatrics recommended that all children receive a daily intake of 400 IU of vitamin D.

See Table 11-11 for MyPlate guidelines for 4- to 8-year-olds.

Meal Patterns and Behaviors

A school-age child cannot consume all the needed nutrients in three child-sized meals. Healthy snacks are necessary to complement the main meals. Likewise, breakfast is essential and should contain one-fourth to one-third of the day's nutrients.

School-age children are generally so active that they may have trouble sitting still. Requiring them to spend 15 to 20 minutes at the table for meals will increase the likelihood that they will eat a complete meal.

Nutrition at School

Nutrition education continues in school, focusing on foods, not nutrients. Interactions with other children and school experiences expose a child to new foods and different cultures.

TABLE 11-10   Indications of Good Nutrition in the School-Age Child

General appearance	Alert, energetic; Normal height and weight
Skin and mucous membranes	Skin smooth, slightly moist; mucous membranes pink, no bleeding
Hair	Shiny, evenly distributed
Scalp	No sores
Eyes	Bright, clear, no fatigue circles
Teeth	Straight, clean, no discoloration or caries
Tongue	Pink, papillae present, no sores
Gastrointestinal system	Good appetite, regular elimination
Musculoskeletal system	Well-developed, firm muscles; erect posture, bones straight without deformities
Neurological system	Good attention span for age; not restless, irritable, or weepy

A program has been developed by four National Institutes of Health called the We Can! (Ways to Enhance Children's Activity and Nutrition) program. The program was developed as a tool for parents, health-care providers, and communities to use in order to help children 8 through 13 years old stay at a healthy weight. We Can! offers tools and resources that can be used by schools to educate children and parents about healthy eating and nutrition, physical activity, and decreased screen time. The resources can be found at: https://www.nhlbi.nih.gov/health/educational/wecan/tools-resources/index.htm.

Because children need nourishment to learn and many come to school hungry, food assistance is available at school. Federally reimbursable school meals programs require participating schools to offer meals free or at reduced prices to eligible children. In 2016, 14.5 million children participated in the School Breakfast Program, and approximately 12 million received their meals free or at a reduced price. See Box 11-4 and Table 11-12 for requirements.

Nutrition in Adolescence

Adolescence is the period that extends from the onset of **puberty** until full growth is reached. For most individuals, adolescence occurs between 12 and 20 years of age. Adolescence is second only to infancy in the nutritional requirements necessary for growth and development. Unfortunately, most adolescents do not meet the daily recommendation for fruits, vegetables, and whole grains; they exceed the daily recommended amount of sodium; and they drink more full-calorie soda per day than milk (Kann et al, 2016). See Box 11-5 for information regarding energy drinks and the adolescent.

Psychosocial Development

Achieving their own **identity** is the developmental task Erikson identified for adolescents, including accepting their capabilities. In this process, teenagers "try on" various identities. Adolescents pick up fads instantly and drop them just as suddenly. Food and eating fads are part of the same pattern.

TABLE 11-11   MyPlate Guidelines for 4- to 8-Year-Olds Based on 1,400 Calories/Day

FOOD GROUP	SERVING SIZE	SERVING SUGGESTIONS
Grains	5 ounces	Make half your grains whole. Aim for minimum of 2½ ounces of whole grains a day.
Fruit	1–1½ cups	Eat a variety of fruit. Choose whole or cut-up fruits more often than fruit juice.
Vegetable	1½ cups	Vary your veggies. Each week aim for the following: Dark green = 1 cup; Red and orange = 3 cups; Beans and peas = ½ cup; Starchy veggies = 3½ cups; Other veggies = 2½ cups
Protein foods	4 ounces	Vary proteins to include seafood, eggs, lean meats, poultry, beans, peas, nuts, and seeds. Keep meat and poultry portions small and lean.
Dairy	2½ cups	Drink fat-free or low-fat (1%) milk. Serve fat-free or low-fat yogurt and cheese. If serving soy products, make sure that they are calcium-fortified and low fat or fat-free.
Fats, sugar, sodium	4 teaspoons oil; Limit saturated fat to less than 16 grams and added sugar to less than 35 grams; Sodium less than 1,900 mg	Serve low-fat dairy. Serve lean proteins. Avoid sugary snacks and beverages. Serve fruits in natural form instead of canned fruits packed in water. Avoid processed foods.

BOX 11-4 ■ School Foods

Federally funded school meals began in 1946 and specify nutritional content to be served (see Table 11-12).

Competitive foods are primary sources of low-nutrient, energy-dense foods that students consume that include items such as candy; chips; noncarbonated, high-sugar drinks; and soda. Federal regulations prohibit access to foods of minimal nutritional value in food-service areas during mealtimes, but schools can sell these foods at other locations during the school day. In the last decade, 39 states have passed law or policy addressing competitive foods and beverages (U.S. Department of Agriculture [USDA], June 7, 2017).

The Institute of Medicine (2010) released standards for items available on school campuses but not part of the federally reimbursable school meals. The purpose of these stricter standards is to promote healthful eating habits. If followed, the standards would make à la carte cafeteria offerings, vending machine products, and fundraising items nearly conform to the Dietary Guidelines for Americans.

Physical Growth and Development

The term *growth spurt* is accurate. Boys and girls differ in the timing and completion of the growth spurt (see Table 11-13). To track an adolescent's growth, BMI-for-age percentile charts (2- to 20-year-old boys and girls) are available at www.cdc.gov/growthcharts.

The peak growth spurt is known to take place between 10 and 14 years in girls and between 12 and 16 years in boys. During the peak of the adolescent growth spurt, the mineral and protein content of the body is increased.

Nutritional Needs and Concerns

For DRIs, see Appendix A. In 2011, the American Academy of Pediatrics endorsed the IOM recommendation that all adolescents receive a daily intake of 600 IU of vitamin D (Golden & Abrams, 2014).

See Table 11-14 for MyPlate recommendations for adolescents 14 years old and older. Current guidelines for distribution of macronutrients can be found in Box 11-6.

Calcium and Iron

Regarding nutrients, adolescent diets are lacking in calcium and iron. Long-term, deficiencies of those minerals may be manifested in osteoporosis or anemia. Short-term, evidence suggests an influence of dietary factors on fracture occurrence. Although rates of fracture vary considerably with age, sex, and maturation, they peak in early puberty. At that time, rates of bone turnover are high, but bone mineral accrual lags behind gains in height and weight. Among the factors impacting pediatric fracture incidence are the following:

- Bone mass and bone mineral density
- Low calcium intake

TABLE 11-12 Federally Reimbursable School Meal Programs

	OPERATING SINCE	STUDENTS SERVED, 2015–2016	FOOD	CURRENT REQUIREMENT
School breakfast	1975	14.5 million	Fruit–1 cup with vegetable substitution	1 cup with vegetable substitution allowed.
			Whole grains	Grades K–6 have 1 oz daily minimum (7–10 oz weekly); grades 6–8 have 1 oz minimum (10–12 oz weekly); grades 9–12 have 1 oz minimum daily (9–10 oz weekly).
			Milk	1 cup Must be fat-free (unflavored/flavored) or 1% low-fat (unflavored)
National school lunch	1946	30.5 million	Fruit/vegetables	¾ cup of vegetables plus ½–1 cup fruit minimum per day. With weekly requirements for dark greens, red/orange, legumes, starchy
			Meat/meat alternate	Grades K–8 have 1 oz daily minimum (grades K–5 require 8–10 oz weekly and grades 6–8 require 9–10 oz weekly); grades 9–12 have 2 oz minimum (10–12 oz weekly).
			Grains	Grades K–5: 1 oz minimum (8–9 oz weekly); grades 6–8: 1 oz minimum (8–10 oz weekly); grades 9–12: 2 oz minimum (10–12 oz weekly) All grains must be whole.
			Milk	1 cup (5 cups weekly for all grade levels) Must be fat-free (unflavored/flavored) or 1% low-fat (unflavored).

Adapted from U.S. Department of Agriculture (June 13, 2017). Available at https://www.fns.usda.gov/nslp/national-school-lunch-program-nslp

<table>
<tr><td colspan="2">BOX 11-5 ■ **Energy Drink Use in Adolescents**</td></tr>
</table>

Energy drinks are beverages that contain higher levels of caffeine than soda and also can contain herbal supplements and vitamins. Energy drinks market the effects of improved energy, reaction time, and improved concentration, which are attractive benefits to some adolescents. There is an increase in energy drink consumption among adolescents in recent years. Studies demonstrated that 30% of adolescents consume energy drinks (Williams Jr., Odum, & Housman, 2017). Adolescents may not be educated on the differences between sports drinks and energy drinks, and use of energy drinks may contribute to a multitude of adverse events, including increased heart rate and blood pressure, arterial stiffness, myocardial infarction, overweight and obesity, renal impairment, diabetes, and dental carries (Children, Adolescents, and Parents, 2014). Adolescents with preexisting conditions or undiagnosed conditions such as heart disease are at increased risk when consuming energy drinks. Education needs to be provided to adolescents while further research is conducted to determine the safety of energy drinks in adolescents.

BOX 11-6 ■ **Macronutrients for Children and Adolescents (4 to 18 years)**

Carbohydrates: 45% to 65% of daily calories
Protein: 10% to 30% of daily calories
Fat: 25% to 35% of daily calories

- Insufficient vitamin D levels
- High body mass index
- Excessive consumption of carbonated beverages
- Lack of weight-bearing physical activity
- Use of corticosteroids

For all children and adolescents, breakfast, or lack thereof, has an impact on overall dietary intake significantly (see Box 11-7). Teens should strive to consume three to four servings of calcium-rich foods fortified with vitamin D daily.

Overenthusiastic Weight Control

Because of the cultural value placed on thinness, adolescents, especially girls, may restrict their dietary intake to achieve a desired slim body. Some use unhealthy practices such as fasting, diet pills, laxatives, and vomiting to remain slim. **Anorexia nervosa** affects 0.5% to 1% of 14- to 18-year-old girls and is covered in Chapter 16. Eating disorders can last for years; malnutrition and dramatic weight loss can affect both short- and long-term growth and development (Rocks, Pelly, & Wilkinson, 2014). Participating in sports that value slimness is a risk factor for both girls and boys (see Box 11-8).

Some adolescents may adopt vegetarianism as a means to control weight and body shape rather than for ecological or spiritual reasons. Regardless of the reason they have

TABLE 11-13 **Adolescent Growth Spurts**

STATUS	AGE IN YEARS	
	Boys	Girls
Age in years	12–17	9.5–14.5
Height gain in year of peak velocity	>10 cm (3.9 in.)	Possibly 9 cm (3.5 in.)
Age at peak growth velocity	13–15	11–13.5
At age 18	2.54 cm growth remains	Slightly less remaining growth than boys Growth 99% complete

TABLE 11-14 **MyPlate Guidelines for 14+-Year-Olds Based on 1,800 Calories/Day**

FOOD GROUP	SERVING SIZE	SERVING SUGGESTIONS
Grains	6 ounces	Make half your grains whole. Aim for 3 ounces of whole grains a day.
Fruit	1½ cups	Eat a variety of fruits. Choose whole or cut-up fruits more often than fruit juice.
Vegetable	2½ cups	Vary your veggies. Each week aim for the following: Dark green = 1½ cups Red and orange = 5½ cups Beans and peas = 1½ cups Starchy veggies = 5 cups Other veggies = 4 cups
Protein foods	5 ounces	Vary proteins to include seafood, eggs, lean meats, poultry, beans, peas, nuts, and seeds.
Dairy	3 cups	Drink fat-free or low-fat (1%) milk. Serve fat-free or low-fat yogurt and cheese. If serving soy products, make sure that they are calcium-fortified and low fat or fat-free.
Fats, sugar, sodium	5 teaspoons oil Limit saturated fat to less than 20 grams and added sugar to less than 45 grams Sodium less than 2,300 mg	Serve low-fat dairy. Serve lean proteins. Avoid sugary snacks and beverages. Serve fruits in natural form instead of canned fruits packed in water. Avoid processed foods.

BOX 11-7 ■ Breakfast Versus No Breakfast Effects

Among children and adolescents, breakfast or lack of breakfast has an appreciable impact on the day's nutritive intake. One significant predictor of adolescent breakfast eating was parental breakfast eating. One study demonstrates that approximately 30% of adolescents skip breakfast every day and up to 60% skip breakfast three to four times per week (Bauer et al, 2015).

On average, children who skipped breakfast did not make up the nutrient deficits during the remainder of the day. Breakfast skipping has also been associated with the development of unhealthy eating habits, weight gain, and obesity. Recent evidence is demonstrating that skipping breakfast is also associated with poor glucose control, and an increased risk of developing type 2 diabetes (Alwattar, Thyfault, & Leidy, 2015). Children who eat breakfast on most days have improved attention spans, concentration, and memory as well has higher intakes of micronutrients. For benefits such as lower weight and greater satiety, breakfast should be consumed daily and consist of low-glycemic, high-fiber carbohydrates and lean proteins.

BOX 11-8 ■ The Female Athlete Triad

Female athletes, who desire athletic success as well as thinness, are at risk for developing a medical condition commonly referred to as the "female athlete triad." The disorder can have a negative impact on athletes' health and performance and is characterized by low energy availability, menstrual dysfunction, and low bone mineral density.

- Low energy availability—occurs from pressure to lose weight and can result in unhealthy dieting practices such as severe calorie restriction, and the use of laxatives or enemas.
- Menstrual dysfunction—cessation of menstrual period related to calorie restriction and/or excess physical exercise.
- Low bone mineral density—osteoporosis can develop from a decreased intake of calcium and vitamin D and from a decrease in estrogen production. All girls and women should be encouraged to participate in sports and physical activities because of the positive benefits, including health benefits, increased self-esteem, and peer socialization. Female athletes should be screened for the triad before participating in sports and educated about the body's need for nutrients.

become vegetarians, these adolescents should have their nutritional status and dietary intake monitored.

Acne and Diet

Acne afflicts more than 17 million Americans, with approximately 80% to 90% of adolescents affected. Acne is triggered by sex hormones stimulating the sebaceous glands. The skin becomes oilier and the ducts to the glands sometimes plug up, permitting the accumulation of harmful bacteria that produce inflammation. The sebaceous glands' production of sebum may be influenced by androgens and hormonal mediators that, in turn, may be stimulated by foods.

There are three dietary components that research has identified as having an influence on the development of acne during adolescence including:

- Hyperglycemic carbohydrates
- Milk
- Saturated and trans fats (Melnik, 2015).

Foods with a high glycemic load (see **glycemic index** in Glossary), such as white bread or potatoes, cause a rapid rise in blood glucose. Foods with a low glycemic index, such as high-fiber cereals or beans, cause a more gradual change in blood glucose. Likewise, dairy has been shown to influence the insulin/insulin growth factor (IGF)-1 pathway that contributes to the increased production of hormones related to development of acne. Higher intake of saturated and trans fats have demonstrated an increase in the production of sebum, which contributes to worsening acne, whereas the consumption of omega-3 fatty acids demonstrated a protective benefit against acne (Melnik, 2015).

Overweight in Children and Adolescents

Childhood obesity has been a concern in the United States for the past 3 decades. Childhood obesity rates have remained consistent for the past decade, affecting 17% of children 2 to 19 years old, which translates to 12.7 million children (CDC, April 10, 2017). Box 11-9 describes the diagnosis and prevalence of overweight and obesity in children and adolescents in the United States. Table 11-15 demonstrates the percentage of children at or above the 95% for weight based on ethnicity.

Obesity is a multifactorial process that includes inactivity, overconsumption of calories, and genetic factors. Over 90% of obesity cases are idiopathic and less than 10% are associated with genetics (Xu & Xue, 2016). One study estimates that there is a 50% to 80% chance that a child with obese parents will become obese (McHugh, 2016). Childhood obesity is associated with obesity as an adult. Those who are overweight or obese have a higher risk of developing:

- Insulin resistance and/or type 2 diabetes
- Hypertension and hypercholesterolemia
- Sleep apnea and/or asthma
- Non-alcoholic fatty liver disease
- Decreased self-esteem
- Increased risk of bullying

Some of the factors contributing to overweight and obesity in children are:

- Unwise food choices
- Inactivity, with television and computer games replacing active play
- Decreased ability to self-regulate energy intake related to overcontrolling parents
- Inability of parents to see child as overweight
- Lower socioeconomic environments
- Genetics

Strategies to prevent overweight are listed in Table 11-16. These approaches cost less than treatment of established obesity and reach the greatest number of children.

Weight management is the subject of Chapter 16. Overweight children require careful supervision to maintain

BOX 11-9 ■ Overweight in Childhood and Adolescence

Technically, obesity refers to fatness, often measured by skinfold thickness, not weight. However, BMI is used as a surrogate measure of obesity because its components, height and weight, are readily available data and the growth charts for comparison are easily obtained. *See "Growth Charts" at www.cdc.gov/growthcharts.*

A BMI between the 5th and the 85th percentile is considered normal for children and adolescents. Values over the 95th percentile have been variously defined in this population as overweight or obese. By late adolescence, the 95th percentile is about equal to an adult BMI of 30, signifying obesity.

Figure 11-6 illustrates the prevalence of obesity in both genders and in all age groups. Table 11-15 shows **NHANES survey** results by gender and ethnic group. Clearly, the distribution varies by ethnicity, but overall the percentage of children and adolescents with BMIs above the 95th percentile continued to increase.

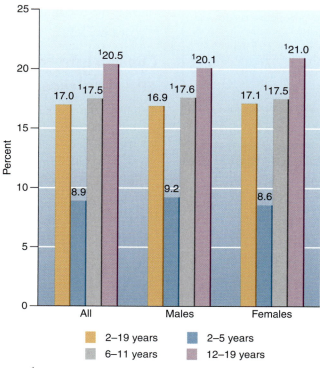

1 Significantly different from those aged 2–5 years.

FIGURE 11-6 Statistics demonstrating the incidence of children, both male and female, at or above the 95th percentile of BMI from 2011 to 2014. *(From Ogden, CL, Carroll, MD, Fryar, CD, and Flegal, KM: Prevalence of Obesity Among Adults and Youth: United States, 2011–2014. NCHS Data Brief, No. 219. National Center for Health Statistics, Hyattsville, MD, 2015. Accessed on August 28, 2017. Available at: https://www.cdc.gov/nchs/data/databriefs/db219.pdf.)*

TABLE 11-15   Percentages of Children Aged 2–19 Years At or Above the 95th Percentile, NHANES 2011–2014

ETHNIC GROUP	MALE	FEMALE
Non-Hispanic white	14.3	15.1
Non-Hispanic black	18.4	20.7
Non-Hispanic Asian	11.8	5.3
Hispanic	22.4	21.4

Source: Ogden, CL, Carroll, MD, Fryar, CD, and Flegal KM: Prevalence of Obesity Among Adults and Youth: United States, 2011–2014. NCHS Data Brief, No. 219. National Center for Health Statistics, Hyattsville, MD, 2015.

normal growth and development while reducing weight and adipose tissue. Treatment of obese children requires a multicomponent program encompassing diet, physical activity, nutrition counseling, and parent or caregiver participation.

The conditions permitting or encouraging overweight among youth have evolved over many years and have become embedded in the dominant culture that involves the food industry and marketing. No single change is going to reverse the trend. Multiple interventions and strategies are needed at all levels: individuals, families, schools, communities, and the nation.

TABLE 11-16 Strategies to Prevent Childhood Overweight

AGE GROUP	STRATEGY	BARRIERS	RATIONALE
Infant	Promote and support breastfeeding	Cultural norms about breastfeeding in general or in public or the workplace	Many health benefits May allow infant to control amount consumed better than with formula feeding
Toddler and preschooler	Implement MyPlate at home and in day care/preschool Limit sweetened drinks Begin 1% or fat-free dairy Encourage daily physical activity	Parents/caregivers may be reluctant to change	Need for full-fat dairy ceases at age 2 Encourage active play each day
School-age and adolescent	Health curriculum Active, appealing physical education for all Offering healthy food and beverages in school	Ingrained curricular models Tendency to emphasize sports that for most youth are spectator events Advertising less healthy foods to youth	60 minutes of moderate to vigorous intensity physical activity each day. Limit screen time Limit carbonated beverages
All ages	Limit TV/computer game time to 2 hours/day Encourage at least 1 hour of physical activity daily Encourage 5 servings of fruits and vegetables daily Eat a healthy breakfast daily Encourage family meals Serve recommended portion sizes Calculate and plot BMIs yearly Advocate for healthful food choices in restaurants Discourage consumption of empty kilocalories Expand access to supermarkets with reasonably priced produce Provide safe environments for physical activity		

Adapted from CDC: Strategies to Prevent Obesity. Updated October 27, 2015. Available at https://www.cdc.gov/obesity/strategies/index.html; USDA: ChooseMyPlate.org. Updated April 19, 2017. Available at https://www.choosemyplate.gov/MyPlate.

KEYSTONES

■ Breast milk is especially suited to the human infant because the protein, fat, and carbohydrate in breast milk are tailored to the infant's digestive capabilities.

■ After the age of 4 to 6 months, semisolid and then solid foods are added to the diet gradually, using carefully selected foods to avoid choking accidents.

■ Nutritional problems in infancy include allergies, colic, and diarrhea, with the latter having the best documented treatment: oral rehydration therapy.

■ Toddlers not only learn to accept new foods but also learn their culture's traditions surrounding food. Common nutritional problems for toddlers are iron deficiency and iron-deficiency anemia.

■ Preschool and school-age children need healthy meals and snacks to sustain growth at a time when parents have less control over the child's eating while away from home.

■ Most adolescents do not consume enough calcium to optimize their growth and development, and most girls lack iron in their diets. Self-prescribed reduction diets and poor choices of food are problems.

■ Pediatric obesity is a major childhood health problem in the United States and the industrialized world, with the potential to spread in developing countries. Consequences are adult pathologies presenting decades early: hypertension, high blood cholesterol, and type 2 diabetes.

CASE STUDY 11-1

Ms. S is a school nurse in an urban elementary school. The principal asked for Ms. S's assistance in improving the students' nutritional and fitness states. A committee was formed that included students, teachers (classroom, home economics, and physical education), cafeteria and kitchen staff, parents, and a dietitian from a nearby hospital. The following plan reflects the program they devised after many meetings.

CARE PLAN

Subjective Data

Focus groups with students revealed their opinions of food and physical activity. ■ A schoolwide survey solicited suggestions for classroom content, menu items, and physical activities.

Objective Data

Analysis of school lunch menus revealed <10% of total calories from saturated fat. ■ Vending machines in and around school offered only high-fat snacks or those with empty kilocalories. ■ Inspection of building usage identified 2 days after school when the gym was empty but other parts of the building were in use. ■ No formal education regarding nutrition and activity.

Analysis

Opportunity to improve students' nutrition and fitness

Plan

DESIRED OUTCOMES EVALUATION CRITERIA	ACTIONS/INTERVENTIONS	RATIONALE
Students will have increased opportunities to choose healthful foods in and around school.	Analyze sample lunch menus monthly to select areas to improve variety in healthy food options while adhering to national standards.	Prioritizing changes is important to budget resources. Feedback to cafeteria staff will help maintain their interest and effort to improve.
	Include fresh fruit and vegetables on every lunch menu.	Fresh fruits and vegetables can offer vitamins, minerals, and fiber as well as decrease the dominance of high-fat items on the menu.
	Use student tasters to develop low-fat versions of popular dishes.	Palatability is critical in devising dishes the students will eat.
	Diversify contents of vending machines to include dairy products, fruit juices, and cereal- and-dried-fruit snacks.	Items must be available to give students the opportunity to choose.
	Collaborate with biology teacher on fruit or vegetable growing as student projects.	Producing food items can stimulate interest in eating their own produce.
Students will demonstrate higher goals for their physical fitness.	Evaluate the place of physical education in the curriculum and campaign for needed changes.	To effectively prepare students for life requires offering skill development for an active life.
	Institute fitness testing in physical education classes.	Feedback to students allows them to track their progress.
	Ensure that 75% of time in physical education class is active.	Inactivity is a major contributor to overweight. Physical education class should not add to the problem.
	Institute activities students suggest, such as ethnic dances and games other than major U.S. sports.	Capitalizing on students' interests will recognize the value of their ideas. Later activities might broaden the scope to activities from other cultures.
	Arrange for supervised activities in the gym after school on the days the building would be open for other events. Vary the activities.	If community or volunteer leaders could be recruited, the cost would be minimized for the school and the students. A variety of activities would attract students other than the usual athletes who are active anyway.

DESIRED OUTCOMES EVALUATION CRITERIA	ACTIONS/INTERVENTIONS	RATIONALE
Students will increase knowledge of healthful eating practices within time and budgetary constraints.	Design and promote a practical course in skills of modern life for both genders.	Practical courses will attract a different student than strictly academic courses do.
	Implement a program such as We Can! to provide nutritional education to students, staff, and families.	Short units would give immediate feedback on the value of the information. Consuming the day's lesson is a bonus.
	Incorporate field trips to grocery stores as appropriate.	Expanding the students' perception of the choices open to them would offer the opportunity to increase variety in their diets.

TEAMWORK 11-1

COMMUNITY COMMITTEE WORK

A committee was formed to improve the area surrounding the elementary school to permit opportunities for daily exercise for the students. Members included YMCA staff, neighborhood business owners, and city officials.

Subjective: *Parents described traffic congestion, lack of sidewalks and bike paths, and suspected undesirable activities occurring around the school.*

Objective: *Police reports of auto-pedestrian accidents, assaults, thefts, and drug arrests indicated increased incidence compared with the district's other elementary schools.*

Analysis: *School's environment a disincentive to walking or bicycling to and from school.*

Plan:

Establish a Neighborhood Watch Program using business owners and nearby families.

Increase numbers of crossing guards and recruit volunteer monitors when students are coming and leaving school.

Improve traffic flow around the school.

Participate in Walk to School and Bike to School programs.

Long-term, construct bike paths and sidewalks to and from the surrounding neighborhoods.

CRITICAL THINKING QUESTIONS

1. What additional interventions might be used to improve nutritional intake and increase physical activity in these students?

2. Identify possible barriers to implementing the outlined program. Suggest strategies to overcome them.

3. It is possible that the committee's goals are not compatible with those of many of the families in this elementary school. How could the families be persuaded to value a more healthful lifestyle?

CHAPTER REVIEW

1. A nurse in a clinic would identify which of the following infants as needing additional assessment of growth?
   1. Baby girl A, 4 months old, birth weight 7 lb 6 oz, present weight 14 lb 14 oz
   2. Baby boy B, 2 weeks old, birth weight 6 lb 10 oz, present weight 6 lb 11 oz
   3. Baby boy C, 6 months old, birth weight 8 lb 8 oz, present weight 14 lb 8 oz
   4. Baby girl D, 2 months old, birth weight 7 lb 2 oz, present weight 9 lb 10 oz

2. Which of the following are advantages of breast milk that formula does not provide?
   1. Less fat and cholesterol
   2. More antibodies and digestive enzymes
   3. More fluoride and iron
   4. More vitamin C and vitamin D

3. Which of the following foods would be appropriate for a 6-month-old infant?
   1. Cocoa-flavored wheat cereal, orange juice, and strained chicken
   2. Graham crackers, strained prunes, and stewed tomatoes
   3. Infant rice cereal, mashed banana, and strained squash
   4. Mashed potatoes, strained beets, and chopped hard-cooked egg

4. Families should be encouraged to provide fortified whole milk for children until the age of
   1. 18 months
   2. 2 years
   3. 36 months
   4. 4 years

5. Which of the following individuals is at greatest nutritional risk?
   1. 3-month-old infant being fed commercial formula
   2. 3-year-old child who drinks 3 cups of milk a day
   3. 8-year-old child who eats four chocolate chip cookies and drinks two glasses of milk after school
   4. 16-year-old girl who is pregnant and attempting weight loss

CLINICAL ANALYSIS

1. Mrs. T is having her 2-month-old son checked in the well-baby clinic. She tells the nurse that the baby is not sleeping through the night yet. Mrs. T's mother advised her to start the infant on cereal to "fill him up" at bedtime. Which of the following statements by the mother would indicate to the nurse the need for further teaching?
   a. "My baby can have solids at 6 months."
   b. "Most babies sleep through the night by age 3 months."
   c. "I will put the infant cereal into a bottle and enlarge the nipple hole."
   d. "I understand that early introduction of foods may increase the risk for allergies."

2. Ms. C has given a 24-hour dietary recall for her 18-month-old son. The nurse is alert to identify common causes of choking. To avoid choking accidents, which of the following foods would be considered safest for a toddler? Select all that apply.
   a. Grapes
   b. Diced peaches
   c. Popcorn
   d. Watermelon chunks
   e. String cheese

3. Ms. K has delivered a 3-lb 8-oz premature infant. She had planned to breastfeed. On which of the following statements should the nurse base her teaching?
   a. Human breast milk can be specially fortified for premature infants to increase its nutritive value.
   b. Because of their larger proportion of body weight as water, premature infants need supplemental water after every feeding.
   c. Formula feeding is advisable because room-temperature feedings are better absorbed than those at body temperature.
   d. Breastfeeding a premature infant offers no advantage to the infant and is difficult for the mother because of the necessary supplements.

Life Cycle Nutrition: The Mature Adult

After completing this chapter, the student should be able to:
- Identify the foods and food groups most likely to be lacking or excessive in the diets of adults.
- Describe the changes in the older adult's body that affect nutritional status.
- Explain how a nutritional assessment of an older adult differs from that of a younger one.
- Illustrate ways in which food can be used to aid in the developmental tasks of adulthood.
- List several suggestions to improve food intake for older people in a variety of living situations.

The life cycle of human growth and development continues throughout the adult years. Both psychosocial and physical developments continue as a person matures. This chapter considers the impact on nutrition of the physiological and psychosocial changes that occur during young, middle, and older adult years. Because much of this book emphasizes the nutritional needs of young and middle-aged adults, the main focus of this chapter is the older adult. One major threat to health in adulthood is inactivity (Box 12-1), which can lead to overweight and obesity, the subject of Chapter 16.

Young Adulthood

Young adulthood spans ages 18 through 39. Not all 18-year-olds are adults, developmentally speaking, nor are all 40-year-olds middle-aged in thought or behavior.

Psychosocial Development

During the early years of young adulthood, the individual may be completing the adolescent task of identity. According to Erik Erikson, the developmental task of young adulthood is **intimacy** (Table 12-1). For example, people who delay commitment to a life partner until their 30s and 40s will probably be working at achieving intimacy; other 40-year-olds may be tackling the next task of generativity.

Nutrition in the Young Adult

Table 12-2 shows MyPlate recommendations for the adult aged 19 to 30 years.

Middle Adulthood

For this section, middle adult years are defined as those between ages 40 and 70 to match the dietary reference intakes (DRI) tables.

Psychosocial Development

Erikson's task of **generativity** involves serving as a mentor to the next generation. Teaching family members to prepare traditional foods, for example, may help a person achieve generativity.

Nutrition in Middle Adulthood

Table 12-3 shows MyPlate recommendations for the adult aged 31 to 50 years.

Older Adulthood

Changes in **life expectancy** and physiology affect the nutrition of older Americans.

Demographics of Aging

People are living longer. Older people constitute a larger proportion of the population. These trends are expected to continue, thus increasing the numbers of frail and dependent elderly people.

Life Expectancy

In 1900, life expectancy at birth was 47 years. By 2014, however, life expectancy at birth was 78.8 years. By ethnic group:

- 81.1 years for white females
- 78.1 years for black females
- 84 years for Hispanic females
- 76.5 years for white males
- 72.0 years for black males
- 79.2 years for Hispanic males (National Center for Health Statistics, 2015)

Proportion of Population

Steady growth is seen in the proportion of the U.S. population older than 65 years. It was:

- 4.1% in 1900
- 6.8% in 1940 (5 years after Social Security was enacted)
- 9.8% in 1970 (5 years after Medicare took effect)
- 14.5% in 2014 (U.S. Census Bureau, 2016)
- Estimated to be 20% by 2030 (Ortman, Velkoff, & Hogan, 2014)

The increase in the aged population is evidence of successful public health efforts: improved sanitation, an increased concern for safety, and control of communicable diseases. In 2015, two major causes of death in adults were heart disease and cancer (Centers for Disease Control and Prevention [CDC], March 17, 2017). Both causes are linked to lifestyle, including diet.

Nursing Home Residency

The CDC (July 6, 2016) reports that in 2014, 1.5 million residents lived in one of the 15,600 nursing homes in the United States.

Psychosocial Development

Erikson's developmental task for older adults is **integrity**, in the sense of being whole or complete. Those who accomplish this task will look back on their lives as being worthwhile.

TABLE 12-2   MyPlate Daily Recommendations for Adults Aged 19 to 30 Years*

FOOD GROUP	WOMEN	MEN
Fruit	2 cups	2 cups
Vegetables	2½ cups	3 cups
Grain	6 oz (3 oz whole grain)	8 oz (4 oz whole grain)
Protein	5½ oz	6½ oz
Dairy	3 cups	3 cups
Oil	6 teaspoons	7 teaspoons

*Servings for those who get less than 30 minutes of moderate exercise each day. Adapted from U.S. Department of Agriculture, ChooseMyPlate.gov (2017).

TABLE 12-3   MyPlate Daily Recommendations for Adults Aged 31 to 50 years*

FOOD GROUP	WOMEN	MEN
Fruit	1½ cups	2 cups
Vegetables	2½ cups	3 cups
Grain	6 oz (3 oz whole grain)	7 oz (3½ oz whole grain)
Protein	5 oz	6 oz
Dairy	3 cups	3 cups
Oil	5 teaspoons	6 teaspoons

*Servings for those who get less than 30 minutes of moderate exercise each day. Adapted from U.S. Department of Agriculture, ChooseMyPlate.gov (2017).

TABLE 12-1   Erikson's Theory of Psychosocial Development in Maturity

STAGE OF LIFE	DEVELOPMENTAL TASK	OPPOSING NEGATIVE TRAIT	USE OF FOOD TO ACHIEVE TASK
Adult	Intimacy	Isolation	Arranging candlelight dinner
Middle adult	Generativity	Stagnation	Teaching someone to prepare family favorite or ethnic dishes
Older adult	Integrity	Despair	Using food fragrances or memories of food to reminisce

A technique to help the older person achieve integrity is reminiscence. Asking an older person to recall special foods can stimulate reminiscence. Familiar food odors often evoke memories.

Socially, older adults must often adapt to the loss of friends and relatives. The death of a spouse demands a tremendous adjustment. The accompanying depression and new responsibility for tasks the spouse performed may significantly affect an older person's food intake.

Physical Changes of Aging

Even without frank disease, the physical abilities of older adults diminish. "Middle-age spread" often gives way to dwindling bulk and waning strength.

The clinical guidelines on overweight and obesity in adults set a body mass index (BMI) of 25 as the upper limit of ideal weight for all adults regardless of age. The CDC reports that obesity is highest among those age 40 to 59 years at 40.2%, and obesity affects 37% of those aged more than 60 years (September 12, 2016). Evidence continues to link overweight and obesity to arthritis, diabetes, coronary heart disease, and other conditions that may have an impact on the older person's quality of life.

Integumentary System

Many changes take place in the skin as a person ages. As subcutaneous fat is lost, the skin becomes dry and wrinkled. Less elasticity is present to spring back after a pinch to the forearm, the usual site assessed for hydration status. The skin of the forehead or over the breastbone is a more reliable site in the elderly client than the forearm.

The older adult also loses some of the ability to synthesize vitamin D from sunshine, so it may take twice as much sun exposure without sunscreens as necessary in a younger person to produce a given amount of vitamin D.

Sensory System

Four senses become markedly less acute as a person ages: vision, hearing, taste, and smell. Because the sense receptors do not deteriorate equally, some of the sense loss is attributed to changes in the central nervous system. Extensive variation exists among individuals.

EYES

Vision is often impaired. The older person sees colors in the red, orange, and yellow spectrum better than blue and green spectrum. Clouding of the lens of the eye—cataract formation—decreases overall vision. Older eyes do not adjust well to glare such as that found in some supermarkets.

These vision changes may make grocery shopping burdensome. The fine-print labels on food items may be illegible to older people. Food preparation may become not only difficult but also hazardous if the person cannot see adequately. Colorful foods with visual appeal and strong contrast might stimulate the appetite in some elderly people.

EARS

The National Institute on Deafness and Other Communication Disorders (NIDCD) estimates that 1 out of 3 people between the ages of 65 to 74 have hearing loss, with half of those older than 75 years experiencing hearing loss (February 13, 2017). The sound receptors in the inner ear deteriorate. First to be lost is the ability to perceive high tones. The older person with age-related hearing loss typically loses the ability to distinguish higher frequencies first, known as **presbycusis**, which results in the ability to hear men's voices better than women's. Hearing aids do not fully compensate for the hearing loss. In fact, they often magnify sideline noise to the point of distracting the wearer. The result may be social isolation when it becomes too laborious to interact with others. Socializing at meals may become embarrassing or frustrating, and older people may avoid such interaction.

NOSE AND TONGUE

For the sense of taste to function well, the sense of smell must also be intact. Food tastes bland when a person has a head cold. After age 60 many people begin to lose some sense of smell. Although the sense of smell is frequently more affected by aging than the sense of taste, both faculties are important to help protect the person from noxious elements in the environment, such as spoiled or burning food or gas leaks.

Chemical taste receptors are concentrated on the tongue's surface but also are located at the base of the tongue, on the soft palate, and in other areas of the nasopharynx. Saliva acts as a solvent to present the foods to the taste buds. If the mouth is dry, taste sensations are indistinct.

Taste receptors have traditionally been known to recognize sweet, sour, salty, and bitter sensations. Receptors have been identified for *umami*, a sensation described as savory or rich. It is caused by the amino acid glutamine in its free form and is associated with monosodium glutamate (MSG). Reported sensory losses are uneven. Unlike sensitivity for bitter and sour that remains intact in older clients, the perceptivity for sweet and salt declines with age, and so many older clients will complain their food tastes bitter. If a person is oversalting his or her food, as a result of a diminished taste sensation for salt, alternate seasonings can be used to decrease sodium consumption; these are listed in Chapter 18. A technique to increase taste sensation in geriatric clients is brushing the tongue as part of oral hygiene.

Gastrointestinal System

Particularly crucial to nutrition is gastrointestinal function. Hundreds of processes are required for the proper digestion, absorption, and metabolism of foods. Many functions of the gastrointestinal system decline significantly in older people.

DENTAL HEALTH

Older individuals are not immune to dental caries. In fact, when exposed by gum disease, the tooth root, lacking enamel, is particularly vulnerable to caries, causing increased occurrence in the elderly population. Contributing factors include the following:

- Inadequate oral hygiene
- Infrequent dental examinations and cleanings
- Salivary gland dysfunction
- Frequent snacking
- Removable partial dentures
- Long-term medication use
- Not receiving fluorinated water

Fluoride applied to the teeth or fluoridated water prevents caries among adults of all ages. Unfortunately, only 28 states met the Healthy People 2010 goal of having 75% of their citizens on public water supplies with fluorinated water (U.S. Department of Health and Human Services [DHHS], June 20, 2017). The goal of Healthy People 2020 is for 79.6% of the population to have access to fluorinated water supplies.

The major cause of tooth loss in the older adult is not dental caries but **periodontal disease,** which affects the gums (gingiva) and the apparatus attaching the tooth to the jaw. Healthy People 2020 also addresses periodontal disease, with the goal of reducing the number of adults with moderate to severe periodontal disease to 40.8% and reducing the proportion of adults aged 65 to 74 years who have lost all of their permanent teeth to 21.6% (DHHS, June 20, 2017). Dentures, like hearing aids, only partially compensate, and so dentures are about 20% as efficient as natural teeth. Advanced gum disease affects 4% to 12% of adults, and 1 out of 5 of adults in the United States aged 65 years or older has lost all of the permanent teeth, a condition called **edentulous** (CDC, July 13, 2016).

Furthermore, a denture cannot be effective if the underlying tissue is in poor condition. Persons with upper dentures that cover the palate containing taste receptors lose some taste sensation and are also subject to impaired swallowing.

The production of saliva decreases sharply in older adults, a condition called **xerostomia.** Chewing and swallowing become more difficult, and food intake may be affected. Also, with age, less mucus and smaller quantities of enzymes are secreted.

OTHER CONDITIONS

Atrophic gastritis, a chronic inflammation of the stomach lining, causes an interruption in the mucous protection of the stomach lining, which leads to atrophy of the stomach wall and decreased gastric acid production. An extreme case is **achlorhydria,** the absence of hydrochloric acid in the stomach. The primary cause of atrophic gastritis is the bacteria *Helicobacter pylori,* known as *H. pylori.* One of the most concerning effects of atrophic gastritis is the increased incidence of stomach carcinoma.

Either of these conditions may interfere with protein digestion and with vitamin and mineral absorption. The stomach atrophy that occurs can interrupt the production of intrinsic factor that is necessary for the absorption of vitamin B_{12}. Vitamin B_{12} may remain locked to the food protein, and less nonheme iron will be absorbed in the more alkaline environment. Intestinal **motility** decreases because of lessened muscle tone. Medications may interfere with electrolyte balance, also diminishing muscle tone.

Urinary System

The size of the kidneys increases until age 40 or 50 years but then decreases. With aging, there is a gradual decline in the weight, or size, of the kidney and a decline in renal blood flow. These age-related changes worsen in the presence of co-morbidities such as hypertension and diabetes. The aging kidney loses some ability to concentrate urine and to conserve sodium. Mild hyponatrenia, the commonest electrolyte imbalance in the older population, is associated with gait and attention deficits, resulting in higher frequency of falls.

This compromised kidney function makes urine samples less reliable for nutrient analyses in elderly people. Two laboratory tests frequently are used to assess renal function: **blood urea nitrogen (BUN)** and serum creatinine. An increase in the BUN level usually indicates a decrease in kidney function. It may also be elevated in dehydration or if excessive protein is presented to the liver for breakdown, as with a high-protein diet or with gastrointestinal bleeding. Because clients with even slightly elevated BUN may not be able to excrete the waste products from protein metabolism, caregivers must be judicious about giving high-protein nutritional supplements to older people with elevated BUNs.

Creatinine, an end product of creatine metabolism, is excreted efficiently by the healthy kidney. The amount of creatinine produced is proportional to the individual's skeletal muscle mass and remains fairly constant in the absence of extensive muscle damage. The serum creatinine test has the advantage over the BUN of being little affected by dehydration, malnutrition, or liver function.

Creatinine levels may not detect decreased kidney function, however, if a slow decline in renal function occurs simultaneously with a slow decrease in muscle mass, as occurs in the aging process. Consequently, both tests may be performed to obtain a more complete diagnostic picture.

Musculoskeletal System

The major loss of body mass in the older adult involves muscle mass. It is estimated that degenerative skeletal muscle loss begins around 35 years of age at a rate of 1% per year, with rates accelerating after age 60 years (Getting a Start, 2017). Because muscle is a more metabolically active tissue than fat, energy needs decline with diminished muscle mass. The losses are reversible, however. Even in elderly people, skeletal muscle protein anabolism can be stimulated by increasing dietary protein to 0.45 to 0.68 grams per pound of body weight (Rethinking Protein Needs, 2015). See Box 12-2 for information regarding sarcopenia.

Nutritional deprivation and catabolic states can affect the muscles of respiration in the chest and diaphragm. Because the older person relies more on the diaphragm than the chest muscles to breathe, a full stomach may impede breathing to a greater extent than in a younger person.

Perhaps more noticeable than the loss of muscle mass in older people is the loss of height. After age 30, bone loss occurs at a rate of about 0.3% to 0.5% per year. A major cause of this loss of height is osteoporosis. Osteoporosis is a chronic skeletal disease that results in decreased bone mass and increases the risk of fracture.

Older joint surfaces are roughened by arthritis. By age 50, half of all adults have some osteoarthritis. The resulting pain and stiffness impairs the use of the hands for opening jars, chopping raw foods, and cutting cooked foods at the table. Arthritis also can affect the mandibular joint of the jaw used for chewing.

Nervous System

For many people, deteriorating brain function is the most feared loss of old age, one that is shared by their loved ones, who may see the person gradually fade from the present with the onslaught of dementia. By the time a person reaches old age, the brain has endured a lifetime of stressors, but some individuals weather the storms better than others. Some significant changes include:

- Brain volume decreases about 0.1% to 0.2% per year between the ages of 30 and 50.
- Blood flow to the brain decreases because of narrowing of the arteries.
- Thirst sensation becomes less operative, increasing the risk of uncompensated dehydration.
- Mortality from heat stroke rises sharply in people older than 60 years.

Several factors influence brain function in elderly people. More years of education, physical exercise, and cognitive stimulation are positively related to better brain function. Nutritional factors of benefit to the aging brain include:

- Vitamins B_6, B_{12}, and folic acid
- High intake of essential fatty acids, both linoleic acid and alpha-linoleic acid (Otaegui-Arrazola et al, 2014)

ALZHEIMER DISEASE

In 2017, it was estimated that Alzheimer disease (AD) affected 5.5 million Americans of all ages, with 5.3 million being aged 65 years or older (Alzheimer's Association, 2017). By 2050, it is estimated that 16 million people will be living with the disease (Alzheimer's Association, 2017). Although the cause of the disease is not fully understood, a significant genetic predisposition is shown in familial AD. Familial AD affects clients aged less than 65 years (Thomas, Thomas, Radcliffe, & Itsiopoulos, 2015). See Genomic Gem 12-1.

Decreased brain levels of docosahexaenoic acid (DHA) are associated with aging and have been shown to be essential for memory and neuroprotection (Schmidt et al, 2015). Consumption of omega-3 fatty acids (particularly DHA, e.g., as obtained in one fish meal weekly) and antioxidants such as vitamin E may lower the risk of AD, but further research is required. Special concerns of nourishing clients with dementia are covered in Clinical Application 12-1.

PARKINSON DISEASE

Another neurological disease that is more common in older people than in younger ones is Parkinson disease (PD). In the United States, 1 million people are thought to live with

GENOMIC GEM 12-1

Alzheimer Disease

Although the cause of Alzheimer disease (AD) has not been fully elucidated, gene mutations may complicate the relation of nutrients to disease risk. Likewise, genetics plays a role in its onset.

One variant of the apolipoprotein E gene, the *APOE4* allele, is the most prevalent genetic risk factor for AD (Li et al, 2016). Clients who inherit one or two copies of the *APOE* gene are at an increased risk of developing AD (National Institutes of Health, June 27, 2017).

The brain is highly metabolic, which makes the organ highly vulnerable to oxidative damage; this can result in protein, lipid, and DNA oxidation, which is associated with AD (Feng & Wang, 2012). The mixed results in studies of the antioxidant vitamin E in relation to AD may result from the varied genomes of the people recruited. Vitamin E from food has been associated with a modest reduction in long-term risk of AD among people without a polymorphism in the apolipoprotein E gene, the *APOE4* allele (Feng & Wang, 2012). There is a correlation between low levels of vitamin D and the onset of AD. Studies have shown that subjects with deficient vitamin D demonstrate a higher risk of developing AD and dementia (Shen & Ji, 2015). Further studies are needed regarding vitamin D supplementation in the prevention of AD.

Screening clients who have symptoms of cognitive impairment can assist the clients and their families prepare for the hardships of life with AD.

CLINICAL APPLICATION

Nutrition and Dementia

Clients with dementia progressively lose the ability for self-care, including feeding. Care of clients with dementia challenges family and health-care providers because eating is fundamental to life. The Edinburgh Feeding Evaluation in Dementia Scale (EdFED) is a screening tool that can be utilized with dementia clients to assess eating and feeding difficulties. The tool can help to identify baseline eating patterns and determine the level of feeding assistance that the client may require.

Managing the client's environment is a major part of the care of the client with dementia.

- Provide quiet, adequately lit dining rooms.
- Offer clients the same seats to achieve familiarity with tables that seat four.
- Serve one course at a time.
- Supply appropriate but limited utensils, large-handled if necessary.
- Select dishes with high sides to enable the client to scoop up the food onto a spoon.
- Serve finger foods that are within the client's capabilities.

Clients with dementia must be reminded of the steps involved in self-feeding:

- Putting the food on the spoon
- Directing it to the mouth
- Swallowing

Verbal cues or guiding the client's hand can get him or her started or keep the process going. Despite the surroundings, common courtesies can be effective in reminding clients of social expectations and in maintaining their dignity. For example:

- Introducing the client to the other people at the table
- Providing a cup rather than a carton for milk
- Offering foods

The effect of music in the dining room is a researched intervention for dementia clients. Selections with a slow tempo—at or below the human heart rate—tend to dampen environmental noises that might startle clients. Because staff members also heard the music, perhaps they also experienced some of the music's relaxing effect.

A multidisciplinary project to improve nutrition in clients with late-stage dementia not only achieved that goal but also decreased the distress of clients and nursing staff caused by the clients' swallowing problems. Among the interventions used were:

- Thickened liquids
- Three levels of dysphagia diets
- Daylong snacks
- Use of nutritional supplements

Enteral nutrition (see Chapter 14) is only recommended for use during periods of acute conditions that cause dysphagia. It is not recommended for dysphagia caused by end-stage dementia (Brooke & Ojo, 2015).

PD, with onset after 50 years of age (American Parkinson Disease Association [APDA], 2017). **Nutraceuticals** are foods or food products that may provide health and medical benefits. The effects of nutraceuticals are being studied to understand their role in the treatment of PD. Nutraceuticals inhibit oxidative stress and inflammation, which can play a role in treatment (Hang, Basil, & Lim, 2016). See the section on vitamins under Nutrition in the Older Adult later in this chapter. Box 12-3 details some nutritional ramifications of the disease.

Endocrine System

The average older person is slowing down. Resting energy expenditure (REE) decreases, especially in the brain, skeletal muscle, and heart. The older adult's REE may be 10% to 12% less than that of a younger person's. Lost muscle mass is replaced, if at all, by adipose tissue that is less active metabolically than muscle.

The pancreas often secretes inadequate amounts of insulin or the body loses its ability to utilize insulin, leading to diabetes mellitus (see Chapter 17). Receptors in the kidney for antidiuretic hormone (ADH) may function poorly to produce a less effective response. Levels of aldosterone also decrease with age. Both of these changes make maintaining correct fluid volume more difficult for an older person than for a younger one.

Cardiovascular System

As the older adult continues to age, cardiac output and heart rate decrease. In response to exercise, the heart rate does not increase as effectively as in youth, nor does it return to normal as rapidly. Because of this diminishment, elderly people are at risk for diseases of the heart. Dietary modifications for heart disease are included in Chapter 18.

BOX 12-3 ■ Parkinson Disease

It is estimated that 30% to 70% of people with Parkinson disease (PD) experience weight loss, which contributes to increased mortality and decreased quality of life (Sharma & Vassallo, 2014). PD is a progressive neurological disorder characterized by degeneration of neurons in the area of the brain that controls movement. This degeneration causes a shortage of dopamine, a neurotransmitter or brain-signaling chemical. Among the signs of the disease are:

- Resting tremors
- Rigidity
- Loss of facial expression
- Gait disorders with postural instability
- Orthostatic hypotension

These changes in movement can affect everyday activities, such as talking, walking, and swallowing. New evidence is emerging that the practice of tai chi can help to improve balance and motor control in clients with PD (Wayne, 2015).

A part of the cardiovascular system, the immune system, is less effective in the older person than in the younger one. T and B cells are lymphocytes with a role in the immune system, and these cells decline in number and activity as a person ages (Pence et al, 2012; Van Epps et al, 2014). In apparently healthy elderly people, micronutrient supplements may enhance the immune response.

At greatest risk of immunodeficiency are persons with protein-kilocalorie malnutrition, which is associated with increased complication rates (mainly infections) and death. Table 12-4 shows some of the effects of aging on **humoral** and **cellular immunity.**

Nutrition in the Older Adult

Table 12-5 shows the MyPlate daily recommendations for people aged 51 and older. MyPlate can be used for assessing and counseling.

MyPlate

MyPlate can serve the older adult well as a guideline for healthy eating. Data have demonstrated that a greater proportion of adults aged 65 or older eat five or more fruits and vegetables daily than do younger adults. In 2013, adults in America consumed fruit 1.1 times per day and vegetables 1.6 times per day (CDC National Center for Chronic Disease Prevention and Health Promotion, 2013). The goal of Healthy People 2020 is to increase the consumption of fruit and vegetable intake in all people greater than age two to 0.93 cups of fruit for every 1,000 calories consumed and 1.16 cups of vegetables for every 1,000 calories consumed. Between 2009 and 2010, 76% of Americans did not meet the recommended fruit intake and 87% failed to meet the recommended vegetable intake (Moore & Thompson, 2015).

A special Modified MyPlate for Older Adults for People Over 50 Years of Age appears as Figure 12-1. The modified MyPlate incorporates the *2015–2020 Dietary Guidelines for Americans* and highlights areas specific for the older adult including:

- Choose herbs and spices and low sodium options.
- Focus on fluid selection of water, fat-free milk, and soup.
- Incorporate healthy oil into the diet.
- Incorporate physical activity into daily life (Tufts, 2017).

TABLE 12-5 MyPlate Daily Recommendations for Adults Aged 51 and Older*

FOOD GROUP	WOMEN	MEN
Fruit	1½ cups	2 cups
Vegetables	2 cups	2½ cups
Grains	5 oz; 3 ounces whole grains	6 oz; 3 ounces whole grains
Protein Food	5 oz	5½ oz
Dairy	3 cups	3 cups
Oil	5 teaspoons	5 teaspoons

Servings for those who get less than 30 minutes of moderate exercise each day.

Energy Nutrients and Energy Balance

Older adults need about 5% fewer kilocalories per decade after age 40 years. Small changes have been recommended in intakes from carbohydrates, fats, and protein. As with younger people, the simplest criterion for the suitability of intake is the maintenance of a healthy body weight. Energy expenditure varies within the elderly population. Table 12-6 summarizes the estimated changes in caloric needs over the life span of the adult based on activity level.

CARBOHYDRATES AND FIBER

Older people should derive 45% to 65% of their kilocalories from carbohydrates. The RDA for carbohydrate, based on its role as primary energy source for the brain, is 130 grams per day, the same as for younger adults.

The AI for fiber is 28 grams per day for men 50 years and older and 21 grams for women in the same age group. Both of the values are less than recommended for younger adults.

FATS

Older people should derive 20% to 35% of their kilocalories from fats, with less than 10% saturated fat. Limiting fats should also increase comfort, because fat absorption is delayed in older people, leading to a feeling of fullness. Particularly among elderly people, rigid application of diet rules may be inappropriate. Restricting fat by eliminating whole milk and eggs, which are easily eaten and relatively inexpensive, could endanger nutrition in the short-term for uncertain long-term benefits.

TABLE 12-4 Some Effects of Aging on Immunity

TYPE OF IMMUNITY	LYMPHOCYTES INVOLVED	FUNCTION	EFFECT OF AGING
Humoral	B cells	Produce antibodies against foreign antigens.	Slightly fewer antibodies produced but less specific and less effective
Cellular	T cells	Protect against viruses, fungi, malignant cells, and foreign tissue grafts without using antibodies; autoimmune reactions are a dysfunction of this mechanism	Declines with age but only after age 90 in healthy people

MyPlate for Older Adults

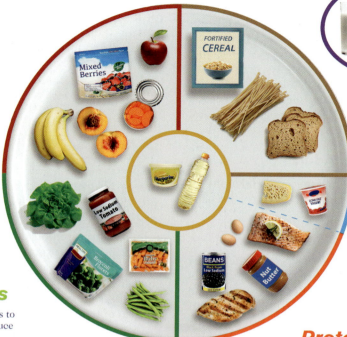

Fruits & Vegetables

Whole fruits and vegetables are rich in important nutrients and fiber. Choose fruits and vegetables with deeply colored flesh. Choose canned varieties that are packed in their own juices or low-sodium.

Healthy Oils

Liquid vegetable oils and soft margarines provide important fatty acids and some fat-soluble vitamins.

Herbs & Spices

Use a variety of herbs and spices to enhance flavor of foods and reduce the need to add salt.

Fluids

Drink plenty of fluids. Fluids can come from water, tea, coffee, soups, and fruits and vegetables.

Grains

Whole grain and fortified foods are good sources of fiber and B vitamins.

Dairy

Fat-free and low-fat milk, cheeses and yogurts provide protein, calcium and other important nutrients.

Protein

Protein rich foods provide many important nutrients. Choose a variety including nuts, beans, fish, lean meat and poultry.

Remember to Stay Active!

Tufts UNIVERSITY   JEAN MAYER USDA HUMAN NUTRITION RESEARCH CENTER AGING   HNRCA   AARP Foundation

FIGURE 12-1 The Modified MyPlate for People Over 50 Years of Age. ("My Plate for Older Adults." Copyright 2016 Tufts University, all rights reserved. "My Plate for Older Adults" graphic and accompanying website were developed with support from the AARP Foundation. "Tufts University" and "AARP Foundation" are registered trademarks and may not be reproduced apart from their inclusion in the "My Plate for Older Adults" graphic without express permission from their respective owners.)

TABLE 12-6   Estimated Calorie Needs per Day

GENDER	AGE	SEDENTARY	MODERATELY ACTIVE	ACTIVE
Female	21–25 years	2,000	2,200	2,400
Female	26–40 years	1,800	2,000	2,400
Female	41–45 years	1,800	2,000	2,200
Female	46–50 years	1,800	2,000	2,200
Female	51–60 years	1,600	1,800	2,200
Female	61+ years	1,600	1,800	2,000
Male	21–25 years	2,400	2,800	3,000
Male	26–40 years	2,400	2,600	3,000
Male	41–45 years	2,200	2,600	2,800
Male	46–50 years	2,200	2,400	2,800
Male	51–60 years	2,200	2,400	2,800
Male	61–65 years	2,000	2,400	2,600
Male	66+ years	2,000	2,200	2,400

Adapted from 2015 Dietary Guidelines for Americans.

PROTEIN

Older people should derive 10% to 35% of their kilocalories from protein. The RDA for protein is 56 grams per day for adult men and 46 grams per day for adult women. Moderately increasing daily protein intake beyond 0.8 gram per kilogram of body weight may enhance muscle protein anabolism and reduce the progressive loss of muscle mass that accompanies aging. Some experts maintain that there is stimulated muscle protein synthesis with an increase in high-quality dietary protein at levels of 1.0 to 1.2 grams per kilogram of body weight (Verreijen et al, 2017). Further research is required on this topic.

Although little evidence links high protein intakes to increased risk for impaired kidney function in healthy individuals, a prudent course would be to assess renal function of older individuals before embracing a higher protein intake.

Although serum albumin levels are used as a measure of body protein stores, for a given individual, serum albumin levels can indicate nutritional status, pathology, or both. It is estimated that 20% to 50% of adults are malnourished on hospital admission, which can contribute to poor client outcomes (National Association of Clinical Nurse Specialists [CACNS], January, 2017). Protein status is an important component in the body's defense system. In seniors with protein-energy malnutrition, decreased functions in all aspects of immunity are strongly related to protein nutritional status.

EXERCISE

Recommendations for exercise in the older adult are the same as for the younger adult; if the person is considered generally fit and has no limiting health conditions, the recommendations are as follows:

- 2 hours and 30 minutes, 150 minutes, of moderate-intensity aerobic activity or 1 hour and 15 minutes, 75 minutes, of vigorous-intensity aerobic activity every week
- Muscle-strengthening activities on 2 or more days a week that work all major muscle groups (CDC, June 4, 2015)

For previously sedentary persons, an exercise routine should be introduced gradually after medical clearance is received. MyPlate recommends that men older than 40 years and women older than 50 years should check with their health-care providers before starting or increasing physical activity.

An objective of Healthy People 2020 is for 24.1% of adults to perform strength-training activities on 2 or more days per week, but only 21.9% achieved this goal in 2008. Strength training decreases muscle mass loss, functional decline, and fall-related injuries. The National Institute on Aging (2016) recommends that all forms of exercise be included in the older adult's exercise plan: endurance, strength, balance, and flexibility.

Vitamins

The RDA/AI for vitamin D is increased for older adults. The RDA for vitamin B_{12} specifies fortified foods or supplements as sources because of the possibility of malabsorption. Mean nutrient intakes from food for older adults are below the RDAs/AIs for vitamins E and K.

VITAMIN E

The RDA/AI for vitamin E is 15 mg per day for all adults. Besides functioning as a scavenger of free radicals, vitamin E has been linked to immune and cognitive functions. Oxidative stress has been shown to contribute to the etiology of dementia. Vitamin E has demonstrated the ability to decrease free-radical damage in neuronal cells, which helps to inhibit dementia progression (Forbes, Holroyd-Leduc, Poulin, & Hogan, 2016).

One difficulty with pinpointing effects of vitamin E is its various forms with differing functions. Tocotrienols possess powerful neuroprotective, anticancer, and cholesterol-lowering properties that are often not exhibited by tocopherols. At minute concentrations, alpha-tocotrienol, not alpha-tocopherol, prevents neurodegeneration.

VITAMIN K

Vitamin K can be depleted relatively more quickly than the other fat-soluble vitamins. Besides its role in blood clotting, vitamin K contributes to bone metabolism and is protective against age-related bone loss. Vitamin K deficiency has been shown to contribute to the occurrence of hip and vertebral fractures in elderly women. As with vitamin E, vitamin K from natural sources is recommended.

Minerals

The 2015 Dietary Guidelines for sodium in the older American is an intake of less than 2,300 mg per day and further reduced for those who have a chronic illness such as hypertension, diabetes, or kidney disease. See Chapters 18 and 19 for more on the relationship of sodium on cardiovascular disease and renal disease.

The AI for calcium has been increased for older persons. The RDA/AI for calcium in women older than 50 years and men older than 70 years is 1,200 mg per day; it is 1,000 mg per day for men aged 51 to 70 years. Calcium is best absorbed by food sources, but studies have demonstrated that the large majority of people do not consume the RDA for calcium, which leads to the recommendation of supplement usage. Whether from food or supplements, calcium intake should be spread out throughout the day, with 600 mg or less being consumed at each meal.

Water

No AI for water has been established for individuals older than 30 years. Healthy older adults need enough fluid intake to produce about 1.5 liters of light yellow urine in 24 hours.

Loss of sphincter muscle tone in women and difficulty urinating in men may prompt older people to limit their fluid intake, a practice that is not recommended. Omitting fluids in the 2 hours before bedtime, however, may help decrease the frequency of nocturia and nighttime incontinence.

One of the early signs of dehydration in elderly people is confusion, which may be difficult to ascertain in clients with dementia or altered consciousness. Signs of dehydration in elderly people are listed in Table 12-7. The increase in pulse rate on standing is an appropriate assessment technique for fluid volume status in elderly clients except when heart disease and its treatments would block the physiological response.

Clients who are immobilized may need as many as 12 to 14 glasses of fluid per day. Immobility increases the calcium loss from bones. The calcium then circulates in the blood until the kidney excretes the excess. A large fluid intake dilutes the urine so that the calcium does not form stones.

Common Problems Related to Nutrition

Although arthritis, osteoporosis, and protein-kilocalorie malnutrition are not unique to elderly people, they do represent special concerns for geriatric clients. Constipation is also a frequent complaint and is covered in Chapter 20. A special food-based recipe to control the symptom of constipation that is effective in nursing home residents is given in Chapter 24.

Arthritis

This group of diseases is characterized by inflammation of various joints, often accompanied by pain, swelling, stiffness, and deformity. **Arthritis** affects an estimated 22% of the U.S. adult population (50 million persons), and 9% (21 million people) reported that arthritis limited their activities. Prevalence was high among:

- Women
- Older age groups
- Obese or overweight individuals
- Physically inactive individuals (CDC, April 13, 2017)

OSTEOARTHRITIS

Formerly known as degenerative joint disease, **osteoarthritis** is characterized by progressive deterioration of cartilage in joints and vertebrae. Osteoarthritis affects more than 30 million adult Americans (CDC, February 2, 2017).

Arthritis of the spine, hips, or knees is more likely to cause disability than that affecting other areas. Risk factors for osteoarthritis include:

- Aging
- Obesity
- Overuse or abuse of joints
- Trauma

Because the force exerted on the knees when walking may be up to six times the body weight, overweight people have a significantly increased risk of osteoarthritis of the knees. Thus, weight control has an important role in the prevention and treatment of osteoarthritis.

RHEUMATOID ARTHRITIS

In contrast to osteoarthritis, which is a local disease, rheumatoid arthritis is a systemic disease, affecting about 2.1 million people in the United States. Because it is a systemic disease, some have tried to modify the disease effects through diet or supplements.

Omega-3 fatty acids, in addition to blocking the formation of inflammatory compounds from omega-6 fatty acids, produce compounds that are less inflammatory and less bioactive than the ones metabolized from omega-6 fatty acids.

Osteoporosis and Fractures

Osteoporosis is covered in detail in Chapter 7. This section examines only the risks for and results of hip fracture (actually a fracture of the femur). Although half as common as reported vertebral fractures, hip fractures are much more likely to be diagnosed and treated. Clinically diagnosed vertebral fractures are estimated to represent just one-third of the total vertebral fractures. The University of Sheffield developed a fracture risk algorithm (FRAX) in 2008 that can predict a person's 10-year probability of hip fracture and is based on the risk factors of age, height, weight, and bone mineral density and is country-, sex-, and race-specific. The FRAX tool can be found at: https://www.sheffield.ac.uk/FRAX/tool.jsp.

INDIVIDUALS AFFECTED

It has been reported that more than 95% of hip fractures are caused by falls. The CDC (September 20, 2016) reports other facts about hip fractures, including the following:

- About 75% of all hip fractures occur in women.
- 300,000 people older than 64 years are admitted for hip fracture annually.
- Hip fracture rates increase with age.

Box 12-4 lists major risk factors for hip fractures.

PREVENTION

The most effective way to prevent fall-related injuries, including hip fractures, is to combine exercise with other fall-prevention strategies. Strength and balance exercise are recommended for all adults to reduce the risk of falls. Weight-bearing exercise for at least 30 minutes per day will

TABLE 12-7	Signs of Dehydration in Elderly People
BODY SYSTEM	**SIGN**
Skin and mucous membranes	Skin warm and dry Decreased turgor; pinch test may be more accurate over the sternum or on the forehead than on the hand Furrowed tongue Elevated temperature
Cardiovascular	Elevated pulse
Urinary	Increased specific gravity Increased urinary sodium
Musculoskeletal	Weakness
Neurological	Confusion

BOX 12-4 ■ Risk Factors for Hip Fractures

Among the risk factors for hip fractures are the following:

- Increasing age
- Female gender
- White race
- History of falls
- Insufficient exercise
- Low body mass index
- Smoking
- Long-term glucocorticoid use
- Inadequate calcium and vitamin D intake

---

help maintain bone strength, balance, and coordination (Swann, 2012). Examples of weight-bearing activities include activities in which the feet touch the ground walking, jogging, or dancing.

Even after sustaining a hip fracture, only a minority of elderly clients receives treatment for osteoporosis to attempt to modify the risk of future fractures. The use of medications such as bisphosphonates reduce the risk of fracture by 50% in women and 25% in men (Rheinboldt, Harper, & Stone, 2014).

Weight Loss and Protein-Kilocalorie Malnutrition

The older person's metabolic rate declines, primarily as a result of less lean body mass or muscle, and so loss of 5% or more of body weight requires aggressive intervention (Morley, 2006). The **anorexia of aging** is described in Box 12-5.

Treatable malnutrition has been reported to occur in 13% to 78% of hospitalized clients worldwide (Shama

---

BOX 12-5 ■ The Anorexia of Aging

Humans and other animals of advanced age have reduced food intake. Physiological factors contributing to anorexia of aging include:

- Changes in taste and smell
- Delayed gastric emptying
- Altered digestion-related hormone secretion and hormonal responsiveness

Healthy elders have been shown to be less hungry at meal initiation and to become more rapidly satiated during a standard meal, compared with younger adults.

Nonphysiological causes include:

- Social (poverty, isolation)
- Psychological (depression, dementia)
- Medical (edentulism, dysphagia)
- Pharmacological factors

Older persons eat more in social situations than when eating alone, even when the person delivering Meals on Wheels just sits with the recipient while dining.

Older adults, who take more than 30% of all prescription drugs, are at increased risk of drug–nutrient interactions, the subject of Chapter 15.

---

et al, 2016), and up to 50% of older adults are malnourished on admission to the hospital. Malnutrition contributes to many complications of illness, such as infections, anemia, and pressure injury (Clinical Application 12-2).

Food Insecurity

The main reason individuals do not consume enough protein or kilocalorie is lack of money (Box 12-6). To rectify the situation for older adults, the federal government, with an amendment to the Older Americans Act, established meal programs for senior citizens. Low-cost meals are offered at central gathering places or are delivered to the homebound and provide one-third of the RDA for elders (Fig. 12-2). The second program offered is the Senior Farmer's Market Nutrition Program (SFMNP), which offers low-income seniors coupons to exchange for fresh produce at farmer's markets and roadside stands.

Dietary Interventions

Enhancing well-consumed menu items with additional kilocalories and protein while maintaining the usual volume of food employs a "food-first" philosophy to counter weight loss. Clients may accept foods more readily than liquid supplements. Oral nutritional supplements (ONS) can be utilized to bridge the gap between a client's nutritional intake and their nutritional requirement, but ONS should be offered as second-line treatment (Blaikley, 2015). Milk-based

---

CLINICAL APPLICATION   12-2

Nutrition and Pressure Injury

The basic cause of **pressure** injury is impaired circulation from the weight of the body on a bony prominence or by shearing forces from pulling on the skin that damages the underlying tissue. Risk factors include:

- Immobility
- Inactivity
- Incontinence
- Impaired consciousness
- Malnutrition

Progression of the ulcer from intact skin to an open, sometimes deep sore increases the challenge to control infection, replenish nutrient losses from the wound, and promote healing.

Pressure injuries may place clients in a hypercatabolic state, which will require an increase in calories to promote healing. Clients with pressure injury will require increased protein to promote growth of granulation tissue (Gould et al, 2016). Protein requirements need to be calculated on an individual basis to ensure that accurate protein requirements are being met but needs can be as high as 1.25 to 1.5 grams of protein per kilogram of body weight if not contraindicated.

Nutritional support is only a part of the overall strategy to combat pressure injuries. The other risk factors must be controlled and diligent nursing care provided to effectively prevent or treat this serious condition.

BOX 12-6 ■ Food Insecurity

Older adults typically are reported as having the highest rate of food security, but data demonstrate an increase in food insecurity among adults aged 65 years and older. In 2015, 2.9 million households with adults aged greater than 65 years experienced food insecurity (Feeding America, 2017). Income has been listed as the risk factor for food insecurity. When looking at demographics in food insecurity, women are affected more than men and African Americans more than whites or Hispanics.

There is emerging evidence that food insecurity can contribute to inflammation in the human body, which can contribute to increased risks of diabetes, hypertension, and cardiovascular disease. Those with food insecurity have been shown to have:

- Lower serum folate levels; folate is needed for immune system activation
- Protein-energy malnutrition (Ihab, Rohana, & Manan, 2015)

Studies demonstrate that adults with food insecurity consumed more total calories, added sugar and empty calories, which resulted in chronic morbidity, such as type 2 diabetes and hypertension, and weight gain (Nguyen, Shuval, Bertmann, & Yaroch, 2015).

Some older adults are forced to make choices between purchasing food, medications, or cigarettes.

Dollars & Sense 12-1

Nutritional Supplements

Substituting Carnation Instant Breakfast® for Ensure® would save 61 cents per serving or $37 for 30 days assuming two servings per day. See calculations below.

To equal the kilocaloric content of Ensure requires a 10-ounce serving of modified Instant Breakfast instead of 8 ounces of Ensure. The protein contents of the Ensure and Instant Breakfast made with whole milk and ice cream are equivalent. The fat, saturated fat, cholesterol, and sodium contents are higher in the homemade recipe. Whether that intake would be a major concern for the client is a clinical judgment. Other nutrients have not been compared.

To implement the Instant Breakfast recipe also requires a refrigerator and freezer and a blender or shaker to mix the one package of instant breakfast, one cup of whole milk, and one-quarter cup of ice cream.

	Ensure	Carnation Instant Breakfast	Whole Milk	Ice Cream
Price	$7.97	$4.84	$3.29	$4.69
Package	8-oz bottles	10 packages of powder	1 gallon	½ gallon
Serving size	1 bottle	1 package	1 cup	½ cup
Cost/serving	$1.33	$0.48	$0.20	$0.29
Kilocalories	250	130	150	137
Protein	9 g	5 g	8 g	2 g
Carbohydrate	40 g	27 g	13 g	16 g
Total fat	6 g	0.5 g	8 g	8 g
Saturated fat	1 g	0 g	5 g	4g
Cholesterol	<5 mg	<5 mg	33 mg	30 mg
Sodium	190 mg	90 mg	120 mg	40 mg

---

supplements that are both nutrient dense and easy to consume might succeed for a person who is losing weight or one who cannot chew.

A more economical choice than prepared supplements may be an instant breakfast preparation. A homemade supplement recipe using ice cream is given in Dollars & Sense 12-1. To prevent dampening of appetite at mealtime, liquid caloric supplements should be given at least 1 hour before a meal.

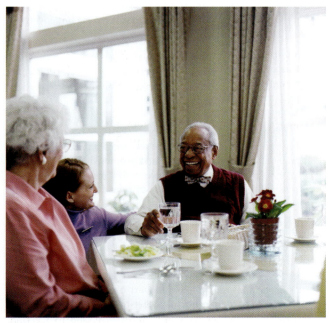

FIGURE 12-2 These older adults partake of an evening meal served at their residence.

To accommodate dentures, the person may reduce his or her intake of meats, fresh fruits, and vegetables. Assistance in selecting appropriate substitute items is in order. A recommended procedure for learning to eat and drink with dentures is explained in Clinical Application 12-3.

Nutritional Care for Elderly People

Box 12-7 lists topics to consider in a nutritional assessment.

Assessment

When assessing elderly people, special care is necessary to ensure that marginal deficiencies are detected before major

CLINICAL APPLICATION 12-3

Learning to Eat With Dentures

Clients should learn to use dentures one step at a time:

1. Practice swallowing liquids with the dentures in place.
2. Practice chewing soft foods.
3. Learn and practice to bite regular foods.

Splitting the process into manageable units decreases frustration.

BOX 12-7 ■ Topics to Be Assessed in Elderly People*

Oral Cavity Function
- Difficulty tasting; changes in taste perception
- Bleeding gums; dry mouth
- Difficulty chewing; toothaches; poorly fitting dentures
- Foods client is unable to eat

Meal Management
- Who shops? Where? Ease of making food decisions?
- Transportation problems?
- Budgeting a concern? Knowledge to make informed choices?
- Who cooks? Knowledge and skill level?
- Refrigeration, storage, and cooking facilities?
- Ability to manage containers: jars, cans, bottles

Psychosocial Factors
- Where are most meals eaten?
- Mealtime companions
- Recent change in living conditions?
- Satisfaction with situation?

*In addition to the normal assessment—that is, appetite or weight changes and bowel habits.

problems occur. Body weight and its stability are critical data in nutrition screening, yet an investigation in three large medical centers revealed that just 65.7% of clients older than 18 years reporting being weighed at admission and only 67% of those not weighed had been asked about their weight.

MINI NUTRITIONAL ASSESSMENT

The Mini Nutritional Assessment (MNA; Fig. 12-3) tool for use with older adults features two parts. The first 6 items provide a screening score and the last 12 items an assessment score that determines if further action is needed. The screening portion has the advantage of incorporating alternative measures for height if the person cannot stand and compensatory calculations for clients with missing limbs. The entire tool is available in many languages. Both a guide to its use and an online scoring program are available. Go to http://mna-elderly.com for more information regarding the tool and for updated resources.

The MNA has been established as a nutritional screening tool for use in a variety of care settings and allows for early detection of malnutrition risk and enables immediate intervention.

NUTRITION SCREENING INITIATIVE TOOLS

Nutritional assessment tools for use with older adults were developed by the Nutrition Screening Initiative. The following is a description of the tools.

- Determine Your Nutritional Health is a self-administered checklist with scoring directions to evaluate risk.
- Level I Screening Tool is to be administered by professionals in health or social service programs and includes directions for appropriate referrals.

- Level II Screening Tool is for use in physicians' offices and health-care institutions and includes a clinical examination, skinfold measurements, and laboratory tests.

Implementation

Some interventions are appropriate regardless of a client's living situation. Others are more focused on older adults living in institutions.

INDEPENDENTLY LIVING ELDERLY PEOPLE

Suggestions to increase the nourishment of elderly clients living in their own homes appear in Box 12-8.

Increasing physical activity according to the client's ability offers benefits beyond weight control. Physical activity helps to:

- Prevent heart disease and hypertension
- Improve bone mineral density
- Enhance balance and strength for activities of daily living
- Promote restful sleep

Many individuals, however, report never having been advised to exercise by their health-care providers. An intervention to enable the client to see improvement (or the need for improvement) is the keeping of an activity log.

HOSPITALIZED ELDERLY PEOPLE

The nurse's role in nourishing hospitalized older clients undergoing diagnostic tests is discussed in Clinical Application 12-4. Obtaining adequate food for such a client may tax the nurse's ingenuity because of timing and the need to entice a fatigued and perhaps fearful client to eat.

INSTITUTIONALIZED ELDERLY PEOPLE

Suggestions to increase the nourishment of older adults living in institutions appear in Box 12-9.

Providing nourishment for frail and ill elderly clients is a monumental task. The nurse must be aware of the client populations who are at greatest risk of undernourishment and those at greatest need for feeding assistance.

- More than half of clients with dementia will develop difficulty with feeding (Ball et al, 2015)
- Trouble swallowing or dysphagia will occur in 37% to 78% of stroke clients (Sivertsen, Graverholt, & Espehaug, 2017).

One study demonstrated that the average time it takes to assist a client with eating a meal averaged 30 to 40 minutes (Buys et al, 2013). This can become overwhelming in a high-paced health-care environment, but the nurse must remain vigilant in ensuring assistance with eating when required.

When asked, nursing home residents recalled that food tasted really good when eating with family and friends, especially in childhood. When staff learn about residents' previously enjoyed foods and occasionally provide those

Mini Nutritional Assessment
MNA®

Nestlé NutritionInstitute

Last name:		First name:		
Sex:	Age:	Weight, kg:	Height, cm:	Date:

Complete the screen by filling in the boxes with the appropriate numbers. Total the numbers for the final screening score.

Screening

A Has food intake declined over the past 3 months due to loss of appetite, digestive problems, chewing or swallowing difficulties?
0 = severe decrease in food intake
1 = moderate decrease in food intake
2 = no decrease in food intake ☐

B Weight loss during the last 3 months
0 = weight loss greater than 3 kg (6.6 lbs)
1 = does not know
2 = weight loss between 1 and 3 kg (2.2 and 6.6 lbs)
3 = no weight loss ☐

C Mobility
0 = bed or chair bound
1 = able to get out of bed / chair but does not go out
2 = goes out ☐

D Has suffered psychological stress or acute disease in the past 3 months?
0 = yes   2 = no ☐

E Neuropsychological problems
0 = severe dementia or depression
1 = mild dementia
2 = no psychological problems ☐

F1 Body Mass Index (BMI) (weight in kg) / (height in m²)
0 = BMI less than 19
1 = BMI 19 to less than 21
2 = BMI 21 to less than 23
3 = BMI 23 or greater ☐

IF BMI IS NOT AVAILABLE, REPLACE QUESTION F1 WITH QUESTION F2.
DO NOT ANSWER QUESTION F2 IF QUESTION F1 IS ALREADY COMPLETED.

F2 Calf circumference (CC) in cm
0 = CC less than 31
3 = CC 31 or greater ☐

Screening score (max. 14 points)

12 - 14 points: Normal nutritional status
8 - 11 points: At risk of malnutrition
0 - 7 points: Malnourished ☐☐

References
1. Vellas B, Villars H, Abellan G, *et al*. Overview of the MNA® - Its History and Challenges. *J Nutr Health Aging*. 2006;**10**:456-465.
2. Rubenstein LZ, Harker JO, Salva A, Guigoz Y, Vellas B. Screening for Undernutrition in Geriatric Practice: Developing the Short-Form Mini Nutritional Assessment (MNA-SF). *J. Geront*. 2001; **56A**: M366-377
3. Guigoz Y. The Mini-Nutritional Assessment (MNA®) Review of the Literature - What does it tell us? *J Nutr Health Aging*. 2006; **10**:466-487.
4. Kaiser MJ, Bauer JM, Ramsch C, et al. Validation of the Mini Nutritional Assessment Short-Form (MNA®-SF): A practical tool for identification of nutritional status. *J Nutr Health Aging*. 2009; **13**:782-788.
® Société des Produits Nestlé, S.A., Vevey, Switzerland, Trademark Owners © Nestlé, 1994, Revision 2009. N67200 12/99 10M
For more information: www.mna-elderly.com

FIGURE 12-3 Geriatric Mini Nutritional Assessment. (© *Nestlé, 1994, Revision 2009, with permission. For further information, go to the MNA® Web site: www.mna-elderly.com.*)

BOX 12-8 ■ Increasing Food Intake in Independently Living Elderly People

Prepare for Mealtime
- Suggest oral hygiene before meals to freshen and moisten mouth.
- Suggest smokers refrain for 1 hour before a meal to increase appetite.

Promote Social Interaction
- Encourage potluck meals with friends for those who live alone.
- Combine meals at the senior center with activities of interest.

Serve Food Attractively
- Suggest varying textures, colors, flavors.
- Suggest raw, crisp-cooked, or marinated vegetables to increase vegetable intake.
- Suggest using attractive dishes and flatware, centerpieces, tablecloths, or placemats.

Provide Nutrient-Dense Foods
- Help the client to select satisfactory meal-replacer supplements, whether commercial canned products or instant-breakfast powders.
- If additional kilocalories are needed, recommend whole milk for beverages and cooking instead of reduced-fat varieties.

Outside Help
- Obtain a home health aide to shop, do basic fix-ahead preparations.
- Provide Meals-on-Wheels for homebound.
- Refer to the social worker for food stamps, surplus commodity programs for those eligible.
- Recommend instructional materials on food purchasing, storage, cooking from county extension services.

BOX 12-9 ■ Increasing Food Intake in Elderly People Living in Institutions

Prepare for Mealtime
- Provide oral hygiene before meals to freshen and moisten mouth.
- Suggest smokers refrain for 1 hour before a meal to increase appetite.
- Manage the environment by removing unsightly supplies or noxious waste.
- Allow 60 minutes to elapse after a significant amount of supplement before serving the next meal.

Promote Social Interaction
- Encourage alert nursing home residents to choose compatible mealtime companions.
- Control the noise in the dining room to avoid overstimulating those with hearing aids.

Serve Food Attractively
- Vary textures, colors, flavors.
- To increase vegetable intake, offer raw, crisp-cooked, or marinated vegetables as appetizers.
- Provide enough nonglaring light so that food can be seen clearly.
- Schedule special events such as musical entertainment to enhance interest in eating.

Provide Nutrient-Dense Foods
- Add powdered milk, margarine, sugar, or ice cream to appropriate beverages and foods.
- Increase the eggs, milk, or cheese in recipes.
- When appropriate, offer 1 ounce of a nutritionally complete supplement every hour and use as "chaser" when administering medications.
- Choose milk-based beverages or beverages with sugar instead of water.
- Avoid use of low-fat or low-sugar foods.

favorites as special treats, residents maintain individuality within their peer group and among staff. Other suggestions to make mealtimes more homelike include:

- Buffet service
- Item selection that permits portion control

CLINICAL APPLICATION   12-4

Hospitalization of Elderly People

Except in obstetrical and pediatric practices, elderly clients dominate as consumers of health care. Eighty percent of elderly people, compared with 40% of individuals younger than 65 years, have one or more chronic diseases. In many cases, elderly clients are admitted to the hospital undernourished, and their nutritive status worsens during hospitalization.

Serving no food to a client because of diagnostic tests is starvation. The conscientious nurse obtains meals or feedings for a client who is *nil per os,* or NPO (i.e., nothing by mouth), for breakfast and lunch. There is nothing magical about the times of 8 a.m., 12 p.m., and 6 p.m. for meals. The committed nurse will arrange for adequate nourishment for clients when their tests are completed and they are permitted to eat. Dietary personnel have no idea when an individual client is finished with tests for the day until notified by the nurse.

- Choice of accompaniments with open seating in the dining room
- Using linen napkins and cups and saucers

Bolstering fluid intake in older adults living in institutions takes planning. Frequent small drinks may be more acceptable to the client than trying to swallow large amounts with meals. See Box 12-10 for strategies to increase fluid consumption.

BOX 12-10 ■ Increasing Fluid Intake in Elderly

- Offer clients sips of fluids frequently and with every contact.
- Leave drinks within the client's reach.
- Provide frequent mouth care.
- Offer preferred beverages.
- Establish client's normal drinking patterns.
- Position the client to a position that facilitates swallowing.
- Develop "happy hour," which can encourage socialization and fluid consumption.

Adapted from Campbell, N: Dehydration: best practice in the care home. *Nurs Residential Care* 14:21, 2012.

KEYSTONES

- Aging has an impact on almost all body systems, affecting food procurement, preparation, consumption, digestion, and metabolism.

- Supplements and fortified foods as sources of calcium and vitamins D and B_{12} are recommended for middle-aged and older adults in recognition of impaired absorption, metabolism, and synthesis as people age.

- Involuntary weight loss in elderly people should stimulate a broad search for causes: physical, environmental, financial, and social.

- Overweight increases the risk for certain diseases such as osteoarthritis and diabetes mellitus.

- The most nutritionally vulnerable adults are nursing home residents who are unable to eat without assistance.

CASE STUDY 12-1

Mr. E is a 70-year-old widower who relies on public transportation. His home is two blocks from the bus route and eight blocks from the nearest supermarket. Mr. E has moderately painful knees from arthritis. He has been taking the bus to the supermarket every other day so that he could manage one package on the way home. He has confided to the nurse in his doctor's office that he is ready to "just give up. It's too much trouble to eat anymore." Mr. E's weight today is 160 lb, 5 lb less than last month.

CARE PLAN

Subjective Data

Dependent on public transportation ■ Painful knees ■ Verbalized discouragement with procuring food

Objective Data

Weight loss of 5 lb in past month

Analysis

Lack of information concerning resources available to maintain senior citizens in their homes

Plan

DESIRED OUTCOMES EVALUATION CRITERIA	ACTIONS/INTERVENTIONS	RATIONALE
Mr. E will acknowledge need for assistance with meals by end of visit today.	Discuss Mr. E's weight change with him. Determine what kind of assistance he would accept.	Clients are likely to change behaviors only if the new behavior is acceptable to them.
Given several options of community support, Mr. E will select one and begin to implement the change within 3 days.	Describe Senior Citizen Nutrition Program, Meals on Wheels, home health aide shopping service, and door-to-door Care-a-Van service, grocery delivery services.	Clients may know about these programs but prefer to remain independent. Allowing the client some time to choose makes the choice more his own.
	Explore social support available from family and less-restricted friends.	Following up with a telephone call shows that the nurse is committed to working through this problem with Mr. E.
	Nurse to follow up with telephone call in 3 days.	During the follow-up telephone call, Mr. E said that he would like information on the Senior Nutrition Program and the Care-a-Van Service.

CRITICAL THINKING QUESTIONS

1. What additional data could be sought in a more comprehensive assessment?

2. What other areas could be investigated to help balance Mr. E's need for assistance with his desire for independence?

3. As you read this case, how would you define the underlying problem?

CHAPTER REVIEW

1. The RDA/AI for which of the following nutrients is increased for older adults compared with younger ones?
   1. Sodium
   2. Calcium
   3. Vitamin C
   4. Vitamin K

2. The decrease in gastric acid that accompanies aging causes concern for the absorption of which of the following nutrients?
   1. Carbohydrate and water
   2. Fat and cholesterol
   3. Vitamins A and E
   4. Vitamin B_{12} and iron

3. A nurse making a home visit routinely screens for dehydration in elderly clients. Which of the following would the nurse assess?
   1. Body temperature and urine specific gravity
   2. Tongue condition, pulse rate, and muscle strength
   3. Skin turgor and heart and lung sounds
   4. Client's intake and output records

4. Which of the following conditions is likely to contribute to vitamin D deficiency in older adults? Select all that apply.
   1. Atrophied skin, dislike for milk, and indoor life
   2. Lack of exercise
   3. Diminished secretion of intrinsic factor
   4. Lactose intolerance
   5. Inability to chew meat

5. Ms. P is a 58-year-old retired cook who tells the clinic nurse that she regrets not having had children and grandchildren. Which of the following activities might assist Ms. P to attain generativity?
   1. Editing a cookbook for her church group
   2. Taking a class in ethnic cooking in preparation for her next trip
   3. Serving on the Meals-on-Wheels advisory board
   4. Volunteering to teach a special recipe at a local school

CLINICAL ANALYSIS

1. Ms. O is a 76-year-old retired schoolteacher who has been admitted to a long-term care facility after surgical repair of a fractured hip.
   While performing the Mini Nutritional Assessment for Ms. O, to calculate the most accurate BMI, the nurse would use the client's height
   a. Listed on her driver's license
   b. At age 50
   c. As determined in the supine position with a tape measure
   d. Using the alternative demi-span measurement

2. Ms. O reports a weight loss of 4 lb in the 3 months before her injury. Her present weight is 125 lb. Which of the following nursing actions is appropriate at this point?
   a. Asking the physician to order an appetite stimulant
   b. Ordering balanced nutritional supplements three times a day
   c. Deferring action until the team conference next week
   d. Instructing the nursing assistants to feed Ms. O

3. Because Ms. O will have limited mobility, providing adequate fluid intake is necessary to prevent complications in the ____ system.
   a. Cardiovascular
   b. Endocrine
   c. Urinary
   d. Integumentary

CHAPTER 13

Food Management

LEARNING OBJECTIVES

After completing this chapter, the student should be able to:
- Describe the conditions under which microbiologic food illnesses can occur.
- Identify foods that are likely to harbor disease-producing microorganisms.
- Teach clients how to prevent foodborne illnesses.
- Discuss the information on food labels.

Effective meal management requires knowledge about food safety, including microbiological hazards, environmental pollutants, and natural food toxins. Reading food labels can help prevent nutritional hazards. How food is handled between the time it leaves the farm and the time it reaches the table affects our health and well-being. How food crops are grown and animals are raised influences health as well. As health care moves from institutions to home care, health-care workers need to understand the vital importance of safe and nutritious food (see Box 13-1).

The Centers for Disease Control and Prevention (CDC), in the Burden of Foodborne Illness findings, estimates that each year, 1 in 6 Americans (48 million people) get foodborne diseases, 128,000 are hospitalized for them, and 3,000 die of them (Centers for Disease Control and Prevention [CDC], September, 2016). Considering the number of people involved in the growth, distribution, preparation, and service of food, our food safety record is excellent. The food supply in the United States is as safe, wholesome, and nutritious as any in the world.

Foodborne illnesses are caused by bacteria, viruses, parasites, mold, toxins, contaminants, and allergens. New strains of pathogens, or disease-producing organisms, are continually evolving; in some cases, these organisms have proven resistant to antibiotics. The development of these resistant foodborne pathogens has been attributed to increased use of antibiotics in hospitals, outpatient facilities, and veterinary applications as well as the home use of antimicrobial products. Antibiotics are widely used to promote growth and prevent infection in livestock. Meat products, which contain antibiotics, are ingested and people are exposed. Animals excrete up to 90% of ingested antibiotics, which causes exposure through fertilizer, groundwater, and surface runoff (Ventola, 2015). Food contamination can happen at any point in the food supply process. Among the goals of the Healthy People 2020 program, a government initiative, is to improve food safety and reduce foodborne illnesses. Education is a key component of the program because proper handling, preparation, and storage of food are critical to ensure food safety (HealthyPeople.gov, 2017).

The following is recommended to reduce the risk of foodborne illness (University of Rhode Island, 2017):

- CLEAN—Wash hands, surfaces, and food.
- SEPARATE—Don't mix raw and cooked foods or use the same cutting board/utensils.
- COOK—Cook foods to safe temperatures, using a thermometer; don't hold foods at temperatures <140°F (<60°C).
- CHILL—Refrigerate foods quickly after purchasing prepared foods or when storing leftovers. Keep refrigerated at 40°F (4.4°C).

Food Irradiation

Food irradiation has been used since 1905 when scientists received patents for food preservation using radiation to kill bacteria in food. It is used to kill parasites, insects, and bacteria in foods such as meat, poultry, flour, vegetables, and eggs. It also is used to delay sprouting (e.g., potatoes) and ripening (e.g., fruit) in foods. When a food has been irradiated, the Food and Drug Administration (FDA) requires the use of a label that states either "Treated With Radiation" or "Treated by Irradiation." The irradiation logo, the Radura, must also be displayed (Fig. 13-1). Foods that are not entirely irradiated but only have ingredients that are subjected to radiation need not have a label. Also, there is no requirement for labeling of irradiated food served in restaurants (Food and Drug Administration [FDA], 2016).

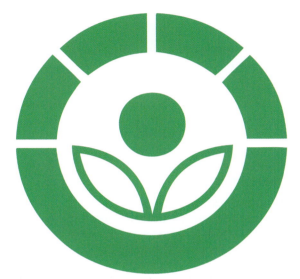

FIGURE 13-1 The Radura symbol for irradiated food labels.

Microbiological Hazards

More than 250 foodborne diseases have been identified. The CDC (September, 2016) defines foodborne illnesses being caused by bacteria, viruses, parasites, toxins, or chemicals. Most foodborne diseases infect the tissues of the digestive tract and cause gastric distress; symptoms range from mild to severe (see Box 13-2). Microorganisms may be carried from one host to another by animals; humans; inanimate objects, including food; and environmental factors, such as air, water, and soil. Many microorganisms cause disease. Under certain conditions, food becomes a vehicle for disease transmission.

   The CDC estimates that top pathogens contributing to domestically acquired foodborne illnesses were the norovirus causing 58%, followed by the following bacteria (CDC, July, 2016):

- *Salmonella nontyphoida*, 11%
- *Clostridium perfringens*, 10%
- *Campylobacter*, 9%
- *Staphylococcus aureus*, 3%

   Of particular concern to pregnant women is the bacterium *Listeria monocytogenes* and parasite *Toxoplasma gondii*, which can cause miscarriage, serious birth defects, and even death of a newborn (FDA, 2017).

Norovirus

Norovirus is normally spread from one person to another through contaminated food, water, or environmental surfaces. Infected kitchen workers can contaminate foods they prepare if they have the virus on their hands. Sewage discharge in coastal growing waters has contaminated oysters before they are harvested (CDC, June, 2016).

   To prevent norovirus, the CDC (June, 2016) recommends:

- Washing hands frequently
- Kitchen workers wearing gloves when working with food
- Cleaning and disinfecting food preparation surfaces and equipment
- No food preparation by individuals who are ill
- Washing fruits and vegetables thoroughly before preparation or consumption
- Cooking shellfish thoroughly
- Washing clothing and table linens thoroughly

Bacterial Foodborne Disease

Bacteria are everywhere: doorknobs, countertops, hands, eyelashes, mouths, some water supplies, and food are a few of the many places where bacteria can be found. Animal and human fluids and waste harbor bacteria and cause many foodborne illnesses. The CDC (September, 2016) reported that the following raw foods contribute to the majority of foodborne illnesses in the United States: foods of animal origin (meats, poultry, eggs, shellfish, and unpasteurized milk), fruits, and vegetables. The following contributes to bacterial contamination of foods:

- Bare-handed food contact by handler/worker/preparer
- Raw product/ingredient contaminates from animal or environment
- Allowing food to remain at room or outdoor temperature for several hours
- Insufficient time and/or temperature during the initial cooking/heat processing

Conditions for Growth

Bacterial growth refers to an increase in the number of organisms. Under ideal conditions, cell numbers can double every half hour: one cell becomes two, two become four, and four become eight (in an hour and a half). A single bacterium can multiply to 33 million after 12 hours. Although bacteria cannot be eradicated from our environment, bacterial growth can be controlled. For this reason, understanding the following conditions necessary for bacterial growth and microbiological food illness to occur is important:

- Source of bacteria—the bacteria must come in contact with the food.
- Food—the food must permit the bacteria to grow (increase in number) or produce a poisonous toxin. Bacteria grow in foods only within a certain pH range. This is why vinegar and lemon juice are frequently used to preserve food, such as cucumbers (pickles) and cabbage (sauerkraut). These ingredients lower the pH and so bacteria cannot grow.
- Temperature—the temperature must be favorable for bacterial growth. The temperature range in which most bacteria multiply rapidly is 40°F (4.4°C) to 140°F (60°C), the range that includes room and body temperature (Fig. 13-2).
- Time—enough time must elapse for bacteria to grow, produce a toxin, or both.
- Moisture—bacteria need water to dissolve and digest food. Foods that contain water support bacterial growth better than do dehydrated foods. This is the reason that dehydration is a food preservation method.
- Ingestion—an unsuspecting person must eat the food or drink the beverage that contains the toxin or bacteria.

Bacteria are frequently odorless, tasteless, and colorless; therefore, laboratory analysis is the only way to tell whether a food will cause illness. Table 13-1 lists pathogens, common food vehicles, and symptoms.

Food Infections

A **food infection** is caused by eating a food containing a large number of disease-producing bacteria.

SALMONELLA

Salmonella is a bacterium that can cause an illness called **salmonellosis.** It is transmitted by the consumption of contaminated foods or contact with an infected person. Some foods support the growth of *Salmonella* better than others. Common food vehicles include raw eggs, unpasteurized milk, and poultry.

CAMPYLOBACTER

Another type of bacteria causing food infections is *Campylobacter jejuni,* which is carried in the intestinal tracts of cows, hogs, sheep, and poultry. The most frequent source of infection is eating undercooked poultry, or foods that have been contaminated with the drippings from the raw chicken. It is the most commonly identified bacterial cause of diarrheal illness in the world (Geissler, Mahon, & Fitzgerald, 2017). Contaminated water or raw manure can spread the organism. For example, an animal can defecate in a vegetable garden and contaminate the produce.

Foods found to be contaminated with *Campylobacter jejuni* include raw milk, fresh mushrooms, and raw hamburger. *Campylobacter* can be controlled by keeping food below 40°F (4.4°C) or above 140°F (60°C) and by maintaining good food-handling practices.

LISTERIA

Another pathogen is *Listeria.* This organism is problematic because the bacteria can grow slowly at refrigerated temperatures (32°F [0°C] to 34°F [1.1°C]) and on moist surfaces. Cooking facilities must be kept clean and dry to prevent the growth of this organism. Chlorine (bleach), one tablespoon per gallon of water, is also effective in inhibiting *Listeria.*

According to the CDC, every year 1,600 Americans become ill with listeriosis, with 260 cases resulting in death. Pregnant women become susceptible to foodborne illnesses because of changes in their immune system. Pregnant women are 10 times more likely to get a *Listeria* infection. Listeriosis can be transmitted to the fetus through the placenta, leading to premature delivery, miscarriage, stillbirth, or other serious health problems for the newborn (CDC, December, 2016). The USDA Food Safety and Inspection Service (FSIS) and the U.S. FDA provide guidelines for pregnant women (foodsafety.gov, see Box 13-3).

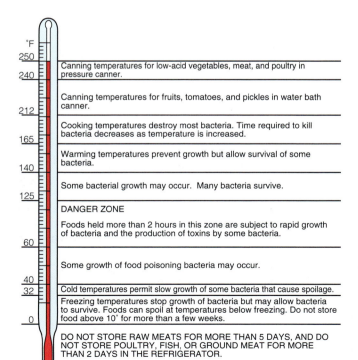

FIGURE 13-2 A temperature guide to food safety.

TABLE 13-1 Pathogens, Common Food Vehicles, and Symptoms (www.cdc.gov)

PATHOGEN	COMMON FOOD VEHICLES (HAZARDOUS FOOD ITEMS)	SYMPTOMS
Salmonella	Raw or undercooked eggs, poultry, or meat; unpasteurized milk or juice; cheese; seafood; fresh fruits and vegetables	May lead to sudden onset of headache, fever, chills, abdominal pain, diarrhea, nausea, and vomiting. Dehydration may be severe, and fever is usually present. May develop into septicemia. Symptoms begin suddenly and last for 12–24 hours (up to 2 weeks in elderly people). See Clinical Application 13-1.
Listeria	Soft cheeses, deli meats, pâté, burritos, ice cream, unpasteurized milk, smoked seafood, deli salads, raw vegetables	Fever, chills, headache, backache, upset stomach, abdominal pain, and diarrhea. May lead to meningoencephalitis and/or septicemia in newborns and adults and miscarriage in pregnant women. Symptoms may appear within a few hours to 3 days. It may take up to 2 months to become ill.
Escherichia coli 0157:H7	Undercooked ground beef, other beef, unpasteurized milk and apple juice, contaminated raw fruits and vegetables, and water	May lead to acute hemorrhagic colitis (cramps, bloody diarrhea, nausea, vomiting, and fever). May result in hemolytic uremic failure or kidney failure. Symptoms can begin 1–9 days after contaminated food is eaten and last 2–9 days.
Campylobacter jejuni	Raw or undercooked poultry, meat, or shellfish, unpasteurized milk, water	May lead to an acute gastroenteritis of variable severity characterized by diarrhea, abdominal pain, malaise, fever, nausea, and vomiting. Guillain-Barré syndrome or meningitis have been seen in severe cases. Symptoms appear 2–5 days after eating and may last 2–10 days.
Norovirus	Produce, raw shellfish, and any other ingredient contaminated by an infected person	May lead to nausea, vomiting, diarrhea, abdominal pain, headache, malaise, and low-grade fever. Symptoms appear in 12–48 hours and usually last 1–3 days but can last 4–6.
Staphylococcus aureus	Poultry, processed meats, milk, cheeses, ice cream, mixed dishes such as potato salad, spaghetti	May cause nausea, vomiting, stomach cramps and diarrhea. Symptoms appear in 30 minutes to 6 hours and last 1–3 days.
Clostridium botulinum	Improperly processed canned food; large masses of food with air-free center	May lead to acute bilateral cranial nerve impairment and descending weakness or paralysis. Double vision, dysphagia, and dry mouth may be present. Vomiting, diarrhea, or constipation may be present initially. Symptoms appear in 18–36 hours but can occur as late as 6 hours to 10 days. Symptoms may last for weeks or months, and some residual problems can last for years. A small percentage (3%–5%) of infected people die.
Clostridium perfringens	Meats, poultry, gravies, and stews in large masses of food such as steam tables or left at room temperature	Abdominal cramping, diarrhea, vomiting, and fever are common. Incubation time is 8–16 hours. Symptoms occur within 16 hours and last for 12–24 hours (up to 1–2 weeks in elderly people).

CLINICAL APPLICATION

13-1

Food Safety and Immunosuppressed Clients

All clients receiving an immunosuppressive agent need counseling on food safety and sanitation. These clients have an inability to fight infections, and so a relatively small number of bacteria could cause illness. **Immunosuppressive agents** are medications that interfere with the body's ability to fight infections. These drugs are used in tissue and organ transplantation procedures, such as a kidney transplant. These are also used as part of the treatment of certain diseases, such as cancer. The neutrophil (white blood cell) count in the blood becomes abnormally low, a condition referred to as neutropenia, making clients susceptible to life-threatening infection. Diet recommendations are to teach basic food safety guidelines to clients who are immunosuppressed. Additionally, these individuals should be careful to do the following:

- Eat foods before expiration date.
- Use a safe water source.

- Wash fruits and vegetables thoroughly before peeling.
- Cook all meet, fish, and poultry well done (165–212°F [73.9–100°C]).
- Do not eat uncooked or undercooked eggs, raw seafood, meats, or unpasteurized milk or dairy products.
- Refrigerate leftovers immediately and do not consume after 3 days.
- Throw away any food that is moldy or has a rotten spot.
- Thaw foods only in the refrigerator.

(University of California San Francisco, 2017; CDC, April, 2015)

Food Intoxication

Food intoxication is caused by the consumption of a food in which bacteria have produced a poisonous toxin.

STAPHYLOCOCCUS AUREUS

One of the most common bacteria producing a poisonous toxin is *Staphylococcus aureus,* commonly referred to as staph. Staph is reportedly in the nasal passages of 30% to 50% of healthy people and on the hands of 20% of healthy people. Infected cuts, boils, and burns harbor this organism.

Heat destroys the bacteria but not the toxins the bacteria have already produced. Because heat does not destroy the toxin, control of temperature alone will not provide protection. Prevention of staph poisoning must include good personal hygiene and keeping foods below 40°F (4.4°C) or above 140°F (60°C) (Bush, 2016).

CLOSTRIDIUM BOTULINUM

Another bacterium producing a toxin is *Clostridium botulinum* and the resulting disease is **botulism**. The organism is found worldwide in soils and the intestinal tracts of domestic animals. Vegetables grown in contaminated soil harbor this organism. Botulin, the toxin produced by *C. botulinum,* is so poisonous that a single ounce is enough to kill the world's population. The spores of *C. botulinum* grow under anaerobic (without oxygen) conditions. Canned foods are processed to be anaerobic, providing an ideal medium for this bacterium's growth. Home-canned, nonacid fruits and vegetables, faultily processed commercially canned tuna, and improperly packaged smoked fish have all transmitted botulism.

Outbreaks of botulism can be avoided by the proper processing and preparation of susceptible foods. For each food, home canners should consult a reliable home-canning food guide regarding proper time, pressure, and temperature required to kill spores. Follow the CDC guidelines for home canning, which includes, "when in doubt, throw it out" (CDC, 2017).

Complicating Factors

The following complicate the risk of foodborne illness:

- The worldwide overuse of antibiotics. Antibiotics kill not only pathogens but also normal flora, which help keep the disease-producing organisms in balance. Pathogens can mutate and become resistant to antibiotics.
- In the United States, the average age of the population continues to increase as life expectancy increases. Older people are more susceptible to pathogenic bacteria than younger people; fewer organisms are needed to produce symptoms in older people.
- Food production has become more centralized, an effect that has both good and bad ramifications. Food inspectors can more closely monitor the sanitation at food-processing plants, but a foodborne illness outbreak affects more people in wider geographical areas.
- As the population becomes highly educated about food safety, illnesses that in the past might have been dismissed as "stomach flu" are increasingly being identified as foodborne illnesses.
- Many foods are imported from countries whose regulatory procedures are not as stringent as those in the United States.
- Consumers are eating more meals away from home and using more convenience foods. Both behaviors increase the number of individuals involved in food handling and the time food is held in the danger zones. For example, a frozen convenience food is held in the temperature danger zone (between 40°F [4.4°C] and 140°F [60°C]) twice, once during assembly in the food-processing factory and a second time when the consumer is reheating it.
- Consumers are eating more raw food and more lightly grilled and sautéed foods, which are sometimes not cooked to proper temperatures.

Box 13-4 discusses how the simple behavior of frequent hand washing minimizes the risk of foodborne disease. Figure 13-3 pictures the correct amount of soap lather needed to cleanse hands.

Infectious Agents

Mad cow disease, also known as **bovine spongiform encephalopathy (BSE),** is related to a disease in humans called variant Creutzfeldt-Jakob disease (vCJD). Humans acquire this disease by eating beef that contains an infective agent (called a prion). A **prion** is a small protein that is resistant to most traditional methods that destroy a protein. BSE has been found in infected brain, spinal cord tissue, retina, dorsal root ganglia (nervous tissue near the backbone), distal ileum, and bone marrow in cattle experimentally infected by the oral route. Cattle acquire the infection when fed

The best defense against foodborne disease is hand washing and keeping the hands away from the mouth. Figure 13-3 demonstrates proper hand washing. Hands should always be washed:

- Before food preparation
- After food preparation
- After using the restroom
- Between touching another person's body, including the hands, and touching the mouth or eating
- After smoking
- Before smoking
- Between touching one person and then another person
- After covering the mouth when coughing or sneezing
- When visibly dirty
- After touching any surface area around any person who is visibly ill
- After changing an infant's diapers or touching any bodily secretion of another person

ground-up carcasses of animals, both sheep and other cattle, which contain the infected prion. As of August 2016, 231 people worldwide have become sick with vCJD (FDA, 2016).

Parasitic Infections

A **parasite** is an organism that lives within, on, or at the expense of a living host without providing any benefit to the host. Several parasites can live in animals that humans use for food. When a person eats an infected animal, he or she also consumes the parasite, and the result is illness. Common parasites are *Trichinella spiralis*, *Toxoplasma gondii*, and tapeworms.

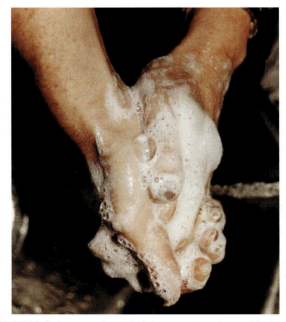

FIGURE 13-3 Amount of soap lather necessary to thoroughly cleanse the hands.

TRICHINELLA SPIRALIS

Although the prevalence of this infection is low in the United States, it is significantly higher in people living in parts of Europe, Asia, and Southeast Asia.

Trichinella spiralis is a worm that becomes embedded in the muscle tissue of pigs. Pigs acquire the worm when fed meat from an animal harboring the worm in its muscle. The worm produces larvae that are protected from animal (including human) digestion. The larvae mature in the animal's stomach in 5 to 7 days. Adult worms then invade the lining of the small intestine, where they reproduce. The larvae enter the bloodstream of the animal and are carried to all parts of the body. They then penetrate the muscles, form cysts, and remain alive and infective for months. The cycle is completed when another animal eats the muscle containing the live *Trichinella spiralis* larvae.

When a human eats the larvae, usually in undercooked pork, he or she develops **trichinosis.** The symptoms of trichinosis usually appear 9 days after the ingestion of infected meat, but the time can vary from 2 to 28 days. This period of time is called the **incubation period**—the length of time it takes to show disease symptoms after exposure to the offending organism. The first symptoms, which mimic food poisoning, are nausea, vomiting, and diarrhea. When the larvae migrate into muscles, including the heart, systemic symptoms develop that include fever, swelling of the eyelids, sweating, weakness, and muscular pain. Death due to heart failure may occur.

TOXOPLASMA GONDII

This is a parasite found in food sources, such as raw or undercooked meat, unwashed fruits and vegetables, contaminated water, dust, soil, and cat feces. Symptoms can be flulike and appear 10 to 13 days after eating, and may last months. Toxoplasmosis can cause miscarriage and birth defects, including hearing loss, intellectual disability, and blindness (FDA, 2016).

TAPEWORMS

Humans acquire tapeworms through the ingestion of raw seafood or undercooked beef and pork. Hogs and steers become intermediate hosts when they graze on sewage-polluted pastures. Tapeworm infestation can occur when human wastes contaminate freshwater streams and lakes, animal pasture, or feed.

Symptoms of a tapeworm infection may be trivial or absent. In some people, the worms attach to the jejunum and hosts develop vitamin B_{12} deficiency, anemia, and massive infections with diarrhea. Obstruction of the bile duct or intestine can be another complication.

Viral Infections

A **virus** is a microscopic parasite that is entirely dependent on the nutrients inside host cells for its metabolic and reproductive needs. Viruses may invade the cells of people, animals, plants, and bacteria to survive and thereby cause disease. Food frequently serves as a vehicle for some viruses, including those that cause influenza and infectious hepatitis.

Food can become contaminated in its growing environment or during processing, storage, distribution, or preparation. Partly for this reason, the federal government requires all food-service workers to wear plastic gloves when handling food.

Some viruses are found in the intestinal tract of infected humans. If an infected person neglects to wash his or her hands after defecation and then handles food, the virus can contaminate the food and be passed on to unsuspecting consumers. The disease varies from a mild illness lasting 1 to 2 weeks to a severely disabling disease lasting several months.

HEPATITIS A VIRUS

The hepatitis A virus causes infectious hepatitis, a liver disease. This virus can be found in water that has been contaminated with raw sewage and in shellfish harvested from fecally contaminated water. During food processing, hepatitis A can be transmitted when polluted water is used or by fecal contamination from insects or rodents. Infected workers can transmit the virus through food they handle. The onset of viral hepatitis A is abrupt, with fever, malaise, anorexia, nausea, and abdominal discomfort. A few days later, the client may develop jaundice.

HEPATITIS E VIRUS

Hepatitis E is believed to be uncommon in the United States, normally only seen with individuals who have traveled to developing countries. The highest rates of disease are seen in regions with the lowest sanitation standards. It is transmitted through:

- Fecal contamination of water
- Foodborne transmission from ingestion of products from infected animals
- Transfusion of infected blood products
- Vertical transmission from a pregnant woman to her fetus

The onset of symptoms, which include jaundice, anorexia, enlarged liver, abdominal pain, nausea, vomiting, and fever, occurs from 2 to 8 weeks after exposure to the virus (CDC, May, 2015).

Substances Made Poisonous by Other Organisms

The consumption of toxic fish and plants can cause illness. Some molds can also produce disease (others are beneficial).

TOXIC SEAFOOD

The tissue of fish and shellfish can be naturally toxic to humans, even when the fish is fresh. The fish may not show any outward signs of illness, and there is usually no way to tell whether the fish is toxic. Because most fish toxins are stable to heat, cooking does not destroy them. **Paralytic shellfish poisoning** outbreaks have been reported involving the consumption of poisonous clams, oysters, mussels, and scallops.

Ciguatera poisoning is a foodborne illness caused by eating fish that is contaminated by ciguatera toxin, affecting approximately 50,000 people annually. The ciguatera toxin is odorless, tasteless, and heat-stable and therefore cannot be killed by cooking or freezing. This intoxication results from eating certain fish that have consumed marine bacteria and algae associated with coastal reefs and nearby waterways. Fish eating the algae become toxic, and the effect is magnified through the food chain so that large predatory fish become the most toxic; this occurs worldwide in tropical areas. Coastal waters are routinely monitored for the presence of the organism that produces ciguatera. If excessive numbers of the organism are found, a "red tide" alert is made. The best prevention is to avoid eating fish caught during a red tide. Symptoms can occur from 2 to 24 hours after ingestion. Symptoms include nausea, vomiting, diarrhea, muscle pain, numbness, tingling, abdominal pain, dizziness, and vertigo (Davis, 2016).

Scombroid fish poisoning is caused by the presence of undesirable bacteria. This poisoning occurs in fish such as tuna, mackerel, bonito, and skipjack. The bacteria produce a toxin on the flesh of fish after the fish have been caught. Scombroid fish poisoning can be prevented by the adequate refrigeration of freshly caught fish and the purchase of fish from reputable sources.

MOLDS

Molds are the most widely encountered microorganism and are spread by air currents, insects, and rodents. Some molds are beneficial, such as those used to make some cheese and soy sauce. Like bacteria, molds are often involved in food spoilage. A number of molds grow well in cold storage but are easily destroyed by heating to 140°F (60°C) or higher.

Molds grow on bread, cheese, fruits, vegetables, preserves, grains, and a wide variety of other products. *Aspergillus* molds produce a series of **mycotoxins** called **aflatoxins** that may be present in peanuts or peanut products, corn, wheat, and oil seeds such as cottonseed. There is a positive association between dietary aflatoxins and liver cell cancer (LCC) (Cornell University, 2015).

The best advice is to discard moldy bread because mold may have penetrated the entire item. Mold on hard, natural cheese can be safely removed (approximately 1 inch should be removed from the cheese) and the remainder of the cheese eaten, because the mold is not likely to have penetrated deeply. Soft cheeses that have mold should be discarded (Ansel, 2015).

Environmental Pollutants

Although environmental pollution is widespread, situations that pose a severe and immediate health danger are uncommon. The Environmental Protection Agency (EPA) regulates the use of **pesticides** and sets tolerance levels to provide a high margin of safety in food.

Chemical Poisoning

Chemical poisoning occurs when people eat toxic substances that may be intentionally or accidentally added to foods during growing, harvesting, processing, transporting, storing, or preparing foods. Two general types of chemical poisoning can occur. They are heavy metal and chemical-product contamination pesticides.

Heavy Metals

Several metals can be toxic. Metals in the soil come from rocks and minerals weathered by water erosion; metals as added ingredients or impurities in fertilizers, pesticides, manure, and sludge; and airborne dust. Airborne dust comes from industrial and mining waste, fossil fuel combustion products, radioactive fallout, pollen, sea spray, and meteoric and volcanic material. This dust eventually settles to the ground and becomes part of the soil. Plants may grow normally but contain levels of selenium, cadmium, molybdenum, or lead that are toxic to humans.

The toxic action of metals is thought to be important in enzyme poisoning. For example, mercury, lead, copper, beryllium, cadmium, and silver have been found to inhibit the enzyme **alkaline phosphatase.** One function of alkaline phosphatase is in the mineralization of bone. Some diseases associated with the consumption of toxic minerals include rickets and bone tumors. Lead ingestion with a subsequent elevation of blood lead levels has been linked to toxic effects, including adverse neurologic, neurobehavioral, and developmental conditions.

Mercury is extremely toxic. It was once an occupational disease of hat manufacturers because mercury was used in the curing of animal pelts used to make hats. Inhalation of the mercury fumes led to mental deterioration, which is the origin of the term "mad hatter." Because mercury can damage the fetal nervous system, the FDA has issued a consumer alert for young children, pregnant and nursing women, and women of childbearing age not to eat large fish types in which mercury may accumulate: shark, swordfish, king mackerel, tuna (bigeye), marlin, orange roughy, and tilefish (FDA, 2017).

Chemical Products

Chemical foodborne illness is also associated with products such as detergents, sanitizers, pesticides, and other chemicals that may enter the food supply. After such toxins have been ingested, symptoms of chemical poisoning appear in a few minutes to a few hours but usually in less than 1 hour. Nausea, vomiting, abdominal pain, diarrhea, and a metallic taste are common complaints with chemical foodborne illnesses, and death is possible (see Box 13-5).

Bisphenol A (BPA) is a chemical used in the production of plastics and is found in some food and drink packaging. It can leach into food from epoxy resin coatings of canned foods and polycarbonate tableware, food storage containers,

---

> **BOX 13-5 ■ Chemical Poisoning**
>
> Chemical poisoning can be prevented by:
>
> - Using each product for its intended use and in the amounts recommended
> - Reading product labels before use
> - Keeping chemicals in their original containers
> - Never storing or transporting chemicals in containers used to store food; they may be mistaken (especially by children) for food or beverages

---

and bottles (including water and baby). To limit exposure, National Institutes of Health (NIH) recommends not microwaving polycarbonate plastic food containers, reducing use of canned foods, and using containers made from glass, porcelain, or stainless steel (National Institutes of Health, 2017).

Pesticides are chemicals used to kill insects or rodents; when accidentally mixed with food, they have caused poisonings in people. In addition, using pesticide-containing aerosols around foods and packaging materials and in food preparation areas can be dangerous. According to the EPA, studies have linked pesticides to problems such as cancer, nerve damage, and birth defects.

Pesticide residues are of great concern to consumers. **Residues** are trace amounts of any substance remaining in a product at the time of sale. Governmental agencies that regulate products that enter the U.S. food supply are:

The Environmental Protection Agency (EPA)
The Food and Drug Administration (FDA)
Food Safety and Inspection Service (FSIS), which is part of the U.S. Department of Agriculture (USDA)

The EPA regulates the use of potentially harmful pesticides in food production. Included among the duties of the EPA is the establishment of tolerance levels for pesticides.

The FDA regulates animal drugs, including food additives, herbicides, and environmental contaminants. The FSIS sets tolerance levels for these chemical residues in edible foods. In setting a **tolerance level,** the FSIS determines the highest dose at which a residue causes no ill effects in laboratory animals. The tolerance level is then divided by a factor ranging from 100 to 1,000 to account for possible differences between animals and humans.

The numbers used assume that humans are 10 times more sensitive than the most sensitive animal species tested. In addition, a further assumption is made that children and older adults are 10 times more sensitive than others. This is the 100-fold safety factor (multiplying 10 times 10). Thus, a large margin of safety is built into residue limits for compounds involved in the production of human food.

The FSIS enforces the residue limits in meat and poultry. The FDA is responsible for foods other than meat and poultry. When an illegal residue is found, the FDA can conduct an investigation and the FSIS can detain future shipments from the violating producer.

Food Additives

Additives may be introduced into food deliberately or accidentally. An **additive** is a substance added to food to increase its flavor, shelf life, or characteristics, such as texture, color, and aroma, and other qualities. In the United States, the FDA regulates food additives under the authority of the Food, Drug, and Cosmetic Act of 1938 and amendments in 1958 and 1960. These amendments include the Delaney Clause, which bans the approval of an additive if it is shown to cause cancer in humans or animals. Before using a new food additive, a manufacturer must petition the FDA for approval. The manufacturer must prove that the additive is not harmful to humans at expected consumption.

Two categories of food additives are not subject to the testing and approval procedure: *prior sanctioned* and *GRAS* (generally recognized as safe) substances. The FDA before the 1958 Food Additives Amendment approved substances appointed as prior sanctioned. GRAS additives are those that have been used extensively in the past with no known harmful effects and are thought to be safe. Substances on the GRAS list have been under review since 1969 and include sugar, salt, and vinegar.

Intentional Use

Additives are intentionally added directly to food during processing for four reasons:

1. To maintain or enhance a food's nutritional value. Vitamins, minerals, and fiber are examples.
2. To maintain a food's quality. Many additives are used to prevent the growth of microorganisms and extend a product's shelf-life. Some additives, called antioxidants, are used to prevent fats in food from deteriorating. Selected antioxidants may be effective in delaying proliferation of some cancers—mainly those related to fat metabolism, such as breast and prostate cancer.
3. To assist in processing, transporting, or holding a food. One additive that helps facilitate the processing of food is an **emulsifier,** to evenly distribute the molecules of two liquids that normally do not mix. Mayonnaise is an example of an emulsified product. Baking soda and baking powder are other commonly used additives. These substances cause such products as cakes to rise and improve their texture and volume.
4. To improve the way a food tastes, looks, or smells. Artificial colors, flavors, and sweeteners all fall into this category.

Types of common food additives are listed in Table 13-2.

TABLE 13-2   Common Food Additives

ADDITIVE	PURPOSE	INGREDIENT
Acidity control agents	Influence flavor, texture, and shelf life	Sodium bicarbonate Citric acid Hydrogen chloride Sodium hydroxide Acetic acid Phosphoric acid Calcium oxide
Antioxidants	Prevent discoloration Protect fats from rancidity	Vitamin C Vitamin E Butylated hydroxytoluene (BHT) and butylated hydroxyanisole (BHA)
Flavors	Food enhancers	Hydrolyzed vegetable protein Black pepper Mustard Monosodium glutamate
Leavening agents	To make dough rise	Sodium acid phosphate Sodium aluminum phosphate Monocalcium phosphate Yeast
Preservatives	To extend shelf life	Sulfur oxide Benzoic acid Propionic acid Ethylenediaminetetraacetate (EDTA) Sodium caseinate Sodium nitrate and sodium nitrite
Stabilizers and thickeners	To enhance texture	Gum arabic Modified starch Pectin

Accidental Use

Some additives enter the food supply accidentally. For example, chemicals may enter food through contact with surfaces that have been cleaned with chemical solutions.

The Food Label

On May 20, 2016, the FDA announced the new Nutrition Facts label, requiring compliance in labeling of foods for July 26, 2018. On June 13, 2017, the FDA announced an extension to allow for additional time for implementation, without providing a new date. The new label is shown in Figure 2-2 and is being implemented to give consumers better information regarding the foods they eat. Changes include increasing the type size for calories, servings per container, and serving size. The number of calories and serving size declaration are highlighted. Serving sizes are being changed to reflect what consumers typically ingest (e.g., a 20-ounce carbonated beverage would be counted as 1 serving, whereas previously 8 ounces was considered as 1 serving). The label reflects updated information about nutrition science regarding nutrients, added sugars (e.g., if orange juice has sugar added, there are values for total and added sugars) to match the *2015–2020 Dietary Guidelines for Americans.* Figure 13-4 provides information on the changes to the new Nutrition Facts panel. The following list describes a food label's contents.

1. *Standardized Format:* Every label has the same layout and design; the nutrition information is titled "Nutrition Facts."

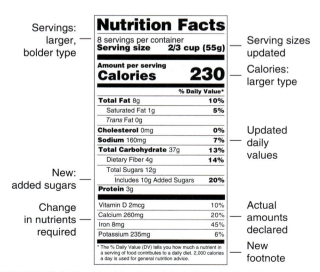

New Label/What's Different

FIGURE 13-4 New Nutrition Facts Label. *(From Food and Drug Administration: Changes to the Nutrition Facts Label. June 2017. Accessed June 2017. Available at www.fda.gov/Food/GuidanceRegulation/Guidance DocumentsRegulatoryInformation/LabelingNutrition/ucm385663.htm.)*

2. *Serving Sizes:* All serving sizes listed on similar products are stated in consistently used household and metric measures to allow comparison shopping.

3. *Daily Values:* Daily values for sodium, fiber, and vitamin D are being updated based on newer scientific evidence. Daily values are reference amounts of nutrients to consume or not to exceed and are used to calculate the percent daily value.

4. *% Daily Values:* The figures for percentage of daily values are based on a 2,000-kilocalorie diet; this schema makes it easier for consumers to judge the nutritional quality of a food.

5. *Health Claims:* A **health claim** describes the relationship between a food or food component and a disease or health-related condition. Food manufacturers are allowed to write health claims on food labels. The FDA has provided guidance (FDA, 2015). For example, if making a claim about sodium and hypertension, the wording should be, "Diets low in sodium may reduce the risk of high blood pressure, a disease associated with many factors."

6. *A Structure/Function Claim:* A **structure/function claim** describes the role of a nutrient or dietary ingredient intended to affect the structure or function in humans or characterizes the documented mechanism by which a nutrient or dietary ingredient acts to maintain such structure or function, for example, "helps promote a healthy heart" or "helps support the immune system."

7. *Descriptors:* Terms such as *low, high,* and *free* used on food labels must meet legal definitions: For example:

Free means less than 0.5 gram of fat per serving and tiny or insignificant amounts of cholesterol, sodium, and sugar.

Low indicates 3 grams of fat or less per serving; also low in saturated fat, cholesterol, and/or kilocalories.

Lean signifies less than 10 grams of fat, 4 grams of saturated fat, and 95 milligrams of cholesterol per serving. (*Lean* is higher in fat than *Low.*)

Extra Lean means 5 grams of fat, 2 grams of saturated fat, and 95 milligrams of cholesterol per serving. (*Extra Lean* is lower in fat than *Lean* but not as low in fat as *Low.*)

Light (Lite) denotes one-third fewer kilocalories or one-half the fat of the original or no more than one-half the sodium of the higher-sodium version.

Cholesterol Free means that the item has less than 2 milligrams of cholesterol and 2 grams (or less) of saturated fat per serving.

High in a nutrient means that the food must contain 20% or more of the Daily Value for that nutrient.

Good Source Of denotes that one serving of a food is considered to be a good source of a vitamin, mineral, or fiber, containing 10% to 19% of the Daily Value for that particular vitamin, mineral, or fiber.

8. Ingredients are listed in descending order by weight. The ingredients list is required on almost all foods, even some standardized ones such as ice cream, mayonnaise, and bread.

KEYSTONES

- The U.S. food supply is as safe, wholesome, and nutritious as any in the world, but there are no guarantees that all food purchased and eaten in the country is safe.

- Thousands of substances besides nutrients are present in foods. Most of these substances are harmless in the amounts typically eaten if the food item is selected, stored, and prepared under recommended conditions.

- The CDC ranks the norovirus as causing the most foodborne illness, followed by pathogenic (disease-causing) bacterial microorganisms.

- Good food-handling methods can control most viral and microbiologic hazards.

- Selecting a wide variety of foods, storing the foods appropriately, and preparing foods correctly all help prevent illness.

- Health-care workers should teach their clients about the use of food labels and the risks of microbiologic and residual chemical hazards of foods.

CASE STUDY 13-1

Ms. N is a 95-year-old woman who is 5 ft tall and weighs 122 lb (dressed without shoes). She has just been admitted to the nursing home. During the routine nursing admission process, Ms. N requested eggnog every night at 8:00 p.m. She stated that she dislikes packaged mixes and would prefer her eggnog made with whole milk, ice cream, and a raw egg. Ms. N's physician has ordered eggnog at HS (Latin for hour of sleep, or just before bedtime) every day. Ms. N stated that she has had a homemade eggnog every night for the past 50 years. The client's daughter has stated that she makes her mother eggnog from raw eggs.

CARE PLAN

Subjective Data

Client stated that she drinks eggnog made with a raw egg each day. ■ Client's daughter stated that she makes her mother such a beverage.

Objective Data

Height: 5 ft 0 in. ■ Weight: admitting 122 lb ■ Age: 95

Analysis

Increased risk of infection related to consumption of raw eggs and client's advanced age.

Plan

DESIRED OUTCOMES EVALUATION CRITERIA	ACTIONS/INTERVENTIONS	RATIONALE
The client will state that raw eggs can make one ill.	Provide verbal and written information to the client and the client's daughter on the relationship between food illness and *Salmonella* infections.	Elderly clients are particularly at risk for salmonellosis.
	Have the client and the client's daughter state that raw eggs are hazardous.	Verbal recognition of a hazard is the first step in behavioral change.
The client will accept and eat another item for her evening snack.	Request that the dietitian provide client with a list of other alternatives for her evening snack and evaluate whether client needs the snack.	Do not offer client an item that is not available from the Food and Nutrition Department.
		The client may need the nutrients in the evening snack.
	Chart acceptance or rejection of the snack.	Refusal to eat substitute snack defeats the purpose of sending the snack.

TEAMWORK 13-1

DIETITIAN'S NOTES

The following Dietitian's Notes are representative of the documentation found in a client's medical record.

Subjective: Spoke with client and her daughter. The risk of Salmonella foodborne disease with the consumption of raw eggs in an older adult was explained to the client and her daughter. A 24-hour dietary recall cross-checked with a food frequency was completed. Client has been eating three times per day, accepts all major food groups, and denies food allergies. Usual intake consists of 6 ounces of protein, 5 servings of starches (3 whole grain), 3 servings of vegetables (including a source of vitamin A), 3 servings of fruit (including a source of vitamin C), and 6 servings of fat. Claims good dentition; denies nausea and vomiting (N/V), constipation, diarrhea.

Objective: Body mass index 23; height 5 ft 0 in.; weight 122 lb; no visual signs of edema or muscle wasting.

Analysis: Usual intake about 1,400 to 1,450 kcal with 67 grams of protein. No evidence of nutritional risk based upon visual observation, diet history, and anthropometrics.

Estimated kilocalorie needs based on maximum ideal body weight (IBW) of 110 lb or 50 kg and 25–35 kcal/kg max equals 1,250–1,750 kcal.

Estimated protein need based on 50 kg and 0.8–1.2 g/kg equals 40–60 grams of protein per day.

Estimated kilocalories in homemade eggnog equals 275 kcal.

After explaining risk with the consumption of raw eggs, client agreed to have one cup of hot cocoa and a banana for her evening snack because she would need the kilocalories from these items to meet her estimated kilocalorie needs. Client's protein intake more than exceeds estimated requirements.

Plan:
1. *Follow-up in 3 days.*
2. *Order evening snack as described above.*

CRITICAL THINKING QUESTIONS

1. What other areas of the home might you inspect to minimize the risk of a foodborne illness?

2. What clients need to take extra precautions to prevent a foodborne illness?

3. Do you think that it is within the scope of practice for a nurse when making a home visit to discuss unsafe food practices?

CHAPTER REVIEW

1. Cold foods should be stored:
   1. At less than 50°F (10°C)
   2. At less than 0°F (−17.8°C)
   3. At less than 40°F (4.4°C)
   4. For no more than 6 hours outside the recommended temperature range.

2. The term *low* on a food label means the product contains:
   1. Less than 3 grams of fat per serving; also low in saturated fat, cholesterol, or kilocalories
   2. Less fat than the original
   3. Less than 10 grams of fat, 4 grams of saturated fat, and 95 milligrams of cholesterol per serving
   4. More fat than a product labeled *extra lean*.

3. Foods commonly contaminated with *Campylobacter* are:
   1. Hard-cooked scrambled eggs
   2. Raw vegetables
   3. Canned foods
   4. Raw poultry

4. The best method to control the spread of foodborne illness is by:
   1. Wearing gloves when handling food
   2. Proper hand washing
   3. Taking food supplements
   4. Avoiding certain foods

5. Farm-raised seafood must be labeled with
   1. Country of origin
   2. Grams of mercury
   3. Kilocalories in one serving
   4. Grams of protein

6. Nutrition Facts will include all except the following: (Select all that apply.)
   1. Total sugars
   2. Added sugars
   3. Potassium
   4. Vitamin A
   5. Sodium

CLINICAL ANALYSIS

1. Mr. P has brought his 35-year-old husband, who has a history of AIDS, to the ambulatory care clinic for treatment for a sudden onset of headache, abdominal pain, diarrhea, nausea, and vomiting. The nurse should:
   a. Document all food consumed during the past 7 days.
   b. Inquire about food practices in the home.
   c. Inspect Mr. P's passport for foreign travel in the past month.
   d. Document the client's immunization status.

2. You are on a committee to help plan the annual hospital picnic. One employee volunteers to make Texas-style chili at home and serve it at the picnic. You have a responsibility to:
   a. Inquire how the chili will be made, transported, and held at recommended temperatures.
   b. Taste the chili on arrival at the picnic for safety.
   c. Check the temperature of the chili on arrival at the picnic.
   d. Review the recipe for the potential use of unsafe ingredients.

3. Mr. J is an 85-year-old man recently discharged from the hospital for a partial bowel obstruction that he had surgically repaired. His wife is getting ready to serve him eggnog made with raw eggs. What would be the most effective way to determine if the client consumed any contaminated food?
   a. Ignore the situation because that is not the purpose of the visit.
   b. Inquire about any gastrointestinal pain Mr. J may have had.
   c. Instruct the wife about the safe preparation of eggs.
   d. Assess the amount of sugar used in the beverage.

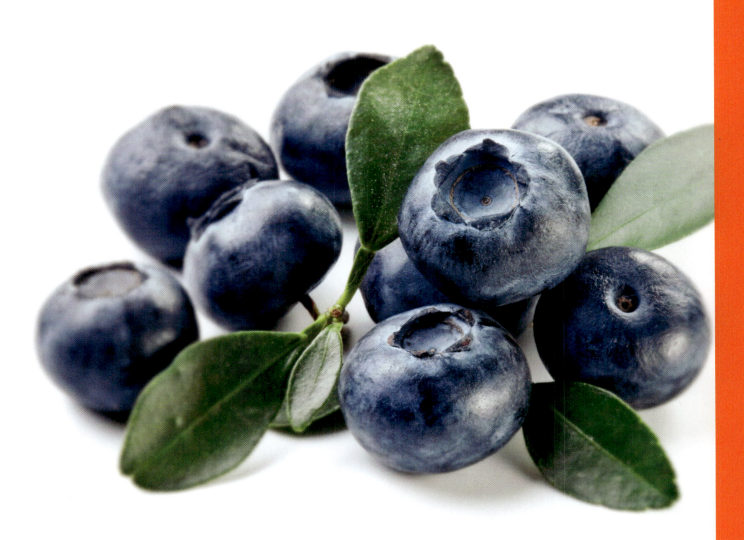

Clinical Nutrition

CHAPTER 14

Nutrient Delivery

LEARNING OBJECTIVES

After completing this chapter, the student should be able to:

- Identify three routes used to deliver nutrients to clients and potential complications with two of these routes.
- Discuss the kinds of commercial formulas available for oral and enteral feedings.
- Discuss why it is important to carefully control the rate of delivery and volume of enteral formula delivered to a client.

- List the reasons for the high incidence of malnutrition in institutionalized clients and the interventions nurses can perform to combat malnutrition.
- Describe suggested procedures for administering medications through feeding tubes.

This chapter introduces the methods commonly used to deliver nutrients to clients: oral, enteral nutrition (EN) via feeding tube, and parenteral nutrition (PN). The major functions of dietetic services in health-care facilities are the preparation and delivery of nutrients via food and supplements and the clinical nutritional care of clients. The nutritional care of clients includes four areas:

1. Assessing the client's need for nutrients
2. Determining the best method for delivering nutrients to the client
3. Monitoring the client's nutrient intake
4. Counseling the client about nutritional needs

High-quality nutritional care helps prevent illness and disease and saves the client's and society's health-care dollars.

Food Service in Institutions

All members of the health-care team need to become familiar with some aspects of the food service in their place of employment. The scheduling of diagnostic procedures, blood work, surgery, and administration of medications is dependent on when the client last consumed food.

Meal Service Patterns

Many institutions serve three meals to clients each day as well as several between-meal feedings. Feedings between meals are available for clients in need of extra nutrients, those who desire extra food, or those who are unable to consume sufficient kilocalories at regular mealtimes. Some institutions offer a room service system, and clients may order food whenever they desire. Specific procedures are necessary to ensure that the provision of medical care is coordinated with meal delivery.

Nutritional Care Services

Institutions vary in the types of nutritional services they offer clients. A large teaching hospital or medical center frequently has nutrition professionals on staff who specialize in treating particular types of clients. A critical care dietitian, for example, has special training to assess, plan, implement, and counsel clients in high-risk stages of trauma, disease, and conditions that affect nutritional support. In such settings, other health-care workers can rely on the critical care dietitian to provide technical support.

At the other end of the spectrum, in a small community hospital or a long-term care facility, a dietitian may be present only part time or as a consultant. In such circumstances, other health-care workers must plan to make the best use of the dietitian's services when he or she is available. In this situation, the nursing staff assumes more responsibility for the nutritional care of clients.

Home- and community-based programs also provide nutritional care services. For example, hospice, home-care programs, and some governmental agencies deliver nutritional care services. Frequently, a dietitian is available through any of these programs for consultation. Third-party payers increasingly cover medical nutritional care, referred to as *medical nutrition therapy* (MNT).

Screening, Assessment, Monitoring, and Counseling

Nutritional care is a responsibility of many health-care team members. The nurse is usually the first team member to interview and assess the client, often before the physician visits the client. The physician and/or physician assistant complete a physical examination of the client, order necessary treatments and diagnostic procedures, and provide either a diagnosis or tentative diagnosis. The diagnosis may change after the diagnostic tests are completed. The nurse, physician, or the physician assistant usually makes referrals to other team members. Institutions frequently require specific team members to assess each client. Figure 14-1 presents an overview of a nutrient-delivery decision-making tree.

Screening

The Joint Commission, which provides accreditation of health-care organizations and programs, requires that a nutritional screening is completed by established criteria

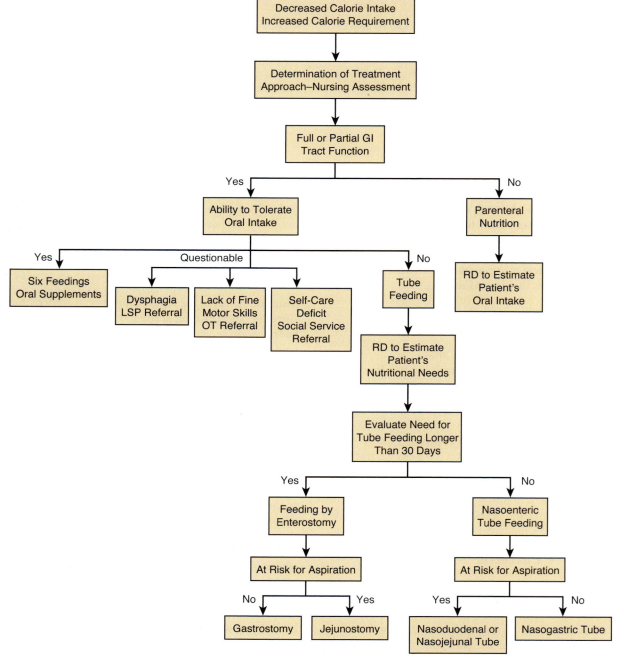

FIGURE 14-1 Nutrient delivery decision-making tree. OT, occupational therapist; RD, registered dietitian; LSP, licensed speech pathologist. *(From Abbott Nutrition Pocket Guide, 2010. © 2011 Abbott Laboratories. Used with permission.)*

within the institution based on the client's needs and conditions, but normally within 24 hours of admission to an acute care facility (The Joint Commission, 2017). The recommendation for critically ill clients admitted to the intensive care unit (ICU) is for immediate nutritional assessment (McClave et al, 2016). A health technician or nurse may use a series of questions, often in the form of a predetermined screening tool, which rates a client's potential nutritional risk. Changes in weight, appetite, or presence of nausea, vomiting, **dysphagia** (difficulty swallowing), and/or disease state (such as diabetes, obesity, hypertension, cancer, etc.) are reviewed. If a client has a positive screen in these areas or there are changes noted, a client may be determined to be at risk nutritionally.

Assessment

Clients found to be at a nutritional risk need to have a complete nutritional assessment by a registered dietitian (RD), which may include the following items:

- Height, weight, body mass index (BMI), and weight history
- Laboratory test values
- Food intake information
- Potential food–drug interactions
- Mastication and swallowing ability
- Client's ability to feed himself or herself
- Bowel and bladder function
- Evaluation for the presence of **pressure injury**
- Food allergies and intolerances
- Any other factors affecting nutritional status, such as food preferences and cultural and religious beliefs about food
- Determination of body composition, including results of a Nutrition Focused Physical Exam, to determine muscle strength and sarcopenia
- Presence of severe burns, trauma, infection, edema, or other physiological stressors that increase nutrient needs and are likely to prolong hospital stay
- Learning barriers such as hearing, mobility, language, need for interpreter, vision, speech, reading/writing skills, inability to follow instructions, cultural and religious barriers, learning disability, learning readiness (requests, accepts, or avoids information), and preferred learning style

The American Society for Parenteral and Enteral Nutrition's (ASPEN) most current Clinical Guidelines for Nutrition Screening, Assessment, and Intervention in Adults defines nutrition assessment as a comprehensive approach to diagnosing nutritional problems that uses medical, nutrition, and medication histories; physical examination; anthropometric measurements; and laboratory data. In addition, "an acute, subacute or chronic state of nutrition, in which varying degrees of overnutrition or undernutrition with or without inflammatory activity have led to a change in body composition and diminished function" is defined as malnutrition (Mueller, Compher, & Druyan, 2011). In this context, nutrition assessment is much more than an initial client screening,

as completed by nursing personnel. A comprehensive nutritional assessment requires data from physical examinations, tests, lab work, and client intake information to be analyzed by the dietitian to determine a nutritional diagnosis and plan of care.

Computer technology and the electronic medical record have greatly facilitated the client assessment process. Information may group clients, such as all those with nutrition-related diagnoses (i.e., diabetes), on specific medications, with low weight for height, and on NPO (nothing by mouth) or on inadequate diets for longer than 3 days, for example. The consolidation of this information allows for a greater number of clients to be identified and targeted for in-depth nutritional assessment and care.

Client care has also become standardized as a result of computer programs and the development of standards of practice. For example, a health-care organization may require clients with a BMI of <18.5 be evaluated by a registered dietitian within 24 hours of admission. A licensed speech pathologist may be required to evaluate all clients with dysphasia before the client is given any food or fluids. A registered nurse may be required to phone a physician immediately on receipt of data showing a potassium level greater than 5.0 mEq/L and document the phone call. The occupational therapist may be required to evaluate clients who are unable to feed themselves.

Regulatory agencies of long-term care facilities require that clients have a nutritional assessment performed by a registered dietitian shortly after admission. An initial assessment or screening identifies clients at nutritional risk. An in-depth assessment as defined by ASPEN requires a care plan by several team members who coordinate services (Mueller, Compher, & Druyan, 2011).

Monitoring

All clients should be reassessed or monitored at appropriate intervals. Most organizations include the required frequency of client monitoring in their standards of practice. Some clients in hospital ICUs require continuous monitoring. Other clients require daily, weekly, monthly, or quarterly reassessment as determined by preset guidelines.

The **client care conference** (interdisciplinary conference) is a productive means of monitoring clients. Before the conference, health-care workers gather information, which impacts the client's nutritional care, including:

- Initial nutritional screen and/or assessment
- Present body weight and weight history
- A record of recent food intake and/or tolerance
- Any changes in medical condition, including diagnoses and test results
- Diet order
- Family support (or lack of)

With this information, health-care workers can more readily determine the reason for most changes in the client's nutritional status. If weight loss is identified, a review of the client's **food acceptance record,** if available, may verify whether such a weight loss is likely a result of poor food intake.

Clients whom health-care providers have determined to be at nutritional risk because of poor food intake should be treated. Treatment may include a nutritional supplement, between-meal feedings, a change in the diet prescription, or a change in feeding status. If, for example, a client can no longer feed himself or herself, the client's feeding status would need to be changed from self-feed to assisted feeding. Many clients require aggressive nutritional treatment that may include EN through a feeding tube, inserted either surgically or nasally, and/or PN. Monitoring the client's weight, laboratory values, and food intake is an important part of delivering high-quality nutritional care.

Counseling

All clients should be evaluated for nutritional counseling. The assumption that a client is not expected to be discharged and therefore is not entitled to education is unjustifiable. Educating the client about nutritional concerns helps the client assume responsibility for his or her own care, thus promoting self-esteem and a sense of worth.

Diet Manuals

Current accreditation standards (both long-term and acute care) require all health-care institutions to have a diet manual available to all team members. Electronic manuals are often used and may be available on an organization's computer system. The diet manual defines and describes all diets used as part of nutritional therapy for clients.

Diet Orders

The physician or designee is responsible for prescribing a diet for the client. Just as a medication cannot be administered to a client without a medication prescription, food or fluids cannot be served to a client without a physician's written diet order.

One of the functions of the diet manual is to define a diet. The diet manual is the first place to look when clients request food items not being served. The diet manual may state, for example, that the food item is restricted or not allowed on the client's prescribed diet.

Special Diets

The purpose of a special or modified diet is to restore or maintain a client's nutritional status by manipulating one or more of the following dietary aspects:

- Nutrients such as protein, calcium, iron, sodium, potassium, and vitamin K may be increased, decreased, or held at a consistent level.
- Kilocalories may be either restricted or increased.
- Texture or consistency of foods may be modified. For example, if a client has dysphagia a minced and moist diet with prethickened liquids may be ordered.
- Fiber may be restricted or increased depending on a client's gastrointestinal (GI) function.
- Fluid may be pushed in the case of dehydration or limited for renal or cardiac diseases.

All modified diets are variations of the general diet; the client nonetheless needs all the essential nutrients. For this reason, each modified diet must be carefully planned to provide each of the essential nutrients or a documented reason for not providing one or more essential nutrients. Physicians determine (normally after recommended by a dietitian) when a specific diet order is medically indicated for a client.

Common Diet Orders

Some common diet orders are for *clear liquid, full liquid, soft,* and *general* or *regular*. A clear-liquid diet is any transparent liquid that can be poured at room temperature. Gelatin, some juices, broth, tea, frozen ices, and coffee are clear liquids. A clear-liquid diet is nutritionally inadequate and normally limited in duration. Clear-liquid nutritional supplements, however, are available.

A full-liquid diet is any liquid that can be poured at room temperature. Milk, custard, all fruit juices, ice cream, strained soups, and all items allowed on the clear-liquid diet are allowed on most full-liquid diets. The major difference between a clear-liquid and a full-liquid diet is that the latter contains milk and milk products (Table 14-1 and Boxes 14-1 and 14-2).

Soft diets vary greatly from one facility to another. For example, a soft, minced, or pureed diet is ordered when the client has only a few or no teeth (edentulous). A soft diet is ordered after surgery when easily digested foods are required.

TABLE 14-1   Composition of Liquid Diets

DIET	PROTEIN (GRAMS)	FAT (GRAMS)	CARBOHYDRATE (GRAMS)	SODIUM (MEQ)	POTASSIUM (MEQ)	KILOCALORIES
Clear liquid	5	Trace	70–95	65	20	375
Clear liquid with three 10-oz servings of Ensure Clear	32	Trace	175–200	215	23.46	915
Full liquid	50	55	205	110	65	1,500

BOX 14-1 ■ Clear-Liquid Diet

Description

The clear-liquid diet provides energy and fluid in a form that requires minimal digestive action.

Indications

The clear-liquid diet is prescribed when it is necessary to limit undigested food in the GI tract and before bowel surgery, diagnostic imaging procedures, and colonoscopic examination. A clear-liquid diet is also used during acute stages of illness to assist with fluid and electrolyte replacement and as a first step in oral alimentation after intravenous feeding, surgery, and GI disturbances.

Adequacy

This diet is inadequate in all nutrients and should be used only in the short-term.

Food Allowed	Foods to Avoid
Coffee and tea	All other food and beverages
Carbonated beverages such as 7UP® and ginger ale	

Fruit-flavored gelatin, Italian ices, and popsicles

Apple, grape, or cranberry juice

Clear fat-free broth and bouillon

Sugar

Recommended to Enhance Nutrition

Nutritional supplement such as Ensure Clear® (Abbott)*
High-protein broth and gelatin desserts are also available.

*Clear-liquid nutritional supplement if client is on this diet for longer than two meals.

BOX 14-2 ■ Full-Liquid Diet

Description

The full-liquid diet provides foods and beverages that are liquid or may become liquid at body temperature.

Indications

This diet is used as a progression between clear liquids and a soft diet and after oral surgery. Acutely ill clients with a chewing or swallowing dysfunction and clients with oral, esophageal, or stomach disorders who are unable to tolerate solid foods because of strictures or other anatomical disorders find this diet useful.

Adequacy

This diet can be adequate in all nutrients according to the Recommended Dietary Allowances. Special care needs to be taken to meet folacin, iron, thiamin, niacin, vitamin A, fiber, and kilocalorie allowances.

Foods Allowed	Foods Not Allowed
Any beverage that pours at room temperature	All others
	Breads, cereals, and grains

All fruit juices — Fruits

Any vegetable juice — Vegetables

Milk — Meats

Butter, margarine, cream, and oils

Custard, ice cream, flavored with gelatin, sherbet, sugar, and popsicles — All others and any made of coconut, nuts, or whole fruit

Special Notes

The use of a complete nutritional liquid supplement is often necessary to meet nutrient allowances for clients who follow this diet for longer than 3 days.

An oral supplement that contains fiber minimizes the potential for problems with constipation and abdominal cramping. However, liquid supplements with fiber are not indicated for all clients on full-liquid diets.

A facility that specializes in treating clients with eye, ear, nose, and throat disorders may have many types of soft diets. A pureed diet usually consists of foods that have been run through a blender or food processor to meet the consistency needs of the client. Table 14-2 lists recommended foods on a pureed, mechanical soft, and soft diet.

A general or regular diet means that the client is on an unrestricted diet. Frequently, an *as tolerated* or *progressive* diet may be prescribed, which means that a clear-liquid diet is to be served initially and the diet advanced (full-liquid to soft to general) as the client is able to tolerate. The nurse may be responsible for determining the client's tolerance for food just before tray delivery. This last-minute determination of client tolerance is necessary for many clients because of fluctuating medical status.

Diets for Diagnostic Procedures

Many diagnostic procedures requiring dietary preparation are performed in hospitals.

Poor Client Preparation

Poor dietary preparation can force a client to have an expensive procedure repeated or postponed (Fig. 14-2). Figure 14-2A is an x-ray film from a poorly prepared client. Feces in the colon block the view of structures within the colon. Figure 14-2B shows the colon of a well-prepared client. In the absence of fecal material, the entire length of the colon can be visualized.

Some x-ray procedures are not only expensive but also uncomfortable. The client must have the procedure repeated if

TABLE 14-2   Consistency Modifications—Recommended Foods

FOOD GROUP	PUREED DIET	MINCED (4 MM) & MOIST DIET	SOFT & BITE-SIZED (1.5 CM) DIET
Soups	Broth, bouillon, strained or blenderized cream soup	Broth, bouillon, strained or blenderized cream soup	Broth, bouillon, cream soup
Beverages	All	All	All
Meat	Strained or pureed meat or poultry, cheese used in cooking	Finely minced, moist meats, or poultry, mashed fish, eggs, cottage cheese	Moist, tender meat, fish, or poultry, eggs, cottage cheese, mild flavored cheese, creamy peanut butter, soft casseroles
Fat	Butter, margarine, cream, oil, gravy	Butter, margarine, cream, oil, gravy, salad dressing	Butter, margarine, cream, oil, gravy, avocado, salad dressing
Milk	Milk, milk beverages, yogurt without fruit, nuts, or seeds, cocoa	Milk, milk beverages, yogurt without seeds or nuts, cocoa	Milk, milk beverages, yogurt without seeds or nuts, cocoa
Starch	Cooked, refined cereal, mashed potatoes	Cooked or refined ready-to-eat cereal, potatoes, pasta, pregelled "soaked" breads	Cooked or ready-to-eat cereal, potatoes, rice, pasta, pregelled "soaked" breads
Vegetables	Strained or pureed, juice	Finely minced, chopped or mashed cooked, without hulls or tough skin (e.g., peas and corn), juice	Soft, steamed, or boiled vegetables
Fruit	Strained or pureed, juice	Cooked or canned mashed fruit without seeds or skins, banana, juice	Cooked or canned fruit, banana, citrus fruit without membrane, juice
Desserts	Gelatin, sherbet, ice cream without nuts or fruit, custard, pudding, fruit ice, popsicle	Gelatin, sherbet, ice cream without nuts or fruit, custard, pudding, fruit ice, popsicle	Gelatin, sherbet, ice cream without nuts, custard, pudding, cake, fruit ice, popsicle
Sweets	Sugar, honey, jelly, candy, flavorings	Sugar, honey, jelly, candy, flavorings	Sugar, honey, jelly, candy, flavorings
Miscellaneous	Seasonings, condiments	Seasonings, condiments	Seasonings, condiments

Based on international dysphagia diet (http://iddsi.org/).

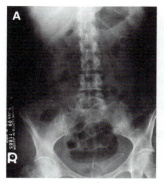 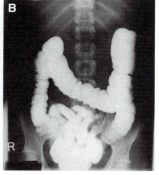

FIGURE 14-2 *A,* Image of a client who was poorly prepared for a barium enema. *B,* Image of a client who was adequately prepared for a barium enema. *(Courtesy Dr. Russell Tobe.)*

necessary bodily structures cannot be visualized. Although the specific dietary preparation for x-ray studies of the colon may vary from one facility to another, dietary preparation is usually somewhat similar. The client may be instructed not to eat or drink anything after midnight on the day of the imaging study. In addition, the client may need to follow a clear-liquid diet for 12 to 48 hours before the x-ray procedure.

Many clients undergo x-ray studies as outpatients. The nurse or medical assistant working in a physician's office is usually responsible for dietary instruction before these procedures.

Misdiagnosis

Poor dietary preparation can lead to a misdiagnosis. For example, a blood sample for a fasting blood glucose (FBS) test should be drawn on a **fasting** individual, that is, one who has not had any food or beverages (with the exception of sips of water) by mouth for at least 8 hours before the blood draw. If the client eats before the procedure, his or her blood glucose level may be elevated, and this elevation may cause a misdiagnosis of diabetes. A misdiagnosis may cause a client unnecessary anxiety, medical treatment, and expense.

Importance of Nutritional Care

Malnutrition associated with acute and chronic disease is common in hospital settings. **Acute** means that the illness has a rapid onset, severe symptoms, and a short course. **Chronic** means that the illness has a long duration.

The presence and importance of malnutrition has been increasingly recognized throughout the world. Malnutrition is one of the most common conditions affecting the care of hospitalized clients. The prevalence of adult malnutrition is estimated to be up to 50% of hospitalized individuals. Malnutrition is associated with a longer length of stay, a higher cost of hospitalization, increased risk for readmission, and increased mortality (Boullata et al, 2016). Malnutrition is associated with a 25% morbidity and a 5% mortality. **Morbidity** is defined as the rate of being diseased. **Mortality** is defined as the death rate. A malnourished client is more likely to be sicker and run a higher risk of death than a well-nourished client with the same diagnosis. Because malnutrition affects morbidity and mortality, it is also associated with a prolonged hospital stay.

Iatrogenic Malnutrition

The term **iatrogenic malnutrition** was first used in 1974 and refers to physician- or institution-induced malnutrition (Butterworth & Blackburn, 1975). Routine hospital practices such as extended periods of food or nutrient deprivation because of treatments, as well as diagnostic tests that interfere with the client's meal schedule or that cause a lack of appetite, are related to the high prevalence of malnutrition. Drug therapy may also affect a client's appetite. Some drugs cause drowsiness, lethargy, nausea, and anorexia. Problems related directly to an illness, such as pain, unconsciousness, paralysis, vomiting, and diarrhea, can also interfere with eating.

Today many institutions have written policies and procedures for clinicians to follow to minimize the likelihood of iatrogenic malnutrition. The tasks that clinical team members should perform to combat institutional malnutrition are discussed in Clinical Application 14-1.

Methods of Nutrient Delivery

Nutrients can be delivered to the client orally in foods or supplements, enterally by feeding tube, or parenterally through veins. **Enteral nutrition** means the feeding of an appropriate formula or liquid via a tube to a client's GI tract. **Parenteral nutrition** designates that nutrients are being provided via an intravenous route.

Figure 14-3 shows two feeding pumps. The feeding pumps are set to deliver a given rate, volume, and amount of both enteral and parenteral feedings to a client. The importance of connecting the enteral feeding to the tube that leads to the client's GI tract and connecting the intravenous solution to the tube that leads directly into the blood stream cannot be overemphasized. Although this is primarily a nursing responsibility, all trained team members should make a habit of checking tube connections every time a client with two feeding routes is visited. The placement of a feeding tube into the wrong lead is called a misconnection.

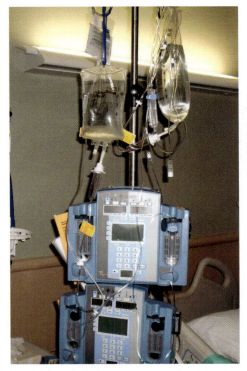

FIGURE 14-3 These two feeding pumps are set to deliver both a tube feeding and parenteral nutrition simultaneously. The client also has lines running for medications. Note how confusing it is to place the lines.

Oral Delivery

Most institutionalized clients are fed orally. Whenever possible, the client should be encouraged to eat foods, because this is an optimal way for the client not only to obtain nutrients but also to experience the normal psychological and physical pleasure associated with eating.

The Menu

An institution's menu can be selective or nonselective. A selective menu is similar to a restaurant menu; clients can choose the specific menu items that appeal to them. Clients eat best when they fill out their own menus or a significant other does so for them. Marking the menu is one way in which a client can participate daily in care planning.

When an institution does not have a selective menu, one kind of meal is prepared and served to all clients. Food and labor required for providing a selective menu is more expensive than for institutions providing a nonselective menu. However, many clients may fail to eat the food from a nonselective menu because they dislike the menu item provided.

Eating Environment

Health-care workers need to create as pleasant an environment as possible immediately before and during mealtime. The room should be checked for objectionable odors, sounds, and sights. Obviously, a full bedside commode or an emesis basin nearby discourages eating. In addition, the client should be prepared to eat when the tray arrives. Cleaning the client's hands and face helps the client become more enthusiastic about eating. The client's bedside table should be cleared of all miscellaneous items, and unnecessary delays in serving the tray should be avoided. The client should be properly positioned to eat. This includes elevating the head of the bed (if his or her condition permits) and positioning the bedside table to the correct height. Assistance with opening food packages or cartons may be required.

Some clients may find the odor of food offensive. For these clients, it is best for the nurse not to uncover the food items directly in front of them, minimizing the risk of nausea. For these individuals, often oncology clients, open food trays in the hallway, or away from the client, to help dissipate the intense odors of hot foods.

Assisted Feeding Versus Self-Feeding

Some clients must be fed. Food should be offered in bite-sized portions and in the order that the client prefers. Clients should not be rushed. Talking with clients while feeding makes mealtime pleasant and signals that they are not being rushed. Personnel are encouraged to sit while feeding clients because this indicates a willingness to spend time with them and encourages relaxation.

Some nursing personnel have found that they can enhance a client's food intake by mimicking normal eating behavior:

- Sit behind the client.
- Place your right arm over the client's arm (if you and the client are right-handed).
- Place a fork or spoon with food in either the client's hand or your own hand (depending on the client's ability to do this maneuver).
- Guide the client's hand to his or her mouth.

In a long-term care facility, a client's ability to feed himself or herself should be reevaluated at regular intervals. Safe feeding temperatures of hot foods should be determined in conjunction with kitchen staff by conducting timed temperature studies of test plates and trays of food, never by touching the food directly.

Assisting the Disabled Client

A client with a disability may require either total or partial assistance with eating. Partial assistance may include opening milk cartons and plastic bags containing condiments and eating utensils, buttering bread, and cutting meat. Visually impaired clients may be able to feed themselves when they know where the food is on the plate. The usual technique is to describe food placement in terms of hours on a clock face.

Some clients can feed themselves but may be slow, clumsy, and messy. A large napkin under the chin may assist in cleanup. Offering hot beverages in small amounts may minimize the likelihood of an accident.

Sometimes the consistency or form of a food may influence whether clients can feed themselves. A thin liquid, for example, may cause some clients to choke. A thicker substance such as yogurt may be better tolerated. Some disabled people are able to manage finger foods such as French fries or hard-cooked eggs. Health-care personnel can learn the food tolerances and preferences of disabled clients by asking or observing. The physician should be notified if a client appears to be choking or coughing while being fed. A licensed speech pathologist (LSP) can be invaluable in determining the optimal solid food and liquid consistency to minimize the risk of aspiration.

Health-care workers should evaluate clients who cannot feed themselves and encourage them to remain as independent as possible in all the activities of daily living, including eating. Some clients' inability to feed themselves may be related to neuromuscular disabilities. The occupational therapist (OT) has special training in the selection and fitting of eating devices to assist such clients.

Supplemental Feedings

Many clients are unable to consume sufficient kilocalories or nutrients because of anorexia, altered GI function, an inability to eat, or an increased need for nutrients. The first step is to offer these clients additional food at or between meals. Any between-meal feedings must adhere to the client's diet order. Closely monitoring a client's food intake, including supplemental feedings, is important. If the client will not accept supplemental feedings, another treatment approach may be needed.

Many clients accept liquid supplementation better than solids. Many debilitated clients seem to feel less full after drinking a beverage than after eating a comparable number of kilocalories and nutrients in foods. Liquid supplements can include:

- Milk
- Milk shakes
- Instant breakfast drinks
- Commercially prepared beverages

Many commercially prepared liquid formulas are available. Increasingly, potentially beneficial nutrients that may enhance immune function such as arginine, glutamine, nucleotides, antioxidants, and fish oils are added to the various formulas and are purportedly shown to reduce infection complications and hospital length of stay. Current evidence does not support these claims (Preiser et al, 2015). Enteral formulas are classified by the U.S. Food and Drug Administration (FDA) as **medical foods,** which means that they are not regulated as either a food or a drug. Although their manufacture must follow safe practices, formulas are exempt from regulations on labeling, including nutrition facts and health claims. The veracity of adult enteral formula labeling and product claims is dependent on formula vendors (Food and Drug Administration, 2016). Infant formula labeling and claims are regulated by the FDA.

Four types of supplements are used for oral and/or enteral feedings:

1. Modular supplements
2. Standard or "polymeric" formulas
3. Elemental and semielemental formulas
4. Disease-specific formulas

MODULAR SUPPLEMENTS

A **modular supplement** contains a limited number of nutrients. Polycose, for example, contains only carbohydrate. Microlipid is an example of a lipid supplement. Modular supplements for protein include Resource Beneprotein® and Pro-Mod Liquid Protein®.

Modular supplements are available in a liquid or powder form and can be added to foods, other types of oral supplements, or tube feedings. Sometimes modular supplements are readily accepted if mixed with food. For example, Beneprotein mixed with hot cereal and mashed potatoes does not change the taste of these foods and adds a significant amount of protein to a client's diet.

STANDARD OR POLYMERIC FORMULAS

A standard or **polymeric formula** is a complete formula used when the GI tract is functional and the client needs all the essential nutrients in a specified volume. Dozens of such products are on the market. A complete supplement, such as Ensure®, Boost®, Jevity®, and Nutren®, should always be used when the formula is the sole source of nutrition.

Some complete nutritional supplements are also designed for tube feedings; the consistency and flavor of a feeding designed to be tube-fed may not be acceptable to the client if fed orally.

Commercial supplements should be used only after the client's requirements for nutrients have been assessed. Excess nutrients are rarely beneficial, and consuming too much of a feeding may be medically harmful. Many organs in the human body are in a stress situation in the poorly nourished client. The client's kidneys or liver may be subjected to unnecessary stress or harm if the nutrients cannot be used efficiently due to illness or disease state (see Clinical Calculation 14-1).

ELEMENTAL AND SEMIELEMENTAL FORMULAS

Another group of oral supplements includes **elemental** and **semielemental.** Examples of such formulas include Peptamen®, Vital®, and Vivonex®. The nutrients in these formulas

CLINICAL CALCULATION 14-1

Calculating an Oral Supplement

1. Place the client on a kilocalorie count.
2. Estimate the client's kilocalorie requirement.
   - Calculate the client's ideal body weight (IBW). Females = 100 pounds for the first 5 feet and 5 pounds for each additional inch ±10%; males = 106 pounds for the first 5 feet and 6 pounds for each additional inch ±10%
   - (1) Use maximum IBW for all further calculations except those who are underweight, for whom use their actual body weight (ABW) to prevent overfeeding. (2) Use ABW for clients within their IBW range.
   - Divide the weight calculated above to obtain the client's weight in kilograms.

- Estimated energy needs for noncritical care clients are 25–35 kcal/kg; energy needs for critical care clients are 20–30 kcal/kg.
- Protein needs for noncritical care clients are 0.8–1.2 grams/kg; protein needs for critical care clients are 1.2–1.5 grams/kg.
- Fluid needs are 1 mL/kg or 30 mL/kg or as tolerated to maintain fluid status.
3. Select an appropriate oral supplement for the client. Some hospitals allow clients to taste several supplements and choose the one most palatable to them.
4. Determine the difference between the client's recorded food intake and kilocalorie allowance.
5. Determine the kilocalorie concentration of the formula. This can be done by referring to either the appropriate table in the

Continued

CLINICAL CALCULATION–cont'd   14-1

diet manual or the supplement's label. Usually formulas are between 1.0 and 2.0 kcal/mL.

6. Determine how many milliliters of formula are needed to meet the client's kilocalorie allowance.
7. Divide the total milliliters needed by the number of feedings to be offered.
8. Check to ensure that the client's protein and fluid needs are within the desired range. If not, select a different supplement.

EXAMPLE

1. Assume that the client ate 550 kcal.
2. Assume that the client is a woman who weighs 132 lb and is 5 ft 2 in. tall. Client's IBW would be 100 lb + 10 lb for her additional 2 in. = 110; ±10% = 100–120. She weighs more than her IBW, and so use her maximum IBW of 120 to compute kilocalorie needs. 120 divided by 2.2 = 54.5 kg.
3. Client's estimated need for kilocalories is 25–35 kcal/kg × 54.5 kg = 1,363–1,908 kcal.
4. Assume that the client has tasted several supplements and prefers Boost 1.0.
5. The client's estimated range for kilocalories is 1,363–1,908. The client ate 300 kcal.
   The difference is a deficit of 1,063–1,608 kcal.
6. Boost contains 280 kcal and 8 grams of protein in 240 mL.
7. The client stated that she would prefer to drink this feeding five times per day, some on each tray, and during two between-meal feedings.

8. Assume from the client's recorded food intake that her diet contains about 10 grams of protein per day. A woman weighing 54.5 kg has an estimated protein allowance of 0.8–1.2 grams/kg.
   54.5 kg × 0.8 gram/kg = 43.6 g of protein to 54.5 × 1.2 grams/kg = 65.4 grams
   Subtract the 10 grams eaten from trays
   43.6 grams – 10 grams = 33.6 grams
   The supplement should provide at least 33.6 grams of protein and no more than 65.4 grams of protein (0.8–1.2 grams/kg of maximum IBW).
9. Five cans of Boost contain 1,400 kcal and 40 grams of protein for a total of 1,200 mL.
10. Eight grams of protein × 5 cans (240 mL each) = 40 grams of protein from oral supplement + 10 g of protein from food = 50 grams.
11. Double check: food intake of 300 kcal + 10 grams of protein + 1,400 kcal from Boost + 40 grams of protein from Boost = 50 grams of protein total + 1,700 kcal total + 1,200 mL fluid total from supplement (client should be encouraged to drink at least 300 mL of water extra per day to meet her fluid needs). This information should be documented and verbally given to the nurse assigned to the client.

---

are easier to absorb because they are in their simplest form, small molecules, which require little digestion. For example, maltodextrins, corn syrup solids, oligosaccharides, and glucose polymers are rapidly hydrolyzed by maltase and oligosaccharidases, which are apt to be present in the small intestine in higher concentrations than lactase.

Protein is either partially or totally hydrolyzed. Partially hydrolyzed protein (small peptides) offer an advantage over totally hydrolyzed protein (single amino acids). Peptides and free amino acids do not inhibit each other's transport across the GI tract, and absorption of nitrogen is actually improved by the inclusion of small peptides. Easier-to-digest fats include medium-chain triglycerides. Partially hydrolyzed fats include monoglycerides and diglycerides.

Elemental and semielemental formulas contain little lactose and residue and may be given orally or enterally through a tube. These formulas are expensive and for use with clients who have limited GI function or metabolic disorders. Because elemental and semielemental formulas are less palatable than **standard feedings,** client acceptance of these as oral feedings is often a problem.

DISEASE-SPECIFIC FORMULAS

The last group of oral supplements includes special formulas designed for clients with specific metabolic problems such as diabetes, kidney, and liver disorders. These formulas are discussed in subsequent chapters.

Oral supplements are also used both in addition to or as a transition from enteral and parenteral feedings. When a client has ceased to consume foods orally for a time, a transition period is always necessary to reacclimate to oral feedings. This process can sometimes take a couple of days to months.

Enteral Tube Feeding

Tube feedings are the second way nutrients can be delivered to clients. EN is the delivery of a formula (which includes breast milk for infants) into a functioning GI tract through a tube. This feeding route should only be considered if the functioning GI tract is sufficient in length for adequate absorption and there is an inability for the client to consume nutrients, either totally or in part, orally. With some medical conditions, oral feeding is impossible, insufficient, or impractical. Several common conditions in which a tube feeding is indicated are listed in Table 14-3.

Tube feeding formulas are commercially prepared to reduce the incidence of contamination. Many medical centers use closed systems for tube feedings in which commercially prepared bags or containers of formula are ready to be hung and fed to clients. Open systems of feeding, if prepared in an aseptic manner, may be done safely in medical centers or at home by clients. Open systems require the filling of a bag or container with liquid formula. This allows the addition of modular components a client may require, such as

TABLE 14-3 Conditions Indicating a Tube Feeding

CONDITION	EXAMPLES
Client has mechanical difficulties that make chewing and/or swallowing impossible or difficult.	Obstruction of the esophagus, weakness or nausea, mouth sores, throat inflammation
Client has an intestinal disease and cannot digest or absorb food adequately.	Malabsorption syndromes
Client refuses to eat or cannot eat.	Esophageal cancer
Client is unable to consume a sufficient amount of food because of a clinical condition.	Coma, serious infections, trauma victims, clients with large kilocalorie requirements

additional fiber or protein. Many of the commercial products described in the previous section can be used for tube feeding.

The American Geriatrics Society does not recommend the use of feeding tubes for individuals with advanced dementia due to its association with agitation, need for a greater use of restraints (chemical and physical), greater health-care costs, and development of pressure injury. Instead, it recommends the careful hand feeding, which has been demonstrated to be similar to a feeding tube for outcomes related to death, aspiration pneumonia, functional status, and comfort (American Geriatrics Society, 2014).

Gastrointestinal Function

The GI tract should always be used to the extent possible. Oral supplements should be considered before tube feeding; tube feeding should always be considered before PN. There is less septic morbidity, fewer infectious complications, and significant cost savings in critically ill adults who receive EN versus PN (McClave et al, 2016). Tube feeding is safer, less expensive, and more closely mimics normal feeding conditions than PN. Nutrients should be supplied intact rather than elemental or semielemental if the client has a normally functioning GI tract. **Intact nutrients** are nutrients that are not hydrolyzed, and so the body must keep producing the secretions and enzymes necessary for digestion, thereby forcing the GI tract to function.

Tube Placement

Feeding tubes can enter the body through the nose or through a surgically made opening. A **nasogastric (NG) tube** runs from the nose to the stomach. A **nasoduodenal (ND) tube** runs from the nose to the duodenum. A **nasojejunal (NJ) tube** runs from the nose to the jejunum. These types of tubes are for short-term use because of client discomfort and tissue irritation.

Long-term feeding devices should be considered when the need for enteral feeding is at least 4 weeks' duration in adults, children, and infants after term age; or when a tube cannot be inserted through the nose (as in throat cancer), an **ostomy** (a surgically created opening) is created. An **esophagostomy** is a surgical opening into the esophagus through which a feeding tube is passed. A **gastrostomy** (called percutaneous endoscopic gastrostomy, or PEG) is a surgical opening in the stomach through which a feeding tube is passed; this is the most common tube insertion method.

A PEG tube can be placed **percutaneously** with the aid of an **endoscope** or surgically if the client is already undergoing abdominal surgery or has a condition that makes working with an endoscope difficult. A PEG tube may be used for feedings ≤4 hours of placement in adults and children. Percutaneous endoscopic jejunostomy (PEJ) tube placement is generally reserved for clients who are not candidates for a PEG. For example, a client who has had a gastrectomy (stomach removal) procedure requires a PEJ tube placement. A PEJ tube is also indicated for clients prone to aspiration. ASPEN recommends that EN feedings should be started within 24 to 48 hours after the onset of critical illness and admission to the ICU (McClave et al, 2016). A critical responsibility of team members is assessment of feeding tube placement, especially with tubes inserted nasally. Radiographic confirmation must be obtained before using a feeding tube to ensure that it is correctly placed. Feeding tubes migrate (after x-ray examination) and may move out of the stomach or jejunum. The acronym MARK can be used to guide the steps for monitoring tube placement. **M** is for marking the tube at the exit with an indelible marker, **A** is for anchoring the tube, **R** is for reassessment of tube placement, and **K** has two meanings, for keeping pressure off the skin and knowledge needed to ensure safe practice of institutional policies (Boullata et al, 2016). Tube migration places the client at risk for aspiration because the tube may move into the trachea. The client is also at risk if he or she regurgitates the feeding. **Regurgitation** means to cause to flow backward. If the feeding backs up into the client's lungs, a lung infection can develop.

When a client has inhaled fluids regurgitated from the stomach, he or she may develop aspiration pneumonia. **Aspiration** is the state in which a substance has been drawn up into the nose, throat, or lungs. Nonsurgically inserted enteral tube feeding increases the risk of aspiration and is associated with the development of nosocomial pneumonia, which significantly increases morbidity and mortality in critically ill clients.

Contamination

All tube feedings provide an excellent environment for growth of microorganisms. When a client's tube feeding becomes contaminated with bacteria, the client receiving the feeding may become ill and suffer from nausea, vomiting, or diarrhea. For this reason, hospitals and nursing homes use only commercially prepared tube feedings that are packaged under sterile conditions. However, commercially prepared formulas can become contaminated if they are not handled properly after opening.

To prevent contamination, first check the can for the correct product, expiration date, and any signs of contamination, such as swelling. If the can is swollen, notify your supervisor. Do not administer a feeding from a damaged can. Other cans in the same shipment should be checked for contamination.

Good personal hygiene is essential. EN formulas must be prepared for client use in a clean environment using aseptic techniques. Sterile, liquid EN formulas should be used in preference to powdered, reconstituted formulas whenever possible. The following recommendations help reduce contamination (Boullata et al, 2016):

- Always properly wash hands and use disposable gloves.
- Shake the container well and wipe down the lid with isopropyl alcohol, allowing it to dry before opening it.
- Transfer the formula into a new administration bag or container.
- Label the administration bag or container and any remaining formula carefully with the client's name, room number, the date and time the formula was opened, the amount in the container, the name of the product, administration route and rate, and other pertinent information. Other information may include whether the formula contains vitamins or other additives.
- Reconstituted formulas made in advance should be refrigerated immediately and, if not used, discarded within 24 hours of preparation; they should be exposed to room temperature for no more than 4 hours when hung for administration.
- Sterile, decanted formula has an 8-hour hang time.
- Sterile, decanted formula or HBM (human breast milk) used for neonates has a limited hang time of 4 hours with administration sets changed at that time.
- Store the formula in the refrigerator in a covered container. When a new supply of formula is received, place it in the rear of the storage area so that the older formula is used first. Check expiration dates carefully to ensure that expired product is not used for tube feedings.
- Administration sets for open system enteral feedings must be changed at least every 24 hours.
- A closed system bag or container is preferable for administering EN and may be hung for 24 to 48 hours per manufacturer guidelines.

Administration

Tube feedings can be administered continuously, intermittently, or by **bolus.** Clogging of the tube occurs significantly more often with continuous rather than intermittent feedings. ASPEN guidelines (Boullata et al, 2016) recommend the following for when administering EN:

1. Evaluate all clients for risk of aspiration.
2. Ensure that the feeding tube is in the proper position before initiating feeding.
3. Client's head should be elevated at a minimum of 30° to 45°.

4. If gastric residual volume (GRV) is checked, feeding should not be held for GRV <500 in the absence of other signs of intolerance. GRV checks are not recommended for ICU clients (McClave et al, 2016).
5. Flush tubes according to guidelines given for the type of feeding.
6. Plan the feeding schedule to maximize delivery of the daily feeding volume required by the client. A volume-based feeding protocol can accommodate interruptions to feeding schedule and give the nurse latitude to meet the client's feeding goal.

CONTINUOUS FEEDING

Continuous feeding is always recommended for formulas delivered directly into the small intestine. Prescribed formula volume is given continuously over 16 to 24 hours (Abbott, 2015). One recommended rate is 30 to 50 mL/hour, increasing daily by 25 mL/hour to the rate necessary to meet energy needs. This gradual increase in the formula's volume gives the client's GI tract a chance to adjust to the formula and helps prevent many complications that occur in tube-fed clients. Children should be started at 1 to 2 mL/kg/hour and advanced by 0.5 to 1 mL/kg/hour every 6 to 24 hours until the goal rate is achieved. For critically ill clients, a conservative recommendation of 10 to 40 mL/hour with advancement to the goal rate in increments of 10 to 20 mL/hour every 8 to 12 hours is recommended by ASPEN guidelines (McClave et al, 2009). Safety precautions for continuous feedings include the following:

1. Flush the tube with 30 mL of water every 4 hours in continuously fed adults and after GRV checks (if any taken) and medication administration; flush with as little water as possible in infants and children. Sterile water should be used with medication administration, in immunocompromised, or in critically ill clients.
2. Allow no more than a 4-hour hang time for each bag of formula (when an open system is used) unless the formula is packaged in a sterilized delivery system (closed system).

These procedures help prevent contamination and bacterial growth. An infusion pump is necessary for precise control of a continuous feeding.

INTERMITTENT FEEDING

An **intermittent feeding** means giving a volume of feeding solution (250 to 500 mL) from a feeding container or bag over 60 to 75 minutes with or without a feeding pump. It is normally used with gastric feedings in stable individuals who have normal gastric function, with a demonstrated tolerance to feeding, and who are able to protect their airway (Abbott, 2015). The tube needs to be flushed before and after each feeding with 30 mL of water to minimize bacterial growth, to prevent contamination, and to minimize the chance the tube will clog (Boullata et al, 2016). Many mobile clients prefer intermittent feedings because they are not continuously attached to the feeding pump. Children may be started with 25% of the goal volume divided by the desired number of feedings. The volume may be increased by 25% per day as tolerated, divided by the number of feedings.

BOLUS FEEDING

Bolus feeding means giving a volume of feeding solution (≥250 mL) by gravity via syringe over approximately 10 to 20 minutes. A client is fed 4 to 6 times per day. Feedings given by this method are frequently poorly tolerated, and clients complain of abdominal discomfort, nausea, fullness, and cramping. Some clients, however, can tolerate bolus feedings after a period of adjustment in which the volume is slowly increased. Bolus feeding is normally used with gastric feedings in stable individuals who are ambulatory, neurologically intact, and able to protect their airway (Abbott, 2015). Children's bolus feedings should be initiated and advanced the same as outlined earlier in the Intermittent Feeding section.

Clients on bolus feedings should not recline for at least 2 hours after the feeding. Tubes should be irrigated (flushed with water) before and after each feeding to prevent contamination and clogging of tube (Boullata et al, 2016).

Potential Complications

Complications fall into three categories:

1. Mechanical
2. Gastrointestinal
3. Metabolic

Table 14-4 reviews these complications and lists system-specific prevention strategies.

TABLE 14-4 Feeding Complications and Prevention Strategies

COMPLICATION	PREVENTION STRATEGY
Mechanical	
Tube irritation	Consider using a smaller or softer tube.
	Lubricate the tube before insertion.
Tube obstruction	Flush tube per instructions.
	Do not mix medications with the formula.
	Use liquid medications if available.
	Crush other medications thoroughly and infuse per instructions.
	Use an infusion pump to maintain a constant flow.
	Feeding should not be started until tube placement is radiographically confirmed.
Aspiration and regurgitation	Elevate head of client's bed 30–45 degrees at all times.
	Discontinue feedings at least 30–60 minutes before treatments where head must be lowered (e.g., chest percussion).
	If the client has an endotracheal tube in place, keep the cuff inflated during feedings.
	If GRV ≥500 mL, a promotility agent should be considered as well as a feeding tube placed in the small bowel.
Tube displacement	Place a black mark at the point where the tube, once properly placed, exits the nostril.
	Replace tube and obtain physician's order to confirm with x-ray imaging.
Gastrointestinal	
Cramping, distention, bloating, gas pains, nausea, vomiting, diarrhea*	Initiate and increase amount of formula gradually.
	Bring formula to room temperature before feeding.
	Change to a lactose-free formula.
	Decrease fat context of formula.
	Administer drug therapy as ordered, e.g., Lactinex®, *kaolin-pectin*, Lomotil®.
	Change to a formula with a lower osmolality.
	Change to a formula with a different fiber content, including soluble fiber and excluding insoluble fiber.
	Practice good personal hygiene when handling any feeding product.
	Evaluate diarrhea-causing medications the client may be receiving (e.g., antibiotics, digitalis).
Metabolic	
Dehydration	Assess the client's fluid requirements before treatment.
	Monitor the client's hydration status.
Overhydration	Assess the client's fluid requirements before treatment.
	Monitor the client's hydration status, evaluate for a higher-caloric, low-volume enteral formula.
Hyperglycemia	Initiate feedings at a low rate.
	Monitor blood glucose levels.
	Use hyperglycemic medication if necessary.
	Select a low-carbohydrate formula.
	Evaluate total kilocalories provided; overfeeding in a critically ill client exacerbates hyperglycemia.
Hypernatremia	Assess the client's fluid and electrolyte status before treatment.
	Provide adequate fluids.
Hyponatremia	Assess the client's fluid and electrolyte status before treatment.
	Restrict fluids.
	Supplement feeding with rehydration solution and saline.
	Diuretic therapy may be beneficial.

(continued)

TABLE 14-4 Feeding Complications and Prevention Strategies (Continued)

COMPLICATION	PREVENTION STRATEGY
Hypophosphatemia	Monitor serum levels. Replenish phosphorus levels before refeeding.
Hypercapnia	Select low-carbohydrate high-fat formula.
Hypokalemia	Monitor serum levels. Supplement feeding with potassium if necessary.
Hyperkalemia	Reduce potassium intake. Monitor potassium levels.

*The most commonly cited complication of tube feeding is diarrhea.

Osmolality

The osmolality of a solution is based on the number of dissolved particles in the solution. The greater the number of particles, the higher the osmolality. At a given concentration, the smaller the particle size, the greater the number of particles present.

Oral supplements and tube feedings with a high osmolality draw body fluid into the bowel, resulting in a fluid imbalance. The symptoms are diarrhea, nausea, and flushing. The osmolality of normal body fluids is approximately 300 mOsm/kg. Hydrolyzed nutrients have a higher osmolality than intact nutrients. An **isotonic** feeding has an osmolality of 300 mOsm, the same as body fluids. A high-osmolality feeding can provide a more concentrated source of nutrients than a feeding of lower osmolality.

Sensitivity to the osmolality of oral supplements and tube feedings varies from one individual to another. All clients need a period of adjustment to a high-osmolality formula. Most clients are able to eventually develop a tolerance to a high-osmolality formula; some clients, however, are more likely to develop symptoms of intolerance. Such clients include those who:

- Are debilitated
- Have GI disorders
- Are preoperative and postoperative
- Have a GI tract that has not been challenged by food for a significant period
- Have newly inserted surgically placed tubes (PEG and PEJ)

Administration of Medications

A pharmacist should always be consulted before administration of medications via a feeding tube. To minimize or prevent complications, all health-care workers should be aware of potential drug–food interactions (see Chapter 15). Clinical Application 14-2 discusses suggested procedures for administering medications through feeding tubes. Medications should *never* be added to the tube feeding formula because they can be physically incompatible with the product because of changes in the feeding's viscosity (thickness) or flow characteristics. Some medications may also cause the feeding to separate, granulate, or coagulate (Boullata et al, 2016).

CLINICAL APPLICATION 14-2

Procedures for Administering Medications Through Feeding Tubes

Procedures for the administration of medications through feeding tubes may vary slightly from one institution to another. Consult a pharmacist to review each medication order (making adjustments as necessary) to determine the safety of enteral administration before delivery of medication. The following procedures, however, are common:

- Do not add medication directly to an enteral feeding formula. Stop formula administration before beginning medication dosing. Restart formula after final flush, or after recommended time as determined by a pharmacist to avoid drug–nutrient interactions.
- If possible, administer drugs in liquid form.
- If the drug is not available in liquid form, consult with the pharmacist; he or she may be able to procure a liquid form or similar drug provided by the American Society of Hospital Pharmacists in Pediatric Extemporaneous Formulation List of the manufacturer's suggestions.
- Exercise caution when calculating equivalent liquid doses. Many liquid dosage forms are intended for pediatric use, and the dose must be adjusted appropriately for adults.
- Administer crushed tablets only when no other alternatives are available.
- If administering crushed tablets, crush the tablet to a fine powder and mix with sterile water. Do not crush any tablet on the list of oral drugs that should not be crushed. Do not crush drugs with a sustained-release action or an enteric coating. If in doubt, consult the pharmacist.
- Administer each drug separately. Do not mix all the medications for one dosing time. Flush with at least 15 mL of sterile water between each medication.
- Flush the tube with at least 15 mL of sterile water before giving the medication and before restarting the tube feeding.
- To avoid causing gastric irritation and diarrhea, dilute drugs that are hypertonic or irritating to the cells that line the GI tract, such as potassium chloride, or those administered with meals, such as indomethacin, in at least 30 mL of sterile water before administration.
- Divide dosing schedules—if necessary—of sustained- or slow-release formulations of drugs used for once-daily dosing when administering in liquid form.

Monitoring

Nutritional status, fluid balance, and GI tolerance should be monitored in tube-fed clients. Whether the client requires daily or weekly monitoring depends on client acuity, duration of feeding, and the practice in the facility.

Nutritional status monitoring begins with a comparison of the client's kilocalorie and protein allowances to the volume and composition of the nutritional product used. Initially the client's kilocalorie and protein allowances are not met because a tube feeding is usually started at a low volume to increase GI tolerance. Changes in the client's medical status and treatment, physical activity, and tolerance to the tube feeding may continually alter the volume and kind of feeding the client requires. Therefore, the caloric and protein content of the tube feeding requires reassessment.

In stable clients, serum levels of sodium, blood urea nitrogen, hemoglobin, and albumin are indicators of fluid status. Urine osmolality can be used to monitor hydration status. Urine osmolality is normally 50 to 1,400 mOsm, with a usual range of 300 to 900 mOsm and an average of 850 mOsm. Decreased osmolality indicates overhydration, and increased osmolality indicates dehydration.

Fluid intake and output need to be recorded daily. Fluid intake should be at least 500 mL greater than output in clients who are neither overhydrated nor underhydrated. This 500-mL surplus is needed to cover insensible losses in feces and from the skin and lungs. Clinical signs of hydration status include skin turgor, presence of axillary sweat, condition of the mucous membranes, and the presence or absence of edema. Constipation is another possible sign of dehydration.

GI tolerance can be assessed by the absence or presence of diarrhea, bowel sounds, nausea, distension, and vomiting. The type of feeding delivered, the volume given, or the delivery rate can cause diarrhea. Diarrhea is frequently caused by medications. Antibiotics, laxatives, H_2 receptor blockers, and antacids with magnesium can cause stools to become watery. Medications that contain sorbitol can also have a laxative effect.

Home Enteral Nutrition

With the increase in home-based health-care agencies, hospitals and nursing homes discharge many clients on EN and follow the clients closely as outpatients.

Parenteral Nutrition

PN, in which nutrients are delivered to the client through the veins (intravenously), is the third means of feeding. PN is normally used in acute care settings in the following circumstances (McClave, 2016):

- In a previously healthy individual admitted to an ICU after 7 days of hospitalization when EN is not feasible.
- If there is high nutrition risk and severe malnutrition, and if it is not possible to feed enterally, PN should begin as soon as possible, beginning at 80% of estimated energy needs but with adequate protein (≥1.2 g protein/kg/d). After stabilization, 100% of energy requirements should be provided.
- If an individual has major GI surgery, and it is anticipated that it will not be possible to feed enterally ≥7 days postsurgically, PN should be initiated 5 to 7 days after the surgery.
- If an individual is unable to meet >60% of energy requirements after 7 to 10 days by enteral route alone.

Peripheral parenteral nutrition (PPN) means to feed the client via a vein away from the center of the body in a line terminating in a peripheral site (Fig. 14-4). In **central parenteral nutrition (CPN),** the client is fed via a central vein. Clients are also fed via a central line that has been inserted peripherally and threaded into the subclavian or jugular veins. This is called a peripherally inserted central catheter, or **PICC line.**

The terminology is confusing. Therefore, note whether the line terminates peripherally or centrally. CPN, PICC lines, and PPN can be used to provide partial or total daily nutritional requirements. Clients who cannot or should not be fed through the GI tract are candidates for CPN, PICC lines, and PPN. See Box 14-3 for appropriate indications for the use of PN.

Peripheral Parenteral Nutrition

Intravenous feeding PPN is routine in some health-care institutions. Intravenous solutions, usually containing water, dextrose, electrolytes, and occasionally other nutrients, are used to maintain fluid, electrolyte, and acid–base balance. Intravenous solutions do contain kilocalories. The calculation of the kilocalorie content of an intravenous solution is demonstrated in Clinical Calculation 14-2.

Amino acids and fat can be supplied peripherally. To prevent ketosis, intravenous lipid emulsions should contribute no more than 60% of the total kilocalories provided. Dextrose concentrations are limited to approximately 10%,

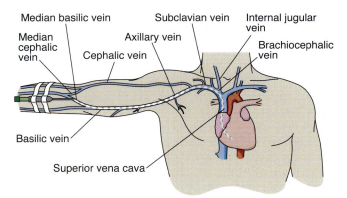

FIGURE 14-4 Correct placement of a peripherally placed central catheter (PICC). *(Modified from Phillips, LD: Manual of IV Therapeutics, ed 5. F. A. Davis, Philadelphia, 2010.)*

CLINICAL CALCULATION   14-2

Calculating Kilocalories in Intravenous Solutions

D_5W means 5% dextrose in water. The subscript following the D tells you the % of dextrose in the solution. Other common concentrations of sugar and water are $D_{10}W$ and $D_{50}W$.

A 5% concentration of dextrose means that 100 mL of water contains 5 grams of dextrose. A 10% concentration of dextrose means that 100 mL of water contains 10 grams of dextrose. A 50% concentration of dextrose means that 100 mL of water contains 50 grams of dextrose. A simple proportion should be used to calculate the number of kilocalories in any given volume of a solution.

The formula is:

percent of concentration/100 mL =
x grams of dextrose/volume of solution client received

For example, a client has received 1,000 mL of D_5W:

5% of dextrose/100 mL =
x grams of dextrose/1,000 =
50 grams of dextrose

Proportions are solved by cross-multiplication and division: (5 grams × 1,000 mL) divided by 100 mL = 50 grams of dextrose. One gram of carbohydrate given intravenously provides 3.4 kcal; thus, 50 grams multiplied by 3.4 kcal/grams = 170 kcal.

because peripheral veins cannot withstand concentrations greater than 900 mOsmol/kg. Thus, PPN has often failed to provide adequate kilocalories and other nutrients for repair and replacement of losses. PPN has been used to supplement a partially successful oral or EN program.

A system for PPN (called all-in-one or three-in-one) has been developed that allows a higher osmotic load (1,200 to 1,350 mOsmol/L) to be delivered peripherally. Lipids, amino acids, dextrose, electrolytes, trace elements, and vitamins are all incorporated into one container. Tolerance of this higher osmotic mixture in peripheral veins might be attributed to the buffering and dilution effects of intravenous fats in combination with the higher pH of the amino acid solutions and the addition of heparin to the mixture.

The use of glutamine in PN therapy is not recommended for routine use in the critical care setting. The safety and efficacy has been brought into question with mortality significantly higher in individuals given glutamine (McClave et al, 2016).

CPN and PICC Lines

When nutrients are infused into a terminal central vein, PN is often referred to as CPN. The **superior vena cava,** one of the largest-diameter veins in the human body, is commonly used for CPN, and CPN can deliver greater nutrient loads because the blood flow in the superior vena cava rapidly dilutes these solutions 1,000-fold. Concentrations for both dextrose and amino acids are determined by the client's needs. A line inserted peripherally but threaded into a central vein is CPN.

INSERTION AND CARE OF A CPN LINE

A physician or certified registered nurse inserts the PICC line, usually to the subclavian vein and into the superior vena cava. The line can be inserted at the client's bedside using strict aseptic technique. CPN solutions and PICC lines need to be sterile. The sterile mixtures consist of dextrose, amino acids, lipid emulsion, electrolytes, vitamins, trace elements, and other additives. The pharmacist usually prepares them in a sterile environment. Careful attention is required to provide vitamins and minerals to clients maintained on CPN/PICC lines to prevent problems such as Wernicke-Korsakoff syndrome (see Chapter 6).

CPN requires close monitoring, and the therapy is costly. The high cost is directly related to the number of highly trained health-care team members required to monitor the client, the laboratory work required for monitoring, and the cost of the solution. A nurse and a dietitian are typically responsible for assessing, monitoring, and educating clients destined for home parental nutrition. The clinical dietitian on the team usually has an advanced degree and special training. The dietitian is responsible for constant nutrition assessment, monitoring, interpretation of data, and calculating formula needs with the physician. The initials CNS (certified nutrition support) indicates that the nurse, pharmacist, or dietitian has had advanced training in the delivery of nutrition orally, enterally, and parenterally.

MONITORING

Careful administration of the central line solution is important. Most institutions have a strict protocol that must be followed by all health-care professionals. A **protocol** is a description of the steps for performing a procedure. Protocols vary widely from one institution to another.

Most PN protocols include the following (Ayers et al, 2014):

- Employ a standardized process for PN ordering and administration, including competent multidisciplinary team members.
- Use a standardized PN order format, preferably using an electronic ordering system.
- Review and verification of orders by pharmacist.
- Standardize labeling for PN formulas.
- Maintenance of a constant rate, unscheduled interruptions in infusion should be avoided because they may contribute to metabolic disturbances and suboptimal nutrient delivery.
- Reduce PN rate appropriately. Adults do not require a gradual reduction in the PN rate (taper-down period); however, pediatric individuals younger than 2 to 3 years are prone to developing rebound hypoglycemia with an abrupt discontinuation and require tapering of the infusion.

Many metabolic complications are possible with CPN. Rapid shifts of potassium, phosphorus, and magnesium from the intercellular compartment to the intracellular compartment result in a lowering of nutrient concentrations in the serum. As a result, initial laboratory tests rapidly fluctuate during the course of treatment. Immediate replacement of potassium, phosphorus, and magnesium is indicated if the corresponding laboratory values of these nutrients fall below normal.

Providing glucose in excess of caloric needs can result in several problems, including carbon dioxide retention with respiratory difficulty. Too high a glucose content in solutions also leads to hyperglycemia. Therefore, glucose levels should be assessed regularly and insulin may be necessary. Liver function test results may become abnormal after an excess glucose load. Excess glucose may also lead to hyperlipidemia and fatty deposits in the liver. Elevated triglyceride levels may indicate too much glucose is being infused.

The avoidance of metabolic complications directly related to a glucose overload is one reason that CPN clients need to be monitored closely. Such complications can be avoided by providing only an appropriate, not an excessive, amount of kilocalories. Box 14-4 lists general recommendations for CPN monitoring.

TRANSITION AND COMBINATION FEEDINGS

Clients need a transition period from CPN to oral feedings. Some physicians prefer to wean clients from CPN by using a tube feeding. This is the situation shown in Figure 14-3. The client has both an enteral feeding line and CPN. Other physicians prefer to avoid the tube and wean clients orally. In the latter case, as the client's oral intake increases, the CPN solution is gradually withdrawn. Expect clients who have been on CPN for a significant time to experience some difficulty with oral feedings. They may need much encouragement to eat.

One of the problems with CPN is that the GI tract does not have to work during CPN administration. Consequently, the GI tract will have undergone some atrophy. Oral foods should be offered slowly during the weaning process. Some physicians avoid this problem by allowing some clients to consume a clear-liquid or light diet while on CPN, if their condition permits.

HOME PARENTERAL NUTRITION

Increasingly, clients are discharged on CPN. These clients need adequate follow-up by either the hospital or a community home-health agency. The pharmacist is responsible for the storage of PN solutions in most institutions. Healthcare organizations that provide nursing services related to home infusion of PN must establish mechanisms for periodic reassessment of knowledge and technique use by clients and caregivers (Ayers et al, 2014).

BOX 14-4 ■ **Monitoring Parenteral Nutrition**

Initial Assessment
- Vital signs (respiration, pulse, temperature)
- Body weight and height
- Serum electrolytes, glucose, creatinine, blood urea nitrogen levels
- Serum magnesium, calcium, phosphorus levels
- Serum triglycerides and cholesterol levels
- Liver function tests
- Serum albumin and prealbumin
- Complete blood count
- Energy (estimated or measured), protein, fluid, and micronutrient needs

Routine Every 4–8 Hours
- Vital signs

Every 24 Hours
- Weight
- Fluid intake and output
- Serum electrolytes, glucose, creatinine, blood urea nitrogen levels; daily for 5 days or until stable, then twice a week

Weekly
- Serum ammonia, SGOT,* serum calcium, phosphorus, magnesium, total protein, and albumin
- Complete blood count
- Reassessment of actual oral, enteral, and PN intake

Other monitors may be indicated depending on the client's clinical condition.

*SGOT (serum glutamic oxaloacetic transaminase) is a liver enzyme that reflects liver cellular damage when elevated (as opposed to liver obstructive disease).

KEYSTONES

- The nutritional care of clients is a joint responsibility of all team members.
- How meals are distributed to clients and meal-service schedules are important for team members to know because they affect the administration of medications and the scheduling of clients for tests and procedures.
- Nutrition screening is an important function of nurses and may determine that a client is at nutritional risk, requiring a nutritional assessment by a dietitian.
- Nutritional care includes four areas: assessing the client's need for nutrients, determining the best method for delivering nutrients, monitoring nutrient intake, and counseling clients about nutritional needs.

- Nutrients can be delivered to clients orally, enterally via a feeding tube, or parenterally.
- One principle is followed when selecting a feeding route: If the GI tract works, use it to maximum capability.
- Oral feedings should be considered before EN.
- EN should be considered before PN.
- PN can be delivered peripherally or centrally.
- Clients on either EN or PN need to be closely monitored.

CASE STUDY 14-1

P was brought to the emergency room by ambulance; his mother accompanied him. The mother stated that her son had been hit by a car while riding his bike. P is 11 years old, 4 ft 11 in. tall, and weighs 89 lb. The client's mother stated that her son was well before the accident. In the emergency room, it was observed that both his eyes were surrounded by contusions, and his throat and the left side of his face were swollen. Communication with the client was at first minimal because it was painful for him to speak. An intravenous solution of 0.9% normal saline was started in the ambulance. He was also shown to have a fractured mandible. Surgery was required, and his jaw was wired. After surgery, the boy was found to have dysphagia, thought to be caused by tissue swelling.

The physician has ordered a nasogastric feeding tube with Nutren 1.0 Fiber®. The order reads:

Day 1 Continuous drip 40 mL/h
Day 2 Continuous drip 60 mL/h
Day 3 Continuous drip 80 mL/h

Nutren 1.0 Fiber contains 1.0 kcal/mL and 40 g of protein per 1,000 mL. The physician states, "The client will remain on a tube feeding until he can consume his kilocalorie requirement orally. This client requires adequate nutrition to enable the mandible to heal properly." P is expected to be discharged on a home enteral tube feeding. His prognosis is good, and he is expected to make a full recovery.

A resident physician inserts the nasogastric tube. The nurse assists at the client's bedside. The client holds the nurse's hand tightly as the tube is inserted. He has a worried look on his face, increased facial perspiration, and increased pulse/respirations during the procedure.

CARE PLAN

Subjective Data
Client held hand tightly during nasogastric tube insertion and appeared worried, apprehensive, and jittery.

Objective Data
Client is a trauma victim who showed increased perspiration and increased pulse/respirations during the tube insertion procedure.

Analysis
Child is showing signs and symptoms of anxiety related to feeding tube placement.

Plan

DESIRED OUTCOMES EVALUATION CRITERIA	ACTIONS/ INTERVENTIONS	RATIONALE
The client's mother will state that he needs the tube feeding to heal his mandible until his jaw is unwired and he is eating to meet his total caloric needs.	Explain enteral nutrition therapy procedures as performed.	A tube feeding is unfamiliar to most clients. Knowledge about the procedure may relax the client and his mother.
	As the client's condition permits, be available for "listening." Give the client a pad of paper and pencil to facilitate communication.	The client needs to vent his feelings about both the tube feeding and the situational crisis (the accident).
Teach client's mother how to safely administer enteral feeding via tube, including the rate, residual check, and proper client placement.	Review home enteral tube feeding instruction sheet, give to client's mother, and have her watch the process of starting the feeding, and if possible practice under the nurse's supervision.	It is important that the individual responsible for the safe handling of the enteral tube feeding understand, see, and, if feasible, practice the process.

TEAMWORK 14-1

DIETITIAN'S NOTES

The following Dietitian's Notes are representative of the documentation found in a client's medical record.

Subjective: *Client not able to provide verbal information. Per client's mother, client was well nourished before accident. No food allergies, intolerances, or food dislikes. Client did not avoid any of the major food groups and ate at least four times a day.*

Objective: *11-year-old child, 4 ft 11 in. tall, weight 89 lb (40.4 kg). Client now being fed 80 mL of Nutren 1.0 Fiber per day every hour times 24 hours. No complaints of nausea, vomiting; last bowel movement this a.m.*

Analysis: *Kilocalorie intake from tube feeding as ordered equals 1,920 per day with 76.8 grams of protein. Client's estimated kilocalorie needs at 30–35 kcal/kg and 40.4 kg equals a maximum of 1,414 kcal. Client's estimated protein needs are 1.0–1.5 g/kg actual body weight or 40.4–60.6. BMI = 17.9. Client is just above the 50th percentile for BMI-for-age percentile. Laboratory values are all within normal limits.*

Client is consuming no food; the tube feeding is the sole source of nutrition.

Plan: *Recommend decreasing the continuous drip rate to 60 mL/hour. This would provide 1,440 kcal, 1,440 mL of fluid, and 57.6 grams of protein. Flush the feeding tube with 78 mL of water 6 times per day to provide fluid requirements.*

CRITICAL THINKING QUESTIONS

1. What would you do if the client pulled out the tube after insertion?

2. After he starts eating, how would you reassess the client's continued need for a tube feeding?

3. How should this client be monitored while on the tube feeding?

CHAPTER REVIEW

1. Parenteral nutrition is usually indicated in the following situation:
   1. Rectal abscess
   2. Cancer of the esophagus
   3. Bowel obstruction
   4. Malnutrition

2. 1,000 mL of a D_5W solution provides ____ grams of CHO and ____ kcal.
   1. 50 and 170
   2. 5 and 20
   3. 50 and 200
   4. 5 and 17

3. Careful administration of central parenteral nutrition includes all of the following except:
   1. A standardized process for ordering and administration
   2. Close monitoring
   3. Abrupt withdrawal
   4. A strict schedule

4. Among the following, diarrhea in a tube-fed client is most likely related to:
   1. Continuous-infusion feeding
   2. Contamination
   3. Fluid deficiency
   4. Insufficient kilocalories

5. Which of the following is not a recommended procedure for administering medications through a tube feeding?
   1. Mix all of the medications together, crush thoroughly, mix with water, and add to the formula.
   2. If at all possible, use medications in the liquid form.
   3. Flush the tube with at least 30 mL of water before giving the medication and before resuming the tube-feeding formula.

2. Ms. L has a jejunostomy. She was discharged from the hospital last week after receiving instructions on home care from the nutrition support service. The local pharmacy is out of the Vivonex formula she has been instructed to use. As the nurse, you recommend that:
   a. She substitute Ensure
   b. She substitute Polycose®
   c. She contact the Nutrition Support Service for instructions
   d. She substitute a standard or polymeric formula

3. Mr. W has been receiving a tube feeding of Ensure via nasogastric tube for 3 weeks via a bolus infusion. He has just started to have loose stools (300 mL each—6 today). You should first suspect the following to be responsible for the diarrhea:
   a. A new medication added to his treatment plan
   b. Bacterial contamination
   c. Intolerance to the bolus delivery method
   d. Lactose intolerance

CLINICAL ANALYSIS

1. Mr. J, 58 years old, visits his physician with a complaint of abdominal pain. He is scheduled for a diagnostic work-up, which will include a **barium enema** (x-ray study of his colon). Before this procedure, the nurse should instruct the client to:
   a. Eat a large breakfast on the day of the examination, such as orange juice, cereal, toast, scrambled eggs, and milk.
   b. Drink ample fluids on the morning of the examination, including at least 12 ounces of juice, 1 cup of gelatin, and broth.
   c. Take nothing orally after midnight on the day of the examination and consume only gelatin; clear broth; tea; coffee; and grape, apple, or cranberry juice on the day before the examination.
   d. Drink milk, juices, and coffee and eat only strained cream soups, ice cream, and gelatin on the day before the examination and take nothing orally after midnight.

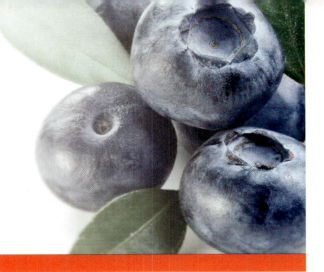

CHAPTER **15**

Interactions: Food and Nutrients Versus Medications and Supplements

LEARNING OBJECTIVES

After completing this chapter, the student should be able to:

- Identify four groups of clients likely to experience food–drug interactions and indicate possible consequences of improper administration or management.
- Describe four ways in which foods, nutrients, drugs, and dietary supplements can interact, and give an example of each.
- Explain why separating grapefruit juice ingestion from oral doses of affected drugs is not an effective strategy for preventing interactions.
- Name the most common food, drug, and dietary supplement to be involved in drug–nutrient interactions.
- List four drugs that should be administered separately from foods and supplements containing calcium, iron, magnesium, and zinc.

- Discuss the tyramine-restricted diet and relate it to the pathophysiology involving monoamine oxidase inhibitors (MAOIs).
- Compare and contrast the regulatory processes for products sold in the United States as dietary supplements with those for products marketed as drugs.
- Relate the mechanism by which *warfarin* achieves anticoagulation to the diet required for therapeutic success.
- Suggest precautions to be used by individuals who wish to use dietary supplements.
- Review principles pertinent to optimizing an athlete's nutrition.

Drug–nutrient–supplement interactions encompass any alteration in the effect of one caused by the interplay with one of the others. Drugs, whether prescription or over-the-counter (OTC), are substances intended for use in the diagnosis, cure, mitigation, treatment, or prevention of disease. OTC drugs can be purchased without a prescription and are approved for safety by the U.S. Food and Drug Administration (FDA) before sale. The complex definition of dietary supplements is explained in a later section of this chapter.

The body does not have separate pathways for food, dietary supplements, and medications. They all share the same organs and systems for digestion, distribution, and elimination. Inevitably those competitions produce winners and losers, the latter often the clients in whose bodies the competitions play out.

Extent of Use

Use of prescribed medications, OTC drugs, and dietary supplements is widespread in the United States. The following figures are derived from various sources.

- Prescription drugs accounted for costs of $297.7 billion in 2014 (Abramowitz & Cobaugh, 2016).

- OTC drug sales in all U.S. outlets amounted to $33.5 million in 2016 (Consumer Healthcare Products Association, 2017).
- Dietary supplements had sales of $28 billion in 2010 and are project to reach $36 billion by 2017 (Axon, Vanova, Edel, & Slack, 2017).

With all those substances in play, the chances of interactions abound.

Some drugs interact with other drugs, foods, nutrients, and supplements in ways that can be beneficial or detrimental, enhancing or inhibiting the action of the other. In no sense is the information in this chapter exhaustive. Emphasis is placed on interactions that illustrate the range of known mechanisms and those that increase the risk of malnutrition or therapeutic failure. Pharmacists and dietitians use computerized databases to elicit possible problem areas. In all cases, pharmaceutical resources should be consulted when administering medications.

As used in this text, the term *drug* includes alcohol and both prescription and OTC medications. As is the usual practice in medical literature, **generic names** are given for drugs.

Some common dietary supplements that may also interact with drugs and nutrients are included later in the

259

chapter. Because of the lack of premarketing regulation and ongoing inspections of manufacturing processes, these substances invite special scrutiny when used by clients.

Because athletes may be tempted to try to gain a competitive edge by using supplements, information on safety and effectiveness of some performance-enhancing supplements as well as food-based interventions for the athlete round out the chapter.

Mechanisms of Interactions

Interactions can be antagonistic or additive; thus, *warfarin*'s effect is impeded by vitamin K and enhanced by vitamin E. Both pharmacokinetics and pharmacodynamics can be involved in interactions with nutrients or supplements.

Pharmacokinetics is the study of the action of a drug, emphasizing absorption time, duration of effect, distribution in the body, and method of excretion. Among the considerations pertinent to pharmacokinetics are:

- **Half-life**—time for a drug's concentration, usually in plasma, to be reduced by one-half.
- **Bioavailability**—proportion of the drug that reaches the systemic circulation. By definition, intravenous drugs and

nutrients administered via parenteral nutrition (PN) are 100% bioavailable.
- **Presystemic clearance**—metabolism of orally ingested compounds before they reach the systemic circulation (formerly known as the **first-pass effect**).

Pharmacodynamics is the study of drugs and their actions on living organisms, as well as their physiologic or clinical effects. Pharmacodynamic effects of interactions that result in toxicities or treatment failures are major concerns of health-care providers.

For instance, *phenytoin*, a drug used to control epileptic seizures, is a folic acid antagonist that competes with the vitamin for binding sites. Its effects can be:

- pharmacokinetic, resulting in lower serum levels of *phenytoin* or
- pharmacodynamic, if seizure activity increases

The interaction works both ways, and so long-term *phenytoin* therapy also can cause folic acid deficiency. Clients should consult with their primary care provider to discuss supplements before taking (see Table 15-1).

Starting at the pharmacy and ending with excretion of the drug or its components, interactions are classified into one of four types.

TABLE 15-1   Nutrient–Drug Interactions

NUTRIENT	DRUG(S)	INTERACTION	INTERVENTION
Calcium	Ciprofloxacin Norfloxacin Ofloxacin Tetracycline	Combines with drugs, yielding insoluble compounds	Separate drug doses from calcium-containing foods
Folic acid	Oral contraceptives Phenytoin Aspirin	Decreased absorption Competition for binding sites Competition for binding sites	Supplementation as needed Monitor blood levels of vitamin and drugs in long-term therapy Monitor blood levels of vitamin in long-term therapy
Iron	Ciprofloxacin Norfloxacin Ofloxacin Tetracycline	Combines with drugs yielding insoluble compounds	Separate drug doses from iron-containing foods
Magnesium	Ciprofloxacin Norfloxacin Ofloxacin Tetracycline	Combines with drugs, yielding insoluble compounds	Separate drug doses from magnesium-containing foods
Niacin	Isoniazid Phenytoin	Drug is structurally similar to niacin Unknown mechanism	Observe for pellagra with long-term therapy Observe for pellagra with long-term therapy
Vitamin B$_6$	Isoniazid Levodopa Penicillamine	Formation of a complex that makes vitamin unavailable (type IIC interaction)	Monitor vitamin status with long-term therapy
Vitamin B$_{12}$	Antacids Nitrous oxide anesthesia Nitrous oxide aerosols	Drugs neutralize gastric acid that normally facilitates separation of vitamin B$_{12}$ from the foods containing it Nitrous oxide oxidizes the cobalt atom in cobalamin to an inactive state Same mechanism	Monitor vitamin status with long-term therapy Take thorough dietary history. Occurred in clients on restrictive vegetarian diets or their breastfed infants Check for abusive use

TABLE 15-1 Nutrient–Drug Interactions (Continued)

NUTRIENT	DRUG(S)	INTERACTION	INTERVENTION
Vitamin D	Carbamazepine Corticosteroids Phenobarbital Phenytoin Rifampin	All interfere with vitamin D metabolism in type III interaction	All: Monitor vitamin status with long-term therapy
Zinc	Ciprofloxacin Norfloxacin Ofloxacin Tetracycline	Combines with drugs, yielding insoluble compounds	Separate drug doses from zinc-containing foods

Type I Interactions

Type I interactions usually occur outside the body:

- In the intravenous or PN solution
- In the syringe where substances are admixed
- In tube feeding reservoirs
- In the respective tubings

No one should rely on visual inspection to identify precipitates that may be

- too small to be seen with the naked eye or
- invisible in opaque solutions

Neither should one ever inject solutions with precipitates into a client. Up-to-date references regarding compatibility should always be consulted. Clinical Application 15-1 offers some insight into the knowledge and skill necessary to administer PN safely. Some of the considerations involved with appropriate administration of tube feedings in conjunction with oral medications appear in Chapter 14.

Type II Interactions

In general, food stimulates gastrointestinal secretions that assist in dissolving solid forms of medication but other drugs are enteric coated with an acid-resistant shell to protect the active ingredient from gastric acid and delay dissolution until the medication reaches the alkaline intestine. Strict adherence to the package administration directions is necessary to maintain the effectiveness of the enteric coating. See Figure 15-1.

Type II interactions occur with oral or enteral intake, producing increased or decreased bioavailability of either the drug or nutrient. Each interaction can impact administration schedules. See Box 15-1 to distinguish delayed from decreased absorption. Factors influencing type II bioavailability include:

- Food intake
- Modification of enzyme activity or transport mechanisms
- Complexing or binding of drugs or nutrients so that one or both are unavailable for absorption

See Type IIC Interactions and Table 15-1.

Food Intake

Some drugs should be ingested into an empty stomach; some should be taken with foods, even specific foods to achieve therapeutic results.

CLINICAL APPLICATION   15-1

Preventing Drug Interactions With Parenteral Nutrition (PN)

PN is a complex formulation of glucose, amino acids, fat emulsion, electrolytes, vitamins, and trace elements. Up to 38 additives may be included, each having individual characteristics that might contribute to interactions. PN has been identified as a high alert medication.

While it is recommended that medications not be added into the PN solution for administration, there are medications that are commonly added, including insulin and heparin. The prolonged exposure of these medications to the PN solution can result in incompatibility reactions, such as forming precipitates, discoloration, and degradation of nutrients or medication. It is also recommended that all PN solutions be administered as a primary infusion. Recommendations advise that co-infusion of medications through the PN tubing be avoided unless impossible in clients who are receiving multiple IV medications or have limited vascular access. If medications are going to be infused as co-infusions with PN, it is essential that the nurse ensure compatibility with the pharmacy before infusion.

Multivitamins should be admixed immediately before infusion. Thiamin and vitamin A are known to have a short stability in PN. Now multichambered bags are available to delay admixing until just before administration. The contents should be mixed by pharmacy staff before dispensing. If being used at home, the client and their family will require thorough training regarding proper mixing.

Interactions may be obvious if changes are noted in the solution or if the catheter becomes plugged, but loss of effectiveness of the drug or the PN can also occur without outward clues.

As with any medication, it is essential that the nurse verify that the ingredients on the PN label match those in the medication order. It is also essential that the nurse follow all institutional policies regarding the administration and monitoring of clients receiving PN to prevent medication administration error.

Adapted from Ayers, P, Adams, S, Boullata, J, Gervasio, J, Holcombe, B, et al: A.S.P.E.N. Parenteral Nutrition Safety Consensus Recommendations. J Parenter Enteral Nutr 38:296, 2014.

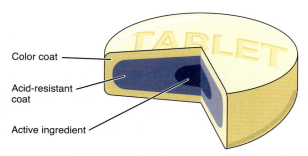

FIGURE 15-1 Enteric-coated tablet. Substances that penetrate the acid-resistant coating defeat the purpose of this type of tablet. *(Reprinted from Clayton, BD, and Stock, YN: Basic Pharmacology for Nurses, ed 9. Mosby, St. Louis, 1989, p. 56, with permission.)*

BOX 15-1 ■ Delayed Versus Decreased Absorption

Some drugs take longer to be absorbed if ingested with food, but the total amount absorbed is unchanged. This delay is the case with *verapamil,* a vasodilator. Therefore, emphasis can be placed on consistency in drug administration in relation to food intake.

However, spacing of doses in relation to food and beverage intake becomes important when a smaller amount of the drug is absorbed in the presence of food than in an empty stomach. In such a situation, correct timing of medication and other intake is necessary. This decreased absorption is the case with *captopril,* an antihypertensive agent.

DRUGS TAKEN ON AN EMPTY STOMACH

Some drugs must be taken on an empty stomach. A strict protocol is used for *alendronate,* a bone resorption inhibitor given for osteoporosis. *Alendronate* must be taken first thing in the morning with plain water 30 minutes before any other medications, food, or beverages. Any intake other than water significantly decreases absorption. Moreover, the person must remain upright for 30 minutes to facilitate passage through the pylorus and minimize risk of esophageal irritation.

The antihypertensive angiotensin-converting enzyme (ACE) inhibitors *captopril* and *moexipril* should be taken with only water, and food intake should be delayed for 1 hour after dosing because food decreases absorption. Other medications that should be taken before or in between meals include *esomeprazole,* a proton-pump inhibitor, and the thyroid medication *levothyroxine.* The antibiotics *doxycycline* and *tetracycline* should also be taken 1 hour before meals or 2 hours after a meal with a full glass of water.

DRUGS TAKEN WITH FOOD

Food increases absorption or bioavailability of several drugs of various classes. The instructions for some drugs specify that they must be taken with food and others that a particular macronutrient is recommended to maximize absorption.

Taking with food increases the absorption of:

- *Cefuroxime,* a second-generation cephalosporin.
- *Ketoconazole,* an antifungal agent that requires an acidic environment to dissolve.
- Lovastatin, an antihyperlipidemic agent.

Taking with food increases the bioavailability of:

- *Atazanavir,* an antiretroviral drug that *must* be taken with food. Taking with food has demonstrated bioavailability 35% to 70% higher than when taken without food.
- *Ritonavir,* an antiretroviral drug.

Meals containing fat favor absorption of certain drugs that require bile salts for optimal absorption. Fat also stimulates the release of cholecystokinin, which slows gastrointestinal motility, thus permitting the drug to remain in contact with the intestinal tissues for a longer time than otherwise. The extra intestinal exposure to the drug enhances its absorption.

Fatty meals are specifically recommended to accompany:

- *Griseofulvin,* an antifungal agent given for infections of the skin such as athlete's foot.
- *Atovaquone,* an antiprotozoal drug given for *Pneumocystis jiroveci* pneumonia.

An example of a special intervention involving a high-fat diet to control epileptic seizures in children appears in Clinical Application 15-2. The ethics of concealing medications in food, which is a separate issue, is briefly discussed in Clinical Application 15-3.

CLINICAL APPLICATION   15-2

The Ketogenic Diet for Seizure Control

About one-third of clients with epilepsy are pharmacoresistant. For a subgroup of this population, both children and adults, the ketogenic diet can be efficacious and should be considered.

Originally used to treat children with **epilepsy** that is poorly controlled with medication, the ketogenic diet (high-fat, low-carbohydrate, and moderate-protein) limits kilocalories and fluid to less than the Recommended Dietary Allowance. Typically 3–4 grams of fat is given for every 1 gram of carbohydrate or protein; although variations of the diet, such as the Modified Atkins Diet, are less strict options. The diet's mechanism of action is unknown and different theories exist. Normally, the brain derives most of its energy from glucose. When deprived of its preferred fuel, the brain uses ketone bodies for energy. Studies have determined that half of children placed on the ketogenic diet will have a 50% reduction in seizure frequency (Sharma & Jain, 2014).

Although the mechanisms underlying the broad clinical efficacy of the ketogenic diet remain unclear, there is growing evidence that the ketogenic diet alters the fundamental biochemistry of neurons in a manner that not only inhibits neuronal hyperexcitability but also induces a protective effect. Unfortunately, the diet has several known complications: kidney stones, gallstones, anemia, and cardiac abnormalities. Nevertheless, the ketogenic diet provides an option for families with a child suffering from difficult-to-control seizures.

The nurse will be responsible for teaching and ongoing assessment, including the monitoring of urine for ketones, renal function, serum glucose, and electrolytes (Southern, Fitzsimmons, & Cross, 2015).

CLINICAL APPLICATION 15-3

The Ethics of Hiding Medications in Food

Nurses' deception of their clients, however well-intentioned, when revealed may cause mistrust of that particular nurse or the health-care system in general. In addition, food universally symbolizes caring. Hiding medications in food is not an action to be taken lightly.

Clients have the right to decline treatment *unless* they are unable to discern the consequences of their decisions. The appropriate assessment of the client's mental fitness is necessary before that right is denied.

If, after deliberation with the client's advocate, colleagues, and the institution's ethics committee, deception is deemed justified, the nurse and pharmacist should ensure that the particular medication, after being crushed and mixed with food, would remain safe and effective.

Changes in Enzyme Activity (Type IIA Interactions)

Cytochrome P450 (CYP450) is a superfamily of more than 50 enzymes found mainly in the liver but also in the gastrointestinal tract, lungs, placenta, and kidneys. Among their functions are the production of cholesterol, the detoxification of foreign chemicals, and the metabolism of drugs. The most significant enzyme is CYP3A4 in the metabolism of medications (Basheer & Kerem, 2015). That function may have evolved to protect the body from toxins.

After uptake by the intestinal epithelial cells (enterocytes), many substances are metabolized by CYP3A4 or returned to the intestinal lumen by a transporter protein, **P-glycoprotein (P-gp)**. Individuals show a wide variation in the amount of CYP3A4 in the liver and the intestine due to genetic, physiological, and environmental factors with resulting differences in the severity of interactions.

GRAPEFRUIT JUICE

An accidental discovery in 1989 that grapefruit juice, used to mask the taste of alcohol in a study, enhanced the absorption of *felodipine* has spurred research into the underlying mechanism. It appears that grapefruit juice's major effect is through the inhibition of intestinal CYP3A4 so that the oral bioavailability of affected drugs is increased dramatically, in some cases as much as fivefold, sufficient to cause drug toxicity and increased side effects or treatment failure. CYP3A4 is responsible for the metabolism of 40% to 50% of current medications that rely on hepatic metabolism for excretion (Takahashi et al, 2015). There is an immediate increased bioavailability when certain medications are taken with even a single serving of grapefruit juice. If the juice is consumed over a period of time, the effects can be long acting.

The components of grapefruit juice vary considerably depending on the variety, maturity and origin of the fruit, local climatic conditions, and the manufacturing process. Furanocoumarin, a component in grapefruit juice, has been shown to cause the interaction (Stohs, Miller, & Romano, 2014). Applying this knowledge to clinical practice is complicated by the fact that even within a given class of drugs, not all agents are metabolized by CYP3A4, and so some medications in the class are affected by grapefruit juice and others are not. The most common medications that are affected by the consumption of grapefruit juice are calcium channel blocker, statins, and anticlotting. Here are some examples.

Of calcium channel blockers, given to manage hypertension and angina pectoris, grapefruit juice increases bioavailability of *felodipine, nicardipine, nifedipine,* and *nisoldipine.*

Similarly, grapefruit juice increases the bioavailability of the benzodiazepines *midazolam, diazepam,* and *triazolam,* but not *clonazepam.*

Likewise, differing effects with grapefruit juice are seen with statin drugs, given to lower cholesterol and prevent ischemic heart disease:

- *Simvastatin* and *lovastatin* had greatly increased blood levels when given with grapefruit juice.
- *Pravastatin* exhibited no effect.

An immunosuppressive agent used to prevent rejection of transplanted organs, *cyclosporine,* is metabolized by intestinal CYP3A4, and elevated blood levels have occurred when administered with grapefruit juice.

In short, avoiding grapefruit juice during oral therapy with affected drugs is well advised. This is particularly true with drugs with a narrow **therapeutic index** and serious side effects that high levels of the drug may evoke.

CRANBERRY JUICE

A similar mechanism but a different isoenzyme is proposed to explain an interaction between the anticoagulant *warfarin* and cranberry juice. *Warfarin* is metabolized by the cytochrome P450 isoenzyme CYP2C9, and cranberry juice contains flavonoids known to inhibit P450 enzymes.

Taking warfarin with cranberry juice increases the effects of the medication, placing clients at a higher risk of bleeding complications. Especially in situations with clear genetic influences, genotype subjects likely would yield more adverse side-effects than the general population (see Genomic Gem 15-1).

LICORICE

Black licorice contains the active ingredient glycyrrhizic acid. Consuming large amounts of glycyrrhizic acid can result in hypokalemia and have potentially serious interactions with some medications. Digoxin, a cardiac glycoside, when taken with licorice can result in fatal heart arrhythmia or myocardial infarction.

Changes in Transport Mechanism (Type IIB Interactions)

A nutrient can also inhibit P-glycoprotein as is the case with water-soluble formulations of vitamin E. Administration of this form of vitamin E to liver transplant recipients and

Genetic Factors in Warfarin Response

Genetic factors explain a higher proportion of variability in *warfarin* response than age, body size, race, concurrent disease, and medications. The identified genes chiefly responsible for the genetic effect are:

- CYP2C9 that codes for an enzyme that metabolizes *warfarin*
- VKORC1 that assists in the production of vitamin K

Clients with mutated CYP2C9 are very sensitive to *warfarin*, displaying over-anticoagulation with standard doses. CYP2C9 enzyme, mainly expressed in the liver, is involved in the metabolism of about 10% of all drugs. A large variation among individuals exists in CYP2C9 activity, which accounts for differences in drug response and in adverse effects. Caucasians are affected more commonly than African Americans (Nagai et al, 2015). When genetic variances of VKORC1 occur, it can cause warfarin sensitivity because it takes a smaller dose of warfarin to affect the clotting mechanism.

healthy volunteers increased *cyclosporine* bioavailability by up to 80%. By the same mechanism, this form of vitamin E increased oral bioavailability of *digoxin* but showed no pharmacodynamic effects, probably because the volunteer subjects were young and healthy.

Hence, a client taking *cyclosporine* could develop toxicity if concurrently consuming grapefruit juice and water-soluble vitamin E, both of which are readily available and, for most people, innocuous. Such a situation demands vigorous and effective client education.

Complexing or Binding of Substances (Type IIC Interactions)

Well-documented interactions involve minerals and mineral-fortified foods, vitamin B_6, and enteral feedings.

MINERALS AND MINERAL-FORTIFIED FOODS

Tetracycline, an anti-infective agent, combines with calcium, iron, magnesium, and zinc to form insoluble compounds. The drug and the nutrient thus bound are both less available for absorption. For this reason, *tetracycline* should be administered 1 hour before or 2 hours after:

- Taking iron or calcium supplements
- Eating iron-containing foods (red meat, egg yolks)
- Consuming milk, other dairy products, or calcium-fortified juices
- Taking antacids, laxatives, or multivitamins containing magnesium, aluminum, calcium, or zinc

Tetracycline should be taken without food or milk to avoid a high risk of treatment failure.

See Table 15-1.

Some *fluoroquinolones* react with metal cations in the same manner as does *tetracycline*. See *ciprofloxacin, norfloxacin,* and *ofloxacin* in Table 15-1. Impaired absorption has been found with enteral feeding, and so withholding tube feedings for 1 hour before and after the dose of medication is usually suggested.

DRUGS INTERACTING WITH VITAMIN B_6

Drugs can have two effects with vitamin B_6. Some drugs will deplete serum vitamin B_6, causing a client to need a vitamin supplement, and other drugs can react with pyridoxine, which causes decreased serum concentration and effectiveness of the drug.

Drugs that decrease serum vitamin B_6 levels include:

- *Isoniazid,* an antibacterial used to treat tuberculosis.
- *Theophylline,* a methlxanthine used to treat respiratory conditions.

Clients taking these drugs or other drugs that decrease serum vitamin B_6 levels in the body may require daily pyridoxine supplements.

Drugs that can have increased metabolism and excretion resulting in less effectiveness when taken in conjunction with pyridoxine include:

- *Phenytoin* and *phenobarbital,* antiepileptic drugs.
- *Levodopa* taken without *carbidopa;* central nervous system agents. Taking levodopa with carbidopa prevents the depletion of B_6. Clients taking these drugs need to be counseled on avoiding the use of pyridoxine unless under the direct supervision of their health-care provider.

ENTERAL FEEDING

Although the exact mechanism is unknown but bearing characteristics of a type IIC interaction, decreased serum levels of the antiepileptic drug *phenytoin* when administered with nasogastric feedings are well documented. Serum levels of the drug rebound when the feedings are discontinued. Initiating enteral feedings on clients previously stabilized on *phenytoin* resulted in a 70% reduction in serum *phenytoin* concentrations.

Interaction with enteral nutrition and *warfarin* has been documented. Studies have demonstrated lower international normalized ratio (INR) values when *warfarin* was administered with continuous enteral feedings. Therefore, continuous enteral nutrition should be withheld for 1 hour before and after *warfarin* administration.

Type III Interactions

Type III interactions occur after the nutrient or drug has reached the systemic circulation that delivers nutrients and drugs throughout the body to be metabolized by multiple organs. Two interactions with pharmacodynamic effects involve *warfarin* and *monoamine oxidase inhibitors* (MAOIs).

Vitamin K and Warfarin

The most commonly prescribed anticoagulant, *warfarin,* is given to prevent blood clot formation in clients with that history, other clotting disorders, and those with mechanical devices in the cardiovascular system.

MECHANISM OF INTERACTION

Warfarin works by competing with vitamin K at its binding sites, thus inhibiting the synthesis of vitamin K–dependent clotting factors II, VII, IX, and X; prolonging clotting time; and "thinning" the blood.

Eating large amounts of foods high in vitamin K during anticoagulant therapy with *warfarin* decreases or may even negate the desired effect of the drug. Clients should not stop eating foods containing vitamin K, but they should avoid large variations in the amounts eaten. A problem might arise if they eat mounds of green leafy vegetables one day and then none for the following several days (see Table 15-2).

Table 15-2 shows a basic diet for *warfarin* therapy. Many health systems have developed protocols for anticoagulation diets. Note that "green leafy vegetables" are not universally interchangeable and that the mode of preparation has an impact on vitamin K content:

- Cooked spinach has 2 times the vitamin K of cooked Brussels sprouts.
- Cooked broccoli has 2.5 times the vitamin K of raw broccoli.

TABLE 15-2 Basic Vitamin K–Controlled Diet

FOODS HIGH IN VITAMIN K	SERVING SIZE	MCG VITAMIN K
Kale, cooked	½ cup	573
Spinach, cooked	½ cup	444
Collards, cooked	½ cup	386
Swiss chard, raw	1 cup	299
Swiss chard, cooked	½ cup	573
Mustard greens, raw	1 cup	144
Turnip greens, cooked	½ cup	426
Broccoli, cooked	1 cup	110
Mustard greens, cooked	½ cup	415
FOODS MODERATELY HIGH IN VITAMIN K		
Spinach, raw	1 cup	145
Turnip greens, raw	1 cup	138
Endive lettuce, raw	1 cup	116
Brussels sprouts, cooked	½ cup	150
Broccoli, raw	1 cup	93
Cabbage, cooked	½ cup	82
Green leaf lettuce, romaine	1 cup	48
Green beans, cooked	1 cup	51
Iceberg lettuce	1 cup	1
Asparagus	4 spears	48

Client's RD will individualize. Consistency is key.
Source: National Institutes of Health, February 11, 2016, United States Department of Agriculture: Agriculture Research Service. USDA Food Composition Database: Nutrient List: Vitamin K. September, 2015. Available at https://ndb.nal.usda.gov/ndb/nutrients/report?nutrient1=430&nutrient2=&nutrient3=&fg=&max=25&subset=0&offset=0&sort=c&totCount=4878&measureby=m

The client's dietitian will individualize the diet prescription to accommodate food preferences. It is important that the food pattern used when the *warfarin* dose is stabilized be continued on subsequent days and weeks. The key to effective *warfarin* therapy is consistent intake of foods containing substantial vitamin K.

Despite its efficacy, *warfarin* remains underused in clinical practice because of its variable dose response, diet and medication interactions, and need for frequent monitoring. Newer classes of low-molecular-weight heparins, such as *fondaparinux* and *enoxaparin,* have been developed that require no dietary restrictions or need for frequent monitoring.

OTHER FACTORS AFFECTING WARFARIN

Abnormal intestinal function and pharmacokinetics of the drug also affect the effectiveness of *warfarin*.

INTESTINAL CONDITIONS. Even a short-term change in physical health can affect *warfarin*'s pharmacodynamics, as has been reported in cases of diarrhea, which may interfere with the absorption of dietary and **endogenous** vitamin K.

Clients taking *warfarin* experiencing diarrhea or decreased food intake should have their INRs monitored more frequently than usual and *warfarin* dosages adjusted accordingly.

PROTEIN BINDING. *Warfarin* is 99% bound to plasma proteins (Mullokandov, Szalkiewicz, & Babayeva, 2014). A client with low levels of serum albumin as a result of malnutrition or disease is at risk for drug toxicity with drugs that are usually highly bound to albumin. The drug that is bound to protein is inactive, whereas the unbound drug circulating in the blood is active and able to exert its intended therapeutic effect. Figure 15-2 sketches two consequences of the competition between drugs and foods or nutrients for protein-binding sites.

Tyramine and Monoamine Oxidase Inhibitors

The usual abbreviation for this group of drugs is **MAOI (monoamine oxidase inhibitor).** Several antidepressants are MAOIs, and some other drugs produce similar reactions with tyramine (see Table 15-3).

MECHANISM OF DRUG ACTION

MAOIs prevent the breakdown of **dopamine** and **tyramine,** chemicals necessary for proper functioning of the nervous system. The drugs' therapeutic effects are to increase the concentration of epinephrine, norepinephrine, serotonin, and dopamine in the central nervous system, thus counteracting depression.

In the peripheral nervous system, MAOIs also prevent the release of the norepinephrine that builds up in the nerves. The stores of norepinephrine become especially high in the nerves that regulate the size of blood vessels. The result is a decreased ability to constrict peripheral blood vessels. The vasodilation thus produced leads to hypotension.

To compound the situation, the drugs also inhibit the body's normal response to a low blood pressure, that is, an increased heart rate. Thus, the individual taking MAOIs

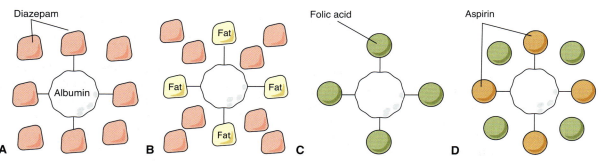

FIGURE 15-2 *A,* Four molecules of diazepam are bound to the albumin molecule, leaving the other four molecules of diazepam free to leave the bloodstream for the central nervous system. *B,* Fat displaces the diazepam from the albumin molecule so that all eight molecules of diazepam are immediately free to exert sedative effects on the central nervous system. *C,* Four molecules of folic acid are attached to the albumin molecule and able to circulate through the kidney intact. *D,* Aspirin displaces the folic acid from the albumin molecule, and the separate molecules of folic acid are likely to be excreted in the urine.

TABLE 15-3   Tyramine-Restricted Diet

DESCRIPTION	INDICATION	ADEQUACY
Restricts food with naturally high levels of tyramine	Used when clients receive drugs classified as monoamine oxidase inhibitors (MAOIs) and those with MAOI activity. Antidepressants: *isocarboxazid* *phenelzine* *tranylcypromine* Anti-infectives: *isoniazid* *linezolid* Antineoplastics: *procarbazine* Antiparkinson: *rasagiline* *selegiline*	Adequate in all nutrients according to the current Recommended Dietary Allowances if the individual makes appropriate food choices

FOOD GROUP	TO AVOID	TO USE MODERATELY
Breads and cereals	None	None
Fruits and vegetables	Avocados Bananas Figs Broad (fava) beans Chinese pea pods Eggplant Fermented soy products Italian flat beans Mixed Chinese vegetables Raspberries Sauerkraut	None
Dairy	Aged cheese (brick, blue, brie, cheddar, camembert, Swiss, romano, Roquefort, mozzarella, parmesan, provolone) Sour cream Yogurt	Gouda cheese, processed American cheese
Meat and fish	Any canned meat Anchovies Beef or chicken liver Sausage (bologna, salami, pepperoni, summer) Fish (caviar, dried fish, salt herring)	
Beverages	Ale, beer, sherry, red and white wines	Coffee, colas, hot chocolate (1-3 cups per day)
Other	Chocolate, bouillon and other protein extracts, protein supplements, meat tenderizer, soy sauce, yeast concentrates	

displays the unusual combination of hypotension and bradycardia.

EFFECT OF FOOD ON MAOIs

Some foods contain **tyramine,** a metabolic intermediate product in the conversion of the amino acid tyrosine to epinephrine. Foods that contain degraded protein, such as aged cheese, are high in tyramine. When a client taking MAOIs consumes foods or beverages high in tyramine, the drugs prevent the normal breakdown of tyramine. The tyramine oversupply consequently leads to excessive epinephrine, producing hypertension. Sometimes the blood pressure is severely elevated, which can cause intracranial hemorrhage.

As with many substances, individuals' responses to tyramine vary. Four factors interact to determine the severity of reaction:

1. The amount of tyramine ingested
2. The type and dose of the MAOI
3. Client susceptibility
4. The time between the drug dose and a tyramine-containing meal

TYRAMINE-RICH FOODS

Many foods contain enough tyramine to create problems for clients receiving MAOIs. The amount of tyramine varies even in different samples of a particular food. Table 15-3 describes the tyramine-restricted diet. Because this interaction can be life-threatening, the best advice to give a client is to avoid all foods capable of causing problems, even though a small amount of the food, or a given batch of a product, might be safe. It is recommended that clients follow low-tyramine diets for several weeks after stopping an MAOI (Hall-Flavin, 2016).

MAOIs, despite proven efficacy for depression, are underprescribed due, in part, to concerns about required dietary and drug restrictions.

Protein Intake and Levodopa

Levodopa is given for Parkinson disease. The amino acids in dietary proteins may compete with the drug for transport across the **blood–brain barrier.** Levodopa is absorbed in the small intestine, and so when the drug is taken with protein rich foods, the drug must compete for absorption. Therefore, it is recommended that levodopa be taken 30 minutes before a meal.

Vitamin D: Multiple Interactions

Corticosteroids increase the **catabolism** of the matrix of the bone, inhibit the osteoblasts from building new bone, and prevent the liver from processing vitamin D. When this lack of vitamin D results in insufficient calcium absorption by the intestine, parathyroid hormone causes withdrawal of calcium from the bones and osteoporosis results. Because of the seriousness of this adverse effect, monitoring of the client's vitamin D status should be ongoing during long-term corticosteroid therapy (see Table 15-1).

Phenytoin and *phenobarbital,* in addition to previously detailed interactions, also affect bone metabolism, reducing bone mineral density and increasing the risk of fractures. The mechanism is presumed to accelerate bone loss through stimulation of cytochrome P450, which increases catabolism of vitamin D (Anwar, Radhakrishna, & Vohora, 2014). By nature a long-term therapy for seizure prevention, *phenytoin* requires conscientious monitoring of the client's bone health and institution of osteoporosis preventive measures. Therefore, clients who are taking anticonvulsant medications are advised to take vitamin D supplements to help reduce long-term effects on bone health. See Table 15-1.

B Vitamins: Multiple Interactions

Water-soluble vitamins are particularly susceptible to drug interactions during long-term therapy.

NIACIN

As with other nutrients, vitamin B_3 can interfere with absorption of some drugs while increasing the effect of other drugs.

Niacin increases the effect of:

- *Warfarin* and *aspirin,* anticoagulants with niacin can increase bleeding risk.
- *Clopidogrel,* an antiplatelet drug with niacin can increase bleeding risk.
- *Ibuprofen* and *naproxen,* nonsteroidal anti-inflammatories with niacin can increase bleeding risk.
- *Doxazosin,* an alpha-blocker with niacin can cause hypotension.

Drugs that have decreased absorption in combination with niacin are:

- *Tetracycline,* an anti-infective
- *Isoniazid,* an anti-infective used in the treatment of tuberculosis

VITAMIN B_{12}

There are several drugs that interfere with vitamin B_{12} absorption and could potentially contribute to the development of anemia, including:

- *Metformin,* a sulfonylurea used in the treatment of diabetes
- *Cimetidine* and ranitidine, H-2-receptor blockers
- *Omeprazole,* a proton-pump inhibitor

Clients on these medications may require monitoring of vitamin B_{12} and may require the use of a supplement.

An uncommon but unique interaction can occur in some clients who have prolonged exposure to *nitrous oxide,* commonly in anesthesia. Vitamin B_{12} deficiency can develop and lead to irreversible neurological destruction if not identified quickly.

Type IV Interactions

Interactions between drugs and nutrients can continue as the kidneys excrete waste products of metabolism.

Sodium, Fluids, and Lithium

Both sodium intake and increased fluid intake affect the mood stabilizer *lithium,* which is one of several drug options for the long-term treatment of bipolar disorder. This drug is absorbed, distributed, and excreted with sodium and may result in the following scenarios.

- Decreased sodium intake with decreased fluid intake may lead to *lithium* retention manifested by slurred speech, decreased coordination, drowsiness, and muscle weakness or twitching.
- Increased sodium intake and increased fluid intake increase the excretion of *lithium,* thus worsening signs and symptoms of mania.

Because of the interaction with salt and water intake, clients who take *lithium* may be taught to monitor the concentration or specific gravity of their urine.

Salt Substitutes and ACE Inhibitors

The ACE inhibitors lower blood pressure by preventing conversion of angiotensin I to angiotensin II, thereby decreasing aldosterone secretion and increasing excretion of sodium and water (see Fig. 8-6) and increasing retention of potassium. Clients receiving ACE inhibitors, such as *captopril, enalapril,* and *lisinopril,* should be monitored for **hyperkalemia.**

Folic Acid Displaced by Aspirin

Plasma proteins can bind with nutrients as well as drugs. When there are insufficient binding sites on the plasma proteins for all of the drug or nutrient, the excess accumulates in the bloodstream as free, small particles. The kidney is likely to excrete these small particles rather than to restore them to the bloodstream.

One common drug that interferes in this manner with a nutrient is *acetylsalicylic acid,* or *aspirin*. It displaces folic acid from its plasma protein. The kidney then excretes the folic acid in the urine (see Fig. 15-2).

Dietary Supplements

Research demonstrates that half of adults in America will consume dietary supplements with only 23% of products being used based on recommendations of a health-care provider (Wang, Gamble, Bolland, & Grey, 2014).

It is estimated that the number of adults who have ever used an herbal preparation or dietary supplement has increased from 50.6 million in 2002 to 53.6 million in 2012 (Wu, Wang, Tsai, Huang, & Kennedy, 2014). Many clients who take prescription medications also use dietary supplements often without reporting supplement use to their health-care provider. Many clients do not consider herbal supplements as a medication or believe that that the use of "natural" substances is safe. As this section details, neither of those assumptions is justified.

Compared with the number of possible interactions between supplements and medications, only a small proportion have been examined or reported. The occurrence and clinical significance of many drug–nutrient interactions remains unclear.

Special Rules

The rules for labeling the nutrient content of foods and drugs in the United States are much more stringent than those applied to dietary supplements.

Before receiving permission to market a new drug, the pharmaceutical company must conduct rigorous tests on animals and on people in randomized, double-blind clinical trials. Randomization requires that participants be assigned by coin toss or equivalent unbiased method to receive the investigative drug or not. **Double-blind** trials are experiments in which neither the subject nor the investigator knows whether a subject is receiving the treatment or a **placebo.**

For foods, label information must be supported by research or scientific agreement, which is not the case with dietary supplements.

Because it is not required by law, research into the effectiveness and adverse effects of dietary supplements is limited. Unlike drugs that can claim treatment, cure, or prevention, dietary supplements may only use one of three claims:

- A health claim
- A nutrient claim
- A structure/function claim (see Box 15-2).

An additional problem pertains to overlapping areas of regulatory responsibility. Food labeling is regulated by the FDA and the U.S. Department of Agriculture, whereas advertising is regulated by the Federal Trade Commission (FTC). The FTC requires that advertising be truthful and claims be substantiated, but the rigor of evidence is less than that of drugs.

Areas of Concern

With botanical products, nature keeps some of the ingredients secret. Not all the constituents of these products have been identified, and they may exert more than one physiological effect in the human body. Therefore, when ingesting one of them, a person takes not only the active ingredient that is purported to have the desired medicinal effect but also other substances in the plant tissue as well.

Among those other substances may be defensive chemicals the plant has evolved to protect itself from predators. Despite a long history of use, little is known about the toxicity of botanical products. Most such knowledge comes from acute cases of toxicity sporadically reported, but recently some scientific studies have been conducted.

Manufacturers and distributors of dietary supplements must record, investigate, and forward to the FDA any reports

---

BOX 15-2 ■ Regulation of Dietary Supplements

The Dietary Supplement Health Education Act of 1994, referred to as DSHEA, created the first regulatory structure for this class of products. The FDA provides primary oversight of dietary supplements along with drugs and most foods.

Under the provisions of DSHEA, dietary supplements can be sold unless shown by the FDA to be unsafe, adulterated, or labeled in a misleading manner. The burden of proof in this case rests with the FDA, not with the manufacturer, and no prior notice from the manufacturer of intent to sell is required unless the product contains a new dietary ingredient. The Bioterrorism Act does require manufacturers to register with FDA before producing or selling supplements, and in 2007, the FDA published comprehensive regulations for Current Good Manufacturing Practices for those who manufacture, package, or hold dietary supplement products (FDA, December 2010).

Under DSHEA (1994), a dietary supplement is defined as a product taken by mouth that

1. Contains a dietary ingredient: vitamin, mineral, herb; botanical, amino acid, enzyme, tissue; or a concentrate, metabolite, or constituent extract from the ingredients previously mentioned.
2. Is in the form of a supplement (meaning tablet, capsule, soft gel, gelcap, liquid, or powder).
3. Is not represented as a food or sole item of a meal or of the human diet.

DSHEA does not limit the serving size or the amount of nutrients in any form of dietary supplement, but its regulations spell out the nature of the claims that can be made for a product on the label and its format. The following types of statements are allowed:

1. Health claims that have substantial scientific support or, if limited support, the claim must contain qualifying statements.

2. Nutrient content claims that describe the level of the nutrient or dietary ingredient in a product compared with an established daily value.
3. Structure/function claims that describe the product's effect on structure or function of the body or on general well-being. These claims must also include the following information displayed prominently on the label:

"This statement has not been evaluated by the Food and Drug Administration. This product is not intended to diagnose, treat, cure or prevent any disease."

Manufacturers of dietary supplements that make structure/function claims on labels or in labeling must submit a notification to the FDA that includes the text of the structure/function claim no later than 30 days after marketing the dietary supplement (FDA, November 23, 2016).

For instance, a structure/function claim could state the product "helps to maintain bone health." If the label said the product is used to treat arthritis, it would be disallowed as a medical claim. The FDA maintains a MedWatch program to receive information about possible adverse effects of dietary supplements. Health-care providers and consumers can report these events online at www.fda.gov/Safety/MedWatch/HowToReport/default.htm or by calling 1-800-FDA-1088. The identity of the client is kept confidential.

DSHEA has supporters of the status quo as well as those calling for regulation of dietary supplements in the same manner as pharmaceuticals. Health-care providers should know the current system and be aware of changes to provide wise counsel to clients.

---

they receive of serious adverse events associated with the use of their products that are reported to them directly (U.S. Food and Drug Administration [FDA], July 5, 2016). Because the FDA's responsibility begins only after the products have been packaged and marketed, the maintenance of quality is the responsibility of the manufacturer.

The FDA lists recalled food and dietary supplements at https://www.fda.gov/food/recallsoutbreaksemergencies/recalls/default.htm. In 2017, in the months of May through June, three dietary supplements were recalled for containing banned ingredients. Two of the supplements contained derivate of anabolic steroids that can result in liver injury, acute kidney injury, and increase the risk of myocardial infarction and stoke, and one contained the banned ingredient Ephedra (FDA, July 6, 2017). Ephedra can increase the risk of myocardial infarction and stroke. Besides the dearth of information and questionable manufacturing practices, issues of standardization, contamination, and interaction with other substances are major concerns.

Lack of Standardization

The potency of herbal products varies with the:

- Climate and soil conditions
- Life cycle of the plants from which they come

Great differences in the quantities of active ingredients have been found, depending on:

- The source
- The species and part of the plant used
- Storage conditions
- Time of harvest
- Method of processing
- Country of origin
- Inclusion of look-a-like plants

Without consistent products, research cannot be generalized as a basis for evidence-based practice.

Botanical products can come to market not containing the ingredients on the label. One study found that 59% of botanical products contained plant species not listed on the label (Starr, 2015).

Contamination With Dangerous Substances

Botanical products have been contaminated with toxic substances. Heavy metals and prescription medications are frequently cited as contaminants. One analysis of 40 products demonstrated that 93% had trace amounts of one or more contaminants, including lead, arsenic, mercury, cadmium, or pesticides (Starr, 2015).

HEAVY METALS

The U.S. Pharmacopoeia (see Box 15-3) limits the presence of heavy metals in nutritional supplements to:

- 3 parts per million (ppm) for arsenic, cadmium, and mercury
- 10 ppm for lead

Additionally, the FDA limits lead to 0.1 ppm in candy likely to be consumed frequently by small children (FDA, June 5, 2015).

DRUGS

Dietary supplements have also been contaminated with prescription medications. Because of the special rules governing the dietary supplement industry, discovery of the contaminants frequently occurs long after the products are first marketed.

While studying natural anti-inflammatory substances in human placental blood, investigators detected an unknown substance. It was subsequently identified as the drug *colchicine,* which is used to treat gout, traced to five women who consumed ginkgo biloba during pregnancy. Further searching located the drug in samples of ginkgo biloba distributed commercially in the area. In 2016, an herbal supplement that claimed weight loss was recalled because it was found to contain sibutramine, a controlled substance that was removed from the market (FDA, December 1, 2016). These are not isolated instances. A search on the FDA Web site in 2017 for seven "undeclared ingredient" yielded hundreds of entries, excluding the FDA archives.

Difficulty Obtaining Reliable Information

Supplement labels are often lacking needed information. It can be difficult not only for the lay public but also for health-care professionals to discern information such as active ingredients and safety concerns. It is prudent for consumers to investigate supplements before consuming.

Reliable information on the quality of dietary supplements is available from:

- FDA at www.fda.gov/Food/DietarySupplements/default.htm
- NIH National Library of Medicine at www.nlm.nih.gov/medlineplus/druginfo/herb_All.html
- NIH Office of Dietary Supplements at http://ods.od.nih.gov/Research/PubMed_Dietary_Supplement_Subset.aspx
- NIH National Center for Complementary and Integrative Health (NCCIH) at http://nccih.nih.gov

Easy to Underestimate Potential Harm

Both the name "dietary supplements" and the ease of procurement can mislead consumers about their possible impact on medications. For those reasons or others, many clients do not inform their health-care providers about their use of dietary supplements. One study determined that 20% to 30% of those using herbal supplements are also using conventional drugs (Choi et al, 2016). These statistics make it essential that the nurse specifically assess for the use of dietary supplements with all clients.

Supplements Reported to Interact With Drugs

Knowledge and caution are necessary to weigh the risks and benefits of dietary supplements (see Fig. 15-3). Although statistics do not predict individual responses, St. John's wort and ginkgo as well as magnesium, calcium, and iron had the greatest number of documented interactions with

---

BOX 15-3 ■ Standards for Health-Care Products

The U.S. Pharmacopoeial Convention (USP), a nongovernment, nonprofit organization, sets standards for drugs, dietary supplements, biologics, and other articles used in health care. Substances listed as USP meet standards of purity and strength as determined by chemical analysis or animal responses to specified doses. A zero tolerance policy for pesticides applies to food and botanicals.

A voluntary verification program for dietary supplements is available to assure consumers of the safety of the products they buy. Certain supplements with known safety concerns are excluded from the program:

- Ephedra
- Kava
- Comfrey
- Chaparral
- Aristolochia

The USP mark on a product verifies the accuracy of the label, the strength and quantity of the contents, the lack of contaminants according to federal standards, and the use of good manufacturing practices (USP Convention, 2017, http://www.quality-supplements.org/).

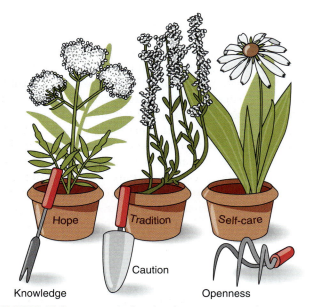

FIGURE 15-3 Because of cultural traditions, many people use botanical products as they seek a measure of self-care and hope. Those who use botanical products, however, need to cultivate knowledge and caution in their choices. They also should practice openness with their health-care providers.

medications (Tsai et al, 2012). Examples of purported mechanisms of action, and experts' advice follow.

St. John's Wort

St. John's wort has been favorably compared to pharmaceutical antidepressants in some studies, but significant interactions with medications have been discovered. Currently there are 95 drugs known to have major interaction with St. John's wort (Mou-Ze et al, 2015). The major interaction of most drugs with St. John's wort is decreasing the efficacy of the drug, which can result in dangerous effects. The medications include:

- Oral contraceptives
- *Warfarin*, anticoagulant
- *Digoxin*, digitalis glycoside used to treat heart conditions
- *Indinavir*, an antiviral used in the treatment of HIV

St. John's wort taken with a class of medications used for the treatment of depression, called selective serotonin reuptake inhibitors (SSRIs), can result in **serotonin syndrome**. Serotonin syndrome results from increased levels of serotonin in the body that can lead to symptoms such as diarrhea, fever, and seizures. This is a potentially life-threatening condition if left untreated. SSRIs include:

- *Paroxetine*
- *Fluoxetine*
- *Citalopram*

Ginkgo Biloba

Ginkgo biloba is promoted to enhance mental functioning through improved cerebral circulation. There is no conclusive evidence that confirms that ginkgo prevents or slows dementia or cognitive decline or helps with memory enhancement (National Center for Complementary and Integrative Health [NCCIH], March 10, 2017).

Ginkgo does not interact with *warfarin* or *aspirin* directly but does have antiplatelet activity. Cumulative effects become apparent when ginkgo is combined with other drugs affecting coagulation. Therefore, there is increased bleeding risk when ginkgo is taken with medications that also have increased bleeding risk, such as *aspirin, warfarin, ibuprofen,* and *naproxen.*

Ginkgo, similar to St. John's wort, can contribute to the development of serotonin syndrome when taken in conjunction with SSRIs. Ginkgo has also demonstrated the effect of lowering blood pressure in some clients, and so caution should be used in clients who are taking antihypertensive medications. The combination could cause severe hypotension.

Garlic

Garlic is promoted for cardiovascular health. Whereas several trials have suggested that garlic has possible blood pressure–lowering effects, a larger number of published studies have reported virtually no effect. It is notable that all positive studies were performed using subjects with elevated **blood pressure** and that, by contrast, almost all negative studies used subjects with normal blood pressure. There is also supporting evidence that using garlic can assist in lowering low-density lipoproteins. Further research is required on both topics.

Garlic has been shown to increase bleeding risk when taken with *warfarin, aspirin,* and *indomethacin.* There is also a decrease in efficacy of the antiviral *saquinavir* when taking in conjunction with garlic.

Glucosamine–Chondroitin

Glucosamine and chondroitin are substances found in the human body in and around cells of cartilage. Consumers sometimes take one or both supplements for osteoarthritis. One study found that 7.4% of older adults take glucosamine–chondroitin, similar to the same percentage of older adults that take acetaminophen (Kantor et al, 2014). Studies are contradictory regarding the effectiveness of the supplement in relationship to the improvement of joint pain and joint structure. Some studies report improvement and others demonstrate no improvement.

As with other supplements, glucosamine–chondroitin, when taken with *warfarin,* can increase the risk of bleeding.

A Prudent Course

Clients at greatest risk of drug–dietary supplement interactions are:

- Children
- The elderly
- People with chronic diseases or impaired organ function
- People taking many medications over a long period of time
- People taking medicines with high risk of interactions (anticoagulants, antiepileptics, antimicrobials)
- Individuals with genetic variants in drug metabolism

The fact that many botanical products have been used for centuries does not negate their dangers. Clearly, "let the buyer beware" holds true. To protect clients, thorough assessment is vital. Often the use of dietary supplements does not come to light until late in the treatment cycle. Did health-care providers ask the clients about use of dietary supplements? If so, was it done in a manner that permitted them to reveal their practices without feeling ridiculed or condemned? Some items to consider when assessing diet supplement use are listed in Clinical Application 15-4.

Education is essential. Without disparaging a client's background, the health-care provider must counter the concept that "everything natural is safe." Substances strong enough to produce the effects attributed to dietary supplements are medicines, no matter what the law currently allows for distribution. Such substances should be treated with respect, including the use of childproof containers.

Enhancing Athletic Performance

Physical training and proper nutrition are vital for success in sports. In general, the diet that is optimal for good health is also optimal for most athletes. Energy and macronutrient

CLINICAL APPLICATION 15-4

Assessment for Dietary Supplement Use

Questions the nurse might ask to determine supplement use:

- What kinds of herbal products, dietary supplements, or other natural remedies do you take?
- Do you give any of them to children?
- Do you find the recommended dose satisfactory?
- Have you changed doses recently?
- Are you taking any prescription or over-the-counter medications for the same purpose? Or for opposite purposes?
- Have you used this product before? For how long?
- Where do you obtain these products?
- Is anyone else in your household taking botanical products?
- Are you allergic to any plant products?
- Are you pregnant, planning to become pregnant, or breastfeeding?

needs, especially carbohydrate and protein, must be met during times of high physical activity to maintain body weight, replenish glycogen stores, and provide adequate protein to build and repair tissue. Sports nutrition has several objectives:

- To foster good health
- To help athletes recover quickly after each training session
- To foster optimal performance during competition

Nutrition for Athletes

As long as competitive sports have existed, athletes have attempted to improve their performance by ingesting a variety of substances. This practice has given rise to a multi-billion-dollar industry. In 2016, 5.67 billion dollars was spent on "sports nutrition supplements" (National Institute of Health [NIH], June 20, 2017).

Ergogenic aids are substances, devices, or practices that enhance an individual's energy use, production, or recovery. They encompass equipment, clothing, training exercises, psychological preparation, and dietary supplements, the topic of this section. For athletes, the aid is any means of enhancing energy utilization, including energy production, control, and efficiency.

Many athletic organizations prohibit the use of certain pharmacological, physiological, and nutritional aids. The World Anti-Doping Agency (2018) lists prohibited substances on its Web site. The National Collegiate Athletic Association (NCAA) (2017) Web site lists banned substances as well as rules governing testing.

Several surveys of supplements available through the Internet and at retail establishments have confirmed that many are contaminated with steroids and stimulants that are prohibited for use in elite sports. Athletes need to be educated regarding banned substances and recognize the risks

of purchasing and consuming unapproved supplements. Some ergogenic aids clearly fall into the classes of nutrients included in Chapters 2, 3, 4, 6, 7, and 8, whereas others do not, although they may be substances with physiological functions. The ergogenic aids included in this chapter are categorized either as nutrients corresponding to those in the above-listed chapters or as nonnutrients.

Nutrients

The Acceptable Macronutrient Distribution Ranges (AMDRs) are broad enough to cover the macronutrient needs of most active individuals, but alternate formulas based on body weight have been developed for athletes (see Clinical Calculation 15-1). These requirements can generally be met by dietary management without the need for supplements.

CLINICAL CALCULATION 15-1

Individualizing Macronutrient Recommendations for the Athlete

Depending on kilocalorie needs and the sport, athletes may need these adjustments in diet.

	GRAMS/KILOGRAM BODY WEIGHT	SUGGESTED DISTRIBUTION RANGE
CHO	5–10	50%–70% of kcal
Protein	1.2–1.7	12%–20% of kcal
Fat	0.8–2	20%–30% of kcal

If an athlete, 70 kg (154 lb), 5 ft 9 in., runs an average of 10 miles per day, lifts weights 3 or 4 times a week, and needs 3600 kcal/day, his suggested intake would be:

CHO

7 grams × 70 kg = 490 grams; 11 grams × 70 kg = 770 grams
490 grams × 4 kcal/gram = 1960 kcal; 770 grams × 4 kcal/gram = 3080 kcal

$$\frac{1960}{3600} = 54\% \qquad \frac{3080}{3600} = 86\%$$

CHO intake = 54% to 86% of 3600 kcal

PROTEIN

1.2 grams × 70 kg = 84 grams; 1.7 grams × 70 kg = 119 grams
84 grams × 4 kcal/gram = 336 kcal; 119 grams × 4 kcal/gram = 476 kcal

$$\frac{336}{3600} = 9\% \qquad \frac{476}{3600} = 13\%$$

Protein intake = 9% to 13% of 3600 kcal

FAT

0.8 grams × 70 kg = 56 grams; 2 grams × 70 kg = 140 grams
56 grams × 9 kcal/gram = 504 kcal; 140 grams × 9 kcal/grams = 1260 kcal

$$\frac{504}{3600} = 14\% \qquad \frac{1260}{3600} = 35\%$$

Fat intake = 14% to 35% of 3600 kcal

CARBOHYDRATE

Carbohydrate is the body's main dietary energy source for:

- **Anaerobic** (1 to 2 minutes) exercise
- **Aerobic** (more than 3 minutes) exercise

Suggested daily intakes of carbohydrate per kilogram of body weight are:

- 5 to 10 grams for the average athlete in training, based on training intensity
- 10 to 12 grams for 36 to 48 hours before prolonged endurance events, greater than 90 minutes in duration
- 7 to 12 grams for 24 hours before activity less than 90 minutes in duration

These amounts exceed the AMDR, which is designed for 97% to 98% of individuals of a given age, gender, or female reproductive status. Athletes should choose healthy carbohydrates, whole grains, legumes, fruits, and vegetables as part of a balanced diet. If an individual has no time to eat before an event, consuming 30 grams of carbohydrate in easy-to-digest foods (grits, bagel, banana, or yogurt) 5 to 10 minutes before it starts may improve performance.

Carbohydrate intake also is necessary after exercise to restore glycogen stores. Ingesting 1 to 1.2 grams of carbohydrate per kilogram of body weight within 30 minutes after exercise is recommended.

Recommended distribution of macronutrients for athletes (see Clinical Calculation 15-1) clearly emphasizes carbohydrate intake.

PROTEIN AND AMINO ACIDS

Because most athletes consume adequate amounts of protein due to high kilocaloric intakes, supplemental protein is unnecessary. Both resistance exercise and endurance training exercise induce protein catabolism during exercise, but protein synthesis predominates in the postexercise recovery period (Moore, Camera, Areta, & Hawley, 2014). Exercise, resistance exercise, and endurance training have an interactive effect with ingested protein, leading to positive muscle protein balance. Milk has repeatedly been shown to acutely increase muscle protein synthesis and to lead to lean mass gains; it may also decrease muscle damage and soreness when consumed after exercise (Papacosta, Nassis, & Gleeson, 2015).

The NCAA (2013) concluded that protein requirements are higher in very active persons than in the general population, suggesting daily amounts of:

- 1.2 to 1.7 grams per kilogram of body weight in resistance athletes
- 1.2 to 1.4 grams in endurance athletes

These amounts are approximately 50% to 100% higher than the RDA, but well within the AMDR of 10% to 35% of daily energy intake given additional kilocalories the athletes require. Meeting these requirements can be easily achieved by consuming natural food sources; protein supplements are not required for athletes in order to achieve recommended intake. A vegetarian diet *per se* is not associated with detrimental effects in athletes, but an optimal protein intake should be achieved through careful planning with an emphasis on protein-rich plant foods. A comparison of three sports protein supplements sold on the Internet by major retailers appears in Dollars & Sense 15-1. The cost for 10 grams of protein from the sampled whey protein supplements exceeds that of 60% of the food items analyzed in Dollars & Sense 4-3.

The questionable efficacy of supplements as well as the expense and possible side effects should encourage an athlete to seek protein in food, not supplements.

WATER

Normal hydration is the goal for athletes. Fluids should be consumed before and during exercise to prevent excessive dehydration (loss of more than 2% of body weight).

Sweat losses vary depending on:

- The activity
- Clothing
- Equipment
- Environmental conditions
- Individual differences in sweat rates

Serious athletes may sweat from 0.5 to 2 liters per hour. Some football players, often with large body weights, reportedly can lose 8 liters of sweat per day in hot weather. It is well documented that inadequate hydration in athletes can contribute to impaired performance.

Dollars & Sense 15-1

Comparison of Sports Powdered Whey Vanilla Supplements

Product	Price	Package	Serving Size	Protein Grams/ Serving	CHO Grams/ Serving	Cost/ Serving	Cost/10 Grams of Protein*
A	$29.99	30.4 oz	1 scoop/27 servings	24	5	$1.11	$0.56
B	$17.99	2 lb	1 scoop/18 servings	30	8	$1.00	$0.33
C	$29.99	2 lb	1 scoop/27 servings	25	2	$1.10	$0.56

*Compare to Dollars & Sense 4-3.

Hydration before, during, and after exercise is essential. See Clinical Application 15-5 for suggestions to maintain hydration. Specially formulated sports drinks are necessary for:

- Intense exercise longer than 60 minutes
- Hot, humid climates
- High sweat rates
- Individuals who have salty sweat

Consuming excessive water, however, can lead to electrolyte imbalances. During long events, an athlete's blood is shunted to the skeletal muscle with less blood flow to the kidneys. If fluids are overconsumed, the kidneys may not be able to excrete the excess fluid producing dilutional hyponatremia. For examples, see Chapter 8.

Nonnutrients

Many ergogenic aids are promoted for athletes, some with little scientific evidence for efficacy and safety. Only four are included here based on availability of information in the medical literature: bicarbonate, creatine, caffeine, and glycerol.

BICARBONATE

Muscular activity generates lactic acid as a waste product with consequent lowering of blood pH. The ingestion of sodium bicarbonate before intense exercise may buffer lactic acid in the muscle cell, which could temper the metabolic acidosis that contributes to fatigue. One study demonstrated that cyclists who took bicarbonate had 11.5% more power than the placebo group in sprints following endurance exercise (Setright, 2015). The current recommendation is 200 to 300 milligrams per kilogram 60 to 90 minutes before exercise. It should be noted that sodium bicarbonate supplementation can result in unwanted gastrointestinal side effects, including reflux, flatulence, and diarrhea. Athletes who benefit most are those who participate in endurance sports with repetitive movements such as cycling.

CREATINE

Creatine is a nonprotein substance synthesized in the body from the amino acids arginine, glycine, and methionine.

CLINICAL APPLICATION   15-5

Hydration Suggestions for Athletes

In amounts:

- Drinking 16 ounces of water 2–3 hours before activity
- Drinking 8 ounces of water 15 minutes before activity
- Drinking 4 ounces every 15–20 minutes during activity
- Drinking 16–20 ounces for every pound lost after activity
- Day before competition, drink enough to ensure adequate hydration.

Source: NCAA (2013). Fueling during exercise. Available at http://www.ncaa.org/sites/default/files/Fueling%20During%20Exercise%20Fact%2

Creatine is produced endogenously, mainly in the liver and kidneys and to a lesser extent in the pancreas, at an amount of about 1 gram per day. Another 1 gram is obtained through the diet predominantly derived from meats and fish (Deminice et al, 2014). When combined with phosphate, the resulting compound, phosphocreatine, serves as a storage form of energy that is released with anaerobic muscle contraction. The mechanisms by which creatine acts in the human body to improve physical and cognitive performance are not clear.

The form of creatine that has been most extensively studied and commonly used in dietary supplements is creatine monohydrate. Studies have consistently indicated that creatine monohydrate supplementation increases muscle creatine and phosphocreatine concentrations by approximately 15% to 40%. Newer forms of creatine have been purported to have better physical and chemical properties, bioavailability, efficacy, and/or safety profiles than creatine monohydrate. However, there is little to no evidence that any of the newer forms of creatine are more effective and/or safer than creatine monohydrate. Creatine supplementation has been shown to reduce the body's endogenous production of creatine; however, levels return to normal after a brief period of time when supplementation ceases. Although at present, ingesting creatine as an oral supplement is considered safe and ethical, it is not recommended for athletes under the age of 18 years.

CAFFEINE

Caffeine mobilizes fat stores and stimulates working muscles to use fat as a fuel, which delays depletion of muscle glycogen and allows for prolonged exercise. The critical period in glycogen sparing appears to occur during the first 15 minutes of exercise, when caffeine has been shown to decrease glycogen utilization by as much as 50%. The effect on performance was a 1% to 3% enhancement in performance during endurance sports (Clark, 2014). Caffeine has been shown to be an effective ergogenic aid for endurance athletes when ingested before and/or during exercise in moderate quantities, 3 to 6 milligrams per kilogram of body weight.

As an ergogenic compound, caffeine raises the heart rate and blood pressure. Consequently, adverse effects, typically manifesting with ingestion of more than 200 milligrams of caffeine, include insomnia, nervousness, headache, rapid heart rate, arrhythmia, and nausea. Caffeine is also on the NCAA Banned Drugs List (2017) if concentrations in urine exceed 15 micrograms/milliliter.

Caffeine is the most common stimulant in energy beverages, a relative newcomer to the market. Regulation of energy beverages, including content labeling and health warnings, differs across countries, with some of the laxest requirements in the United States. Energy drink consumption in the United States increased from 26 million gallons in 2001 to 354 million gallons in 2009 (Treloar et al, 2017). Hundreds of different brands of energy beverages are now marketed, with caffeine content ranging from a modest 50 mg to an alarming 505 mg per can or bottle. By comparison, an 8-oz cup of coffee contains:

- 110 to 150 milligrams for drip
- 65 to 125 milligrams for percolated
- 40 to 80 milligrams for instant.

GLYCEROL

To increase tolerance for fluid loss during exercise, athletes may attempt to hyperhydrate by consuming extra fluid before exercise. Because a large fluid intake is typically accompanied by diuresis, hyperhydrating is difficult. Enter glycerol with the capacity to enhance body fluid retention. Glycerol-induced hyperhydration has been shown to increase endurance performance that starts declining at a dehydration level (loss of >2% of body weight). Glycerol hyperhydration can increase body water by one liter or more.

Advice for Athletes

Products marketed to athletes to provide the macronutrients needed before, during, and after exercise are not superior to ordinary foods but may have some advantages. They are portable and premeasured, thus convenient. Trying them out in training, not during competition, is wise. Before using any supplements, the athlete, with the advice of a health-care provider, parents, and coach, should evaluate the supplement carefully. Although most of the supplements described herein appear safe when using the recommended dose, the effects of higher doses (as often taken by athletes) on indices of health remain unknown, and further research is warranted.

The same advice given for the general dietary supplements applies to those marketed for athletes. Just because they are available OTC does not ensure safety. The list of prohibited substances of the World Anti-Doping Agency classifies the administration of several steroids in sports as doping. As mentioned earlier in the chapter, several supplements have been recalled for containing steroid derivatives that were not listed on the label. Every attempt should be made to ascertain quality of supplements and ingredients. Athletes should seek advice from qualified nutritionists. Sports nutrition is a specialty practice for dietitians who often assist professional and college athletes maximize their performances in their chosen activity through individualized nutrition prescriptions.

Some basic suggestions for fueling the body for high-energy expenditure sports appear in Table 15-4. The timing and distribution of nutrients is intended to ensure adequate glycogen levels and to maximize protein synthesis and recovery.

Responsibilities of Health-Care Professionals

The standards for hospital accreditation and client safety by The Joint Commission address existing or potential food–drug interactions, specifically considering the reduction of harms by anticoagulant therapy in the National Patient Safety Goals 2015 and 2016 (2016 National Patient Safety Goals, 2016). Preventing or modifying pharmacodynamic effects of drug–nutrient–supplement interactions is a team effort involving physicians, pharmacists, dietitians, and nurses. Health-care agencies often assign the client teaching to certain members of the team to ensure that no one will be missed. For instance, pharmacists may be responsible for teaching clients receiving *warfarin* therapy and dietitians for teaching those receiving tube feedings. Nurses often do the discharge teaching and follow-up with a telephone call to field questions after the client returns home.

TABLE 15-4 CHO and Water Fueling Basics for Athletes*

TIME	CHO	WATER	EXAMPLE
3–4 hours before exercise	3–4 grams per kilogram of body weight	5–7 milliliters per kilogram of body weight	1 cup steel cut oatmeal with blueberries and walnuts (45 grams of CHO), 1 cup low-fat milk (13 grams CHO), 1 chicken wrap (65 grams CHO), fruit smoothie (45 grams of CHO), 1 ounce pretzels (31 grams of CHO).
2 hours before exercise	2 grams per kilogram of body weight	16 ounces	2 cups granola, 1 cup skim milk with ¼ cup powdered milk (130 grams CHO)
1 hour before exercise	1 gram per kilogram of body weight	8 ounce 15 minutes before exercise	1 large banana (35 grams of CHO)
Within 45 minutes and for the first 4 hours after exercise	1–1.2 grams per kilogram of body weight also include 7–20 grams of protein postexercise	16 ounces per pound of weight lost	2 cups 1% fat chocolate milk (52 grams CHO)

*Depending on athlete's size, the sport, environmental conditions, and so on.
Adapted from NCAA (2013). Fueling during exercise. Available at http://www.ncaa.org/sites/default/files/Fueling%20During%20Exercise%20Fact%20Sheet.pdf; NCAA (August 6, 2013). Fueling for performance: how proper timing of meals affects both sport and academic performance. Available at http://www.ncaa.org/health-and-safety/nutrition-and-performance/fueling-performance-how-proper-timing-meals-affects-both

Persons at highest risk for food and drug interactions are those who:

- Take many drugs, including alcohol
- Require long-term drug therapy
- Have poor or marginal nutrition
- Are critically ill
- Receive enteral or parenteral nutrition

The main predictors of drug–nutrient interactions in a client are:

- Increased age
- Multiple chronic illnesses
- Current use of multiple medications and supplements

The most commonly cited substances in interactions from three categories are:

- Among supplements, St. John's wort
- Among drugs, *warfarin*
- Among foods, grapefruit juice

Polypharmacy, the concurrent use of a large number of drugs, is a risk factor for untoward reactions, particularly if the person is treated by many prescribers. Elderly people are particularly vulnerable because they take more than 30% of prescription drugs that presumably are more potent than OTC drugs.

Elderly people are likely to be on long-term regimens for chronic diseases, further increasing the risk of adverse effects, as exemplified in Figure 15-4. Other groups at risk of food and drug interactions are infants and adolescents because of high nutrient needs and immature detoxification systems. Clinical Application 15-6 reviews triggers that should prompt a further search for drug–nutrient interactions.

The consequences of improper scheduling of drugs and foods or nutrients can be:

- Treatment failure
- Toxicity
- Increased expense

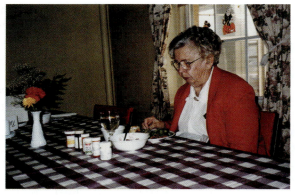

FIGURE 15-4 This woman has several risk factors for drug–nutrient interactions. She is elderly, is on a multiple-drug regimen, and takes some of her medications with a meal.

CLINICAL APPLICATION   15-6

Screening Clients at Risk for Drug–Nutrient Interactions

Further nutritional assessment may be in order if a client:

- Reports a recent weight change.
- Abuses alcohol.
- Consumes a modified diet, prescribed or self-imposed, including one with significant changes in protein content.
- Receives tube feedings.
- Takes many medications or dietary supplements, some with meals, some known to interfere with nutrition.
- Shows worsening of signs and symptoms of disease.
- Displays laboratory values indicating nutrient depletion.

Health-care providers should keep up with the scientific findings to counsel clients appropriately. Overbroad prohibitions should be avoided because some complementary and alternative medicine therapies may improve the client's well-being. The possibility of identifying the client's inherent ability to metabolize drugs to the best advantage offers exciting opportunities to individualize treatment and minimize interactions.

KEYSTONES

- Persons at risk for food–drug interactions are those who take many drugs, require long-term medication therapy, have immature or impaired metabolic systems, or receive enteral or parenteral nutrition, any of which can result in treatment failure, drug toxicity, or nutritional deficiency.

- Interactions can take place in the delivery device (type I) or within the body by affecting absorption and bioavailability (type II), cellular or tissue distribution (type III), or disposition by the liver or kidneys (type IV).

- Separating grapefruit juice from drugs metabolized by CYP3A4 is an inadequate intervention because the juice and drug do not interact directly. Rather the juice inhibits intestinal CYP3A4, causing the excessive bioavailability of the drug to last several days until the intestine produces more of the enzyme.

- The most commonly cited interactions, sometimes life-threatening, involve grapefruit juice, *warfarin*, or St. John's wort interacting with each other or with another food, drug, or dietary supplement.

■ To avoid the formation of insoluble compounds with calcium, iron, magnesium, and zinc, the following drugs should be separated from substances containing those metal cations: ciprofloxacin, norfloxacin, ofloxacin, and tetracycline.

■ When a client taking MAOIs consumes foods or beverages high in tyramine, the drugs prevent the normal breakdown of tyramine, which leads to excessive epinephrine that produces hypertension, sometimes severe. A tyramine-restricted diet limits selected foods in every food group except grains.

■ In the United States, prescription and OTC drugs are tested in randomized, double-blind clinical trials before being marketed. Food label information must be supported by research or scientific agreement. In contrast, dietary supplements can be sold without testing unless shown by the FDA to be unsafe, adulterated, or labeled in a misleading manner.

■ *Warfarin* achieves anticoagulation by competing with vitamin K at its binding sites, thus inhibiting the synthesis of vitamin K–dependent clotting factors. To attain therapeutic goals, the client should avoid large swings in the intake of foods high in vitamin K, mainly green leafy vegetables. Elimination of food is unnecessary; consistency of intake is key.

■ Persons taking dietary supplements should be aware of the risks associated with their production, not assume "natural" products are inherently safe, obtain as much credible information as possible, and always inform their health-care providers of their use.

■ Athletes should consume a healthy diet emphasizing appropriate proportions of carbohydrate and protein for their body and sport, take care to hydrate appropriately, and, if dietary supplements are desired, select those certified to contain labeled ingredients and no substances prohibited for athletes.

CASE STUDY 15-1

Mr. K, a 48-year-old accountant, is admitted to the hospital for treatment of deep vein thrombosis (DVT) and correction of INR of 1.2, signifying almost no therapeutic effect of his prescribed *warfarin*. His treatment of DVT includes intravenous administration of the antithrombotic heparin until oral *warfarin* level becomes therapeutic between 2.0 and 3.0. (See Type III Interactions for mechanism.) His admitting nurse recorded a previous episode of thrombophlebitis 5 months ago, for which he has been medicated with *warfarin* and monitored with blood work to prevent recurrence.

The factors possibly contributing to his current illness relate to a road trip Mr. K took to his 30th high school reunion. He drove 13 hours, virtually nonstop, both going to the reunion and returning. In addition, Mr. K described his food intake on his trip as significantly different from usual. He "pigged out" on Southern cooking, consuming large amounts of cooked greens at least twice a day over the 4-day reunion. "But I didn't eat any of the salads," he said. He could not recall specifics of the dietary instruction he had received during his initial bout with thrombophlebitis except that he needed to equalize intake of green, leafy vegetables.

A vitamin K–controlled diet was ordered for him and a consultation with the registered dietitian (RD) scheduled. On the basis of these data and his observations, the admitting nurse prepared a care plan. The portion of it pertinent to food and drug interactions appears below.

CARE PLAN

Subjective Data

Takes prescribed *warfarin* at same time each day ■ Faithful in reporting for blood work and keeping follow-up appointments ■ Significant change in vitamin K–containing foods in the past 10 days

Objective Data

Wearing *warfarin* Medic Alert bracelet
INR = 1.2 in doctor's office before admission

Analysis

Lack of correct information regarding self-care related to food–drug interaction as evidenced by described recent food intake contributing to DVT

(Continued on the following page)

Plan

DESIRED OUTCOMES EVALUATION CRITERIA	ACTIONS/ INTERVENTIONS	RATIONALE
Client will understand requirements of diet related to *warfarin* therapy by discharge.	Schedule RD consultation.—Done. Observe food intake on actual vitamin K–restricted diet.	RD will individualize diet prescription. Current practices should clarify educational needs.
Client will prepare for dietitian's consultation by listing food preferences related to vitamin K content.	Provide writing materials if necessary. Prompt with questions about usual daily intake.	Review of current practices may stimulate questions to ask the dietitian.
Client will state that the key to successful *warfarin* therapy is day-to-day consistency of vitamin K intake.	Emphasize that RD will individualize diet plan to accommodate preferences. Stress that consistency of intake of foods high in vitamin K is essential to successful *warfarin* therapy.	Advance preparation will maximize effect of RD's instruction. Review and redundancy enhances learning.

TEAMWORK 15-1

DIETITIAN'S NOTES—NEXT DAY

The following notes are representative of the documentation found in a client's medical record.

Subjective: *Had been classifying any raw green vegetable as forbidden by his diet. Thought cooking destroyed vitamins, including vitamin K, and therefore cooked vegetables would be safe to eat as desired. Favorite vegetables include broccoli, Brussels sprouts, cabbage, "and greens if someone cooks them."*

Objective: *INR today 1.5*

Nurse's note states that he did not eat the tossed salad with broccoli and lettuce served for dinner, stating, "They're not on my diet." Reminded that he was served a vitamin K–controlled diet.

Analysis: *Faulty understanding of diet for warfarin therapy*

Plan: *Client will demonstrate 100% proficiency at identifying amounts of vegetables represented by food models.*

Client will demonstrate 80% proficiency at sorting preferred foods with significant vitamin K content into a quasi-exchange daily dietary pattern.

Client will report to RD by telephone the result of his first postdischarge INR and his progress regarding dietary intake.

CRITICAL THINKING QUESTIONS

1. What other information about meals might the RD have obtained that would bear on the ability of this client to maintain a vitamin K–restricted diet?

2. In light of the anticoagulation failure just described, do you believe that this client is motivated to improve his lifestyle to avoid future occurrences of thrombophlebitis? Why or why not?

3. Would this situation be likely to have developed in the same way if the client had been a woman? Why or why not?

CHAPTER REVIEW

1. Which of the following clients is at greatest risk for food–drug interaction?
   1. A 50-year-old man with no current disease who takes one baby aspirin daily to prevent heart disease
   2. A 75-year-old woman taking medication for several chronic diseases
   3. A 39-year-old man who usually consumes two cocktails before dinner
   4. A 25-year-old pregnant woman who is taking a prenatal vitamin supplement and calcium tablets

2. For which of the following items is there most agreement that athletes require increased amounts compared with more sedentary individuals?
   1. Creatine
   2. Glucosamine
   3. Glycerol
   4. Protein

3. Which of the following statements by a client prescribed simvastatin would indicate that he understood the instructions?
   1. "One glass of grapefruit juice a day is as much as I can have."
   2. "I can have grapefruit juice for breakfast since I take the pill at bedtime."
   3. "I won't drink grapefruit juice while I am taking this drug."
   4. "I can start with 1 ounce of grapefruit juice and work up to 4 ounces over a month's time."

4. A client taking lithium is most likely to experience increased mania with:
   1. Decreased fluid intake and decreased sodium intake
   2. Decreased fluid intake and increased potassium intake
   3. Increased sodium intake and decreased potassium intake
   4. Increased sodium intake and increased fluid intake

5. Individuals following a vitamin K–controlled diet as outlined in the text may have three servings per day of all of the following except:
   1. Cooked collards or spinach
   2. Raw broccoli or spinach
   3. Endive or Romaine lettuce
   4. Asparagus and leaf lettuce

CLINICAL ANALYSIS

1. Mr. A is being admitted to a long-term care facility. He is a 45-year-old posttrauma client. The motor vehicle accident in which he became paralyzed below the waist also killed his wife and daughter. The accident occurred 6 months ago. In the meantime, he has been treated at a rehabilitation center. He is depressed and freely shares his feelings of guilt and loss. The depression has interfered with his progress toward rehabilitation and also contributed to a 20-pound weight loss since the accident. After many trials of various antidepressants, he is now receiving *phenelzine*. The following questions relate to his care.
   Close attention to Mr. A's diet is essential. Which of the following foods will he have to avoid completely?
   a. Baked beans, dates, and roast beef
   b. Sugar, molasses, and maple syrup
   c. Bologna, cheddar cheese, and wine
   d. Green beans, whole-wheat bread, and oranges

2. When teaching nursing assistants about the dietary restrictions needed by Mr. A, the nurse should be sure that the nursing assistants understand that:
   a. The potential complication can be life-threatening.
   b. Mr. A is to be kept unaware of the seriousness of his condition.
   c. As time goes on, the forbidden foods can be added to the diet slowly, one at a time.
   d. If Mr. A does not cooperate in his dietary care, his paralysis is likely to worsen.

3. Ms. O is seeking advice at a clinic before becoming sexually active. She is leaning toward the use of oral contraceptives. She tells the nurse that she takes some herbal products "to keep my strength up and get me through the day." Which of the following products would raise the greatest concern for the nurse?
   a. Natural vitamin C from rose hips
   b. Ginger
   c. St. John's wort
   d. Protein supplement for athletes

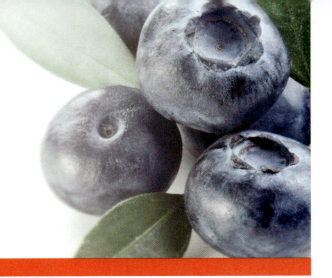

Weight Management

Weight management is a concern not only from a personal viewpoint but also from a societal perspective. Consequences of excessive body weight cause many individuals to suffer economically, socially, mentally, and physically (see Dollars & Sense 16-1).

Studies have repeatedly shown that, at any one point in time, more than 40% of the population describe themselves as trying to lose weight. Approximately 85% of those who lose weight will regain their original weight within 5 years. Although this sounds dismal, it also means that 15% of all people who lose weight are successful over the long-term. Weight management, although difficult, is not impossible, and the financial and health benefits of weight control, both to the individual and society, are enormous.

Terminology and Classification

Historically the classification of people as underweight, normal weight, overweight, and obese has been a challenge for practitioners. Yet how a person is classified is becoming more important. Third-party payers (insurance companies and state and federal governments) want an individual to meet specific criteria before they will grant financial approval for treatments. Percentage body fat is the true measure of how to classify clients, but there are problems with this measurement. Therefore, body mass index (BMI) and waist circumference are the most commonly used methods for classifying clients (Table 16-1).

Percentage Body Fat

An individual's percentage body fat is associated with her or his health risk. The most accurate definition for obesity is a body fat content greater than or equal to 32% for women and greater than or equal to 25% for men. The exact percentage is defined differently by various professional groups. The optimal fat content for females is 25% to 31%. The optimal fat content for males is 18% to 24%. Women tend to present with about a 10% higher body fat composition than men. However, percentage body fat is expensive to measure accurately.

Techniques used to measure body fat involve underwater weighing, tissue x-ray examinations, ultrasonography, electrical conductivity, computed tomographic scans, and magnetic resonance imaging scans. Electrical impedance is used by some health-care workers, but this method is gaining disfavor because of a lack of consistent results. Limitations include less accuracy in extremely obese persons; overhydration and underhydration; hormone abnormalities; and the need for a qualified technician. Thus, measurement of body fat is of limited usefulness for persons trying to lose weight. The other procedures previously mentioned are expensive and not available in clinical settings.

Dollars & Sense 16-1

Costs of Obesity

According to a national study, costs associated with obesity demonstrated a cost of $1,429 more for obese clients compared to those of normal weight and total annual health-care costs of $147 billion in associated costs related to obesity in 2008 (CDC, 2017). Approximately one-half of these costs were paid for by Medicaid and Medicare. These costs do not include the indirect costs attributed to obesity such as absenteeism and decreased productivity.

TABLE 16-1   Classification of Overweight and Obesity by BMI, Waist Circumference, and Associated Disease Risks

	BMI (kg/m²)	Obesity Class	DISEASE RISK* RELATIVE TO NORMAL WEIGHT AND WAIST CIRCUMFERENCE†	
			Men ≤40 in. (102 cm) Women ≤35 in. (88 cm)	Men >40 in. (102 cm) Women >35 in. (88 cm)
Underweight	<18.5		—	—
Normal	18.5–24.9		—	—
Overweight	25.0–29.9		Increased	High
Obesity	30.0–34.9	I	High	Very high
	35.0–39.9	II	Very high	Very high
	≥40.0	III	Extremely high	Extremely high

*Disease risk for type 2 diabetes, hypertension, and cardiovascular disease.
†Increased waist circumference also can be a marker for increased risk, even in persons of normal weight.
Source: Data from American Association of Clinical Endocrinologists [AACE] and American College of Endocrinology [ACE]. 2016. Clinical Practice Guidelines for Comprehensive Medical Care of Patients with Obesity—Executive Summary. Available at https://www.aace.com/files/guidelines/ObesityExecutiveSummary.pdf

Body Mass Index

The National Institutes of Health (NIH) recommends and encourages all health-care professionals to use BMI to classify clients as underweight, normal weight, overweight, and obese in clinical settings. The classification of an individual as underweight, normal weight, overweight, and obese is defined according to BMI:

- Underweight, <18.5
- Normal, 18.5 to 24.9
- Overweight, 25 to 29.9
- Obese class 1, 30 to 34.9
- Obese class 2, 35 to 39.9
- Obese class 3, >40 often referred to as "severe" or "extreme" obesity

Individuals can calculate their own BMI using Clinical Calculation 16-1. Or they can use a Body Mass Index Chart (Table 16-2) to determine BMI without doing any calculations. The more complex calculation for BMI is weight in kilograms divided by height in meters squared. There are also online calculators that calculate BMI by simply entering height and weight at https://www.cdc.gov/healthyweight/assessing/bmi/adult_bmi/english_bmi_calculator/bmi_calculator.html.

Although BMI correlates with the amount of body fat a person has, it does not measure body fat. Some athletes may have a BMI that identifies them as overweight, but they do not have excessive amounts of body fat. The extra pounds are lean body mass (LBM) acquired from rigorous training.

Similarly, a teen with a normal BMI may have all the health-related consequences of obesity if the client has a high body fat content of greater than 33%. The teen may have a history of minimal physical activity and poor food choices. The health-care professional should carefully evaluate the results of any BMI measurement along with other nutritional assessments (laboratory data, physical examination, and diet history).

Waist Circumference

Waist circumference is also used to classify fat distribution and central obesity. Waist circumference should be used in conjunction with BMI for evaluating risk of obesity-related diseases. Women with a waist circumference greater than 35 inches and men with a waist circumference greater than 40 inches are at a higher health risk than those with a lower waist circumference (Centers for Disease Control and Prevention [CDC], May 15, 2015).

Prevalence and Incidence of Overweight and Obesity

The prevalence of obesity in the United States has had a startling increase since the mid-1970s. Figure 16-1 illustrates these trends more dramatically than words. **Prevalence** means the total number of cases of a specific disease divided by the number of individuals in the population at a certain time.

Many experts are concerned about the incidence and prevalence of obesity in the nation's children. **Incidence** is

CLINICAL CALCULATION   16-1

Steps in Calculating BMI

BMI can be calculated in three easy steps.

1. Multiply weight in pounds by 703.
2. Multiply height in inches by height in inches.
3. Divide the product of step 1 by the product of step 2.

For example, for a 166-pound person who is 5 ft 6 in. (i.e., 66 in.) tall:

1. $166 \times 703 = 116{,}698$
2. $66 \times 66 = 4{,}356$
3. $116{,}698$ divided by $4{,}356 = 26.8$

TABLE 16-2   Body Mass Index Chart

BMI	19	20	21	22	23	24	25	26	27	28	29	30	31	32	33	34	35	36
Height (Inches)									Body Weight (Pounds)									
58	91	96	100	105	110	115	119	124	129	134	138	143	148	153	158	162	167	172
59	94	99	104	109	114	119	124	128	133	138	143	148	153	158	163	168	173	178
60	97	102	107	112	118	123	128	133	138	143	148	153	158	163	168	174	179	184
61	100	106	111	116	122	127	132	137	143	148	153	158	164	169	174	180	185	190
62	104	109	115	120	126	131	136	142	147	153	158	164	169	175	180	186	191	196
63	107	113	118	124	130	135	141	146	152	158	163	169	175	180	186	191	197	203
64	110	116	122	128	134	140	145	151	157	163	169	174	180	186	192	197	204	209
65	114	120	126	132	138	144	150	156	162	168	174	180	186	192	198	204	210	216
66	118	124	130	136	142	148	155	161	167	173	179	186	192	198	204	210	216	223
67	121	127	134	140	146	153	159	166	172	178	185	191	198	204	211	217	223	230
68	125	131	138	144	151	158	164	171	177	184	190	197	203	210	216	223	230	236
69	128	135	142	149	155	162	169	176	182	189	196	203	209	216	223	230	236	243
70	132	139	146	153	160	167	174	181	188	195	202	209	216	222	229	236	243	250
71	136	143	150	157	165	172	179	186	193	200	208	215	222	229	236	243	250	257
72	140	147	154	162	169	177	184	191	199	206	213	221	228	235	242	250	258	265
73	144	151	159	166	174	182	189	197	204	212	219	227	235	242	250	257	265	272
74	148	155	163	171	179	186	194	202	210	218	225	233	241	249	256	264	272	280
75	152	160	168	176	184	192	200	208	216	224	232	240	248	256	264	272	279	287
76	156	164	172	180	189	197	205	213	221	230	238	246	254	263	271	279	287	295
Height (Inches)									Body Weight (Pounds)									
58	177	181	186	191	196	201	205	210	215	220	224	229	234	239	244	248	253	258
59	183	188	193	198	203	208	212	217	222	227	232	237	242	247	252	257	262	267
60	189	194	199	204	209	215	220	225	230	235	240	245	250	255	261	266	271	276
61	195	201	206	211	217	222	227	232	238	243	248	254	259	264	269	275	280	285
62	202	207	213	218	224	229	235	240	246	251	256	262	267	273	278	284	289	295
63	208	214	220	225	231	237	242	248	254	259	265	270	278	282	287	293	299	304
64	215	221	227	239	238	244	250	256	262	267	273	279	285	291	296	302	308	314
65	222	228	234	240	246	252	258	264	270	276	282	288	294	300	306	312	318	324
66	229	235	241	247	253	260	266	272	278	284	291	297	303	309	315	322	328	334
67	236	242	249	255	261	268	274	280	287	293	299	306	312	319	329	331	338	344
68	243	249	256	262	269	276	282	289	295	302	308	315	329	328	335	341	348	354
69	250	257	263	270	277	284	291	297	304	311	318	324	331	338	349	351	358	365
70	257	264	271	278	285	292	299	306	313	320	327	334	341	348	355	362	369	376
71	265	272	279	286	293	301	308	315	322	329	338	343	351	358	365	379	379	386
72	272	279	287	294	302	309	316	324	331	338	346	353	361	368	375	383	390	397
73	280	288	295	302	310	318	325	333	340	348	355	363	371	378	386	393	401	408
74	287	295	303	311	319	326	334	342	350	358	365	373	381	389	396	404	419	420
75	295	303	311	319	327	335	343	351	359	367	375	383	391	399	407	415	423	431
76	304	312	320	328	336	344	353	361	369	377	385	394	402	410	418	426	435	443
BMI	37	38	39	40	41	42	43	44	45	46	47	48	49	50	51	52	53	54

To use the table, find the appropriate height in the left-hand column. Move across to a given weight. The number at the top of the column is the BMI at that height and weight. Pounds have been rounded off.

defined as the frequency of occurrence of any event or condition over time and in relation to the population in which it occurs. Asian American children have the lowest incidence of obesity. Native American children have the highest incidence of obesity. Data comparing obesity rates between years 2011 to 2012 and years 2013 to 2014 demonstrated that obesity rates remained relatively consistent at the following percentages for children aged 2 to 19 years (Ogden, Carroll, Frayar, & Flegal, 2015):

- For non-Hispanic Asian males, the prevalence of obesity is 11.8%.
- For non-Hispanic white males, the prevalence of obesity is 14.3%
- For non-Hispanic black males, the prevalence is 18.4%

- For Hispanic males, the prevalence is 22.4%
- For non-Hispanic Asian females, the prevalence is 5.3%.
- For non-Hispanic white females, the prevalence is 15.1%.
- For non-Hispanic black females, the prevalence is 20.7%.
- For Hispanic females, the prevalence is 21.4%.

Basic Science of Energy Imbalance

To understand the science of energy imbalance, think of the human body as a machine. Tens of thousands of researchers have spent years studying how the human body reacts to a kilocalorie imbalance. It is not adequate to say people weigh too much or too little because they overeat and do not exercise enough or vice versa. We need to ask: Why does someone's

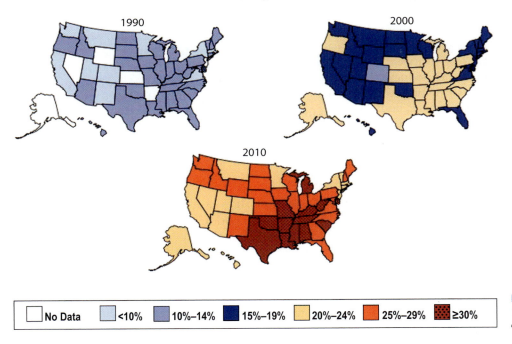

Obesity Trends* Among U.S. Adults
BRFSS, 1990, 2000, 2010
(*BMI ≥30, or about 30 lbs. overweight for 5'4" person)

| No Data | <10% | 10%–14% | 15%–19% | 20%–24% | 25%–29% | ≥30% |

FIGURE 16-1 U.S. Obesity Trends 1990 to 2010 (*www.cdc.gov/obesity/data/trends.html*).

body seek or not seek food or exercise, when the human machine has adequate or inadequate energy available? What is not working? First, a brief outline of the science of energy imbalance follows.

Energy Imbalance

Energy imbalance results when the number of **kilocalories** eaten does not equal the number used for energy. An individual can determine whether food intake is meeting energy needs by monitoring his or her weight. If more kilocalories are eaten than are used by the body, weight gain will occur. If fewer kilocalories are eaten than are used by the body (and protein intake is adequate), weight loss will occur. (A low protein intake over an extended period will eventually lead to fluid retention and a subsequent weight gain from the fluid retained. In this situation, energy imbalance is difficult to ascertain by body weight alone.) Anyone can determine whether he or she is in energy balance by monitoring his or her weight over time. (This assumes normal hydration.)

There are two basic principles of energy imbalance. First, it takes a specific number of kilocalories to gain or lose a pound of body fat. Second, the body stores energy and uses that stored energy in a highly specific manner.

The Five-Hundred Rule

To lose 1 pound of body fat per week, an individual must eat 500 kilocalories fewer per day than his or her body *expends* for 7 days. To gain 1 pound of body fat per week, the

individual must eat 500 kilocalories more per day for 7 days than his or her body expends. The gain or loss of body fat need not occur during the course of a week; the kilocalorie surplus or deficit may occur over a month or year. The principle is the same. The total number of kilocalories required to gain or lose a pound of body fat is 3,500. Too many kilocalories from any source of carbohydrates, fat, and/or protein promote weight gain. The 500 rule means that weight loss is independent of diet composition.

The key term here is *expend*. As you learned in Chapter 5 on energy balance, the human body has some small subtle internal mechanisms that cause more or fewer kilocalories to be expended in some situations. The human body also has some small subtle internal mechanisms that cause the individual to eat more or less food in some situations.

Body Fat Stores

Excess kilocalories from any source (fat, carbohydrate, or protein) are stored as body fat in adipose fat tissue, which can accumulate in unlimited amounts. This accumulation can lead to overweight and, eventually, obesity. During a kilocalorie deficit, the body first seeks the energy necessary to sustain body functions in glycogen stores, which are limited. When a kilocalorie deficit occurs for longer than about 1 day, the body seeks the energy necessary to sustain its functions in both body fat stores (adipose tissue) and protein stores (organ and muscle mass). Weight loss always includes some loss of LBM. How much LBM is lost depends on how the weight loss is achieved.

Energy Imbalance and Body Composition

Weight loss affects body composition, and body composition affects health. The human body's two largest components (after water) are fat and lean mass that includes protein. Protein is stored primarily in muscle tissue, organs, and certain body chemicals. Preservation of LBM and optimal health go hand in hand. A loss of structural body content (e.g., heart and respiratory muscles, kidney, liver, body chemicals) is undesirable. Exercise can preserve and somewhat increase LBM. Weight gain increases body fat content. Weight loss decreases both body fat and LBM. An understanding of the difference between body fat content and LBM content is crucial to understanding the science of energy imbalance. The health benefits of weight loss are all related to a loss of body fat and not a loss of LBM (see Genomic Gem 16-1).

Loss of Fat Versus Loss of Water and Protein

Most people, especially the overweight, can lose only about 2 pounds of body fat a week by eating less. Any weight loss beyond that is probably due to loss of water and/or lean muscle tissue. There is always some loss of body protein along with body fat during weight loss. This loss occurs because LBM is more metabolically active and therefore burns more kilocalories than fat tissue. The loss of body protein from reduced food intake is greater than the loss of body protein from a combination of reduced food intake and regular exercise. Thus, physical activity during weight loss protects LBM. Also, the greater the rate of weight loss, the more LBM is lost.

Severity of Obesity and LBM

Weight loss affects body composition of lean and obese people differently. The amount of LBM an individual loses during weight reduction depends on the degree of severity of the obesity. Obese animals tolerate starvation better than

thin ones, and the same is true of humans. *Tolerate* means that they conserve body protein during weight loss. This means that overweight and mildly obese individuals are at a higher risk of becoming protein-depleted during rapid weight loss. Rapid weight loss (0.5 to 1.0 pounds per day), if sustained for many weeks, is associated with an excessive loss of LBM and protein depletion of the heart. Malnutrition of the heart muscle can lead to sudden death. As an individual loses more and more fat during rapid weight loss, the ability to conserve LBM decreases. Thus, the length of time an individual diets as well as his or her beginning total body fat content have an impact on the amount of LBM lost.

Consequences of Obesity

Obesity can lead to many adverse consequences. For example, the distribution of body fat affects a person's susceptibility to medical problems, and the **psychological** ramifications of obesity are significant. Clients are commonly enmeshed in a tangle of societal, cultural, prejudicial, and psychological issues. Many clients find great difficulty in breaking the cycle of behaviors that contribute to obesity. With an understanding of the issues, health-care providers can educate overweight and obese clients about the need for weight loss and encourage these clients to lose weight.

Social

The social consequences of obesity are connected to cultural expectations and the documented prejudice many obese people experience.

Cultural Expectations

Culture, in this context, refers to the convictions of a given people during a given period. Currently, many Americans perceive leanness as being attractive and desirable and fatness as being unattractive and undesirable. Some studies have demonstrated that culture can affect attitudes toward thinness. One study found that African American women with larger body figures reported higher satisfaction and a more positive attitude than Caucasian women (Webb, Webb, Fults-McMurtery, & Fuller, 2014). Yet what is and has been considered attractive has changed over time. Leanness has not always been the preferred body build. For example, during the 1800s, an overly fat body was considered the most attractive. Carrying excess weight meant that the person was well-to-do—that he or she could afford to overeat. Our society is slowly changing perceptions of what is attractive. For example, many perceive women with well-developed muscles as being more attractive than their lean, not-so-muscular counterparts. The increased numbers of female bodybuilders demonstrate this attitudinal shift.

In the United States, obese people have been under intense pressure to lose weight. Evidence of this pressure is the billions of dollars spent on weight-reduction programs

GENOMIC GEM 16-1

Obesity Genetic or Environmental?

Research has demonstrated that children with obese relatives are associated with a higher risk of obesity regardless if the family members live together or apart (Trier et al, 2014). This does not mean that a child with a high complement of susceptibility genes will inevitably become overweight, but his or her genetic endowment gives them a stronger predisposition. Our environment gives children unprecedented opportunities to overeat and be sedentary. Therefore, nutritious food and participation in daily physical activity should be provided to counterbalance the effect of genetics and help should be given to those who are more susceptible to obesity.

and special foods each year. In an effort to be more attractive, many obese clients try to lose weight. Over time, however, most people regain the weight they have lost and commonly gain an additional few pounds. Thus, a self-defeating cycle begins. Clients generally need to be reminded that, although body weight is important, health and wellness are even more important.

Documented Prejudice

Research has documented that health-care professionals, including both physicians and nurses, often have biases toward obese clients. Studies have demonstrated that many health-care providers may hold strong negative attitudes and stereotypes about obese clients that can result in prejudice, derogatory comments, and poor treatment in the health-care setting (Phelan et al, 2015). Health-care workers need to try to understand their own feelings about fatness, obesity, and obese persons. Sometimes, health-care workers unconsciously insult obese clients. For example, comments made in front of clients, such as "It will take three of us to move this client," are hurtful. Health-care providers should treat obese clients with respect, kindness, and patience.

Psychological

Obesity can be associated with a range of psychological problems, which may result from food restriction. One important psychological consequence of obesity is body image disturbances.

Body Image Disturbances

Body image is the mental picture a person has of himself or herself. A disturbed body image can manifest itself in two ways. First, people with distorted body images are usually dissatisfied with their bodies. Chronic complaints, demands for extra attention, and frequent negative statements made by clients about the way they look may be signs of an underlying body image disturbance.

Second, persons with distorted body images frequently do not view their bodies realistically. For example, people may view themselves as having certain body parts larger than they actually are. A later section in this chapter discusses clients with anorexia nervosa, a mental health disorder, who frequently have body image disturbances. Very thin clients who have this condition frequently view themselves as overweight despite valid evidence to the contrary.

Medical

Obesity is considered a major health problem in the United States and is also considered a chronic medical condition. People who are overweight or obese are more likely to develop health problems such as:

- Hypertension
- Dyslipidemia (e.g., high total cholesterol or high levels of triglycerides)

- Type 2 diabetes
- Coronary heart disease
- Stroke
- Gallbladder and liver disease
- Osteoarthritis
- Sleep apnea and respiratory problems (CDC, March 5, 2018)

The distribution of body fat affects risks. **Abdominal obesity**, in which excess weight is between the client's chest and pelvis, is more dangerous than gluteal-femoral obesity. Clients with abdominal obesity are said to be shaped like an apple and are especially vulnerable to chronic disease risks associated with excessive body weight. A man's waist should measure less than 40 inches (102 cm), and a women's waist should measure less than 35 inches (88 cm).

There continues to be an increase in the prevalence of abdominal obesity in U.S. adults, which increases the risk of developing hypertension, diabetes, and cardiovascular disease (Chia et al, 2016). In **gluteal-femoral obesity**, the excess weight is around the client's buttocks, hips, and thighs. Clients with gluteal-femoral obesity are said to be pear-shaped and are not as susceptible to chronic disease risks associated with excessive body fat.

The **waist-to-hip ratio** measures central distribution of fat. Waist-to-hip ratio is calculated by dividing waist circumference by hip circumference. A ratio of 1.0 or more in men and 0.85 or more in women indicates increased abdominal weight compared with total body fat, which is a risk factor for obesity-related medical conditions.

Factors Influencing Food Intake

Lifestyle behaviors, appetite, satiety, and, questionably, macronutrient energy distribution influence food intake.

Lifestyle

These factors affect how much is eaten and influence kilocalorie consumption:

- Variety—The greater the variety of food served, the more kilocalories consumed.
- Taste—The better food tastes, the more is eaten.
- Weekend activity—Eating at regular times and planning non–food-related activities for weekends may assist in weight control.
- Skipping breakfast—People who regularly skip breakfast are more likely to be obese. Those eating four or more times daily are less likely to be obese. The fourth meal should be a small snack. Skipping meals is not a good weight-control strategy.
- Eating out—Eating meals away from home is associated with increased energy intake and lower nutritional quality (U.S. Department of Agriculture [USDA], December 30, 2016).
- Speed—The faster food is eaten, the more is consumed because it takes a little longer for satiety signals to reach the

brain. The more foods need to be chewed, the fewer kilocalories are eaten because it takes time to chew the food.

■ Soda intake—The consumption of sweetened soda is associated with excess added sugar and energy intake (World Health Organization, January 10, 2017).

■ Dietary fat—High dietary fat foods tend to be higher energy-dense foods.

Lifestyle behaviors that are responsible for *decreased* energy expenditure also increase body weight.

■ Sedentary activities—The more hours spent on screen time—watching television, playing video games, or being on the computer—the less time is spent being physically active.

■ Changes in energy expenditure—Small daily increases in energy expenditure, such as getting up to change the channels on the television and opening the garage door manually, may be significant over the course of a year.

Physiology

Numerous hormones and neuropeptides that stimulate or inhibit food intake through central and peripheral mechanisms have been identified. Molecules that affect metabolic rates and energy expenditure are also an area of current research. Figure 16-2 illustrates multiple molecules and pathways involved in the internal regulation of food intake. In general, there is redundancy and counterbalance among these pathways so that, for instance, the inhibitory effect of one molecule is dampened by another. This intricate redundancy and counterbalance makes effective treatment of obesity complex. Perhaps as researchers learn more about the human energy balance system, more effective and safe treatments for imbalances may be available.

The brain, stomach, small intestine, and fat cells are all part of this complex energy balance system. The stomach, small intestines, and fat cells send messages to the brain to turn on or turn off eating. The triggers that influence food intake include satiety signals and hunger signals. When the brain, for instance, receives a satiety signal, animals stop eating.

Peptide hormones produced from the gastrointestinal tract are considered regulators of appetite, including both satiety and food intake (Nguo, Walker, Bonham, & Huggins, 2016). Ghrelin is one example of a gastric-made polypeptide that stimulates growth hormone and regulates food intake. Serum ghrelin increases before a meal and decreases after a meal (Yang, Liu, Yang, & Jue, 2014).

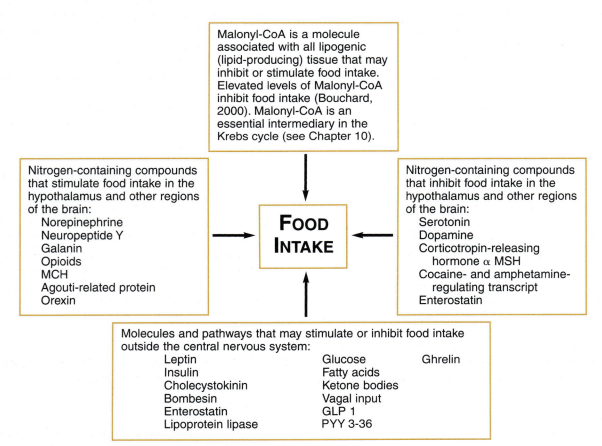

FIGURE 16-2 The hormones, molecules, and pathways that influence food intake through central or peripheral mechanisms. *(Adapted from Bouchard, C: Inhibition of food intake by inhibitors of fatty acid synthase. N Engl J Med 343:25, 2000.)*

Neuropeptide Y is one example of a polypeptide in the brain that results in increased food intake. This chemical causes carbohydrate cravings, initiates eating, decreases energy expenditure, and increases fat storage. All of these actions favor positive energy balance and weight gain. Leptin, a protein made by fat cells, is a hormone that acts on the hypothalamus to decrease food intake. Leptin acts on receptors to counteract effects of feeding stimulants secreted by cells in the gut and in the hypothalamus. Interestingly, blood leptin levels are generally increased in obese individuals and are proportional to the total amount of adipose tissue in the body (Ghouse, Barwal, & Wattamwar, 2016). This is a short summary of the many ways the body has evolved to cope and survive during repeated cycles of feast and famine. Appetite can also be influenced by gastrointestinal distention to decrease food intake and contractions of an empty stomach to increase food intake. Satiety signals are sent from this area to the brain.

Macronutrient Energy Composition

Researchers have conducted many studies on the role of macronutrient composition in energy balance. Following is a brief summary of this research. Protein has been found to be the most satiating macronutrient (Chungchunlam, Henare, Ganesh, & Moughan, 2015) followed by carbohydrate and then fat. The brain appears to need some carbohydrate (delivered as glucose) for an individual to achieve satiety. In addition, fiber expands the stomach to assist in counteracting the release of polypeptides that increase food intake. In summary, eating a well-balanced meal that is planned to provide the energy nutrients within the accepted macronutrient distribution range (AMDR) is the best approach to weight management.

Glycemic Index

A low-glycemic diet may also help with weight management, although studies are still producing conflicting findings. Some experts believe that eating carbohydrates that have a low glycemic index (GI) may result in a spontaneous reduction in food intake. GI is a measure of how much the blood glucose level increases after consumption of a particular food that contains a given amount of carbohydrate. A slice of white bread or glucose is the reference food. All other foods' GIs are set in comparison to white bread or glucose and are ranked according to their potential to raise blood glucose compared with the reference white bread or glucose. Foods with a low GI are thought to promote satiety and decrease food intake. The glycemic index of mixed meals is not known. Following are some examples of the glycemic index of selected foods. Note: The reference food is white bread:

- White bread, 100
- Glucose, 138
- Fructose, 26
- Honey, 126
- Whole-wheat bread, 100
- Rye (whole grain, pumpernickel), 88
- Cornflakes, 121
- Banana, 84
- Baked potato, 116
- Kidney beans (canned), 74
- Ice cream, 69
- Sucrose, 83
- White rice (polished, boiled 10 to 25 minutes), 81
- Oatmeal, 85
- All-bran, 74
- Plum, 34
- Sweet potato, 70
- Lentils (green, canned), 74
- Skim milk, 46
- Orange, 59
- Orange juice, 71
- Yogurt, 52
- Soybeans (canned), 22

If the reference food is glucose, the numbers will be different, but not wrong. Many factors influence a food's GI. The rate of consumption and the time of day a food is eaten may increase or decrease a particular food's GI. Other components in a food besides carbohydrate influence a food's GI, including fat, fiber, and protein content and starch characteristics. How a food is prepared and processed influences GI. Physiological effects, including pregastric hydrolysis, gastric emptying rate, intestinal response, hydrolysis and absorption, pancreatic and gut hormone response, and colonic effects, influence a food's GI. Nondietary factors that influence a food's GI include medications taken, stress, physical activity, and overall health status.

Clinical use of GI as a guide to food selection may provide a health benefit and appears to be without adverse effects. Hints to incorporate the GI into the diet include these suggestions:

- Keep it simple—substitute whole grains and fresh fruits and beans for higher-GI foods.
- If eating a food with a high glycemic index, combine with a low-glycemic-index food to balance effects on blood sugar (American Diabetes Association, May 14, 2014).
- Do not worry about foods that contribute 5 or fewer grams of carbohydrate in a serving. Some nutritionally dense foods, such as carrots, have a higher GI but contain a low amount of CHO in a serving.

Theories About Obesity

Theories about obesity are plentiful. Box 16-1 discusses one theory: the malfunctioning hypothalamus.

Efficient Metabolism

Some obese individuals actually require fewer kilocalories for normal body functions than do lean individuals. Some obese individuals thus use kilocalories very efficiently.

Brown Fat

Brown fat, a special type of fat cell, accounts for less than 1% of total body weight. Brown fat burns kilocalories and then releases the energy as heat. Energy released as heat is not stored as body fat. Some obese people may have defective brown fat or less brown fat than lean people.

Set Point Theory

The set point theory argues that each individual has a unique, relatively stable, adult body weight based on biologic factors. Hence, an obese person may have a higher set point than a lean counterpart.

Number of Fat Cells

Obese individuals have many more fat cells than do their lean counterparts. A kilocalorie deficit can reduce the fat in each cell but cannot break down the cell. Once manufactured, a fat cell exists until death. Empty fat cells release a chemical messenger that travels to the brain and sends a message to the reduced obese person to fill the depleted fat cells. As a result, the reduced obese person must learn to constantly ignore internal hunger signals. Ignoring such pains can be done for a short period, but long-term adaptation to hunger is difficult.

Enzymes in the Metabolic Chain

Lipoprotein lipase is an enzyme that is involved in the uptake of fatty acids for the manufacture of fat in individual fat cells. Research has shown that the activity of this enzyme increases during weight reduction. This action makes fat cells even more efficient in synthesizing fats.

Obesogens

Research has emerged regarding **obesogens**. Obesogens are chemicals in the environment that are thought to mimic or block the action of hormones responsible for the development of fat tissue and energy homeostasis (Konkel, 2015). Known and suspected obesogens include the following:

- Diet: monosodium glutamate
- Smoking: nicotine
- Industrial chemicals: bisphenol A (BPA) and perfluorooctanoic acid (PFOA)
- Organophosphate and organochlorine pesticides

Federal Guidelines

There are clear advantages to weight loss for overweight and obese clients. The primary reason should be to decrease the risk of disease. Treatment is also indicated for persons who have an obesity-related disorder. Options offered to clients should depend on their degree of overweight and obesity.

Advantages of Weight Loss

Federal clinical guidelines for identifying overweight and obesity in adults focuses on the medical benefits to be derived from weight loss. This panel recommends:

- Weight loss to lower blood pressure in overweight and obese persons with high blood pressure
- Weight loss to lower elevated levels of cholesterol, low-density lipoprotein cholesterol, and triglycerides and to raise low levels of high-density lipoprotein cholesterol in overweight and obese persons with dyslipidemia (see Chapter 18)
- Some weight loss to lower elevated blood glucose levels in overweight and obese persons with type 2 diabetes

Determining Overweight and Obesity

According to U.S. federal guidelines, practitioners should use the BMI and waist circumference to classify the degree of energy imbalance in clients. Body weight alone can be used to follow weight loss and to determine efficacy of treatment (U.S. Department of Health and Human Services [HHS], National Institutes of Health [NIH], National Heart, Lung, and Blood Institute [NHLBI], 2017a).

Treatment of Energy Imbalances

Federal guidelines address goals for weight loss, how to achieve weight loss, goals for weight maintenance, how to maintain weight loss, and special treatment groups.

Goals for Weight Loss

The initial goal of weight loss should be to reduce body weight by 10% from the baseline (current weight). With success, further weight loss can be attempted, if indicated. Safe weight loss occurs at about 1 to 2 pounds per week for a period of 6 months, with the subsequent strategy based on the amount of weight lost (HHS, NIH, NHLBI, 2017b).

Achieving Weight Loss

The approach to weight loss should depend on professional evaluation and the client's BMI, waist circumference, and other factors. These are some of the weight-loss treatment options for clients:

- Dietary therapy (also called medical nutrition therapy)
- Physical activity
- Behavior therapy
- Pharmacotherapy
- Weight-loss surgery
- Combined therapy (some or all of the above)

Diet Therapy

A weight-loss diet should include a reduction in total kilocalories averaging 500 to 750 kcalories per day decrease while maintaining a daily consumption of 1,000 to 1,500 kcalories per day. Diets must maintain adequate amounts of all nutrients and should provide at least:

- 45% of kilocalories from carbohydrate
- 20% of kilocalories from fat
- 10% of the kilocalories from protein or 0.8 gram/kg, whichever is higher
- Remaining 25% of kilocalories open to negotiation with the client
- 25 to 35 grams of fiber
- All essential vitamins and minerals

The meal plan should be one the client can and will follow. When clients are given a standardized meal plan, weight loss is not usually successful. However, when behavior modification, nutritional counseling, and exercise recommendations support the meal plan, weight loss can be more successful.

Different clients need different types of dietary directions. A few clients want to be told what to eat and will follow through with appropriate behaviors. Some clients prefer receiving simplified instructions and do not want to learn a complicated diet. Following ChooseMyPlate Guidelines and using a SuperTracker (USDA, 2017) dietary plan may work well for the latter type of client (provided behavior modifications and the need for exercise are also discussed). Portion control must be emphasized.

There are also numerous smartphone and computer applications available for the more technologically advanced client. Certain applications allow clients the ability to track their daily intake of calories and nutrients and log exercise minutes. The program also allows the client the ability to scan bar codes on packaged food items to enter nutrient data. Online and mobile applications give clients objective, visual cues that can assist in holding the client accountable for their weight loss goals.

Sometimes clients are unable to make drastic changes in their food intake and become discouraged. In this situation, nutritional counselors should encourage clients to make major behavioral changes in their eating habits slowly. The goal in weight-reduction counseling is to help the client make permanent lifestyle changes.

Physical Activity

Population studies conducted in the United States, Great Britain, and France suggest that the rapidly increasing prevalence of obesity in recent decades may be largely due to increasing sedentary behaviors, perhaps to a greater extent than dietary excesses. Some nutrition counselors advocate a nondieting approach to weight control. Exercise and healthy eating is encouraged instead of adherence to a rigid diet plan (Fig. 16-3).

Physical activity should be part of any comprehensive weight-loss and weight maintenance program because it:

- Modestly contributes to weight loss in overweight and obese adults
- May decrease abdominal fat
- Increases cardiopulmonary fitness
- Increases LBM

Initially, adults should participate in moderate levels of exercise for 150 minutes, or 2 hours and 30 minutes, each week as well as performing resistance training 2 to 3 days per week. The person who is attempting to lose weight should gradually increase the duration of their exercise with some adults having to participate in 300 minutes of exercise a week to achieve their weight loss goals.

To identify individuals at risk for heart disease, a healthcare provider should screen all clients before making exercise recommendations. Clients with known heart, lung, or metabolic disease should have a physician-supervised stress test before beginning an exercise program.

Behavior Modification

Behavior modification is a useful adjunct to weight loss and maintenance plans. It is assumed that eating and exercise are learned behaviors, and with lifestyle modification long-term changes to physical activity levels and dietary habits can occur (Stoutenberg, Stanzilis, & Falcon, 2015). A client's

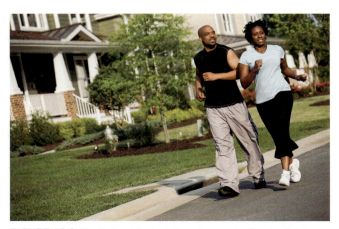

FIGURE 16-3 Physical activity is an important part of maintaining a healthy weight.

motivation to enter weight-loss therapy and his or her readiness to implement a plan require evaluation. Permanent weight loss can result only from a permanent change in eating and exercise behaviors. See Box 16-2 for common weight-reduction strategies.

Pharmacotherapy

According to federal guidelines, U.S. Food and Drug Administration–approved weight-loss medications may be used as part of a comprehensive weight-loss program, which includes diet and physical activity, for clients with a BMI equal to or greater than 30 and no concomitant obesity-related risk factors or diseases. For clients with a BMI equal to or greater than 27 and concomitant obesity-related risk factors or diseases, medications may also be indicated.

BOX 16-2 ■ Behavior Modification Techniques to Share With Clients

These behavior-change tips can help facilitate a weight-loss program.

Self-Monitoring
- Keep a food diary and record all food and fluid intake.
- Keep a weekly graph of weight change.
- Keep an exercise diary.

Stimulus Control
- At home, limit all food intake to one specific place.
- Plan food intake for each day.
- Rearrange your schedule to avoid inappropriate eating.
- Sit down at a table while eating.
- Use a smaller dinner plate.
- At a party, sit a distance from snack foods, eat before you go, and substitute lower kilocalorie drinks for alcohol.
- Decide beforehand what you will order at a restaurant.
- Have the restaurant bag half the meal to go before serving the meal.
- Save or reschedule everyday activities for times when you are hungry.
- Avoid boredom; keep a list of activities on the refrigerator.
- Remove high-fat food from the home.

Slower Eating
- Drink a glass of water before each meal. Drink sips of water between bites of food.
- Swallow food before putting more food on the utensil.
- Try to be the last one to finish eating.
- Pause for a minute during your meal and attempt to increase the number of pauses.

Reward Yourself
- Chart your progress.
- Make an agreement with yourself or a significant other for a meaningful reward.
- Do not reward yourself with food.

Cognitive Strategies
- View exercise as a means of controlling hunger.
- Practice relaxation techniques.
- Imagine yourself ordering a side salad, diet dressing, low-fat milk, and a small hamburger at a fast-food restaurant.
- Reframe negative thoughts with positive thinking.
- Enhance social support.

Medications should never be used without lifestyle modification. Medication therapy for obesity should be continually monitored for efficacy and safety and discontinued if the client does not lose weight. Medication therapy should only be used for 3 to 6 months. Table 16-3 lists weight-loss medications, actions, and adverse effects.

Surgery

Weight-loss surgery is an option for selected clients with clinically extreme or severe obesity (BMI >40 or >35 with comorbid conditions) when less-invasive methods of weight loss have failed and the client is at high risk for obesity-associated morbidity or mortality.

There are currently four FDA-approved devices for the treatment of obesity:

- Gastric band—band placed around upper portion of stomach to decrease stomach size.
- Electrical stimulation system—device placed in abdomen to block nerve activity between the stomach and the brain.
- Gastric balloon—balloon placed in stomach to take up space.
- Gastric emptying system—tube used to empty stomach contents after eating (U.S. Food and Drug Administration, May 8, 2017)

Numerous surgical procedures are used to treat obesity. A **jejunoileal bypass** involves the removal of a part of the small intestine. Clients lose weight after this procedure because they cannot absorb all the food they eat, although this places these clients at a nutritional risk. The jejunoileal bypass procedure is rarely performed currently; however, health-care providers are likely to encounter clients who have had this procedure.

Two of the most commonly performed surgeries for weight management are **gastric banding** and **gastric bypass (Roux-en-Y).** Diagrams of these procedures are shown in Figure 16-4.

Gastric banding involves the placement of an adjustable band to create a small stomach pouch. When the stomach is smaller or reduced, only a limited amount of food can be consumed at one feeding. This induces weight loss from reduced kilocalorie intake. The Roux-en-Y gastric bypass procedure results in the creation of a small gastric pouch. Before surgery, the surgeon specifies a diet, and the client must make an enormous commitment to follow the diet exactly and choose foods carefully.

Another surgical option is the **gastric sleeve** procedure. During the procedure, the surgeon removes approximately 75% to 80% of the stomach until it resembles a tube or sleeve. This surgical approach will also result in strict, postprocedure, dietary changes.

Postprocedure dietary changes include not only a reduction in the volume of food that can be consumed but also limitations on the variation of foods that are acceptable to consume. Clients who have undergone either the Roux-en-Y or the gastric sleeve procedure will begin a diet

TABLE 16-3 Weight-Loss Medications

DRUG	ACTION	ADVERSE EFFECTS
Naltrexone sustained-release and bupropion sustained-release (Contrave)	Norepinephrine and dopamine reuptake inhibitor and opioid receptor antagonist	Headache Dizziness Constipation Caution use in congestive heart failure
Liraglutide (Saxenda)	Glucagon-like peptide 1 receptor agonist	Nausea Diarrhea Fatigue Increased lipase
Orlistat (Xenical)	Inhibits pancreatic lipase, decreases fat absorption	Decrease in absorption of fat-soluble vitamins Soft stools and anal leakage Possible link to breast cancer
Lorcaserin (Belviq)	Serotonin receptor agonist	Insomnia Dry mouth Constipation Fatigue
Phentermine and extended-release topiramate (Qsymia)	Norepinephrine, dopamine, and serotonin reuptake inhibitor	Increased heart rate Increased risk of birth defects Tingling of hands and feet Insomnia Dry mouth

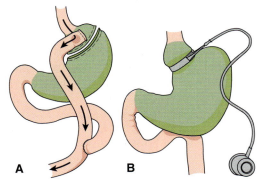

FIGURE 16-4 Surgery for weight loss. *A*, Roux-en-Y stomach bypass: large portion of stomach and duodenum are bypassed. *B*, Adjustable gastric banding: stomach opening can be tightened or loosened over time to change the size of the passage.

with specific dietary progression guidelines that must be followed. The diet for both procedures begins with small sips of clear fluids and advances slowly, increasing the volume and texture of food.

Bariatric surgeons usually depend on team members to screen and monitor clients, who typically have several sessions with the team before the procedure is done. Most surgeons screen and monitor clients because the liability risk is great if clients are not screened and educated.

Clinical Application 16-1 discusses problems that clients often encounter after gastric surgery and suggests general guidelines for these clients to follow. Clients should be followed carefully postoperatively because of risks for deficiencies such as iron, folic acid, and vitamin B$_{12}$. Clients are also at risk for maladaptive eating behavior. Clinical Application 16-2 discusses nutrition guidelines for these clients postsurgery.

CLINICAL APPLICATION 16-1

Complications of Gastroplasty and Gastric Bypass

There are many potential acute complications of gastric surgery for weight reduction. These include:

- Nausea, vomiting, bloating, and/or heartburn: These signs and symptoms can be caused by overeating, not chewing food well, eating too quickly, drinking cold or carbonated beverages, using drinking straws, or eating gassy foods.
- Obstruction: An obstruction is the blockage of a structure. In this case, a blockage can occur close to the area stapled. A frequent cause of obstruction is poorly chewed food. The result is stomach pain, nausea, and vomiting.
- Dumping syndrome: Intake of concentrated sweets and large quantities of fluids causes quick dumping of food into the small intestine. Abdominal fullness, nausea, diarrhea 15 minutes after eating, warmth, weakness, fainting, racing pulse, and cold sweats are symptoms of this syndrome.
- Among the long-term risks is osteoporosis, due to decreased calcium absorption.

Expected results from gastric surgery procedures should always be explained to clients. No permanent effects can be promised, and having the surgery does not mean that afterward the client can overeat without weight gain. Ninety percent of weight loss occurs in the first year, and clients typically begin to gain weight again in the second and third years. The client should view the procedure as a tool to be used in conjunction with behavioral training—the small pouch helps clients learn to reduce and slow down food intake. After the first year, because of pouch stretching or intestinal adaptation, much of the effect of the surgery can be negated, and

CLINICAL APPLICATION 16-2

Post–Gastric Surgery Nutrition Guidelines

These strategies can help clients adjust after surgery:

- Eat three to six small meals per day.
- Eat slowly.
- Chew food thoroughly.
- Eat very small quantities.
- Stop eating when full.
- Do not eat longer than 30 minutes at a time.
- Drink most fluids between meals.
- Select a balanced diet high in lean proteins.
- Take a chewable multivitamin–multimineral supplement.
- Exercise regularly.

BOX 16-3 ■ Weight Management in Children

These are three ways in which individuals and communities can help children enjoy the physical activities that can aid in weight management.

Develop appropriate activities—The enjoyment of physical activity should start young. Children aged 2 to 5 years should engage in active play several times a day. Examples of appropriate activities for young children include ballet lessons, tricycle or bike riding, walking daily with a family member, swimming lessons, and sledding.

Develop play areas—Communities need to develop safe play areas for children. Local school districts should be encouraged to offer more opportunities for young people to be active in a noncompetitive environment.

Encourage noncompetitive activities—A totally sedentary child who is uncomfortable in a competitive situation will gain important health benefits from physical activity. Children aged 6–17 should engage in 1 hour of physical activity each day at a moderate to vigorous aerobic intensity.

the lost weight may be regained. Studies have shown that 30% to 97% of clients who underwent a surgical intervention for weight loss will experience long-term weight gain, and 37% will experience excessive weight gain defined as gaining greater than 25% of weight lost (Conceicao et al, 2016).

Weight-Loss Maintenance

Weight regain typically occurs after weight loss. A program of dietary therapy, physical activity, and behavior therapy enhances the likelihood of weight-loss maintenance. Drug therapy can also be used according to the guidelines published by the National Institutes of Health; however, drug safety and efficacy beyond 1 year of total treatment have not been established.

The National Weight Control Registry (NWCR) was founded in 1994 to investigate people who have had long-term successful weight loss and maintenance. There are currently 10,000 people registered, and they report the following behaviors as contributing to their continued weight loss success:

- Have maintained diets low in calories.
- Have maintained diets low in fat.
- 78% report eating breakfast daily.
- 75% weigh themselves at least weekly.
- 62% watch less than 10 hours of television each week.
- 90% exercise, on average, 1 hour per day (The National Weight Control Registry, 2017).

The Role of Nutrition Educators

Appropriate roles for nutrition educators include:

- Providing accurate information
- Assisting children to prevent unhealthy weight gain (see Box 16-3)
- Warning against dangerous practices, such as self-imposed starvation diets that eliminate one or more of the major food groups and encourage the intake of only one food group (see Table 16-4)

- Guiding clients to understand the risks and benefits of weight loss and weight-loss programs, products, medicines, and procedures
- Teaching clients to evaluate the risks and benefits of surgery for themselves
- Referring clients to health-care professionals, including physicians and dietitians, when appropriate
- Helping clients set realistic goals (see Box 16-4)
- In states that have regulations, assisting in efforts to enforce these standards for safe weight loss

Reduced Body Mass

Clients with a reduced body mass are as difficult, if not more difficult, to treat as overweight or obese clients. Body fat has important roles in insulation and protection of body organs. A client with a low body fat content usually has a loss of LBM as well, and loss of this functioning tissue concerns clinicians. Women may cease to ovulate and menstruate when the percentage of body fat falls below 15% to 17%. The client may experience cardiac abnormalities and become more prone to infections. These clients are at risk for osteoporosis in the long-term.

Classification

A person with a BMI below 18.5 should be evaluated before being classified as underweight. A man with a body fat content less than 15% and a woman with a body fat content less than 18% (if known) need to be evaluated and assessed before being classified as having a reduced body mass. The only reliable method to determine if the individual is at a nutritional risk is to do a complete nutritional assessment.

Consequences

Long-term follow-up of studies indicates that excessive leanness is associated with increased mortality and decreased life expectancy. However, the causes of mortality are different

TABLE 16-4   Weight-Loss Diets in the Popular Media

Fad diets come and go. Typically, fad diets limit a person to a few specific foods or food combinations and do not provide kilocalories within the acceptable macronutrient range and the nutrient density so necessary for optimal health. For example, the brain needs sufficient carbohydrate (CHO) for optimal function. One hundred and thirty grams of CHO is the average minimum amount of glucose used by the brain, and the acceptable macronutrient range for CHO is 45% to 65% of kilocalories. The following describes three popular diets, along with the diet author's rationale. Studies have failed to demonstrate long-term safety of modified-carbohydrate diets. These diets are not widely endorsed by the health-care community; however, health-care professionals should know which diets their clients may be following.

NAME OF DIET	RATIONALE OF DIET'S AUTHOR	DESCRIPTION
Atkins	Claims that processed CHO and insulin rather than excess kilocalories are responsible for weight gain and obesity.	Four phases: • Phase 1: Induction—eat protein, healthy fat, and vegetables with 20–25 g net CHO. • Phase 2: Ongoing weight loss—continue phase 1 foods and increase CHO by 5 g week until 25–50 g net CHO. • Phase 3: Premaintenance—eat phase 2 foods and introduce fruits, legumes, breads, and grain by adding 10 g CHO each week. 50–80 g net CHO • Phase 4: Lifetime maintenance—eat phase 3 foods and increase CHO to 80–100 g net CHO.
Gluten-free diet	Gluten-free diets are for the treatment of celiac disease clients, but over the last several years theories have emerged regarding gluten and weight gain. Some believe that gluten stimulates the appetite, causing a person to consume more calories, and others believe that limiting gluten limits dietary choices, which causes a person to eat less.	Avoid foods containing wheat, barley, and rye; soy sauce; whey products; and alcohol. Choose low-fat dairy. Choose monounsaturated or polyunsaturated fats. Choose low-fat protein sources. Make half the plate fruits and vegetables. Gluten-free products should contain less than 30% of calories from fat.
Paleo Diet	The author suggests that when humans were hunter-gathers their diets consisted of meat, vegetables, and seasonal fruit and now diets are dependent on grains such as breads and pastas. Following the Paleo Diet works because the author claims that it is the only diet that works with your genetics to keep you lean and fit.	Diet is high in saturated fats, moderate in animal protein, and low to medium carbohydrate. Foods to consume include grass-fed meats, fresh fruits and vegetables, eggs, nuts and seeds, and healthful oils. Foods to avoid include cereal grains, legumes, dairy, refined sugar and vegetable oils, potatoes, processed foods, and salt. Encourage to eat only when hungry.

BOX 16-4 ■ Realistic Goals

Health-care and wellness professionals can assist clients in setting realistic goals for weight reduction and encourage loss of modest amounts of weight. Typically, clients have an unrealistic weight-loss goal. Despite considerable professional agreement that weight losses of 5% to 10% from baseline are successful for reducing comorbid conditions associated with obesity, obese clients often desire weight losses two to three times greater than this. For example, a weight-reduction diet may be planned to allow for a 1-pound-per-week weight loss. The client may expect to lose 5 pounds per week. A female client may expect to be able to eventually to wear a size 5 dress as a result of dieting. This expectation is not realistic for some clients with large bones. Health-care workers provide a valuable service when they teach clients, especially those who are overweight, how to set achievable goals that will allow for maintenance and prevent future weight gain.

from those associated with excess weight. An excessively lean person is almost twice as likely to succumb to respiratory diseases, such as tuberculosis. In addition, these clients have greater difficulty maintaining body temperature during cold weather. Infections and disturbances of the gastrointestinal tract are more likely in an underweight person, as is fragile bone structure and osteoporotic changes.

Causes

A person may be underweight because of genetic factors or because of a long-term or recent weight loss. A recent weight loss can often be related to a recent new medical diagnosis (such as trauma), a psychological diagnosis, or socioeconomic issues.

Rapid Loss Increases Risk

The greater the rate of weight loss, the more the client is at a nutritional risk. **Rate** means loss per unit of time. For example, a 20-pound weight loss in 2 weeks is an excessive weight loss. Such a client has lost a large amount of LBM. However, a 20-pound weight loss during a 20-week period could be attributed mostly to a loss of body fat with a minimal loss of LBM. If the client began with surplus body fat stores, a loss of 20 pounds may not place this client at a very high nutritional risk. If the client had a reduced body mass, even a slow weight loss may place him or her at a high nutritional risk. Laboratory data are useful to determine a client's nutritional risk level.

Not all changes in body weight are caused by insufficient kilocalorie intake. For example, a client may lose several pounds of body weight over the course of a single day as a result of diuretic therapy. The weight loss in this instance would be due to water loss and not to body fat or protein loss (see Box 16-5).

Eating Disorders

There are numerous theories to the cause of the development of eating disorders, but most agree that the cause is a combination of biological, sociocultural, and psychological factors. Many experts are concerned about the prevalence of anorexia nervosa, bulimia, and binge-eating, which may all result in nutritional problems. In the United States, as many as 20 million females and 10 million males have suffered from a significant eating disorder during some point in their life (NationalEatingDisorders.org, 2016).

Anorexia Nervosa

Anorexia nervosa is a medical condition that results from self-imposed starvation. Symptoms include:

- Recent unplanned weight loss of 5% or more
- Decreased resting energy expenditure (REE)
- **Amenorrhea** (cessation of menstruation)
- Constipation
- Excessive hair loss
- Abnormal sleeping patterns
- Preoccupation with food
- Body image disturbance
- Misconception about physical status
- Intake of only 500 to 800 kilocalories per day
- Slow eating
- Increased physical activity
- Social isolation
- Intense fear of becoming obese
- Poor muscle tone

The disorder appears in 1 out of every 250 females and 1 out of every 2,000 males (El-Radhi, 2015). The client may resort to a variety of methods to lose weight, including starvation, vomiting, and laxative use. The disorder may be life-threatening.

Bulimia

Bulimia is more common than anorexia nervosa, especially during adolescence and young adulthood. The mean age for females at diagnosis was 23 years. An estimated 1.1% to 4.2% of females have bulimia nervosa in their lifetime. The condition is rare in males.

Bulimics binge and purge. **Binging** involves the consumption of as much as 5,000 to 20,000 kilocalories per day. **Purging** is the intentional clearing of food out of the system by vomiting and/or using enemas, laxatives, and diuretics. Individuals with bulimia often have disordered eating patterns that combine binging and purging with episodes of food restriction either before or after binge episodes in order to maintain weight. Athletes such as ballerinas and gymnasts sometimes are bulimic. The female triad is a serious syndrome comprising three interrelated components (see Chapter 11):

- Disordered eating
- Amenorrhea
- Osteoporosis

Binge-Eating Disorder

Binge-eating disorder (BED) is recognized as a distinct eating disorder in the *Diagnostic and Statistical Manual of Mental Disorders, Fifth Edition* (DSM-5). Binge-eaters eat large amounts of high-fat and high-sugar foods in short periods of time; unlike the bulimic, binge eaters do not follow a binge with a purge. BED is the most common eating disorder in the United States, with 3.5% of adult women, 2% of adult men, and 1.6% of adolescents experiencing the disorder at some point in their lives (Brownley, Peat, La Via, & Bulik, 2015). Clients with BED may be overweight or obese and often experience feelings of shame and guilt after episodes of binging. Binge-eaters can often associate eating at times of stress or emotional distress, experience lack of control, and eating until they are uncomfortably full. BED can contribute to the development of obesity and obesity-related conditions.

Treating Eating Disorders

The treatment of eating disorders requires a multidisciplinary approach, including nutritional counseling; psychotherapy, which can include behavioral therapy, family therapy, and group therapy; psychopharmacology therapy and the use of antidepressants; and medical therapy to correct complications related to the illnesses. It is important to help the client discover the reason why he or she chooses to eat, not eat, binge, or purge. Some of these clients have symptoms such as a fixation on food, weight, physique, or exercise (see Box 16-6).

BOX 16-5 ■ Is the Client Eating Enough?

One method for determining whether a client is eating enough food is to monitor his or her food intake. Kilocalorie intake is monitored by recording actual food consumption and calculating the kilocalories eaten. Using programs such as the USDA's SuperTracker provides a user-friendly way to assist with calculations and developing dietary plans. The program can be found at www.supertracker.usda.gov/default.aspx.

BOX 16-6 ■ Treating Eating Disorders in the Hospital Setting

Some clients may be admitted to the hospital for treatment if they require medical stabilization or weight regain (Smith et al, 2016). Careful recording of kilocalories consumed and expended is indicated. Close monitoring of clients is often indicated during meals and until 2 hours after meals because these clients may attempt to hide food in their clothes, mouth, bedding, or anywhere else. It is sometimes necessary for the nurse to accompany these clients to the bathroom. Clients with eating disorders have been known to flush their food down the toilet or engage in purging activities such as self-induced vomiting after a meal. Clients will require daily weights.

KEYSTONES

- Energy imbalance results from an inequality of energy intake and expenditure.

- The reason an individual eats more or fewer kilocalories than needed to maintain a stable body weight is only partially understood.

- Reasons a person may be in energy imbalance are both internal and external.

- Weight loss decreases both body fat and lean body mass (LBM).

- Care needs to be taken to minimize the loss of LBM during weight reduction.

- Exercise should be encouraged because it helps minimize the loss of LBM during weight reduction.

- Exercise, a well-balanced diet, and behavior modification are all essential components of a sound weight-reduction program.

- The prevention of energy imbalance is the key to decreased health-care costs nationally.

- Medications and surgical interventions may be indicated for individuals who meet the criteria set by the guidelines.

- Treating the client who has a reduced body mass is a concern for health-care workers.

CASE STUDY 16-1

The client arrives at the physician's office for a routine blood pressure check. Her blood pressure is 150/95. Her medications include 100 mg metoprolol daily and 25 mg hydrochlorothiazide daily. The client works nights as a cashier at a service station and days at a dry cleaner. Her BMI is 28. She recently had a stress test that was considered normal. The doctor would like the client to lose weight to help lower her blood pressure.

CARE PLAN

Subjective Data

Client stated, "I can barely afford my blood pressure medication, and the doctor has encouraged me to lose about 14 pounds. I know I need to eat less and exercise more. I need to spend less money on medications. I know I'm not too smart because I only completed the sixth grade in school." A food frequency record showed that this client usually eats four times each day. Her usual pattern includes 3 cups of low-fat milk, 8 carbohydrates (mostly refined), ½ cup of vegetables, 1 piece of fruit, 6–8 ounces of meat, 5 fats, 1 dessert, and an occasional beer. She eats fast food two nights each week and has pizza weekly for lunch. "I am desperate and will do anything to lose weight." The client has health insurance that will pay for one wellness program per year.

Objective Data

Blood pressure 150/95 ■ height 5 ft 6 in. ■ BMI 28; waist circumference 36 ■ stress test was normal.

Analysis

Energy imbalance ■ kilocalorie intake greater than kilocalorie expenditure. Overweight as evidenced by BMI of 28 and waist circumference of 36, probably contributing to hypertension.

Plan

DESIRED OUTCOMES EVALUATION CRITERIA	ACTIONS/ INTERVENTIONS	RATIONALE
Increase physical activity.	Recommend Mrs. R monitor her exercise behaviors and try to walk at least 30 minutes three times per week and increase to 7 days per week as able.	Self-monitoring of lifestyle behaviors promotes behavioral change. Sedentary individuals receive the most health benefit from even small amounts of exercise.
Consume foods in appropriate portions following the MyPlate Guide.	Review MyPlate model with Mrs. R with emphasis on whole grains, fruits and vegetables, lean proteins, and the limiting of fats. Review portion sizes indicated on this teaching tool.	The MyPlate Guide is a good tool to use for clients with a lower reading level and promotes a high-fiber, low-fat diet.

(Continued on the following page)

DESIRED OUTCOMES EVALUATION CRITERIA	ACTIONS/ INTERVENTIONS	RATIONALE
Client will state why a weight loss of 1–2 pounds per week may reduce her blood pressure.	Explain to the client that the rate of weight loss is important and why.	A 1–2-pound per week weight loss will minimize the loss of lean body mass. Self-starvation rarely results in long-term weight loss for overweight clients.
Refer client to the local hospital's wellness center that incorporates diet, behavior modification, and exercise in the program.	Explain to the client why you are referring her to this particular program.	The best wellness programs include diet, exercise, and behavior modification.

TEAMWORK 16-1

FOLLOW-UP NOTE FROM HOSPITAL'S WELLNESS PROGRAM

Thank you for your referral to our program. Client has met with our registered dietitian, exercise physiologist, and psychologist during group sessions. She has attended most sessions and has done remarkably well. She has lost a total of 5 pounds at the rate of 1 to 2 pounds per week for the past 8 weeks. We were also able to arrange a scholarship for her to attend the program for 8 more weeks. She keeps good food and exercise records. She has made several friends in the class and says that she looks forward to this night out with her new friends. Thank you again for this referral.

Cordially,

Wellness Program Director

CRITICAL THINKING QUESTIONS

1. What foods does this client need to eat less, and what foods does she need to eat more?

2. What would you tell the client if after 1 week she gained a pound, even though she had given up her daily dessert and had increased her vegetable intake to 5 servings each day?

3. What other dietary modifications would you recommend?

CHAPTER REVIEW

1. To lose 2 pounds of body fat per week, an individual must eat ____ fewer kilocalories each day for 7 days without a change in energy expenditure.
   1. 1,000
   2. 1,500
   3. 2,000
   4. 2,500

2. A very rapid rate of weight loss (1 pound per day) in an adult who is slightly overweight:
   1. Usually encourages permanent changes in behavior
   2. May lead to sudden death in some clients
   3. Will preserve lean body mass
   4. Fosters long-term weight maintenance

3. An obese client should be enrolled in a weight-management program and meet the following criteria before medications are tried:
   1. BMI of 20 and waist circumference of 30 inches
   2. In a male, waist circumference of at least 35 inches and BMI of 27
   3. BMI of 27 and no concomitant obesity-related risk factors
   4. In a female, waist circumference of at least 35 inches and BMI of 30 or greater

4. A client with anorexia nervosa:
   1. Has an increased resting energy expenditure
   2. Frequently complains of constipation
   3. Is not likely to have a body image disturbance
   4. Typically seeks the company of others

5. An elderly overweight smoker should first be encouraged to:
1. Lose weight
2. Quit smoking
3. Lose weight and quit smoking using any means possible
4. Be evaluated to determine if weight loss is indicated and bone health is adequate

---

CLINICAL ANALYSIS

1. Mrs. D is a 40-year-old mother of three. She has arthritis in both knees. She weighs 180 pounds, has a medium frame, and is 5 ft 3 in. tall. Her BMI is 32. Her physician has told her to lose weight to help reduce her knee pain. According to Mrs. D, she never thought that she was overweight until she was 24 years old. At this time, her weight started increasing. When she weighed 140 pounds, she started to diet. One time she lost a total of 25 pounds, which she promptly regained plus an additional 5 pounds. The client described four additional **weight cycles.** Mrs. D claims that she cannot exercise because "it is too painful on my knees." She has tried every conceivable type of diet, including a comprehensive medically supervised weight-control program. Mrs. D states that for the past year, no matter how little she eats, she cannot lose weight even on a 1,200-kilocalorie diet. Mrs. D:
a. Has knowledge of weight loss strategies, because she has successfully lost weight before
b. Knows very little about foods, because she always regained the weight she lost
c. Lacks motivation, because she has an inability to follow through with the appropriate behavior
d. Should be discouraged from further attempts to control her weight

2. Mrs. M had a slow weight gain for about 10 years. She asks for advice concerning how to best manage her weight. Mrs. M lives a sedentary lifestyle, eats three well-balanced meals each day, and enjoys going out to dinner with her husband one night each week. Her BMI is 27. Mrs. M would most likely benefit from:
a. Decreasing her meal frequency
b. Increasing her physical activity
c. Taking a medication to lose weight
d. Not going out to dinner with her husband each week

3. Mr. P wants to lose weight and has a BMI of 30 and a waist circumference of 41. Initially, the nurse should advise Mr. P to:
a. Follow a 1,200-kilocalorie diet.
b. Ask his doctor for a medication to assist in weight reduction.
c. Self-monitor and write down his food intake and physical activity.
d. Refer the client to a surgeon for an evaluation.

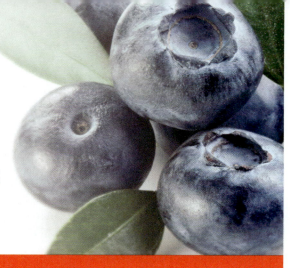

CHAPTER 17

Diet in Diabetes Mellitus and Hypoglycemia

This chapter introduces the importance of nutrition in diabetes mellitus (simply referred to as diabetes throughout the rest of this chapter) and hypoglycemia. These two diseases are associated with insulin secretion and/or resistance to insulin accompanied by characteristic long-term complications. Diabetes is caused by the low secretion and/or use of insulin. Hypoglycemia is seen in suboptimal treatment of diabetes and in other causes such as gastric surgery, some medications, and hormone and enzyme deficiencies. The Centers for Disease Control and Prevention (CDC) estimates the prevalence of diabetes in the United States for all ages to be 29.1 million, or 9.3% of the population, while 25% of adults who have diabetes remain undiagnosed (Beckles & Chou, 2016; Centers for Disease Control and Prevention [CDC], 2016b). Nationally, diabetes is the seventh leading cause of death (CDC, 2016a). Type 2 diabetes is frequently not diagnosed until complications occur. It is estimated that as many as 1 in 3 U.S. adults could have diabetes by 2050. Over 20% of health-care spending is for individuals with diagnosed diabetes (CDC, 2016a). Nutrition is integral to the management of diabetes.

Definition and Classification

Diabetes can be defined as a group of disorders with measurable persistent hyperglycemia, which results from defects in insulin production, insulin action, or both. **Hyperglycemia** means an elevated level of glucose in the blood. Definitions and classifications for the various subclasses of diabetes have been standardized. Diabetes may produce symptoms of excessive urine production, thirst, excessive hunger, blurred vision, and, in some cases, weight loss (American Diabetes Association [ADA], 2015).

Diagnosis

Diabetes is diagnosed and defined by laboratory analysis of the blood. A glycosylated hemoglobin (A1C) of 6.5% or higher is used as a diagnosis for diabetes mellitus in adults; the test should be repeated for a definitive diagnosis. A1C levels indicate the level of blood glucose control an individual has had over approximately 2 to 3 months. If blood glucose is high, the excess attaches to the hemoglobin, causing the A1C level to be high.

Advantages of using the A1C test include:

- Fasting is not required for the blood test
- Levels reflect an average level of blood glucose over time
- Greater preanalytical stability
- Less impact during periods of stress and illness

Disadvantages of using the A1C test include:

- Greater cost associated with the test
- Decreased availability in remote regions of the country and world
- Controversy in differences of normal levels in different race/ethnicity groups
- Uncertainty exists with the usage in children
- Unable to use in individuals with abnormal red cell turnover, such as that occurs in pregnancy, with recent blood loss or transfusion, and in some forms of anemia
- Identifies ⅓ fewer cases than using the fasting glucose

For individuals who cannot be diagnosed by using A1C levels, the diagnosis of diabetes must be done using blood glucose levels. This is an accurate method used to diagnosis diabetes.

Fasting glucose levels of at least 126 milligrams per **deciliter** (mg/dL) are required for a diagnosis of diabetes in nonpregnant adults. Fasting is defined as no kilocalorie intake for at least 8 hours. A fasting blood glucose level of 100 to 125 is diagnosed as prediabetes or **impaired fasting glucose.** Casual or random blood glucose (RBG) greater than 200 mg/dL plus classic symptoms (increased urination, increased thirst, weight loss) are also an established method for diagnosing diabetes in adults and children. A test result, which is diagnostic of diabetes, should be repeated to confirm the diagnosis. A random blood glucose between 140 and 199 mg/dL is diagnostic of prediabetes. Random means that the blood sample is tested without regard to time of day, prior diet, and physical activity (ADA, 2016). Refer to Clinical Application 17-1 for an explanation of common tests used for diabetes.

Classification

There are four clinical classes of diabetes: type 1, type 2, gestational (GDM), and other, secondary causes. The two major forms are **type 1** and **type 2.**

Prediabetes occurs in individuals with impaired glucose tolerance but who are not yet diagnosed with diabetes. This

CLINICAL APPLICATION   **17-1**

Laboratory Tests for Diabetes Mellitus

Biochemical tests for diabetes include fasting blood sugar, glucose tolerance test, urine tests, and glycosylated hemoglobin.

FASTING BLOOD SUGAR

A measurement of a **fasting blood sugar (FBS)** is performed routinely on most diabetic clients. In preparation, the client should be instructed not to smoke, eat, or drink for 8 hours before the test. Water is the exception because it will not interfere with test results. The test ideally should be done after at least 3 days of unrestricted diet (150 grams of carbohydrate per day) and unlimited physical activity. The individual should remain seated throughout the test. If the client usually takes insulin or a hypoglycemic agent, the medication should not be taken or given until the blood test is done. Normal FBS should be less than 100 mg/dL. A finding of 126 mg/dL or greater is diagnostic of diabetes.

GLUCOSE TOLERANCE TEST

In the **glucose tolerance test,** 75 grams of anhydrous glucose dissolved in water is given orally or intravenously after a fasting blood sugar sample has been drawn. Blood samples are then drawn at specified intervals. The client's ability to process glucose can be evaluated by this means. A blood glucose value above or equal to 200 mg/dL at 2 hours and at least one other sample at less than 2 hours are required for the diagnosis in nonpregnant adults. A normal 2-hour blood sample would have an upper level of 140 mg/dL. Values between 140 and 199 mg/dL are indicative of impaired glucose tolerance or prediabetes. In the absence of unequivocal hyperglycemia, these criteria should be confirmed by repeat testing on a different day (ADA, 2016).

Clients may need to discontinue certain drugs for 3 days before the test and follow a high-carbohydrate diet of 300 grams of carbohydrate per day. The client should be given written instructions explaining the pretest dietary requirements. An inadequate diet before the glucose tolerance test may diminish carbohydrate tolerance and cause high glucose levels, creating a false-positive result. During the test period, the client should be instructed not to have anything by mouth except water. Tobacco, coffee, and tea can alter the test results.

URINE TESTS

For most people, when blood glucose reaches 180–200 mg/100 mL, the kidneys begin to spill glucose into the urine. This point of spillage is called the **renal threshold.**

At one time, this test was assumed to reflect the glucose content of the blood, but the renal threshold varies from individual to individual. The renal threshold may also change in a given individual with decreasing kidney function. Although urine tests are used as screening tests, they are less reliable than the blood glucose tests available for home use.

URINE ACETONE

As a consequence of the body's inability to metabolize glucose, fat is partially broken down for energy. The intermediate products of fat breakdown are ketone bodies. These ketone bodies build up in the blood because the quantity of fat being catabolized exceeds the body's capacity to process these intermediate products effectively. As this occurs, ketone bodies begin to spill into the urine. One of the ketone bodies is acetone, which can be measured in urine. The presence of acetone in the urine is called **ketonuria,** a sign that the diabetes is out of control. Clients may be taught to test for urinary ketones if their blood glucose level exceeds 240 mg/dL. When a client exhibits ketonuria, the physician and diabetes educator should be consulted for changes in the diet prescription and/or insulin dosage.

GLYCOSYLATED HEMOGLOBIN (A1C)

Glucose attaches to the hemoglobin molecule in a one-way reaction throughout the 120-day life of the red blood cell. In a high-glucose environment, a greater percentage of the hemoglobin is glycosylated. This blood test is performed on a random blood sample; the client does not have to fast. The result is not influenced by exercise or diabetic drugs.

Because the **glycosylated hemoglobin** value reflects the average blood glucose level for the preceding 2–3 months, it is a good test of the effectiveness of long-term therapy. A client cannot follow the prescribed regimen for just a few days before a doctor's visit and claim otherwise. Glycosylated hemoglobin values between 5.7% and 6.4% is considered prediabetes. An A1C greater than 6.4% confirms a diagnosis of diabetes.

Testing for A1C is recommended at least two times a year for people in good control and quarterly in clients who are not meeting glycemic goals or whose therapy has changed (ADA, 2016).

is an important group to diagnose and treat because they are more likely to be diagnosed with diabetes.

Prediabetes

Impaired glucose tolerance (IGT) and impaired fasting glucose (IFG) refer to a metabolic state intermediate between normal with glucose homeostasis and diabetes. The ADA encourages the use of the term *prediabetes*. Individuals who have A1C level of 5.7% to 6.4% or a fasting glucose level of greater than 100 mg/dL but less than 126 mg/dL on more than two occasions meet the criteria for IGT or IFG. IGT may represent a step in the development of types 1 and 2 diabetes, heart disease, and stroke. The CDC estimates that a third of Americans, approximately 86 million individuals, have prediabetes and 90% don't know it. People who participate in structured lifestyle change programs can reduce their risk of developing diabetes by 58% (CDC, 2016).

IGT and IFG are associated with abdominal obesity, dyslipidemia, and hypertension and are indicative of **metabolic syndrome,** which increases the risk of developing diabetes, discussed in Chapter 18 (National Institutes of Health [NIH], 2016).

Type 1

Type 1 diabetes has also been called **insulin-dependent diabetes mellitus (IDDM),** juvenile-onset diabetes, and type I diabetes. This form of diabetes accounts for 5% to 10% of those with diabetes. This type of diabetes normally results from a cellular-mediated autoimmune destruction of the β-cells of the pancreas, which produce insulin. The rate of the destruction is variable. Although mostly found in children and adolescents, it can occur at any age. Clients with this disorder cannot survive without daily doses of insulin because the pancreas does not produce sufficient insulin for glucose uptake. This situation results in elevated blood glucose. After treatment starts, clients on medications that lower their blood glucose levels may have problems with blood glucose levels that are too low. These variations in blood glucose levels make clients prone to two conditions.

1. The first condition is **ketoacidosis.** The signs of ketoacidosis are hyperglycemia and excessive ketones. Ketoacidosis is discussed later in this chapter.
2. The second condition is **hypoglycemia,** or a low blood glucose level.

Individuals with type 1 diabetes are more prone to other autoimmune disorders such as Graves disease, lymphocytic thyroiditis (Hashimoto thyroiditis), Addison disease, vitiligo, celiac disease, autoimmune hepatitis, myasthenia gravis, and pernicious anemia. Some, but few, individuals with type 1 diabetes have no evidence of autoimmunity. It is thought that their diabetes is strongly inherited, seen mostly in African or Asian ancestry. Their need for insulin replacement therapy may come and go (ADA, 2016).

Type 2

Type 2 diabetes has also been called **non–insulin-dependent diabetes mellitus (NIDDM),** adult-onset diabetes, and type II diabetes. Most of these clients are obese, and weight reduction usually improves their ability to process glucose. These individuals have insulin resistance and may have varying degrees of insulin deficiency. Initially, and sometimes throughout the course of the disease, insulin injections are not required. However, some clients do require insulin injections because of persistent hyperglycemia. Clients with type 2 diabetes can manufacture some insulin but often do not make enough or cannot use insulin efficiently. The risk of developing type 2 diabetes increases with age, obesity, lack of physical activity, in women with previous GDM, and individuals with dyslipidemia and is associated with a strong genetic component (see Genomic Gem 17-1). Ninety percent to 95% of people with diabetes in the United States have type 2 (ADA, 2016).

The onset of this disorder is gradual, with the severity often not enough for individuals to notice any symptoms. However, during this undiagnosed period, macrovascular and microvascular complications may occur (ADA, 2016). Table 17-1 summarizes the differences between type 1 and type 2 diabetes.

Gestational Diabetes

Gestational diabetes (GDM) occurs in approximately 7% of all pregnancies. GDM carries risks for the mother, fetus, and neonate. Guidelines recommend that all women be assessed for their risk of GDM at their first prenatal visit. If a woman has the risk factors for diabetes such as obesity, a personal history of GDM, a family history of diabetes, or glycosuria, testing for diabetes should be done as soon as possible. Women not known to have diabetes should undergo one of two tests at 24 to 28 weeks of gestation (ADA, 2016):

1. A one-step 75-gram oral glucose tolerance test (OGTT). The following blood levels must be met or exceeded for a diagnosis of GDM:
   - 92 mg/dL fasting plasma glucose (FPG)
   - 180 mg/dL 1 hour after glucose load
   - 153 mg/dL 2 hours after glucose load

GENOMIC GEM 17-1

Maturity-Onset Diabetes in the Young

Maturity-onset diabetes in the young (MODY) is a term used to describe a diabetes disorder that is found in clients younger than 25 years. This condition is genetic with a defect in the gene involved in the stimulation of the pancreatic ß cells to produce insulin. A parent with MODY has a 50% chance of passing on MODY to his or her children. Clients with MODY do not always need insulin treatment and can often be treated with oral agents and a weight-reduction diet.

TABLE 17-1 Type 1 and Type 2 Diabetes Mellitus Comparisons (ADA, 2016)

	TYPE 1	TYPE 2
Cause	Beta cells damaged	Tissues resist insulin
Most common age at onset	Younger than 20 years	Older than 45 years
Medication	1. Insulin injections or pump 2. Insulin injections or pump and oral agents 3. Insulin drip during critical illness	1. None 2. Oral agents 3. May require insulin injections to attain optimal blood glucose levels 4. Insulin drip during critical illness
Usual body build	Thin, underweight	Obese
Nutrition therapy	Integration of insulin therapy, activity, and food intake Consistent timing of insulin to food intake	Achievement of near-normal glucose, lipid, and blood pressure goals Weight loss through diet and increased activity is desirable; bariatric surgery may be considered in extreme cases with BMI >35

2. A two-step approach using a 50-gram (nonfasting) screen followed by a 100-gram OGTT for those with a positive screen (blood glucose ≥140 mg/dL after 1 hour). The diagnosis of GDM is made based upon the following criteria:
   - 95 mg/dL fasting plasma glucose (FPG)
   - 180 mg/dL 1 hour after glucose load
   - 155 mg/dL 2 hours after glucose load
   - 140 mg/dL 3 hours after glucose load

Immediately after pregnancy, approximately 10% of women with GDM are found to have diabetes, usually type 2. Women with GDM have a 35% to 60% chance of developing diabetes in the next 5 to 10 years (Man, 2016).

Other/Secondary Diabetes

Most diabetes results from a primary failure of insulin production or use. Other conditions can cause diabetes, such as genetic defects, surgery, medications, infections, pancreatic disease, and other illnesses. The term **secondary diabetes** is sometimes used when one of these disorders is responsible for hyperglycemia. Examples include:

- Pancreatitis
- Cystic fibrosis
- Down syndrome
- Surgical removal of the pancreas
- Cushing disease
- Maturity-onset diabetes of the young (MODY)
- Pharmacological doses of glucocorticoids (e.g., prednisone) or other hormones or drugs

The diabetes may be resolved if the cause is alleviated (such as discontinuation of drugs or resolution of pancreatitis). If the cause is not correctable, secondary diabetes is treated similarly to other forms of diabetes (ADA, 2016).

Functions of Insulin

Every cell in the human body depends somewhat on glucose to meet energy needs. The brain and the rest of the nervous system depend almost exclusively on glucose for energy. Normally blood glucose levels decrease and increase within a given range pre- and postfeeding. Levels are lower before eating and higher after eating. Insulin is the only hormone that lowers blood glucose. A person normally secretes insulin in response to an elevated blood glucose level. Insulin decreases blood glucose by accelerating its movement from the blood into the cells. As glucose enters the cells, it may be metabolized to yield energy, may be stored as glycogen, or may be converted to fat (Table 17-2).

The ultimate fate of glucose once it is inside the cell depends on the body's need and the amount of glucose that enters the cell. The cells' energy needs will be met first. If cells have available glucose over and above immediate energy needs, the excess glucose is stored as glycogen. Insulin stimulates the storage of glucose as glycogen. Once the glycogen stores are filled to capacity, any remaining glucose is converted to fat. The body can store about 0.4 pound of glycogen, which is equal to 800 kilocalories.

Insulin influences the metabolism of protein and fat, and stimulates entry of amino acids into cells and enhances protein formation. It also enhances fat storage in adipose tissue and indirectly inhibits the breakdown of fat for energy. If the body has ample glucose available for energy, protein and fat need not be broken down to meet energy needs. If the body does not have glucose available for energy, it will use dietary protein or break down internal body protein stores to meet its immediate need for energy.

TABLE 17-2 Metabolic Activities Promoted by Insulin

ACTIVITY	METABOLIC PATHWAY
Movement of glucose into cells	None
Energy production from glucose	Glycolysis
Manufacture of glycogen	Glycogenesis
Fat formation from carbohydrate and protein	Lipogenesis

Note: "Genesis" means forming of.

Insulin levels fluctuate in the blood. Normally, blood insulin levels increase as the blood glucose level increases. A high level of insulin in the blood signals the cells not to break down stores for energy (Table 17-3). An anabolic, or building, state exists when metabolism is normal and glucose and insulin levels are high. Normally insulin levels decrease as the blood sugar level decreases. A low level of insulin in the blood indirectly signals the body to begin to break down body stores for glucose. Figure 17-1 illustrates glucose use by the cells.

Other Hormones

Glucagon and somatostatin assist in coordinating the storage and mobilization of the energy nutrients: carbohydrate, fat, and protein. Glucagon increases blood glucose levels and stimulates the breakdown of body protein and fat stores. Somatostatin acts locally within the Islets of Langerhans to depress the secretion of insulin and glucagon. Evidence has shown that these hormones may not be at optimal levels in some clients with diabetes.

Cellular Sources of Glucose

Cells obtain glucose from both food that is eaten and internal glucose stores. Almost all carbohydrate eaten (except fiber), about 50% of protein eaten, and about 10% of fat eaten enter the blood as glucose. The internal body stores that can be converted to glucose are glycogen, some protein, and the glycerol portion of triglycerides. Body fat is stored as triglycerides in adipose tissue. To understand diabetes, it is necessary to know how the body coordinates all internal and external sources of glucose to maintain a normal blood glucose range.

Blood Glucose Curve

Given the vital need for every cell to have an uninterrupted supply of energy, the human body has evolved to allow an uninterrupted energy supply to reach cells without continuous eating. The blood glucose level increases after eating and decreases in the fasting state. Figure 17-2 illustrates the normal blood glucose curve.

Causes of Diabetes

When the β cells of the pancreas cannot make enough insulin, or when the body's cells are resistant to the insulin, blood glucose cannot be transported into cells for their use. The result is hyperglycemia. The major causes of diabetes include genetic factors, lifestyle, autoimmune diseases, and viral infections. Some susceptibility to diabetes is genetic. However, not everyone with susceptible genes develops clinical diabetes. Before diabetes becomes apparent, this genetic susceptibility is often triggered by the individual's lifestyle or other environmental factors. A healthy lifestyle is particularly important for the *prevention* of diabetes in genetically susceptible clients. Excessive body fat, inactivity, and stress are risk factors for type 2 diabetes. A loss of body fat alone is sometimes sufficient to balance the insulin produced with

TABLE 17-3	Metabolic Activities Inhibited by a High Level of Insulin
ACTIVITY	**METABOLIC PATHWAY**
Movement of glucose from noncarbohydrate sources, e.g., glycerol and amino acids	Gluconeogenesis
Release of glucose from glycogen	Glycogenolysis
Breakdown of fat from adipose tissue	Lipolysis

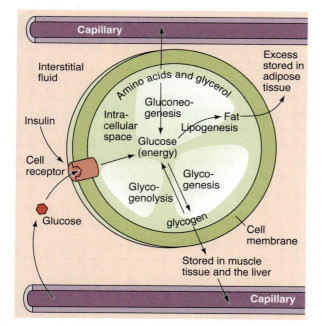

FIGURE 17-1 Insulin is necessary for glucose to gain entry into a cell. Once inside the cell, glucose can meet several fates: it can be burned as energy or stored as glycogen, or the glycerol portion of a fat molecule or some amino acids can be broken down into glucose. Some amino acids will be converted to glucose if the cell requires glucose.

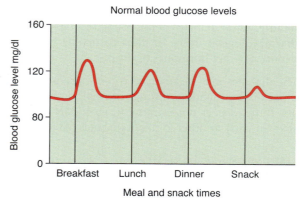

FIGURE 17-2 A person's blood glucose level normally goes up after food consumption and then down between feedings.

a modified food intake. Sometimes emotional or physical stress is the stimulus that causes hyperglycemia. The body's stress response involves the release of epinephrine from the adrenal glands. One action of epinephrine is to raise the blood glucose level so the person has energy for the "fight or flight" response.

Signs and Symptoms

The classic triad of signs and symptoms includes:

1. **Polyuria** (increased urination)
2. **Polydipsia** (increased thirst)
3. **Polyphagia** (increased appetite and weight loss)

The triad is most commonly seen in type 1 diabetes. The following section describes these and other signs and symptoms commonly seen in persons with diabetes.

Classic Triad

In diabetes, glucose cannot optimally move from the intravascular space across a cell membrane into the intracellular space. This is why the blood glucose level of people with diabetes remains elevated after eating. Under normal circumstances, the blood glucose level does not increase excessively because excess glucose undergoes glycolysis and is readily converted to adipose tissue or stored as glycogen inside the cell. As the glucose-rich blood circulates through the kidneys, these organs reabsorb as much glucose as they can. After this point is reached, glucose enters the urine. **Glycosuria** means an abnormally high amount of glucose in the urine. As the glucose exits the body in urine, water is pulled out also, as a result of the osmotic effect of glucose. This results in polyuria, or a large urine output. The large loss of water causes excessive thirst, polydipsia, and prompts the person to drink fluids.

When glucose is not available for energy inside the cells, the body begins to break down protein and fat for energy. In untreated type 1 diabetes, the body's cells are starving. These starving cells send a message to the brain to turn on the person's appetite. The person responds by eating to satisfy the craving for food. The third most common symptom or sign of diabetes is **polyphagia,** an abnormal increase in appetite.

Other Signs and Symptoms

The abnormal carbohydrate metabolism of diabetes and its effects on the body's tissues cause other problems. Weight loss is more commonly seen in clients with type 1 diabetes than in clients with type 2. Clients with both types of diabetes may show these signs and symptoms:

- Blurred vision
- Fatigue
- Infection
- **Vaginitis** (inflammation of the vagina)
- Bladder infections
- Poor wound healing
- Impotence in men
- Kidney disorders

Complications

Both acute and chronic complications occur with diabetes. Acute complications require immediate care. Chronic complications include diseases of the eye, kidneys, heart, and nervous system. Chronic complications are responsible for the increased death rate among individuals with diabetes and the diminished quality of life that many of these clients' experience.

Acute Clinical Situations

Three acute complications are seen in clients with diabetes:

1. **Diabetic ketoacidosis (DKA)**
2. Hyperglycemic hyperosmolar nonketotic syndrome
3. **Hypoglycemia**

Ketoacidosis

Individuals with type 1 diabetes who experience a profound insulin deficiency may progress to ketoacidosis. The three main precipitating factors in ketoacidosis are:

1. A decreased or missed dose of insulin
2. An illness or infection
3. Uncontrolled disease in a previously undiagnosed person

Ketoacidosis is a complex, life-threatening condition that demands emergency treatment. The predominant clinical manifestations and general principles of treatment are discussed next.

DEHYDRATION

Without insulin, glucose cannot be transferred across the cell membranes into the cells. A greatly increased number of glucose molecules (300 to 800 mg/dL) in the blood exert an osmotic effect, causing water to move from within the cells to the intravascular space and producing cellular dehydration. The body excretes the excess water, glucose, and electrolytes in urine.

ACIDOSIS

Unaware that the problem is not lack of glucose but lack of insulin, the body proceeds to increase blood glucose by mobilizing protein and fat from the tissues to be converted to glucose by the liver. Because the human body can use only the glycerol portion of the triglyceride molecule for glucose, the fatty acid portion is processed into ketones. Normally ketones are metabolized and excreted as carbon dioxide and water.

Under conditions of ketoacidosis, however, the body cannot metabolize this overload of ketones rapidly enough to maintain homeostasis. The client has excessive ketones in the blood (ketonemia) and spills ketones into the urine (ketonuria). Acetone is one of the ketone bodies for which urine is tested. The ketone bodies are acid, and thus the term *ketoacidosis*.

ELECTROLYTE IMBALANCES

Clients with severe ketoacidosis may excrete 6.5 liters of fluid and 400 to 500 milliequivalents of sodium, potassium, and chloride in 24 hours. A fluid loss of 15% of body weight is not unusual. Most critical in the treatment of electrolyte imbalances in diabetic ketoacidosis is the body's level of potassium. As the cells are being catabolized for fuel, the intracellular potassium is transferred to the intravascular space.

Serum potassium levels can be low, normal, or elevated in the person with ketoacidosis, depending on the body's current coping mechanism. Regardless of the serum concentrations of potassium and sodium, the pathological process of diabetic ketoacidosis depletes these electrolytes. Either hypokalemia or hyperkalemia can lead to cardiac arrhythmias and must be carefully managed in clients with ketoacidosis.

TREATMENT

Clients with severe diabetic ketoacidosis are critically ill. Treatment includes supplemental insulin, fluid and electrolyte replacement, and medical monitoring. Serum electrolyte levels change dramatically once treatment commences. Intensive care is necessary to provide the careful monitoring and frequent adjustments in therapy required as the fluids and electrolytes are being replaced. Intravenous regular insulin will permit the use of carbohydrate for energy and will halt the body's excessive use of fat, which has produced the ketone bodies. Insulin drives glucose back into the cells. Potassium too moves from the intravascular space to the intracellular space, necessitating frequent measurement of the serum levels of both glucose and potassium. When the client recovers, identification of the precipitating factor for the ketoacidosis and education focused on preventing additional occurrences are essential.

Hyperglycemic Hyperosmolar Nonketotic Syndrome

The four signs of **hyperglycemic hyperosmolar nonketotic syndrome (HHNS)** are:

1. Blood glucose level >600 mg/dL
2. Absence of or slight ketosis
3. Plasma hyperosmolality
4. Profound dehydration

This life-threatening emergency is usually seen in older people with diabetes, more often in type 2 diabetics, and is normally brought on by an illness or infection. HHNS is like DKA except that the insulin deficiency is not as severe, so increased **lipolysis** (the breakdown of body lipid stores) does not occur. Because these clients do not have symptoms of vomiting, nausea, and acidosis brought on by severe ketosis, as do clients with type 1 diabetes, they often do not seek prompt medical help. Their blood sugar levels

are higher and their dehydration more severe than is seen in ketoacidosis.

In these clients, prolonged osmotic diuresis and dehydration secondary to hyperglycemia lead to decreased renal blood flow and allow blood glucose to reach very high levels. Medications that cause an increase in blood glucose levels, chronic disease, and infection may contribute to this condition. Treatment includes correction of the electrolyte imbalance, hyperglycemia, and dehydration.

Hypoglycemia

In both type 1 and type 2 diabetes, an individual can develop hypoglycemia, which is defined by a blood glucose level <70 mg/dL. Hypoglycemia may be caused by:

- Too much insulin (accidental or deliberate)
- Too little food intake; or a delayed meal
- Excessive exercise
- Alcohol (especially in the fasting state)
- Medications such as oral hypoglycemic agents

Symptoms may include:

- Confusion
- Headache
- Double vision
- Rapid heartbeat
- Sweating
- Hunger
- Seizure
- Coma

The treatment of hypoglycemia is discussed later in this chapter.

Chronic Complications

Clients with both type 1 and type 2 diabetes of sufficient duration are vulnerable to serious complications involving the eyes, kidneys, and nervous system.

Diabetic **retinopathy** is a disorder that involves the retina. Diabetes is a leading cause of blindness and vision loss in the adult U.S. population. The blurred vision reported by these clients is related to retinopathy. These clients are also at a higher risk for cataracts.

Diabetic **neuropathy** is a chronic complication of diabetes. Clients may complain of a lack of sensation in their extremities. They may puncture, cut, or burn their feet and not feel any pain. A wound may become infected and heal poorly. Gangrene, or tissue death, may follow. The treatment for gangrene is amputation. **Neuropathy** can affect gastric or intestinal motility, erectile function, bladder function, cardiac function, and vascular tone.

Gastroparesis (paralysis of the stomach with delayed gastric emptying) may occur and alter the absorption of meals, which makes glycemic control problematic.

Cardiovascular disease (CVD) is more common in clients with diabetes than in the nondiabetic population of the same age and gender. This is related in general to the fact that diabetes is a small-vessel disease and the critical end arteries in the heart muscle are small vessels.

Diabetic **nephropathy,** or kidney disease, is another common complication in clients with diabetes.

Tragically, some clients with diabetes do not take the threat of chronic complications seriously until much damage has occurred.

Management

The American Diabetes Association advocates a client-centered approach to the management of diabetes. A team of clinicians should work with the client to determine his or her level of engagement to successfully develop a joint, comprehensive plan of disease self-management to include lifestyle changes (ADA, 2016). The goals of the treatment plan for management of the client's diabetes should be developed by the team in conjunction with the client to ensure the plan is reasonable and understandable. The client's age, work and/or school schedule, physical activity, eating habits (which include social and cultural factors), as well as other medical conditions must be taken into account when developing diabetes self-management education for clients. The two primary methods for health-care providers and clients to assess the effectiveness of the diabetes management plan are through **self-monitoring of blood glucose** (SMBG) and testing A1C levels. Table 17-4 presents glycemic goals recommended by the American Diabetes Association (ADA, 2016).

All health-care workers should assist the general population in the early detection of diabetes and prevention of complications. As Figure 17-3 emphasizes, the three cornerstones of the management of diabetes after diagnosis are:

1. Physical activity
2. Medication
3. Nutritional management

Self-monitoring of blood glucose levels enables the client to assess how each of these factors interacts.

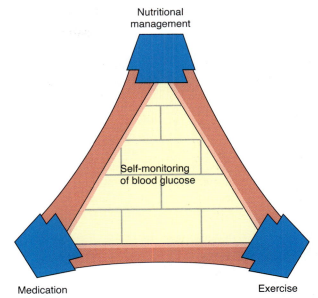

FIGURE 17-3 Nutritional management, medication, and exercise are the three components of treatment for diabetes. Each of these cornerstones has an influence on blood glucose levels. An individual can identify how each of these cornerstones affects his or her blood glucose level by self-monitoring blood glucose.

Self-Monitoring of Blood Glucose

Clients' self-monitoring of blood glucose (SMBG), using a blood glucose meter, is an important tool for determining the effectiveness and adherence to a treatment plan. For individuals using multiple insulin injections or an insulin pump, SMBG should be done multiple times per day. For some clients, this requires testing 6-10 times per day, but needs vary. Increased daily frequency of SMBG is associated with lower A1C and fewer complications.

Individual response to medication, diet, and exercise can be determined with SMBG and can be performed using a single drop of blood. The client obtains the drop of blood from a finger with either a lancet or a spring-loaded device. The blood sample is placed in the meter,

TABLE 17-4   Glycemic Goals for Individuals With Diabetes

GLYCEMIC RECOMMENDATIONS	ADULTS	CHILDREN 0-6	CHILDREN 6-12	ADOLESCENTS 13-19	GDM	GDM/PRE-EXISTING DM
Bedtime and overnight (mg/dL)	N/A	110-200	100-180	90-150	N/A	60-99*
Preprandial mg/dL	70-130	100-180	90-180	90-130	≤95	60-99*
1 hour postprandial mg/dL	<180	†	†	†	≤140	100-129
2 hour postprandial mg/dL	<180	†	†	†	≤120	100-129
A1C %	<7.0	<8.5	<7.0	<7.5	N/A	<6.0

*If achievable without excessive hypoglycemia.
†Postprandial blood glucose levels should be measured when there is a discrepancy between preprandial blood glucose values and A1C levels to help assess glycemia in those on basal/bolus regimens.

called a glucometer, and the test results are available in less than 1 minute. The client can then adjust insulin dose and food and exercise behaviors accordingly. Many experts consider SMBG to be the most important development in diabetes management since the discovery of insulin.

SMBG has allowed clients to try to normalize their blood glucose levels throughout the day. Health-care workers need to teach clients carefully how to interpret the results of SMBG. Continual reassessment of the client's technique and blood glucose records is necessary to guide treatment decisions. SMBG helps evaluate the need for changes in diet or medications. Continuous glucose monitoring (CGM) devices are available to measure blood glucose and have alarms when low or high levels are measured (ADA, 2016).

Physical Activity

Exercise plays a key role in the management of diabetes. All individuals with diabetes are encouraged to perform at least 150 minutes per week of moderate-intensity aerobic physical activity. Strength training should also be performed, if there are no contraindications. Children should have at least 60 minutes of physical activity every day (ADA, 2016). People with diabetes who exercise should be encouraged to follow these guidelines:

1. Wear proper footwear and use other protective equipment if necessary.
2. Avoid exercise in extremely hot or cold environments.
3. Inspect feet daily and after exercise for open areas, blisters, punctures, swelling, and redness; report any of these signs to the physician immediately.
4. Avoid exercise during periods of poor metabolic control (blood glucose levels that are <70 or >240 mg/dL levels).
5. Wear a diabetes ID badge or bracelet.
6. Carry a source of glucose in case of a decrease in blood glucose because exercise decreases blood glucose levels.
7. Ingest additional carbohydrate pre-exercise if using insulin, or insulin secretagogues, if blood glucose levels are less than 100 mg/dL before exercise (ADA, 2016).

Exercise and Type 1 Diabetes

The ADA strongly endorses an exercise program for people with type 1 diabetes because of the potential for improving cardiovascular fitness and psychological well-being. Exercise involves some risk for individuals with type 1 diabetes because it changes insulin requirements in sometimes unpredictable ways for more than 24 hours after the exercise. Retinopathy, neuropathy, and renal disease may worsen in some clients with type 1 diabetes who exercise. Blood pressure may also become elevated. For this type of client, self-monitoring of blood glucose should be incorporated into a modified exercise program tailored to individual needs and limitations. The client should demonstrate the ability to self-treat a hypoglycemic episode.

Exercise and Type 2 Diabetes

Physical activity is widely endorsed for persons with type 2 diabetes. Physical activity increases the number and binding capacity of insulin receptors, assists in lowering blood glucose levels, and reduces insulin requirements in persons who use insulin. Improved blood lipid levels occur in some clients who engage in regular exercise. This improvement helps delay or prevent the CVD complications commonly seen in these clients. Exercise also assists in weight control and improves muscle strength and flexibility.

Exercise, SMBG, and Food Intake

Clients with type 1 diabetes who exercise and all type 2 clients who engage in nonroutine exercise should monitor their blood glucose levels before, during, and after exercise. It is best to exercise 60 to 90 minutes after meals, when the blood glucose level is highest. If the blood glucose level is greater than 100 mg/dL before exercise, no additional food is usually needed if the planned exercise is of short duration and low intensity. Exercise of long duration and high intensity generally requires more kilocalories. Snacks with an additional 15 to 30 grams of carbohydrate-containing food should be ingested for every 30 to 60 minutes of exercise. Good choices for snack foods include:

- Fruit
- Starch
- Dairy

To prevent wide swings in blood glucose levels, care should be taken not to overeat. Too much food will cause the blood glucose level to go up too high and subsequently to drop too low.

Medications for Diabetes

Two primary types of medications are used with diabetic clients:

1. Insulin
2. Oral hypoglycemic agents

Clients with type 1 diabetes require insulin. Clients with type 2 diabetes may not require any medication, or may need to have an oral hypoglycemic agent and/or insulin prescribed. Frequently, clients with type 2 diabetes are able to discontinue or reduce medications after a significant loss of body fat.

Insulin

Almost all the insulin used in the United States is human. Human insulin is manufactured by recombinant-DNA technology (biosynthetic). Human insulin (**Humulin**) produces few allergic reactions. Insulin cannot be taken orally because the gastrointestinal tract enzymes will digest it before absorption. Insulin must be administered by needle either

subcutaneously (beneath the skin) or intravenously (IV). Only regular insulin is given IV. The substances used to delay absorption of intermediate- and long-acting insulins are not designed for IV administration. Regular insulin is usually administered IV only for the severely hyperglycemic or hospitalized client.

Insulin can also be administered with an insulin pump. These pumps are designed to provide a small inflow of insulin continuously and large inflows before eating, mimicking normal insulin secretion. Continuous subcutaneous insulin infusion (CSII) or insulin pumps have been available for nearly 25 years but have become more widely used.

Medications are described according to the onset, peak, and duration of action. A bolus dose of insulin is short acting and designed to cover needs for one meal. A basal dose of insulin is longer acting and usually injected once or twice a day. Table 17-5 lists the times of onset, peak, and duration of insulin. Variation in duration makes it possible to inject insulin in a pattern that is as close as possible to normal insulin activity. Ideally, the medication is planned around the diet, not vice versa. It is for the client's benefit, and long-term quality of life, to change a medication to cover food/meal ingestion for the greatest flexibility.

TABLE 17-5 Times of Onset, Peak, and Duration of Action for Insulins

TIMES IN HOURS

	Onset	Peak	Duration
Insulin Bolus (Short Acting)			
Humalog® or lispro	15–30 minutes	30–90 minutes	3–5 hours
NovoLog® or aspart	10–20 minutes	40–50 minutes	3–5 hours
Regular	30–60 minutes	2–5 hours	5–8 hours
Apidra® or glulisine	20–30 minutes	30–90 minutes	1–2½ hours
Basal Insulin (Intermediate-Long Acting)			
Lantus®*	1–1½ hours	None	20–24 hours
NPH	1–2 hours	4–12 hours	18–24 hours
Novolog 70/30®†	10–20 minutes	1–4 hours	Up to 24 hours
Lente	1–2½ hours	3–10 hours	18–24 hours
Ultralente	30 minutes–3 hours	10–20 hours	20–36 hours
Levemir®	1–2 hours	6–8 hours	Up to 24 hours

*Lantus® is a long-acting insulin that is designed to be given at HS (Latin for hour of sleep, commonly used to mean just before bedtime). Lantus® has no pronounced peaks, with a relatively constant level over 24 hours. The Food and Drug Administration approved Lantus® in early 2000 and Levemir® in 2005.
†Mixture is a premixed insulin with intermediate-acting and short-acting insulin in one bottle or insulin pen.

Oral Hypoglycemic Agents

Oral hypoglycemic agents lower blood glucose levels in type 2 diabetes. These drugs stimulate insulin release from the pancreatic beta cells, reduce glucose output from the liver, and increase the uptake of glucose in tissues. Many oral agents are being prescribed in the United States (Table 17-6). Metformin is the preferred initial oral medication given to individuals with prediabetes and diabetes, unless there is a contraindication (such as reduced kidney function or severe GI side effects). Commonly prescribed oral hypoglycemic agents include glipizide, glyburide, glimepiride, acarbose, and glitazones. Oral agents are frequently used in combinations to help get diabetics to their recommended glycemic levels without hypoglycemia. Many of the oral agents work on different cell receptor sites (ADA, 2016).

Management of Hospitalized Clients

Increased lengths of stay and adverse outcomes are seen in hospitalized clients with hyperglycemia. In the hospitalized population with hyperglycemia, when blood glucose levels are greater than 180 mg/dL, treatment with insulin is recommended, along with checking the A1C levels so that individuals with existing diabetes can be distinguished from those with hyperglycemia triggered from acute stress. Oral diabetes medications should be discontinued during most acute hospitalizations and resumed as appropriate after discharge. Because hospitalized individuals may have a rapidly changing condition, and/or be NPO (no food by mouth) for treatment and tests, flexibility in insulin therapy is critical. A basal and bolus insulin therapy that helps prevent periods of hyper- and hypoglycemia is recommended. The three components to this type of therapy include basal insulin, which is long acting and given once per day; mealtime bolus insulin, which is fast acting and helps prevent postprandial rises in blood glucose and is given before a meal and withheld if the client is NPO; and correction insulin, which is also fast acting and given to lower hyperglycemic blood glucose levels not caused by nutritional hyperglycemia (ADA, 2016).

Medical Nutritional Management of Diabetes

Diabetes is directly related to how the body uses food. Nutrition is thus an essential component of management for all persons with diabetes. Clients who participate in Diabetes Self-Management Education (DSME), in which making informed nutritional decisions is an essential component, experience improved health; better control of body weight; improved control of blood glucose, blood pressure, and lipid levels; and better prevention of complications of diabetes when they adhere to dietary recommendations. Clients who receive individualized medical nutrition therapy (MNT) by a registered dietitian show a decrease in A1C of 0.3% to 1% in type 1 and 0.5% to 2% in type 2 diabetes (ADA, 2016).

TABLE 17-6   Diabetes Oral Medications and Major Actions

CLASSIFICATION	MAJOR ACTIONS	GENERIC NAME (TRADE NAME)	COMMENTS
Sulfonylureas	Stimulate insulin release by the pancreas and may help decrease liver glucose production.	Glipizide (Glucotrol®, Glucotrol® XL) Glyburide (DiaBeta®, Micronase®, Glynase PresTabs®) Glimepiride (Amaryl®)	Glipizide must be taken on an empty stomach. Glyburide can be taken with food or on an empty stomach. Low toxicity. Use caution with elderly.
Biguanides	Decrease liver production of glucose. Increase glucose uptake into tissues.	Metformin (Glucophage®)	Given in 2–3 doses per day with meals. Not metabolized.
Meglitinide	Stimulates immediate insulin release from pancreas as needed for meals.	Repaglinide (Prandin®) Nateglinide (Starlix®)	Given in 2–4 doses per day 15–30 minutes before meals.
Alpha-Glucosidase Inhibitors	Slow the rate of digestion of starches and complex sugars.	Acarbose (Precose®)	Given in 3 doses per day with meals. 98% not absorbed. Rest excreted by kidneys.
Thiazolidinedione	Decreases insulin resistance.	Pioglitazone (Actos®) Rosiglitazone (Avandia®)	Clients need to be monitored for fluid retention and weight gain.

Clients' nutritional goals need to be determined individually. There is no "diabetic diet" or "ADA diet," but several meal-planning approaches are widely endorsed by the ADA and the Academy of Nutrition and Dietetics (see Dollars & Sense 17-1).

Nutritional Goals

The goal of medical nutritional therapy is to educate the client with diabetes so that he or she can make changes in food and exercise habits that lead to improved metabolic control. Specifically, the client needs assistance with:

1. Attaining and maintaining near-normal blood glucose levels as feasible by the coordination of food intake, **endogenous** and **exogenous** insulin and/or hypoglycemic agents, and physical activity. This goal is a challenge in some clients who have fluctuating endogenous insulin production.
2. Attaining and maintaining optimal serum lipid levels and blood pressure
3. Providing adequate kilocalories to:
   - Attain and maintain a healthy body weight for adults and normal growth and development for children
   - Recover from illnesses
   - Meet the metabolic needs of pregnancy and lactation
4. Preventing and treating the acute and chronic complications of diabetes, such as renal disease, autonomic neuropathy, hypertension, and CVD.

Dollars & Sense 17-1

Dietetic Foods

Clients with diabetes do not need to buy special foods labeled "dietetic." Many clients find they actually save money because they eat less by consuming more nutrient-dense foods.

5. Improving overall health through good nutrition. Clients must be given support to make informed self-management choices within their individual preferences, needs, and values. *MyPlate* and *USDA 2015-2020 Dietary Guidelines for Americans* illustrate and summarize nutritional guidelines for all Americans. These resources may be used to demonstrate different healthy eating styles the client may choose to use as a basis for positive dietary changes.

Goal Priority

The medications prescribed, the type of diabetes the individual has, and the client's desire to change behavior determine goal priority. A high priority for the person taking insulin is to facilitate consistency in the timing of insulin to cover meals and snacks to prevent wide swings in blood glucose. This priority requires coordination among exercise, insulin, and food intake.

A high priority for the individual with type 2 diabetes is achieving glucose, blood pressure, and lipid goals. To achieve these goals, diet is a cornerstone of treatment. Weight reduction for these clients usually improves short-term glycemic levels and long-term metabolic control. The client's motivation to lose weight needs to be carefully assessed by the health-care educator.

Meal Frequency

Meal spacing is more crucial in type 1 than in type 2 diabetes. Consistent timing of medication type and administration and meal size assist in stabilization of blood glucose levels in type 1 diabetes. In general, people with diabetes benefit from eating on a regular basis (every 4 to 5 hours), but this must be individualized based on the client's lifestyle and/or medical condition.

Client Readiness to Change

Food and physical activity behaviors are difficult to change. Although some clients with diabetes do successfully change or alter food and activity behaviors to enhance their outcomes, many clients do not, will not, or cannot change harmful behaviors. Modification of harmful behaviors involves progression through five stages: precontemplation, contemplation, preparation, action, and maintenance. Individuals typically recycle through these stages several times before terminating negative behaviors. Following is a brief description of each stage:

1. *Precontemplation:* Individuals exhibit no intention to change behavior in the foreseeable future.
2. *Contemplation:* Individuals know they have a problem and are seriously thinking about overcoming the harmful behavior but are not ready to take action.
3. *Preparation:* Individuals plan to take action in the near future, may have taken action unsuccessfully in the past, and may report small behavioral changes.
4. *Action:* Individuals modify their behavior, experiences, and environment to overcome the harmful behavior. This stage requires considerable commitment of time and energy.
5. *Maintenance:* Individuals continue to work to prevent relapse and to consolidate gains.

Health-care workers can assist clients in the precontemplation and contemplation stages by attempting to raise clients' consciousness about the benefits of behavioral change. Stimulus control and reinforcement also help clients become more aware of the need to alter behaviors (see Chapter 16). The most challenging clients for the health educator are at the precontemplation phase. Clients at the action stage are associated with better diabetes self-management (Holmen et al, 2016).

A technique called motivational interviewing (MI) that can be used by health-care workers helps determine what the client's interest in disease management and education is and can strengthen the client's desire to make positive changes. If the client wishes to gain better blood glucose control, the clinician working with that individual would help explore how he or she wishes to do so. Options using diet, medications, and/or exercise should all be discussed and assistance with the client's goal provided. Consulting a dietitian, pharmacist, and/or physical therapist may be helpful for the client to reach and maintain his/her goal. MI has been shown to improve treatment outcomes; client quality-of-life, engagement, and retention; and staff satisfaction (Case Western Reserve University, 2017).

The health-care educator needs to consider carefully how much information the client desires and how ready he or she is to change behaviors. For example, an educational tool that takes 3 to 4 hours to review with a client is inappropriate for someone who is willing to devote just a few minutes to learning about his or her diet. In contrast, the client who wants to learn everything he or she can about self-care will not be satisfied with an elementary meal plan.

Meal-Planning Approaches

The ADA (2016) advocates several meal planning tools available for use with clients including:

- MyPlate
- Dietary Guidelines for Americans
- Carbohydrate Counting

Many hospitals and private practitioners provide comprehensive educational programs to achieve optimal blood glucose and lipid control. Different tools for meal-planning are discussed later in the chapter. Figure 17-4 illustrates a dietitian providing nutrition counseling.

Energy Nutrient Distribution

The distribution of energy nutrients refers to the percentage of total kilocalories that should be derived from carbohydrate, fat, and protein as well as to the division of carbohydrate, fat, and protein among the day's meals/feedings. Total energy requirements for an individual with diabetes do not differ from those for individuals without diabetes. Twenty to 35 kcal/kg, depending on the client's level of physical activity, nutritional status, desire for weight loss or gain, and body weight, is

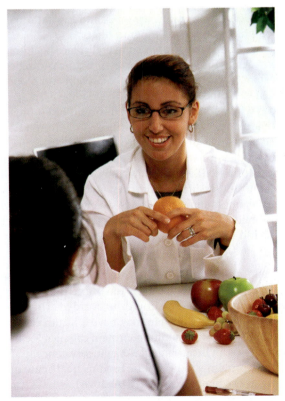

FIGURE 17-4 A diabetes educator providing nutritional counseling. The use of food models facilitates the learning process and teaches portion control.

usually a good starting point to estimate a need for kcal. The client should eat a set amount of kcal for a few weeks and compare body weight before and after the given kcal level is consumed. Adjustments based on the treatment goals can be made, as necessary. If weight loss is desirable, the rate of loss should be 1 to 2 pounds per week. The only way to more accurately determine a client's need for energy is by indirect calorimetry and this equipment is not widely available.

Macronutrient Distribution

The acceptable macronutrient distribution recommended for the general population is also recommended for clients with diabetes. There is no one optimal mix of carbohydrate, protein, and fat that must be followed by every person with diabetes. This should be individualized based upon each client's lifestyle, preference, and comorbidities (ADA, 2016).

CARBOHYDRATE

Dietary Guidelines for Americans recommends all people choose a variety of fiber-containing food, such as whole grains, fruits, and vegetables, because they provide vitamins, minerals, fiber, and other substances that optimize health. The contribution of carbohydrate to total kilocalorie intake should be individualized based on nutrition assessment, laboratory results, and weight and treatment goals.

The ADA guidelines that pertain to carbohydrates include the following (ADA, 2016):

- A dietary pattern that includes carbohydrate from fruits, vegetables, whole grains, legumes, and low-fat milk with an emphasis on foods higher in fiber.
- Sugar-sweetened foods, which may displace healthier, nutrient-dense foods, should be avoided. Avoiding sugar-sweetened beverages helps control weight and reduce the risk of CVD and fatty liver.
- Foods with a lower glycemic load should be emphasized.
- Individuals on a flexible insulin schedule should be educated on using carbohydrate counting.
- Individuals on fixed insulin dosing should be informed that a consistent intake pattern of carbohydrates (time and amount) results in improved glycemic control.
- Sugar alcohols and nonnutritive sweeteners are safe when consumed within the daily levels established by the U.S. Food and Drug Administration.

PROTEIN

The need for protein in the diabetic population is the same as for the general population if renal function is normal. Excessive dietary protein should be avoided. The concept that excessive dietary protein may have a health risk is discussed in Chapter 4. In addition, protein can increase insulin response without increasing plasma glucose concentrations. Therefore, protein should not be used to treat acute or prevent nighttime hypoglycemia (ADA, 2016).

FAT

Data on the ideal total dietary fat content for individuals with diabetes are inconclusive; however, an eating plan emphasizing a Mediterranean-style diet rich in monounsaturated fats may improve glucose metabolism and lower CVD risk. Additionally, ADA recommends (2016):

- Consume foods rich in long-chain omega-3 fatty acids, such as fatty fish, nuts, and seeds.
- Do not consume omega-3 fatty acid supplements as science does not support any benefit.

Carbohydrate Counting

Carbohydrate (CHO) counting is another frequently used menu-planning tool. Because CHO is the energy nutrient that has the greatest influence on blood glucose levels, some clients adhere to nutritional recommendations more closely with this approach and SMBG. Clients can readily see the effect that diet has on blood glucose levels throughout the day when combined with SMBG. The advantages of the carbohydrate-counting meal plan concept include:

- Single-nutrient focused
- More precise matching of food and insulin
- Flexible food choices
- A potential for improved blood glucose, and client-controlled treatment

Challenges for the client who uses this system may include:

- The need to weigh and measure food
- Maintenance of extensive food records
- Monitoring of the blood glucose before and after eating
- The need to read food labels and calculate grams of carbohydrate consumed
- The need to maintain healthful eating and weight management

Knowledge of carbohydrate counting is often a prerequisite before consideration of insulin pump therapy. It is also a prerequisite for clients who want to learn how to calculate insulin-to-carbohydrate ratios. This type of teaching is usually done by a certified diabetes educator (CDE) and is considered advanced teaching.

In carbohydrate counting, approximately 15 grams of carbohydrate equals approximately one serving. Food labels, tables of food composition, and smart phone apps are some of the tools clients can use to determine the carbohydrate content of a particular food. Following is a typical meal plan for a client who has been taught to count carbohydrates:

Breakfast: 3 carbohydrates
Example: 1 whole bagel and 8 ounces (oz) skim milk
Lunch: 3 carbohydrates
Example: ⅔ cup plain yogurt (or sweetened w/an artificial sweetener), 1 fresh orange, and ¾ ounce whole-wheat crackers (2 to 5)
Dinner: 3 carbohydrates
Example: 1½ cups pasta
Snack: 1 carbohydrate (range, 8 to 22 grams)
Example: 8 oz skim milk

Protein and fat intake are not counted with this meal-planning system but should be given some consideration. Clients are usually counseled to eat about the same amount of protein each day and choose foods that contain healthy fats.

MyPlate for Diabetes

Figure 17-5 is the MyPlate for individuals with diabetes. This is an easy way to get started eating for diabetes. Half of the dinner plate should be filled with nonstarchy vegetables, such as spinach, carrots, lettuce, greens, cabbage, green beans, broccoli, cauliflower, tomatoes, cucumber, beets, mushrooms, onions, and peppers. The second half of the plate should be separated in half. One of these halves should be filled with starchy foods, such as whole-grain breads, rice, pasta, tortillas, cooked beans, peas, corn, potatoes, or low-fat crackers, snack chips, pretzels, and fat-free popcorn. The last section of the plate should have low-fat proteins, such as poultry without the skin, fish, seafood, lean cuts of beef and pork, tofu, eggs, or low-fat cheese. To this plate, an 8-ounce glass of nonfat or low-fat milk or 6-ounce container of low-fat, no-sugar-added yogurt should be added. For dessert, a small piece of fruit, or $1/2$ cup of no-sugar-added fruit salad can be added for a complete meal (ADA, 2016).

Mediterranean Diet

The Mediterranean diet is based on the way people who live in Italy, Spain, and other countries in the Mediterranean region have eaten for centuries. The diet consists of (U.S. Department of Agriculture, 2015):

- Plant-based meals with small amounts of meat and chicken when they are used
- Whole grains, fresh fruits and vegetables, nuts, and legumes
- Fish and seafood, limited red meat
- Olive oil as the main source of fat

Glycemic Index and Glycemic Load

Not all carbohydrates affect blood glucose levels in the same manner. The glycemic index (GI) was discussed in the previous chapter and can be an important tool in the improvement of diet management in diabetes. Foods with a GI less than 55 are low, 56 to 69 are moderate, and 70 to 100 are high (diabetes.org). In general, the more processed a food is, the higher the GI. However, the determination of GI was based on the same portion of a food item and not necessarily that in a normal portion size. It is important to take the portion size into consideration when evaluating a food; in doing this, the glycemic load (GL) of the food item is calculated. GL is the GI of the food multiplied by the carbohydrate per serving, divided by 100. A food with a low GL is less than 10, medium is 11 to 19, and high is greater than 20 (Harvard Health Publications, 2015). There can be wide variability in the calculated values of different foods. The University of Sydney, where the research on GI and GL was pioneered, lists a value for the GI of an 80-gram serving of carrots based on their state of preparation from raw, to peeled, boiled and ground, to unspecified. In this example, clients may be told to consume only raw carrots. But if the GL is calculated, based on the carbohydrate content in a serving, the GL is 1, 4, and 6, respectively (Table 17-7), all of which are considered low-GL food items (www.glycemicindex.com).

When discussing the GI or GL of a food item, the following should be kept in mind as affecting the overall glycemic effect of foods (Kirpitch & Maryniuk, 2011):

- The more processed a food, typically, the higher its GI/GL.
- Combining foods in a mixed meal (cheese, white rice, and nonstarchy vegetables) will minimize the overall glycemic effect of one food that has a high GI/GL. In general, protein and fat have little glycemic impact, and adding the cheese to the rice will lower the overall GI/GL of the meal.
- Fiber (insoluble) from whole grains, fruits and vegetables, and seeds provides a physical barrier slowing the breakdown of the carbohydrate and therefore have a lower GI/GL.

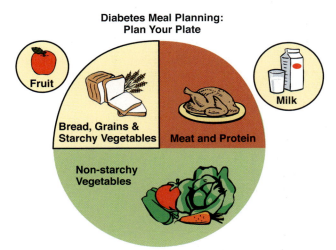

Diabetes Meal Planning: Plan Your Plate

Fruit

Bread, Grains & Starchy Vegetables

Meat and Protein

Milk

Non-starchy Vegetables

FIGURE 17-5 MyPlate for people with diabetes shows the division of a typical plate of food, which should comprise vegetables, whole-grain starchy foods, and lean proteins.

FOOD	SERVING IN GRAMS	GI	CHO GRAMS/ SERVING	GL
TABLE 17-7 Glycemic Load (GL) Calculation of Carrots				
Carrots, raw	80	16	8	1
Carrots, peeled, boiled, and ground	80	60	6	4
Carrots, unspecified	80	92	6	6

CHO, carbohydrate; GI, glycemic index.

- Fiber (soluble) from beans and oats is more viscous and tends to have a lower GI/GL in its more unprocessed form.

Because eating foods with a lower GI/GL lowers the glycemic response by the body, there is a lower insulin response. It has been shown that following a low-GI/GL diet has the following benefits for people with diabetes (Kirpitch & Maryniuk, 2011):

- Lower A1C by 0.5%
- Decrease in hypoglycemia
- Reduce the incidence and risk for microvascular complications
- May be helpful in improving lipid profiles by lowering low-density lipoprotein and raising high-density lipoprotein cholesterol levels and therefore reducing the risk for cardiac disease
- May facilitate weight loss, which may improve insulin sensitivity

Special Considerations

People with diabetes frequently ask questions about nutritional problems related to supplements, alcohol, acute illness, eating out, and delayed meals.

Supplements

There is no clear evidence that people with diabetes benefit from vitamin or mineral supplementation solely because they have diabetes. Routine supplementation with antioxidants, such as vitamins E and C and carotene, is not advised because of lack of evidence of efficacy and concern related to long-term safety. Benefit from chromium supplementation in individuals with diabetes or obesity has not been clearly demonstrated and are not recommended (NIH, 2017). All supplements should be assessed for interactions with other drugs. A pharmacist should be consulted with any questions.

Alcohol

Moderate use of alcohol does not adversely affect diabetes in well-controlled clients. Recommendations are as follows (ADA, 2016):

- If people with diabetes choose to drink, daily intake should be limited to one drink per day or less for women and two drinks or less per day for men.
- May cause delayed hypoglycemia in both insulin users and insulin secretagogues; people with diabetes who choose to drink should be educated regarding recognition and management of delayed hypoglycemia.

Nutrition During Acute Illness

Colds and flulike symptoms can be fatal for some people with diabetes unless precautions are taken. Secretion of both glucagon and epinephrine increases during illness and contributes to an increase in blood glucose levels. This action may lead to a loss of glucose, fluid, and electrolytes. Dehydration, electrolyte depletion, and a loss of nutrients may follow. Acute illnesses can lead to DKA in type 1 and to HHNS in type 2 diabetes.

Dehydration is more rapid when electrolytes and fluids are not replaced. Vomiting, diarrhea, and fever all result in fluid loss. During acute illness, the individual should be instructed to monitor his or her blood glucose level every 2 to 4 hours until the symptoms subside. Urine ketone levels should be checked. The following guidelines are recommended by the ADA (2016):

- Ingestion of 15 to 20 grams of glucose is the preferred treatment for hypoglycemia, although any form of CHO that contains glucose may be used.
- The response to treatment of hypoglycemia should be apparent quickly. Plasma glucose should be tested again in 15 minutes because additional treatment may be necessary. This may need to be repeated several times until the blood glucose is greater than 70 mg/dL.
- Once blood glucose returns to a level greater than 70 mg/dL, if the next meal is more than an hour away, a snack should be eaten.

Increased fluids reduce the risk of dehydration. Clients who are vomiting or nauseated and are unable to tolerate regular food should drink liquids that contain carbohydrate or electrolytes (Table 17-8). A general guideline is that approximately 15 grams of carbohydrate should be consumed every 1 to 2 hours. Some clients have an individually calculated sick-day menu based on the carbohydrate content of their regular diet.

Other meal-planning tips that may prove helpful during periods of acute illness include the following:

- Increase water intake, even for clients who can eat regular foods.

TABLE 17-8	Carbohydrate-Containing Foods for Sick Days	
FOOD	AMOUNT	GRAMS OF CARBOHYDRATE
Regular cola	1/2 cup	13
Ginger ale	3/4 cup	16
Milk	1 cup	12
Apple juice	1/2 cup	15
Grape juice	1/3 cup	15
Orange juice	1/2 cup	15
Pineapple juice	1/2 cup	15
Prune juice	1/3 cup	15
Regular gelatin	1/2 cup	20
Sherbet	1/2 cup	30
Tomato juice*	1/2 cup	5

*High in sodium.

- Eat smaller, more frequent meals.
- Eat soft, easily digested foods.

During acute illnesses, testing plasma glucose and urinary ketones, drinking adequate amounts of fluids, and ingesting carbohydrates are all important (ADA, 2016).

Hypoglycemia in Diabetes

The immediate treatment goal for a glucose level of less than 70 mg/dL is to increase blood glucose to within a normal level as rapidly as possible. Take care not to overtreat hypoglycemia. If the client is monitoring his or her blood glucose level, at the first sign or symptom of hypoglycemia, he or she should measure the blood glucose level. If the blood glucose level is less than 70 mg/dL, 15 grams of glucose should be consumed, after 15 minutes, blood glucose should be measured. If blood glucose is not yet above 70 mg/dL, another 15 grams of glucose should be consumed, and blood glucose should be rechecked. This should be repeated until blood glucose is normal. The individual should then consume a snack or meal to prevent recurrence of hypoglycemia (ADA, 2016). Fifteen grams of carbohydrate should be consumed, such as:

- 3 to 4 glucose tablets
- 1 serving of glucose gel
- 5 to 6 pieces of hard candies
- 4 to 6 ounces of fruit juice
- 1 cup of milk
- 1 tablespoon of sugar or honey

Teaching Self-Care

People with diabetes ultimately treat themselves. The better educated the individual is about diabetes, the greater the likelihood of his or her avoiding the acute and chronic complications of this disease. Many public health departments, hospitals, and clinics hold classes for clients with diabetes. Newly diagnosed clients with diabetes need to learn DSME.

Because of the genetic predisposition toward diabetes, many newly diagnosed clients have relatives who have suffered from the acute and chronic complications of diabetes. Hearing about such complications firsthand often creates fear in newly diagnosed clients. They need time to accept their condition. Clients grasp the principles of self-care at various levels and reinforcement may be necessary. During hospitalization, it is extremely difficult to effectively educate clients. Follow-up with a certified diabetes educator (CDE) and a registered dietitian (RD) is crucial.

Hypoglycemia Not Related to Diabetes

There are two types of hypoglycemia not related to diabetes, reactive and fasting. The symptoms are the same as those experienced by diabetics with hypoglycemia.

Reactive hypoglycemia is hypoglycemia that occurs within 4 hours after a meal. The causes are uncertain but may be related to an individual's sensitivity to the body's release of epinephrine or deficiency in glucagons secretion. Other causes may include gastric surgery (causing the rapid passage of food into the small intestine) and enzyme deficiencies early in life (hereditary fructose intolerance).

Fasting hypoglycemia is defined as a blood glucose level less than 70 mg/dL after an overnight fast, between meals, or after physical activity. Causes include some medications (large dose salicylates, sulfa medications, pentamidine, and quinine), alcoholic beverages (especially binge drinking), critical illnesses (affecting the liver, heart, or kidneys), hormonal deficiencies (shortages of cortisol, growth hormone, glucagons, or epinephrine), tumors (in the pancreas), and infancy and childhood conditions (hyperinsulinism, enzyme, or hormonal deficiencies) (Desimone & Weinstock, 2016).

The dietary management of reactive hypoglycemia consists of avoiding simple carbohydrates and sometimes taking small, frequent feedings. Previously mentioned meal patterns for diabetes offer a reasonable guide to meal planning.

KEYSTONES

- Diabetes is caused by an undersecretion or underutilization of insulin and/or receptor or postreceptor defects.
- Diabetes is actually a group of disorders with a common sign of hyperglycemia.
- The two major types of diabetes are type 1 and type 2. Impaired glucose tolerance or impaired fasting glucose, secondary diabetes, and gestational diabetes are other categories of this disease.
- People with diabetes suffer from acute and chronic complications.
- Treatment involves medication, nutrition management, and exercise.
- Nutrition is a fundamental part of treatment.
- Hypoglycemia, a rarer condition than diabetes, is caused by oversecretion of insulin and is also treated with dietary manipulation.

CASE STUDY 17-1

Mrs. S, a 45-year-old woman, came to your doctor's office because she had a sore that would not heal on her leg. She is 5 ft 5 in. and weighs 200 lb (body mass index [BMI] = 33.5). Vital signs are temperature 98.6°F, pulse 70 beats per minute, respirations 16 breaths per minute, and blood pressure 160/95 mm Hg.

Mrs. S reports a gradual increase in her weight since her third child was born 20 years ago. That baby weighed 12 lb. Two previous pregnancies produced infants weighing 10 and 11 lb. She has no known allergies. None of the children live at home. Mrs. S lives with her husband, who works as a construction laborer. She has been seasonally employed as a hotel maid at a nearby resort. Health insurance coverage is sporadic. They have a new insurance policy now.

Mrs. S is the oldest of six children. Her father died of a heart attack at age 60. Her mother died of a stroke at age 62. Both parents reportedly "had a little sugar." The sister who is closest to Mrs. S in age developed diabetes 3 years ago and is being treated with oral medication. Their youngest sister was diagnosed with type 1 diabetes at age 18 after an episode of mumps.

Mrs. S reports a good appetite and a fluid intake of about 3 quarts per day. Her favorite beverage is iced tea with sugar and lemon. She does most of the grocery shopping and cooking.

Mrs. S hit her left ankle with the screen door about 2 months ago. The resulting sore has not healed but has gotten worse. Mrs. S knows that a sore that does not heal is a sign of cancer, which is why she sought medical attention. The ankle now has an open lesion 5 cm in diameter over the lateral ankle bone. The entire foot is swollen to twice the size of the right foot. The bandage over the sore had greenish-yellow drainage on it. A random blood glucose test 3 hours after her last meal shows a glucose level of 400 mg/dL. Her urine glucose was negative for ketones. The physician diagnoses Mrs. S with type 2 diabetes.

The physician prescribed the following care for Mrs. S:

- Bed rest with left leg elevated
- Diet assessment and teaching
- Multivitamin, 1 capsule daily
- Culture and sensitivity of drainage from left leg
- Cefuroxime, 250 mg, orally every 12 hours
- Warm, moist dressing to left leg ulcer four times per day
- Fasting blood sugar (FBS), electrolytes
- Metformin, 500 mg with breakfast and dinner

The nurse constructed the following Care Plan for Mrs. S.

CARE PLAN

Subjective Data
Family history of diabetes mellitus ■ Large appetite ■ Large fluid intake ■ Delay in seeking medical attention

Objective Data
Obesity: ht 5 ft 5 in ■ wt 200 lb ■ Newly diagnosed type 2 diabetes ■ Possible hypertension (only one reading given) ■ Open lesion 5 cm diameter over left lateral ankle ■ purulent discharge

Analysis
Lack of knowledge of disease process related to new diagnosis with type 2 diabetes. Through interviewing, client is willing to attend a diabetes class.

Plan

DESIRED OUTCOMES EVALUATION CRITERIA	ACTIONS/ INTERVENTIONS	RATIONALE
Client will understand type 2 diabetes	Briefly discuss type 2 diabetes causes, effects on the body, and tools for management of the disease.	The more a client understands about the disease, the more likely she is to become part of the treatment process.

DESIRED OUTCOMES EVALUATION CRITERIA	ACTIONS/ INTERVENTIONS	RATIONALE
Client will verbalize self-care measures related to type 2 diabetes	SMBG will be taught using a glucometer. A blood glucose log will be given to client and asked to bring to next appointment. Refer to dietitian for nutritional assessment and education.	Client needs to become aware of blood glucose goals and self-management techniques to manage her diabetes. One of the cornerstones of treatment of type 2 is weight loss. Clients with diabetes essentially need to learn to treat themselves as much as possible and know when to seek medical treatment. The American Diabetes Association recommends all clients with diabetes learn DSME.
Client will verbalize willingness to continue nursing/medical regimen.	Ask the client what her interests are for her management of the diabetes, help her set achievable goals that she can work on (motivational interviewing). Refer to social worker for sources of food and medical attention when uninsured (or underinsured). Teach principles of wound care, including effect of high blood sugar on infection. Reinforce dietitian's instruction. Have Mrs. S review MyPlate for diabetes and the reason why it is important to follow. Have Mrs. S describe the meal plan she follows. Request physician's referral to diabetes class.	The client will feel more empowered and is more likely to work toward goals she help set. This can be done over time if the client is able to return for follow-up. Social workers are most familiar with community resources. If Mrs. S understands that high blood sugar feeds the bacteria causing the infection, she may be more willing to work hard to control the diabetes. Knowledge usually precedes behavior change. Short periods of instruction are most effective; frequent review of the material will help the client master it. Insurance companies will more likely cover outpatient educational programs if ordered by a physician.

TEAMWORK 17-1

DIETITIAN'S NOTES

The following Dietitian's Notes are representative of the documentation found in a client's medical record:

Subjective: *Spoke with client, who was tearful throughout our session. Client describes an uncontrollable thirst and hunger and inability to prepare food while her husband is at work. Claims her husband left her a thermos of coffee and snacks before he left for work. Snacks included bread, a jar of peanut butter, and a jar of jelly. Generally, she claims to have eaten the jars of both the peanut butter and jelly every day, along with half the loaf of bread. She didn't eat the whole loaf because she knows too much bread is bad for anyone. For dinner, her husband usually brought home fast food from the burger store (hamburgers and French fries) or pizza. Denies daily consumption of milk, fruits, and vegetables.*

Objective: *Diagnosis: Type 2 diabetes (newly diagnosed) with open lesion over left ankle with drainage.*

Analysis: *Inappropriate carbohydrate (CHO) intake related to diabetes and food and nutrition knowledge deficit as evidenced by blood glucose greater than 400 and diet history. Body mass index (BMI) is 33.5. Ideal body weight based on maximum ideal body weight of 100 lb for the first 5 ft and 4 lb for each additional inch equals 120; plus or minus 10% equals 108–132 lb. 132 pounds divided by weight in kilograms (2.2) equals 60 kg, and this is the weight used to estimate kcal and protein needs.*

Estimated kcal needs based on maximum ideal body weight and 25–35 kcal/kg equals 1,500–2,100. A 50% acceptable macronutrient distribution range was used to determine carbohydrate needs per meal: 12.5 portions/day or 3 per feeding and 3–4 for an evening snack.

Estimated protein needs based on 1.0 grams/kg equals 60 grams per day. Estimated protein needs on the high side to provide enough protein for wound repair.

Education: *Reviewed carbohydrate counting with client. Will need much encouragement to follow through with healthful behavioral changes.*

Plan:
1. *Recommend to client three carbohydrate (CHO) portions per meal and three to four carbohydrate portions at bedtime.*
2. *Recommend referral to diabetes class for more education.*
3. *Concur that social worker would be helpful to determine eligibility for home-delivered lunch and transportation assistance to diabetes class.*

TEAMWORK **17-2**

SOCIAL WORKER'S NOTES

The following Social Worker's Notes are representative of the documentation found in a client's medical record.

Arrangements have been made for the client to receive a hot lunch daily and a cold boxed dinner 5 days per week. Will contact meal delivery program.

Arrangements have also been made to provide client with transportation to and from the diabetes class.

CRITICAL THINKING QUESTIONS

1. What symptoms in Mrs. S led to her diagnosis with type 2 diabetes?

2. Why is a home delivery of meals beneficial for Mrs. S?

3. Why is a referral to a certified diabetes educator crucial for this client?

CHAPTER REVIEW

1. If a client has a history of ketoacidosis, he or she most likely has which type of diabetes:
    1. Type 1
    2. Type 2
    3. Pituitary
    4. Gestational

2. Which of the following statements is true?
    1. Acute illness lowers blood glucose levels.
    2. Fluid and electrolyte replacement is essential during episodes of acute illness in all persons with diabetes.
    3. Persons with diabetes who have an acute illness require a vitamin and mineral supplement.
    4. Persons with diabetes should never eat forms of simple sugar.

3. Dietary guidelines for people with diabetes include:
    1. One serving of alcohol daily
    2. Consume no more than 2,000 milligrams of sodium each day
    3. Restrict fat intake to less than 10% of total kilocalories
    4. Consume at least 20–35 grams of fiber each day

4. For most clients, the cornerstone of treatment of type 2 diabetes is:
    1. Stress management
    2. Meal planning
    3. Strict adherence to five planned meals per day
    4. Hypoglycemic drugs

5. The diet for reactive hypoglycemia includes the following features:
    1. Small, frequent meals with restricted simple sugars
    2. Three meals with ample simple sugars and high complex carbohydrate
    3. Four to six small meals that are high in fat
    4. Three high-carbohydrate meals that are moderate in fat

CLINICAL ANALYSIS

1. Ms. N, a 14-year-old, was diagnosed 1 year ago with type 1 diabetes mellitus. Her blood sugar levels have been stable on intermediate-acting insulin and a 370-gram CHO diet. The teenager is now being seen in the doctor's office for routine follow-up. The nurse is reviewing Ms. N's knowledge of self-care.

    To assess knowledge, the nurse asks how the client would handle a day when the client could not eat solid foods. Which of the following answers would show understanding of the usual procedure?
    a. Skip insulin that day.
    b. Call the doctor after missing one meal.
    c. Replace the carbohydrates in the meal plan with liquids containing equal amounts of carbohydrate.
    d. Take half her usual insulin dose and double the usual fluid intake.

2. The client plays volleyball for the high school team and is moderately active during practices and games. Self-monitoring blood glucose (SMBG) records indicate a daily glucose level of between 120 and 140 mg/dL before the time she usually plays volleyball. Which of the following behaviors are appropriate for her before playing?
    a. No additional food is indicated
    b. Increase intake by 15 grams of carbohydrate
    c. Decrease intake by 15 grams of carbohydrate
    d. Increase intake by one vegetable exchange and one fat exchange

3. The client states, "I am getting tired of pricking my finger several times a day. Why can't I manage my diabetes with urine testing like my grandmother?" Which of the following responses by the nurse would be most appropriate?
    a. "The urine test is more accurate in older people."
    b. "The point at which sugar is spilled in the urine varies even for one individual. Therefore, the blood test is more accurate."
    c. "Urine tests are more costly."
    d. "The blood test is the newest thing. Your grandmother's doctor must be old-fashioned."

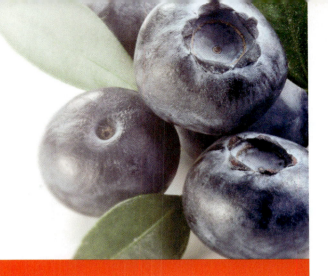

CHAPTER 18

Diet in Cardiovascular Disease

LEARNING OBJECTIVES

After completing this chapter, the student should be able to:
- Discuss the relationship between diet and the development of cardiovascular disease.
- Identify strategies that are most likely to reduce the risk of cardiovascular disease.
- Compare and contrast dietary modifications for clients with myocardial infarction, heart failure, and stroke.
- Describe the DASH diet.
- List several flavorings and seasonings that can be substituted for salt on a sodium-restricted diet.

The cardiovascular system includes not only the heart and blood vessels but the blood-forming organs as well. This chapter covers common diseases of the heart and blood vessels that can be influenced by dietary modification.

Occurrence of Cardiovascular Disease

Heart disease and stroke remain the first and fifth leading causes of death in the United States, respectively. More than 92.1 million American adults suffer from cardiovascular disease (CVD) or effects of stroke. Direct and indirect costs are estimated to total more than $316 billion (heart.org, 2017). The American Heart Association (AHA) goals for 2020 include improving the cardiovascular health of all Americans by 20% while reducing deaths from CVD and strokes by 20% through healthy diets; exercise; decreasing dyslipidemia, blood pressure, and body weight to normal levels; and eliminating smoking (heart.org, 2017).

Underlying Pathology

Two major pathological conditions contribute to cardiovascular disease:

1. Atherosclerosis, the most common form of **arteriosclerosis**
2. Hypertension, included here as contributing to pathology and later in the chapter as a risk factor for cardiovascular disease

Atherosclerosis

In **atherosclerosis,** fatty deposits of cholesterol, fat, or other substances accumulate inside the artery, accompanied by inflammation. Initially, the deposited material, or plaque, is soft, but later it becomes fibrosed or hard. This disease process interferes with the pumping of blood through the artery in two ways:

- The deposits gradually make the lumen smaller and smaller.
- The fibrosis makes it progressively harder for the artery to constrict or dilate in response to the tissues' needs for oxygenated blood (Fig. 18-1).

When the lumen, or opening through the artery, is 70% blocked by atherosclerotic plaque, the person is likely to show symptoms of impaired circulation distal to the obstruction.

Hypertension

Blood pressure (B/P) is the force exerted against the walls of the arteries by the pumping action of the heart. Blood pressure is recorded in two numbers, for example, 120/80. The top number, **systolic pressure,** is the pressure when the heart beats. The bottom number, **diastolic pressure,** is the pressure between beats. Both pressures are reported in millimeters of mercury (mm Hg). Normal blood pressure is less than 120/80 mm Hg. In November 2017, the American College of Cardiology Foundation and the AHA published new high blood pressure clinical practice guidelines (Whelton, 2017).

Diagnosis of Hypertension

Hypertension is defined as:

- Elevated blood pressure—A systolic reading of 120 to 129 mm Hg, and a diastolic reading less than 80 mm Hg.
- High blood pressure (stage 1)—A systolic reading of 130 to 139 mm Hg, or a diastolic reading of 80 to 89 mm Hg.

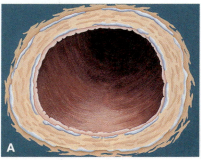
Normal artery

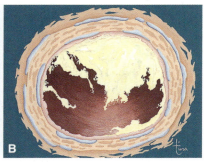
Atherosclerotic artery

FIGURE 18-1 Cross section of a normal coronary artery (*A*) and an atherosclerotic artery (*B*). Note both the narrowed diameter and the roughness within the lumen in the diseased artery. (*Reprinted from Scanlon, VC, and Sanders, T: Essentials of Anatomy and Physiology, ed 5. FA Davis, Philadelphia, 2007, p. 280, with permission.*)

- High blood pressure (stage 2)—A systolic reading greater than 140 mm Hg, or a diastolic reading greater than 90 mm Hg.

Several readings (2 to 3) are taken on various days to eliminate the possibility of excitement or nervousness or incorrect positioning of client causing a transient elevation. Hypertension is classified as stage 1 or 2 (Table 18-1). A person with hypertension may not feel sick, so blood pressure screening is often offered as a community service (Fig. 18-2). Along with temperature, pulse, and respirations, blood pressure is a vital sign that is usually taken at every health-care visit.

Types of Hypertension

Depending on the cause, hypertension is labeled primary or secondary. About 90% of hypertensive clients have primary or **essential hypertension.** There is no single, clear-cut cause for this high blood pressure.

Secondary hypertension occurs in response to another event or disease in the body. One such event is pregnancy, during which hypertension may occur (see Chapter 10). Medications also can cause secondary hypertension. Birth control pills that contain progesterone stimulate the production of renin (see Fig. 8-6), which may result in an elevation in blood pressure.

As mentioned in Chapter 15, the combined intake of monoamine oxidase inhibitors (MAOIs) and tyramine-rich foods or beverages can cause hypertension. Secondary hypertension can also result from diseases of the kidney, adrenal glands, or nervous system.

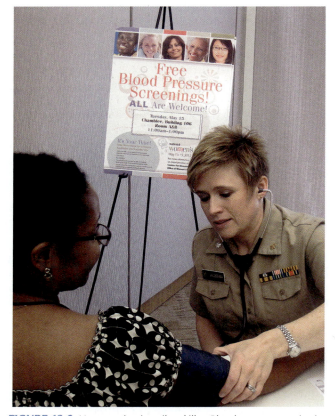

FIGURE 18-2 Hypertension is a silent killer. Blood pressure monitoring is a part of most health-system visits.

Positive Feedback Cycle

Many cardiovascular conditions have interlocking causative factors. The interaction between atherosclerosis and hypertension is an example of a **positive feedback cycle.** In this situation, the presence of the second condition worsens the first. Atherosclerosis narrows the lumen of the arteries, and the smaller opening increases blood pressure. Then the higher blood pressure forces more lipids into the arterial wall, worsening the atherosclerosis, and the cycle is repeated.

TABLE 18-1	Classification of Blood Pressure for Adults	
CLASSIFICATION	**mm Hg SYSTOLIC**	**mm Hg DIASTOLIC**
Normal	<120	and <80
Elevated blood pressure	120–129	and <80
Stage 1 hypertension	130–139	or 80–89
Stage 2 hypertension	>140	or >90

Source: Whelton (2017).

End Result of Pathology

Most affected people do not have either atherosclerosis or hypertension. More commonly, they have both conditions. Although many organs are likely to be damaged by atherosclerosis and hypertension, the major concern is the effect on the heart and brain, as described in the following sections on coronary heart disease and cerebrovascular disease.

Coronary Heart Disease

When the coronary arteries that supply the heart muscle with blood become blocked, the result is **coronary heart disease (CHD)** or coronary artery disease (CAD). If the blockage is temporary, due to increased activity and the body's increased demand for oxygen, the person may experience **angina pectoris,** or severe pain and a sense of constriction about the heart. Rest and the administration of vasodilating medications commonly produce relief, but changes in diet and lifestyle are necessary to stave off heart damage.

However, if the vessel is blocked by atherosclerotic plaque, by a **thrombus** (blood clot), or by an **embolus** (a circulating mass of undissolved matter), the heart tissues beyond the point of obstruction receive no oxygen or nutrients. When this happens, the person exhibits signs and symptoms of a **coronary occlusion,** or a heart attack. When the blood supply cannot be restored quickly, myocardial cells in the affected area die. The medical diagnosis then becomes **myocardial infarction.**

Heart Failure

When the heart cannot keep up with the demands on it, **heart failure (HF)** occurs. The AHA estimates that 6.5 million people in the United States have HF and that by 2030 eight million people 18 years of age or older will have HF (American Heart Association [AHA], 2017). Heart failure is any clinical syndrome that results from any structural or functional impairment of ventricular filling or ejection of blood (National Institutes of Health [NIH], 2015). Causes may include the following:

- Atherosclerosis
- Hypertension
- Myocardial infarction
- Obesity
- Diabetes

The right side of the heart normally collects the blood returning from the body and pumps it to the lungs to excrete carbon dioxide and absorb oxygen. If the right ventricle is failing, usually due to lung disease, the blood backs up into the veins that empty into the right atrium, and the client has the signs of peripheral edema. If the client has excessive fluid volume and edema of the small bowel, the client suffers from anorexia and nausea.

The left side of the heart normally receives the oxygenated blood from the lungs and pumps it out to the body.

If the left ventricle is failing, usually after a myocardial infarction, the blood that cannot be pumped effectively to the body backs up in the blood vessels of the lungs. Next, the fluid from the blood is forced into the lung tissue. The client will display shortness of breath and moist lung sounds and will expectorate frothy pink sputum.

In addition, if the heart cannot pump enough blood to maintain blood pressure, the body implements the renin response. Angiotensin II constricts the blood vessels, raising blood pressure. Aldosterone causes the kidneys to conserve sodium, and with it, water. More fluid fills the blood vessels. The higher blood pressure pushes this fluid out into the interstitial spaces, causing edema.

Obviously, one side of the heart cannot function long if the other side is failing. Therefore, the health-care worker learns to look for early signs of heart failure in the extremities in right-sided failure or in the lungs in left-sided failure.

The incidence of HF increases in people over 65 years of age due to a weakened heart muscle and other comorbidities; blacks are more likely to have HF than other races; overweight individuals due to comorbidities; and those who have had a myocardial infarction (NIH, 2015).

There is a lower risk of developing HF by following these healthy lifestyle recommendations:

- Regular exercise
- Follow a heart-healthy diet with only moderate alcohol intake
- Manage stress
- Aim for a healthy weight
- Quit smoking

HF treatment includes:

- Treating underlying causes such as hypertension, CHD, and diabetes
- Treating sleep apnea
- Treating depression

Cerebrovascular Accident

When a blood vessel in the brain becomes blocked by atherosclerosis (ischemic stroke), the tissue supplied by that artery dies. This pathology causes about 87% of strokes or **cerebrovascular accidents (CVAs)** in the United States (Centers for Disease Control and Prevention [CDC], 2017). Strokes also can be caused by an embolus or by a ruptured blood vessel. Cerebrovascular accidents are usually secondary to atherosclerosis, hypertension, or a combination of both.

Each year, approximately 795,000 strokes occur in the United States. Someone in the United States has a stroke approximately every 40 seconds. Stroke accounts for 1 of every 20 deaths in the United States (AHA, 2017). The Centers for Disease Control and Prevention (CDC) reports that it is the fifth leading cause of death in the United

States. One in four stroke survivors has another stroke within 5 years (CDC, 2017),

Stroke is called a "brain attack" and early treatment can minimize the long-term effects of ischemic stroke, but people often ignore initial signs and symptoms or fail to react appropriately. The American Stroke Association (ASA) states that anyone can have a stroke and everyone should be ready to ensure quick treatment. Their acronym FAST was developed to trigger awareness of symptoms (http://www.strokeassociation.org/STROKEORG/):

- Face drooping
- Arm weakness
- Speech difficulty
- Time to call 911

The ASA estimates that approximately 80% of strokes can be prevented by following a healthy lifestyle. This includes:

- Monitor and normalize blood pressure
- Exercise daily
- Eat a heart-healthy diet rich in fruits, vegetables, whole grains, cereal fiber, and fatty fish
- Stop smoking

These are the same principles used to prevent cardiovascular conditions resulting from atherosclerosis. A heart-healthy diet may also be a head-healthy diet. The AHA's 2020 goal is to improve the cardiovascular health of all Americans by 20% while reducing deaths from cardiovascular diseases and stroke by 20%. It recommends that an adult consuming 2,000 calories per day should consume:

- Fruits and vegetables: at least 4.5 cups per day
- Fish (preferably oily fish): at least two 3.5-ounce servings/week
- Fiber-rich whole grains: at least three 1 ounce equivalent servings/day
- Sodium: less than 1,500 mg/day
- Sugar-sweetened beverages: no more than 450 calories/week
- Nuts, legumes, and seeds: at least 4 servings/week
- Processed meats: no more than 2 servings/week
- Saturated fat: less than 7% of total energy intake

Risk Factors in Cardiovascular Disease

The occurrence of cardiovascular disease in a person cannot be predicted with certainty. Many attributes and behaviors interact to produce the illness (see Table 18-2).

Unmodifiable Risk Factors

Risk factors that cannot be changed to prevent atherosclerosis and hypertension are:

- Age
- Gender

TABLE 18-2   Risk Factors for Cardiovascular Disease

UNMODIFIABLE	MODIFIABLE
Age	Hypertension
Gender	High blood cholesterol
Race	Obesity
Heredity	Diabetes mellitus
Family history	Physical inactivity
Prior medical history	Alcohol intake, cigarette smoking

- Race
- Family history
- Personal medical history

Age, Gender, and Race

Hypertension usually develops at about age 50 to 60, and coronary atherosclerosis becomes problematic more frequently in individuals older than 40.

Risk for coronary heart disease increases in men after age 45 and women after age 55. Until menopause, women have less atherosclerosis and coronary heart disease than men, but women postmenopausal and younger diabetic women are stricken with coronary heart disease just as often as men are.

Non-Hispanic blacks have a higher risk for hypertension and hypertension-related complications than non-Hispanic whites and Mexican Americans (AHA, 2017).

Family and Prior Medical Histories

Genetics is one thing the family shares, but also important are lifestyle and home environment. Individuals growing up in a household of sedentary smokers who consume fast food may negatively influence the risk factors (such as hypertension and hyperlipidemia) for heart disease (Harvard Health Publication, 2016). See Genomic Gem 18-1 for more information about genetics and CVD risks.

GENOMIC GEM 18-1

Premature CVD Risk

A family history of premature cardiovascular disease (CVD) in a parent or sibling increases a person's risk of the disease. Premature CVD is a myocardial infarction or a coronary artery procedure before age 55 in men and 65 in women. Siblings of those with premature CVD increase their chances of developing CVD by 40% and children by 60%–75%. Identical twins had an increase in the hazard ratio of death from CAD by 3.8–15 times if an identical sibling died of CAD before 75 years of age. The risk was three times higher for identical than fraternal twins (Kolber & Scrimshaw, 2014).

Modifiable Risk Factors

The major modifiable risk factors for CAD are:

- Hypertension
- Elevated serum cholesterol
- Obesity
- Physical inactivity
- Diabetes mellitus
- Alcohol intake
- Cigarette smoking

Hypertension

According to the AHA, hypertension is a leading risk factor for CAD as well as the most important risk factor for stroke. People with normal blood pressure have about half the lifetime risk of stroke compared with those with high blood pressure. Hypertension affects approximately 46% of American adults (AHA, 2017). Only 54% of those with hypertension have it controlled. Elevated blood pressure (previously referred to as prehypertension), the precursor to hypertension, affects 1 in 3 American adults. The costs of hypertension to the nation, health-care services, medications, and lost days of work are estimated to be $46 billion annually. By reducing sodium in the diet to the recommended Dietary Guidelines to 2,300 mg per day, it is estimated that there would be a reduction of 11 million cases of hypertension and save 18 billion in health-care dollars annually (CDC, 2016). See Table 18-1 for the classification for blood pressure levels in adults.

HIGH SALT INTAKE

Blood pressure values increase with age everywhere except in extremely remote areas of the world and are significantly related to salt intake. Approximately 30% to 50% of hypertensive people and smaller percentages of normotensive people are salt-sensitive, meaning that their blood pressure goes up in response to ingesting sodium. Salt sensitivity is more common in blacks, the elderly, individuals with high blood pressure, and those with comorbidities such as chronic kidney disease (CKD), metabolic syndrome, and diabetes. These groups account for more than 50% of the U.S. population (Whelton, 2017).

It is estimated that the average American consumes 3,400 mg of sodium per day. The *2015-2020 Dietary Guidelines for Americans* recommend that everyone decrease their sodium intake. Table 18-3 lists the daily adequate intake (AI) of sodium for individuals by age group. The tolerable upper intake level (UL) was set for all individuals 14 years and older at 2,300 mg of sodium per day.

Americans are consuming more sodium in part because they consume more food, eat out more, and use more processed foods, which are higher in sodium (CDC, 2016). Frequent consumption of the following foods contributes the indicated percentage of sodium intake of Americans (*2015-2020 Dietary Guidelines for Americans*):

- Burgers and sandwiches (21%)
- Snacks and sweets (8%)

TABLE 18-3	Daily Adequate Intake (AI) of Sodium for Individuals by Age Group
AGE IN YEARS	**AI/DAY (MG)**
1–3	1,000
4–8	1,200
9–50	1,500
51–70	1,300
≥71	1,200

- Pizza (6%)
- Rice, pasta, and grain dishes (7%)

POTASSIUM INTAKE

Potassium influences blood pressure because it promotes urinary excretion of sodium. Potassium also helps reduce the tension in blood vessel walls, which helps lower blood pressure. The AHA (www.heart.org) recommends a diet rich in potassium-containing fruits and vegetables as one component of a healthy eating pattern for controlling blood pressure in individuals who have healthy kidney function (AHA, 2016).

A higher intake of certain foods, such as fruits, vegetables, and low-fat dairy, has been correlated with a decrease in CVD occurrence. The AHA does not recommend taking supplements for cardiovascular health; no definitive studies demonstrate evidence of their benefits (AHA, 2016).

Elevated Blood Cholesterol

Despite its categorization as a risk factor for cardiovascular disease, **cholesterol** serves vital functions in the body. Cholesterol is a component of:

- The nerve tissue of the brain and spinal cord
- The tissues of the liver, the adrenal glands, and the kidneys
- Bile

In addition, cholesterol serves as a precursor of adrenal hormones and the sex hormones.

Although some cholesterol contributes to a healthy body, blood cholesterol levels are measured to monitor risk, to promote health, and to prevent disease (see Boxes 18-1 and 18-2).

RELATIONSHIP TO DIET

About 1,000 milligrams of cholesterol is synthesized in the body per day, and a healthy adult consumes approximately

---

BOX 18-1 ■ Cholesterol Screening Goals

A national health objective of Healthy People 2020 is to screen 82.1% of adults aged 18 years and older for blood lipid screening. Blood lipids should be screened in adults every 5 years.

Between 2009 and 2010, approximately 69.4% of U.S. adults 20 years of age and older met the goal. In 2009, of the 96 million health-care office visits, only 9.2% included cholesterol screening (CDC, 2015).

BOX 18-2 ■ Screening Children's Cholesterol

Universal screening of children's cholesterol is recommended for all children at two time points, once between 9 and 11 years of age and once between 17 and 21 years of age. Nonfasting total cholesterol and high-density lipoprotein cholesterol (HDL-C) are recommended for the initial lipid screening test. Children with elevated cholesterol or low HDL-C who fail at lifestyle changes of diet and exercise should be considered for pharmacological treatment at age 10 (de Ferranti and Washington, 2012; National Heart Lung and Blood Institute, 2013). The need for screening at a younger age is determined by family history of cardiovascular disease, unknown history (i.e., adopted children), or presence of other risk factors. For these children, the first screening should take place after 2 years of age but no later than 10 years of age. Screening before 2 years of age is not recommended (Daniels & Greer, 2008; National Heart Lung and Blood Institute, 2013).

A survey was conducted in 2013–2014 looking at pediatrician compliance with pediatric cholesterol screening guidelines. The results were based upon 451 responses and indicated that 18% conducted universal screening in those aged 9–11 years and 31% in those aged 17–21. In those with a risk factor (obesity or family history of high cholesterol, heart attack, or stroke), 67% aged 9–11 years and 78% aged 17–21 were screened (Rodday, 2015).

Children who do have elevated serum cholesterol levels have to be managed carefully so that sufficient food is provided to support growth.

300 milligrams of cholesterol from the diet, exclusively from foods of animal origin. Nearly all of the body's tissues can synthesize cholesterol, with the liver and the intestine producing the greatest amount. Most people can produce less cholesterol or increase its excretion in response to high levels of dietary cholesterol but others respond weakly. This is thought to be genetically based and seems to be caused by synthesis occurring in the liver (https://themedicalbiochemistrypage.org/cholesterol.php).

Consumption of substances other than dietary cholesterol can also influence serum cholesterol levels. *Trans* unsaturated fatty acids in vegetable oil products are a risk factor for cardiovascular disease because they raise low-density lipoprotein cholesterol (LDL-C) levels and lower high-density lipoprotein cholesterol (HDL-C) levels.

MEASUREMENT OF BLOOD CHOLESTEROL

Lipids such as triglycerides (the major form of dietary fat and of stored body fat) and cholesterol (a sterol with fat-like properties) cannot dissolve in water. To travel in the bloodstream, they are bound to lipoproteins. See Table 18-4 for the functions and significance of the four main classes of lipoproteins: **chylomicrons, very low-density lipoproteins (VLDL), low-density lipoproteins (LDLs), and high-density lipoproteins (HDLs).**

Blood tests for serum cholesterol are reported as total cholesterol, LDL-C, or HDL-C based on cholesterol's association with the two major transport lipoproteins. Serum cholesterol itself is neither good nor bad, but the lipoproteins are associated with greater or lesser risk of CHD.

A client may be prescribed pharmacological and non-pharmacological treatments. The AHA recommends that therapeutic lifestyle changes (TLC) remain an essential modality in clinical management, which includes a heart-healthy diet, exercise, avoiding cigarette smoke, and maintaining a healthy weight (AHA, 2017). Table 18-5 describes a cholesterol-lowering diet. Cholesterol-lowering medications are added to a healthy lifestyle, not substituted for it.

Obesity and Inactivity

The location of the body fat is significant: abdominal obesity is related to cardiovascular disease and diabetes mellitus more than is **gluteal-femoral obesity.** Abdominal obesity is associated with increased triglyceride levels and decreased HDL-C levels. Abdominal obesity, or having an "apple shape," is one of the risk factors of metabolic syndrome. Weight loss contributes to improvement in lipid level, blood sugar, and blood pressure (NIH, 2016).

Lack of exercise contributes to many other risk factors for cardiovascular disease. For instance, activity is inversely

TABLE 18-4 Functions and Significance of Various Lipoproteins

LIPOPROTEIN	FUNCTION	CLINICAL SIGNIFICANCE
Chylomicrons	Transport exogenous triglycerides from intestines to blood stream	Formed in small intestine; present in blood only after a meal
VLDL-C	Main transporter of endogenous triglyceride	Synthesized by liver from free fatty acids, glycerol, and carbohydrate
LDL-C	Transports cholesterol to body cells	Evolves from VLDLs as body's cells remove triglyceride from them and attach cholesterol Carrier of about 60% of total serum cholesterol The higher the LDL-C level, the greater the risk of CHD Major target of cholesterol-reducing therapy
HDL-C	Transports cholesterol from body cells to liver to be excreted Inhibits atherosclerosis through anti-inflammatory, antioxidant, and antithrombotic actions (Hausenloy & Yellon, 2008)	Synthesized by liver and intestines The higher the HDL-C level, the lower the risk of CHD Aerobic exercise increases HDL-C levels

CHD, coronary heart disease; HDL-C, high-density lipoprotein cholesterol; LDL-C, low-density lipoprotein cholesterol; VLDL-C, very low density lipoprotein cholesterol.

TABLE 18-5   Cholesterol-Lowering Diets

DESCRIPTION	INDICATION	ADEQUACY
These diets limit lipids and, for many clients, sugars and sodium.	These diets are prescribed when clients have elevated serum cholesterol. Consultation with a registered dietitian is essential to individualize a dietary plan based upon a client's interest in change, culture, and lifestyle. A dietitian will help give the client the tools to make healthy choices.	The diets are adequate in all nutrients with the possible exception of iron because of the restriction on red meat. Clients must be encouraged to consume an energy level to obtain and maintain a healthy body weight.

related to blood pressure independent of being overweight in both sexes and across all ages. As well, increased physical activity has been accompanied by increased HDL-C levels with its attendant lessening of risk.

Metabolic Syndrome

A particular constellation of signs and symptoms labeled **metabolic syndrome** is used to designate a cluster of risk factors for cardiovascular disease. Clients with this condition display three or more of the following signs: glucose intolerance, hypertriglyceridemia, low HDL-C, hypertension, and abdominal obesity (NIH, 2016). Specific criteria are:

- Fasting blood glucose ≥100 mg/dL
- Triglycerides ≥150 mg/dL
- HDL-C <40 mg/dL in men; <50 mg/dL in women
- Blood pressure >130 mm Hg systolic; >85 mm Hg diastolic
- Waist circumference >40 inches in men; >35 inches in women
- Insulin resistance or glucose intolerance

Diabetes Mellitus

Diabetic individuals have a two to three times higher risk of atherosclerosis than other people. Diabetic women lose the preventive advantages usually associated with premenopausal women regarding cardiovascular risk.

Insulin is required to maintain adequate levels of **lipoprotein lipase,** an enzyme that breaks down chylomicrons. When lipoprotein lipase is inadequate, chylomicrons and VLDL particles accumulate in the blood. After the diabetes is controlled, serum lipid levels decrease.

Lipoprotein lipase activity is greater in physically active subjects and increases with exercise, a valuable concept in the management of type 2 diabetes.

Alcohol Consumption

Moderate alcohol intake has been linked to lower occurrence of cardiovascular events. In small amounts, alcohol seems to cause vasodilation, whereas at high doses it acts as a vasoconstrictor. The incidence of heart disease in moderate drinkers is lower than that in nondrinkers; however, with increased intake of alcohol, there is an increased risk of hypertension, obesity, and stroke. Current evidence does not justify encouraging nondrinkers to begin imbibing (AHA, 2015). See Dollars & Sense 18-1 for estimated savings from moderating alcohol intake.

Dollars & Sense 18-1
Drink Less, Save Money, and Health

A couple drinks a bottle of wine (two glasses for her, four for him) every night with dinner and dines in a restaurant twice a week. Assuming modest tastes in wine, $8 per bottle at the grocery and $4.50 per glass in the restaurant, their current annual outlay is $2,808 for restaurant wine and $2,080 for home wine.

If they implemented the cardioprotective diet plan and reduced their alcohol intake by one-half, they would save $2,444 in a year while lessening the risk of cardiovascular disease.

Cigarette Smoking

Among the major coronary risk factors, cigarette smoking has been shown to be particularly harmful to the heart and blood vessels, whether from active or secondhand smoke. The exact toxic components among the thousands of pharmacologically active substances present in tobacco smoke and their mechanisms affecting cardiovascular dysfunction are largely unknown. The AHA summarizes that smoking increases the risk of CHD by decreasing tolerance for physical activity, decreases HDL-C, and increases tendency for blood clots (AHA, 2016).

Dietary Measures in Prevention and Treatment

Major lifestyle changes have proven to be effective in reducing cardiovascular risk. Dietary changes that may help are listed in Table 18-6. Many of the recommendations in the table were proven effective in controlling hypertension by the DASH (Dietary Approaches to Stop Hypertension) diet, which is still recommended for hypertension control (NIH, 2015). Lifestyle changes are the initial steps in management of hypertension (Alexander et al, 2017).

Implementing Dietary Changes

The AHA recommends a diet to help control blood pressure:
Rich in:

- Fruits
- Vegetables
- Whole-grains
- Low-fat dairy products
- Skinless poultry and fish

TABLE 18-6 Dietary Changes That May Reduce Cardiovascular Risk

ACTION	RATIONALE	CONCERNS
Consume fatty fish (salmon, herring, trout, sardines, tuna) twice a week.	Omega-3 fatty acids are associated with a decreased risk of death from cardiac events.	Recommended for clients with and without CHD Beware of mercury hazards (see Chapter 10)
Consume 1 tbs canola or walnut oil, 0.5 tbs ground flaxseed	Plant-based sources of omega-3 fatty acids	Conversion of alpha-lipoic acid in the body produces modest amounts of docosahexaenoic acid
Take omega-3 supplements in consultation with physician	If food sources unacceptable to client for lipid management	Especially for clients with documented coronary heart disease Do not appear to lower blood pressure
Substitute 25 grams of soy protein (isolated soy protein, textured soy, tofu) daily for animal protein	May reduce LDL-C by 10%	If not contraindicated by risks or harms FDA approved a health claim for soy foods Minimal evidence of direct cardiovascular benefit Indirect benefit if reduce saturated fat and cholesterol intake Isoflavones not proven to be beneficial
Consume 5 ounces of nuts (walnuts, almonds, peanuts, macadamia, pistachios, pecans) per week.	Contain beneficial fatty acids May reduce LDL-C 6%–29%	Substitute for equal kcal from other sources to avoid weight gain.
Increase fruit and vegetable servings to 10–12 daily.	Good sources of antioxidants and potassium	Beta-carotene and vitamin C and E supplements have shown no cardioprotective benefit. Potassium intake <DRI is associated with increased B/P
Select whole oats and foods high in psyllium (e.g., Bran Buds).	Soluble fiber lowers serum LDL-C without affecting HDL-C and triglyceride concentrations.	FDA approved health claims for whole oats and foods containing psyllium seed husk. Consume adequate fluids.

CHD, coronary heart disease; LDL-C, low-density lipoprotein cholesterol; DRI, daily recommended intake; HDL-C, high-density lipoprotein cholesterol.
Adapted from American Dietetic Association (2008a, 2008b); AHA (2013); Lichtenstein et al (2006); Theuwissen & Mensink (2008); Harvard Health Publication (2015).

- Nuts and legumes
- Nontropical vegetable oils

Limit:

- Saturated and trans fats
- Sodium
- Red meat (if you do eat red meat, compare labels and select the leanest cuts available)
- Sweets and sugar-sweetened beverages

See Box 18-3 for information on coffee and tea consumption with heart disease.

The DASH Diet

Features of the DASH diet are shown in Table 18-7. The example is based on a 2,000-kilocalorie diet. The daily nutrient goals of the DASH diet for this caloric level are as follows: no more than 27% fat (with no more than 6% saturated fat, and 150 mg cholesterol), 18% protein, 55% carbohydrate, no more than 2,300 mg sodium (1,500 mg is better for individuals with high BP, African Americans, and middle-aged and older adults), 4,700 mg potassium, 1,250 mg calcium, 500 mg magnesium, and 30 g fiber.

Foods Not Supplements

Atherosclerosis is thought to be related to oxidative stress. One might conclude that antioxidant supplements would

> **BOX 18-3 ■ Coffee, Tea, and Heart Disease**
>
> Current research indicates that moderate consumption of both coffee and tea provides health benefits (Harvard School of Public Health, 2017; AND, 2017). Coffee consumption was associated with a reduced risk of stroke and CHD. Black tea consumption is associated with a reduction in the incidence of heart attack and green tea with lower total cholesterol, LDL-C and triglycerides, and a higher HDL-C.
>
> The exact ingredient or mechanism that is attributable to the benefit of these beverages has not been definitively determined. The benefit may come from the caffeine (though some studies show a benefit with decaffeinated products), the naturally occurring antioxidants, or other substances not yet discovered.
>
> Other health benefits of coffee may include a reduction in Parkinson disease, type 2 diabetes, liver diseases, and gallstones.

be effective in preventing atherosclerosis. Antioxidant-rich fruits, vegetables, and whole grains have been associated with reduced disease risk. However, beta-carotene and vitamin C and E supplements have not protected against cardiovascular events or mortality and, in fact, may increase health risks in smokers (Natural Medicines, 2017).

Reducing Saturated Fat Intake

About two-thirds of saturated fatty acids in the U.S. diet come from animal fats. Using nonfat or low-fat dairy

TABLE 18-7   The DASH Diet (based on a 2,000-kilocalorie diet)

FOOD GROUP	DAILY SERVINGS	SERVING SIZES	EXAMPLES AND NOTES	SIGNIFICANCE OF FOOD GROUP TO DASH DIET
Grains and grain products (whole grains are recommended)	6–8	1 slice bread ½ cup dry cereal ½ cup cooked cereal, brown rice, or pasta	Whole-wheat bread, English muffin, pita bread, bagel, cereals, grits, oatmeal	Major sources of energy and fiber
Vegetables	4–5	1 cup raw leafy ½ cup cooked 6-oz juice	Tomatoes, potatoes, carrots, peas, squash, broccoli, turnip greens, collards, kale, spinach, artichokes, sweet potatoes, beans	Rich sources of potassium, magnesium, and fiber
Fruits	4–5	6 oz juice 1 medium fruit ¼ cup dried fruit ½ cup fresh, frozen, or canned fruit	Apricots, bananas, dates, oranges, grapefruit, mangoes, melons, peaches, pineapples, prunes, raisins, strawberries, tangerines	Important sources of potassium, magnesium, and fiber
Low-fat or nonfat dairy foods	2–3	8 oz milk 1 cup yogurt 1.5 oz cheese	Skim or 1% milk, skim or low-fat buttermilk, nonfat or low-fat yogurt, part-skim mozzarella cheese, nonfat cheese	Major sources of calcium and protein
Meats, poultry, and fish	6 or fewer	3 oz cooked meat, poultry, or fish	Select only lean; trim away visible fat, broil, roast, or boil instead of frying; remove skin from poultry	Rich sources of protein and magnesium
Nuts, seeds, and legumes	4–5 per week	1.5 oz or ⅓ cup nuts ½ oz or 2 tbsp seeds ½ cup cooked legumes	Almonds, filberts, mixed nuts, peanuts, walnuts, sunflower seeds, kidney beans, lentils	Rich sources of energy, magnesium, potassium, protein, and fiber
Fats and oils	2–3	1 tsp	Canola, olive, peanut oils	Contain mainly monounsaturated fatty acids

Adapted from NIH (2012).

products is recommended by the AHA as a way to reduce fat in the diet. To lower saturated fats, the AHA recommends selecting lean cuts of meat, trim all visible fat, broil rather than fry meats using a rack to facilitate draining off fat, remove skin from poultry before cooking, and limit the consumption of processed meats such as sausage and luncheon meats (AHA, 2017). Techniques to reduce fat in meat are shown in Figure 18-3.

Plant Sterols

Specialty foods containing plant sterols may be recommended *in prescribed amounts*. These foods are marketed as table spreads (butter substitutes), juices, yogurts, and salad dressings. **Plant sterols** (phytosterols) are compounds that structurally resemble cholesterol but are not absorbed in the human body to any extent. In the gastrointestinal tract, plant sterols bind with bile and cholesterol, increasing their excretion in the feces. For maximum effectiveness, 1 to 2 grams daily of foods containing plant sterols should be consumed to lower LDL-C 6% to 14% in 4 weeks (Joslin Diabetes Center, 2017).

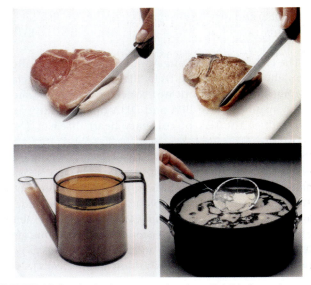

FIGURE 18-3 Selecting lean meat, trimming off visible fat, and skimming fat from meat juices reduce the amount of fat consumed. *(From the National Live Stock and Meat Board, 444 North Michigan Avenue, Chicago, IL 60611, with permission.)*

Despite their occurrence in foods, plant sterols should be monitored by the health-care provider as are drugs.

Omega-3 Fatty Acids

The regular consumption of foods rich in marine omega-3 fatty acids, **eicosapentaenoic acid (EPA)** and **docosahexaenoic acid (DHA),** may:

- Decrease occurrence of arrhythmia and sudden death
- Lower plasma triglycerides
- Slightly raise HDL levels
- Reduce homocysteine levels
- Lower blood pressure
- Reduce blood clotting tendencies

Fish containing omega-3 fatty acids that are low in mercury include the following (*2015-2020 Dietary Guidelines*):

- Anchovies
- Herring
- Mackerel (Atlantic and Pacific, not king mackerel)
- Pacific oysters
- Rainbow trout
- Salmon
- Sardines

Vegetarian sources of omega-3 fatty acids include (Consumer Lab, 2017):

- Algal oil (from algae)
- Ground flax
- Chia seeds
- Oils: canola, soy, and walnut

Individuals who have hypertriglyceridemia should follow therapeutic lifestyle change (TLC), which include the dietary recommendations outlined in the *2015-2020 Dietary Guidelines*, and may be given a prescription for fish oil supplements providing 2 to 4 grams of purified DHA/EPA (NIH, 2016).

The U.S. Food and Drug Administration (FDA) allows supplements containing DHA/EPA to have a label claim stating, "Supportive but not conclusive research shows that consumption of EPA and DHA omega-3 fatty acids may reduce the risk of coronary heart disease" (NIH, 2016).

Clinical studies suggest that tissue levels of long-chain omega-3 fatty acids may be depressed in vegetarians, particularly in vegans. Vegetarian diets, especially the vegan, are relatively low in alpha-linolenic acid (ALA) and provide little, if any, eicosapentaenoic acid (EPA) and docosahexaenoic acid (DHA). Vegetarians are encouraged to consume algae, flaxseeds, walnuts, canola oil, and soy in their diets as good sources of ALA (Academy of Nutrition and Dietetics [AND], 2016).

Conversion of ALA by the body to the more active longer-chain metabolites is less than 5% to 10% efficient for EPA and 2% to 5% for DHA. Thus, total omega-3 requirements may be higher for vegetarians than for nonvegetarians. Moreover, the balance between omega-3 and omega-6 fatty acids

impacts the conversion rate. Thus, it may be wise to consult a dietitian if the client:

- Is at risk for cardiovascular disease
- Has increased need for EPA and DHA (pregnant or lactating women)
- Is likely to poorly convert ALA to EPA and DHA (persons with diabetes or neurological disorders, premature infants, elderly)

More research is needed to show a cause-and-effect relationship between alpha-linolenic acid and heart disease (NIH, 2016). Figure 18-4 shows fatty acids with their common food sources.

Psyllium

Psyllium is a gelatinous substance, which is a soluble fiber. It was previously thought to be very effective in lowering LDL-C if 10.2 grams per day was consumed, lowering LDL-C on average 7%. However, various studies had mixed conclusions. Psyllium is thought to have "modest but significant" improvement in total and LDL-C levels (Consumer Lab, 2015). The FDA has permitted a health claim on the labels of foods containing psyllium seed husk (e.g., Kellogg's All-Bran Buds). The health claim states that the food, *as part of a diet low in saturated fat and cholesterol*, may reduce the risk of coronary heart disease.

To qualify, the food must provide at least 1.7 grams of soluble fiber in an amount customarily consumed. To obtain the result achieved in the controlled studies on which the FDA approval was based, a person would have to consume four servings per day (U.S. Food and Drug Administration [FDA], 1998).

Soy Protein

Soy is a high-quality plant protein that is a source of all essential amino acids, as well as dietary fiber and iron. Clinical trials have shown that consumption of soy protein compared with other proteins, such as those from milk or meat, can lower total and LDL-C levels. The key is to replace some of the animal protein with soy protein. Consuming 25 grams of soy protein daily has been found to lower cholesterol by approximately 10% (Harvard Health Publication, 2015).

In 1999, the FDA approved a health claim for soy-containing foods stating that including soy protein in a diet low in saturated fat and cholesterol may reduce the risk of CHD by lowering blood cholesterol levels. Because 25 grams of soy protein daily in the diet is needed to show a significant cholesterol-lowering effect, to qualify for this health claim, a food must contain at least 6.25 grams of soy protein per serving (Sports, Cardiovascular, and Wellness Nutrition, 2012; FDA, 1999). Figure 18-5 shows the many choices available using soy with MyPlate.

Because soy contains phytoestrogens, clients should discuss the feasibility of adding soy products to their diets as a cardioprotective strategy with their health-care providers.

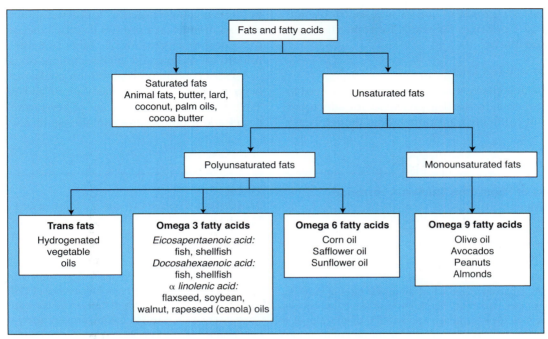

FIGURE 18-4 Fatty acids and their common food sources. Omega-3 fatty acids are particularly desirable in a heart-healthy diet. *(Adapted from Din, JN, Newby, DE, and Flapan, AD: Omega 3 fatty acids and cardiovascular disease—fishing for a natural treatment. BMJ 328:30, 2004.)*

HOW SOY FITS INTO THE USDA'S MYPLATE

The Dietary Guidelines for Americans gives science-based advice on food and physical activity choices for health. To see the full Dietary Guidelines, go to http://health.gov/dietaryguidelines/dga2010/DietaryGuidelines2010.pdf. Soyfoods can be an important part of a healthy diet as prescribed by the USDA MyPlate. Most soyfoods contain no cholesterol, little or no saturated fat, high quality protein and dietary fiber. Many soyfoods also provide essential vitamins and minerals, such as B vitamins, vitamins A and D, calcium, iron and potassium.

Grains
- Soy cereal
- Soy grits
- Soy waffles
- Soy pasta
- Soy bread
- Soy flour

Consuming at least three or more ounce-equivalents of whole grains per day can reduce the risk of several chronic diseases and may help with weight maintenance. Soy flour is part of this group. Substitute up to one-fourth of the total flour in your favorite baked product recipe.

Vegetables
- Green soybeans (edamame)
- Canned soybeans
- Soynuts

One-half cup of green soybeans (edamame) contains 10 grams of soy protein. All soybeans are a good source of dietary fiber and isoflavones.

Oils
- Soybean oil (also called vegetable oil)

Soybean oil is rich in polyunsaturated fat and contains only minimal saturated fat. Soybean oil is a rich source of omega-3 fatty acids. Soybean oil, labeled "vegetable oil," is a source of the antioxidant Vitamin E.

Milk
- Soy beverage
- Soy cheese
- Soy yogurt
- Soy ice cream

According to the USDA food guidelines, protein choices for those who do not consume milk products include calcium-fortified soy beverages, soybeans, soy yogurt, soy cheese and tempeh. Soy ice cream products are a part of this group, but do not contain as much calcium or protein as other options.

Meat & Beans
- Soy burgers
- Soy hot dogs
- Soy nuggets
- Soy burger-type crumbles
- Tofu
- Soynuts
- Canned soybeans
- Green soybeans (edamame)
- Soynut butter

According to the USDA food guidelines, protein choices in this category include all of the above listed soyfoods. Soybeans are a source of high quality protein and include all eight of the essential amino acids.

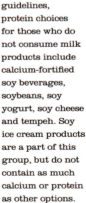

FIGURE 18-5 How Soy Fits into the U.S. Department of Agriculture's MyPlate *(United Soybean Board [USB] 2012 Soybean Guide, with permission.)*

Not all research is easily or quickly interpreted. Clinical Application 18-1 describes the search for connections between diet and disease.

Sodium-Controlled Diets

Individuals with hypertension or heart failure may need to control their sodium intake. The preference for salty foods is learned and culturally transmitted, even though heavy salting is no longer necessary for preservation of food. After about 3 months on a sodium-restricted diet, most individuals lose their appetite for salt. Table 18-8 lists the legal definitions for sodium and salt descriptions on labels.

Unseen contributions to sodium intake may come from beverages, over-the-counter medications, and drinking water. Table 18-9 lists sodium content of beverages. Many toothpastes and mouthwashes contain significant amounts of

---

CLINICAL APPLICATION   18-1

The Limits of Population Studies: A Historical Perspective

Research is sometimes misinterpreted or applied prematurely. Rarely does a single study merit widespread changes in diet in the pursuit of health.

FAT INTAKE

In the 1960s, Japan and Greece had the lowest rates of heart disease among seven countries. People in those two countries were very different in their fat consumption: 10% of kilocalories in Japan and 40% on the island of Crete. On the face of these findings, fat intake might be dismissed as irrelevant to heart disease. But the Greeks derived less than 10% of kilocalories from animal protein and 33% of their kilocalories from olive oil, which is 82% monounsaturated.

MULTIPLE CAUSATION

Since 1976, Spain has experienced a decrease in cardiovascular mortality, despite increased intakes of dairy products and meat, particularly pork and poultry. If attention focused only on those foods, the rationale for the decreased mortality would be missed.

Most of the decrease in cardiovascular mortality was due to a decline in stroke mortality. Improved hypertension control, including decreased intake of salt and salt-cured foods, is thought to have influenced this trend. Other contributing factors were increased consumption of fruit and fish, reduction in cigarette smoking, and expanded access to clinical care, including a major increase in the use of aspirin as a platelet inhibitor (Serra-Majem et al, 1995).

RED WINE

Consumption of red wine is credited with conferring some protection against coronary heart disease (CHD). The "French Paradox" refers to the observation in the early 1990s that despite the high intake of saturated fats in their diet, there was a low incidence of CHD in the French population. This was thought to be because of the red wine intake of the French (Brannon, 2011; Catalgol, Batirel, Taga, & Ozer, 2012; Ferrieres, 2004). Resveratrol is one compound found in abundance in red wine that has been identified and studied as the potential beneficial substance contributing to red wine's benefit. Resveratrol has been the subject of many studies that have shown it to potentially have cardiovascular benefits, including lowering systolic blood pressure, triglyceride levels, LDL cholesterol oxidation, hgb A1C, and platelet aggregation; improved liver function and insulin sensitivity; and increasing levels of HDL-C levels (Brannon, 2011; Consumer Lab, 2012; Natural Medicines Comprehensive Database, 2012). More controlled studies are necessary to make any definitive conclusions regarding the role of resveratrol in health (Catalgol et al, 2012).

IRON

Men in eastern Finland have one of the highest recorded incidences of mortality from CHD. An association was reported between high levels of stored iron (as assessed by serum ferritin levels or ratio of serum transferrin receptor to serum ferritin) and increased risk for acute myocardial infarction (Salonen et al, 1992; Tuomainen, Punnonen, Nyyssönen, & Salonen, 1998). Iron overload thus was hypothesized to cause the higher occurrence of CHD in men compared with women. A study in Greece also correlated high dietary iron intake with increased risk of coronary artery disease in men and women 60 years of age or older (Tzonou et al, 1998).

A more detailed study found no association between total iron intake and risk of myocardial infarction after adjustment for age and gender, but the study did find high dietary intake of heme iron associated with occurrence of and mortality from myocardial infarction (Klipstein-Grosbusch et al, 1999). A reanalysis of Salonen's data associated increased iron intake with increased consumption of red meat (AHA, 2000).

HOMOCYSTEINE

More than 30 years ago, extensive atherosclerosis was found on autopsy of individuals with elevated plasma homocysteine levels due to errors of metabolism. This autosomal recessive genetic disease, homocystinuria, occurs in about 1 of 300,000 live births with a higher prevalence in Ireland and New South Wales (Refsum et al, 2004).

When untreated, homocystinuria results in thromboembolic events in 50% of the clients and a 20% mortality rate before the age of 30 (Nygård et al, 1997). Extending investigations to general populations found plasma homocysteine levels related to heart failure (Vasan et al, 2003), risk of stroke (Tanne et al, 2003), but also cancer mortality and all-cause mortality as well as cardiovascular mortality (Vollset et al, 2001).

Consequently, the early enthusiasm for reducing cardiovascular risk by reducing homocysteine levels has waned. Homocysteine appears to be a marker, rather than a cause, of cardiovascular disease. Therefore, routine screening for and treatment of elevated homocysteine levels to prevent cardiovascular disease is not supported by the evidence (Wierzbicki, 2007). Clinically, there is little justification for using folic acid or B vitamins in clients with established cardiovascular disease, whether or not they have elevated homocysteine levels (O'Callaghan, 2007). The AHA recommends that individuals obtain their folic acid and B vitamins from foods, consuming fruits and green, leafy vegetables daily (AHA, 2012).

Thus, evidence accumulates slowly and must be interpreted cautiously. The many correlations found in large studies are often statistically significant but do not prove causation and may not be clinically useful. Advice to clients should be evidence based from clinical practice guidelines.

TABLE 18-8 Labeling Regulations for Sodium Content Descriptions

TERM	LEGAL DEFINITION
Free	Less than 5 mg of sodium per serving
Salt-free	Must meet the criteria for free
Very low* sodium	Less than 35 mg of sodium per serving. For meals and main dishes: 35 mg or less per 100 g
Low* sodium	Less than 140 mg of sodium per serving. Meals and main dishes: 140 mg or less per 100 g
Reduced or less	This term means that a nutritionally altered product contains 25% less sodium than the regular, or reference, product. However, a reduced claim cannot be made on a product if its reference food already meets the requirement for a "low" claim.
Light in sodium or lightly salted	May be used on food in which the sodium content has been reduced by at least 50% compared with an appropriate reference food.
Unsalted or no added salt	Must declare "This is not a sodium-free food" on information panel if the food is not sodium free.

*Synonyms for "low" include "little," "few," and "low source of."

TABLE 18-9 Examples of Sodium Content of Beverages*

| Beverage† | REGULAR | | DIET | |
	Sodium (mg)	Kilocalories	Sodium (mg)	Kilocalories
Club soda			75	0
Coffee	4	0		
Cola	15	151		
With aspartame			21	2
With saccharin			75	2
Gatorade	39	123		
Ginger ale	25	125	130	4
Kool-Aid	0	150		
With aspartame			0	6
Lemonade	12	150		
Lemon-lime soda	41	149	70	4
Pepper-type	38	151	70	0
Root beer	49	152	170	4
Tea	2	0		

*Serving size is 12 fluid ounces.
†Sodium content may vary depending on the source of water.

Clients who require a diet containing less than 2 grams of sodium may elect to use bottled, distilled, deionized, or demineralized water for drinking and cooking to consume preferred sodium-containing foods. Some clients prefer a daily allotment of salt in a shaker to be used as desired. If this strategy is adopted, the foods high in sodium must be limited to a greater extent than for a standardized sodium-controlled diet (Fig. 18-6).

Many salt substitutes are available. Some substitute potassium for sodium and may be unsuitable for clients with kidney disease or those taking potassium-sparing diuretics or angiotensin-converting enzyme (ACE) inhibitors. Clients should consult their health-care providers about using these salt substitutes. These products are for table use only and are not appropriate for cooking because they turn bitter. Other salt substitutes are made up of different herb and spice blends and exclude salt and are excellent for enhancing the flavor of food and making low sodium cooking more palatable.

In clinical practice, diet orders such as "no-added-salt diet" or "low-sodium diet" require clarification. Usually, a facility's diet manual defines the terms. A "no-added-salt diet" may be calculated as 4 grams of sodium and a "low-sodium diet" as

sodium and should not be swallowed. Over-the-counter medications that may contain significant amounts of sodium include analgesics, antacids, antibiotics, antitussives, laxatives, and sedatives.

Softening water can increase its sodium content.

■ Sodium in city water supplies has varied from 1.2 milligrams per liter in Seattle to 100 milligrams per liter in Phoenix.
■ "Mineral waters" contain from 8 to 172 milligrams of sodium per liter. "Read the label" is appropriate advice.

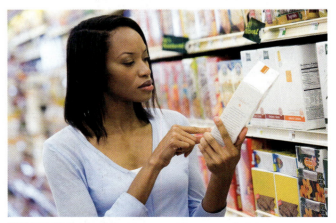

FIGURE 18-6 When clients are on sodium-controlled diets, it is important that they read labels carefully to ensure that they are selecting low-sodium foods.

2 grams in one facility but differently in another. Diet prescriptions should be written in milligrams or grams of sodium to be clear.

Modifications for Common Conditions

Persons with heart attacks, heart failure, or stroke may require modifications in diet. Referral to the dietitian should be made.

Myocardial Infarction

After a heart attack, the client may be in shock. One adaptive response of the body is to slow gastrointestinal function. Thus, the client may receive nothing by mouth while the shock persists. Fluid is given intravenously to maintain fluid balance and to keep an access site open for intravenous medications.

As the client recovers, the diet may progress from a 1,000- to 1,200-kilocalorie liquid diet to a soft diet of small, frequent meals. Large meals can increase the workload of the heart. The diet prescription begins to implement the principles of a cardioprotective diet. As soon as possible, client education should start.

Heart Failure

For clients in heart failure, the diet order may read "as tolerated" but sodium and fluid restriction is common. Energy needs are increased due to the workload of the heart and respiratory system. Undernutrition should be assessed by

the dietitian to ensure that the client is receiving an adequate diet (AND, 2017).

Food for the client with heart failure should be nutrient-dense, easily eaten, and easily digested. An hour's rest before meals conserves energy. Large meals, which would exert upward pressure on the chest, are undesirable. Liquid formulas, some special low-volume, nutrient-dense preparations, can be used to provide nutrients while moderating the feeling of fullness. It may be necessary to provide supplements of water-soluble vitamins and minerals that may be lost as excess fluid is excreted through treatment.

Stroke

Clients who have had a stroke may have trouble seeing their food as well as problems chewing, swallowing, and manipulating utensils. Generally, thicker, rather than thinner, liquids are easier to manage for a person with swallowing difficulty. Dry, chunky, or sticky foods are best avoided. Nurses feeding clients with hemiplegia should place the food on the unaffected side of the tongue. Turning the client's head toward the weak side while he or she is sitting upright may help with swallowing. In addition, stroke clients may be aphasic and unable to communicate their needs or desires. A speech pathologist is skilled in assessing function and restorative therapy using adaptive devices for clients with dysphagia and aphasia and should be consulted before feeding a client to ensure a proper diet order (see Chapter 9 for more information on dysphagia).

KEYSTONES

- Major modifiable risk factors for cardiovascular disease are hypertension, hypercholesterolemia, obesity, physical inactivity, diabetes mellitus, alcohol consumption, and cigarette smoking.
- Dietary modifications in cardiovascular disease most often involve cholesterol-lowering and/or blood pressure-controlling measures.
- The major target of cholesterol-lowering measures is low-density lipoprotein cholesterol (LDL-C).
- Lifestyle changes effective for hypertension control include reducing sodium intake and, if necessary, body weight.
- Dietary treatment of chronic heart failure focuses on fluid balance and preventing malnutrition.

CASE STUDY 18-1

Mr. Z is a 59-year-old man who was admitted to the acute-care hospital with a diagnosis of possible myocardial infarction. Subsequent testing proved Mr. Z did not have an infarction. His medical diagnoses are stage 2 hypertension and myocardial ischemia. He is being readied for discharge to home.

Mr. Z is vice president for sales of a large manufacturing company. His business activities involve luncheon and dinner meetings at which alcohol consumption is common. He stated that he has "at least one cocktail, usually two" with lunch and with dinner.

The clinical dietitian visited Mr. Z to evaluate his food behaviors as requested by the physician. After the dietitian left, Mr. Z said to the nurse, "That diet is impossible for my situation. She just doesn't understand the business world. I don't believe there's anything wrong with my heart anyway. It was just indigestion."

Providing client care is a dynamic process. Based on the above information, the nurse added the following modifications to Mr. Z's care plan.

CARE PLAN

Subjective Data

Reported alcohol intake of two to four drinks per day ■ Perceived incompatibility of prescribed diet with current lifestyle ■ Stated disbelief in medical diagnosis

Objective Data

LDL-C 158 ■ B/P 150/96 ■ BMI 27

Analysis

Denial of illness and negative perception of treatment regimen as evidenced by statements to nurse.

Plan

DESIRED OUTCOMES EVALUATION CRITERIA	ACTIONS/ INTERVENTIONS	RATIONALE
Client will acknowledge effect of lifestyle on health by hospital discharge.	Review pathophysiology of hyperlipoproteinemia and atherosclerosis with client. Analyze with the client the possibility of partial compliance. Refer to dietitian for repeat visit to prioritize actions and individualize diet plan. Obtain the client's permission to discuss lifestyle changes with significant other. Inform physician of extent of intended compliance with treatment regimen.	Repeated information reinforces learning. Perhaps the many changes required are overwhelming Mr. Z. One or two alterations might be acceptable as a starting point. Enlisting a support person might, over time, give Mr. Z reason to reconsider his options. These statements will affect the success of treatment. It is appropriate to notify the physician and record it on the client's medical record.

The following day, the physician showed Mr. Z his laboratory results and reviewed his diagnosis and risks.

TEAMWORK 18-1

DIETITIAN'S NOTES

The clinical dietitian revisited Mr. Z and wrote the following:

Subjective: *Able to repeat the information given by physician. Does not smoke. Eats three servings of vegetables most days, some of them fried. No exercise program. Usually eats two weekday meals in a restaurant. Client consumes one to two servings of alcohol daily or twice daily. Client perceives that it is impossible to make dietary changes when he eats in restaurants.*

Objective: *B/P 150/96, LDL-C 158, HDL-C 36*

Analysis: *Harmful beliefs/attitudes about food or nutrition-related topics related to stage 2 hypertension and myocardial ischemia as evidenced by client's reports.*

Plan: *Use local area restaurant menus to illustrate healthy meals—Done.*

Mr. and Mrs. Z agreed to referral to Heart Healthy Support Group to help refocus Mr. Z's view of his health. Gave contact information to client should he decide he wishes to have further dietitian education after participating in support group.

CRITICAL THINKING QUESTIONS

1. How could additional assessment data regarding family history be helpful in interpreting this client's reaction? Would you expect his reaction to be different if the diagnosis of myocardial infarction had been confirmed?

2. What additional interventions have the potential to achieve the stated outcome after hospital discharge?

3. When more genomic information becomes available in the future, how might this scenario change?

CHAPTER REVIEW

1. The DASH diet to reduce hypertension emphasizes:
   1. Increased amounts of fruits, vegetables, nuts, seeds, and legumes
   2. Specialty formulas as meal replacements
   3. Carbohydrate control and counting similar to that used in diabetes mellitus treatment
   4. Increased amounts of protein through low-fat dairy products and large servings of meats

2. The first action a hypertensive client should take to lower blood pressure is to:
   1. Restrict fluid to 1,500 mL per day
   2. Eliminate saturated fat from the diet
   3. Lose weight if necessary
   4. Limit sodium intake

3. Lifestyle changes that are recommended to reduce cardiovascular disease risk limit saturated and *trans*-fat intake to _____ % of daily kilocalories and cholesterol to _____ milligrams per day.
   1. 45, 450
   2. 30, 300
   3. 15, 250
   4. 7, 200

4. Which of the following seasonings are permitted on a sodium-controlled diet?
   1. Catsup, horseradish, mustard, and tartar sauce
   2. Chili powder, green pepper, and caraway seeds
   3. Celery seeds, seasoned meat tenderizer, and teriyaki sauce
   4. Dry mustard, garlic, and Worcestershire sauce

5. Which of the following lifestyle changes would have the greatest effect in reducing risk of atherosclerotic cardiovascular disease?
   1. Limiting cholesterol intake to the recommended amount
   2. Consuming plant sterols in recommended amounts
   3. Limiting alcohol intake to one (women) or two (men) standard drinks per day
   4. Eating five servings of fruits and vegetables daily

6. By having a parent with early onset CAD, one's likelihood of developing CAD is increased by:
   1. 40%
   2. 70%
   3. 10%
   4. 60-75%

CLINICAL ANALYSIS

1. Mr. A is a 55-year-old man being seen in a health clinic for hypertension. His blood pressure was 152/98 three months ago when he was first diagnosed. It has remained below that level but has not returned to normal. Today his blood pressure is 146/100.

   Mr. A is 5 ft 9 in. tall and weighs 173 lb. He has a medium frame. When first diagnosed, he weighed 178 lb. A weight-loss diet with no added salt was prescribed, but progress has been slow.

   Now the physician is prescribing a 2-gram sodium diet and starting Mr. A on a mild potassium-wasting diuretic. The clinic nurse is responsible for instructing the client. Before he or she instructs Mr. A, which of the following actions by the nurse would best ensure his compliance with the diet?
   a. Doing a financial analysis to see if Mr. A can afford the special foods on his new diet
   b. Finding out which favorite foods Mr. A would have most difficulty giving up
   c. Listing the possible consequences of hypertension if it is not controlled
   d. Asking to see Mrs. A to instruct her on the preparation of foods for the new diet

2. Which of the following breakfasts would be best for Mr. A?
   a. Applesauce, raisin bran, 1% milk, and a bagel with cream cheese
   b. Canned pears, cornflakes, whole milk, and a cholesterol-free plain doughnut
   c. Cooked prunes, instant oatmeal, 2% milk, and raisin toast with margarine
   d. Orange juice, shredded wheat, skim milk, and whole-wheat toast with jelly

3. Mr. A has agreed to limit his alcohol intake to two drinks per week. He asks the nurse to recommend beverages compatible with his diet. Which of the following is the best choice?
   a. Tomato juice and bouillon
   b. Buttermilk and club soda
   c. Plain tea and fruit juice
   d. Gatorade and lemonade

CHAPTER 19

Diet in Renal Disease

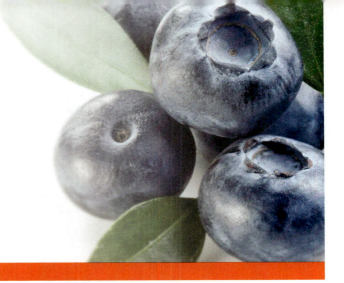

Chronic kidney disease (CKD) is gradual loss of kidney function over time. The National Kidney Foundation estimates that 14% of Americans have CKD. Diabetes and hypertension are two leading causes of CKD (National Institutes of Health [NIH], 2016).

Diet therapy for clients with kidney disease depends on an understanding of the normal function of the kidneys and basic concepts of pathophysiology of renal diseases. **Renal** means pertaining to the kidneys. The nutritional care of clients with renal disease is complex. These clients frequently must learn not just one diet in which one to seven nutrients are controlled but several different diets as their medical condition and the treatment approach change. The failure to adhere to necessary dietary changes can result in death. One aspect of working with clients with renal disease is that inattentiveness to dietary modifications can be measured objectively in weight changes or changes in blood chemistry.

Anatomy and Physiology of the Kidneys

The kidneys perform multiple functions. These functions are possible because of the kidneys' internal structure.

Internal Structure

The functioning unit of the kidney is the **nephron.** Each kidney contains about a million nephrons. Figure 19-1 shows an individual nephron. Each nephron has two main parts. The first part, **Bowman capsule,** is the cup-shaped top of the nephron. Inside Bowman capsule is a network of blood capillaries called the **glomerulus** (plural, *glomeruli*). The second part of the nephron is the **renal tubule.** (A tubule is a small

tube or canal.) The renal tubule is the ropelike portion of the nephron. This ropelike structure ends at the collecting tubule. Several nephrons usually share a single **collecting tubule.**

Functions

The kidneys assist in the internal regulation of the body by performing the following functions:

1. *Filtration:* The kidneys remove the end products of metabolism and substances that have accumulated in the blood in undesirable amounts during the **filtration** process. Substances removed from the blood include:
   - Urea
   - Creatinine
   - Uric acid
   - Urates

   Also filtered from blood are excessive amounts of:

- Chloride
- Potassium
- Sodium
- Hydrogen ions

   The **glomerular filtration rate (GFR)** is the amount of fluid filtered each minute by all the glomeruli of both kidneys and is one index of kidney function. This rate is normally about 125 milliliters per minute (Fig. 19-2).

2. *Reabsorption:* Previously filtered substances (e.g., water and sodium) needed by the body are reabsorbed into the blood in the tubules.

3. *Secretion of Ions to Maintain Acid–Base Balance:* Secretion is the process of moving ions from the blood into the

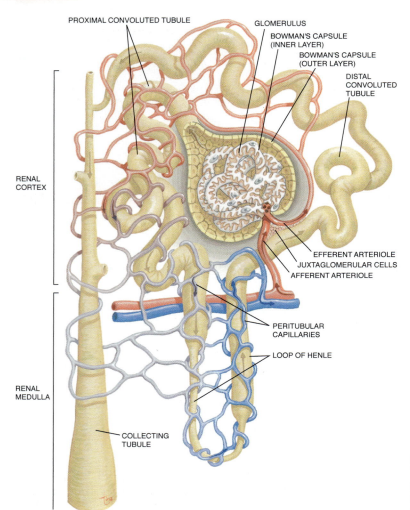

PROXIMAL CONVOLUTED TUBULE

GLOMERULUS

BOWMAN'S CAPSULE
(INNER LAYER)

BOWMAN'S CAPSULE
(OUTER LAYER)

DISTAL
CONVOLUTED
TUBULE

RENAL
CORTEX

EFFERENT ARTERIOLE
JUXTAGLOMERULAR CELLS
AFFERENT ARTERIOLE

PERITUBULAR
CAPILLARIES

LOOP OF HENLE

RENAL
MEDULLA

COLLECTING
TUBULE

FIGURE 19-1 A nephron with its associated blood vessels. The arrows indicate the direction of blood flow. *(Reprinted from Scanlon, VC, and Sanders, T: Essentials of Anatomy and Physiology, ed 5. FA Davis, Philadelphia, 2007, p. 423, with permission.)*

urine. Secretion allows for the amount of a substance to be excreted into the urine in concentrations greater than the concentration filtered from the plasma in the glomeruli. The kidneys regulate the balance between bicarbonate and carbonic acid by the secretion and exchange of hydrogen ions for sodium ions.

4. *Excretion:* The kidneys eliminate unwanted substances from the body as urine.
5. *Renal Control of Cardiac Output and Systemic Blood Pressure:* The kidneys adapt to changing cardiac output by altering resistance to blood flow both at the beginning of the glomerulus and at the end.
6. *Calcium, Phosphorus, and Vitamin D:* The kidneys produce the active form of vitamin D, **calcitriol.** Activated vitamin D regulates the absorption of calcium and phosphorus from the intestinal tract and assists in the regulation of calcium and phosphorus levels in the blood.
7. *Erythropoietin:* The kidneys produce a hormone called **erythropoietin,** which stimulates maturation of red blood cells in bone marrow.

Kidney Disease

Because the kidneys perform so many metabolic functions, kidney disease has serious consequences.

Causes

Renal disease can be caused by many factors, including:

- Trauma
- Infections
- Birth defects
- Medications
- Chronic disease (e.g., atherosclerosis, diabetes, hypertension)
- Toxic metal consumption
- See Genomic Gem 19-1.

Diabetic nephropathy is the most common cause of renal failure. A physiological stress such as a myocardial infarction (MI; commonly called a heart attack) or an extensive burn can precipitate renal disease by decreasing the perfusion of the kidney or markedly increasing catabolism.

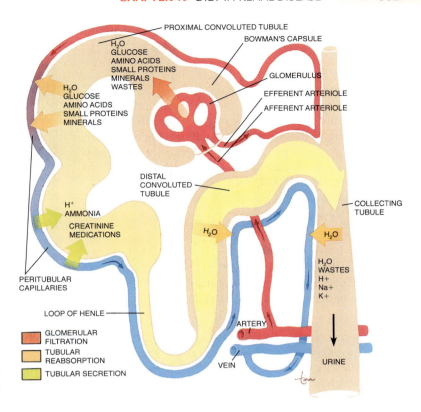

FIGURE 19-2 Schematic representation of glomerular filtration, tubular reabsorption, and tubular secretion. The renal tubule has been uncoiled, and the peritubular capillaries are shown adjacent to the tubule. *(Reprinted from Scanlon, VC, and Sanders, T: Essentials of Anatomy and Physiology, ed 6. FA Davis, Philadelphia, 2011, p. 455, with permission.)*

GENOMIC GEM 19-1

Genetic Mutations

Some kidney diseases are caused by errors in the genetic code. A genetic mutation can make it possible that a particular disease will happen. For example, high blood pressure is strongly associated with a selection of minor mutations plus lifestyle choices in diet, exercise, smoking, other environmental exposures, and kidney disease.

CLINICAL APPLICATION 19-1

Renal Response After a Myocardial Infarction

Immediately after a myocardial infarction (MI), blood flow through the systemic circulation is diminished. Systemic circulation refers to the blood flow from the left part of the heart through the aorta and all branches (arteries) to the capillaries of the tissues. Systemic circulation also includes the blood's return to the heart through the veins.

After an MI, blood flow to the myocardium (heart muscle) is decreased, impairing myocardial function. Less blood is delivered to the tissues. The kidneys sense the decreased cardiac output and try to compensate by reabsorption of additional water. This may lead to a fluid overload and edema. For that reason, clients who have had an MI may be on fluid restriction.

Clinical Application 19-1 describes the renal response after MI and the effect of reduced renal blood flow. Catabolism causes an increase in nitrogenous products and potassium, which must be excreted, overworking the kidneys. Renal disease is a feared complication of many pathologies and treatments—including radiocontrast materials used in diagnostic procedures, some antibiotics, and some pain medications.

Three common conditions increase the risk of renal disease:

1. Obesity
2. Poorly controlled diabetes
3. Hypertension

Losing weight may reduce the severity of diabetes and hypertension, the two leading causes of kidney failure, and helps prevent those conditions in people who have not developed them. Normalization of blood glucose and lipid levels along with blood pressure control also decrease the risk of renal disease. The Diabetes Control and Complications Trial (DCCT) and Epidemiology of Diabetes Interventions and Complications (EDIC) observational study of the DCCT participants have shown that intensive diabetes therapy can significantly reduce the progression of microvascular complications in people with diabetes. It is recommended that an A1C level of 7% should be the target for individuals (Betonico et al, 2016).

Hypertension is one of the leading causes of CKD. Those with CKD over the age of 65 have a 69.6% incidence of cardiovascular disease CVD compared to 34.7% among those who do not have CKD (NIH, 2016).

Glomerulonephritis

A general term for an inflammation of the kidneys is referred to as **nephritis.** This is the most common type of kidney disease. Inflammation of the glomeruli is called **glomerulonephritis,** which can be either acute or chronic. This condition may be caused by infections such as strep and various autoimmune diseases such as lupus (National Kidney Foundation [NKF], 2015). Symptoms include:

- Nausea
- Vomiting
- Fever
- Hypertension
- Blood in the urine (**hematuria**)
- Decreased output of urine (**oliguria**)
- Protein in the urine (**proteinuria**)
- Edema

Recovery is usually complete. However, in some clients the disease progresses and becomes chronic. This leads to a progressive loss of kidney function. Some clients develop **anuria,** which is a total lack of urine output. Without treatment, this condition is fatal.

Specific Tubular Abnormalities

A structural problem in the renal tubules may result in abnormal reabsorption or lack of reabsorption of certain substances by the tubules. The result of a tubular abnormality is ineffective cleansing of the blood.

Nephrotic Syndrome

The result of a variety of diseases that damage the glomeruli capillary walls is called **nephrotic syndrome.** Signs of nephrotic syndrome include:

- Proteinuria
- Severe edema
- Low serum protein levels
- Anemia
- Hyperlipidemia

Usually the higher the hyperlipidemia, the greater the proteinuria.

The disease is caused by the degenerative changes in the kidneys' capillary walls, which consequently permit the passage of albumin into the **glomerular filtrate.** Water and sodium are retained. Edema is sometimes so severe that it masks tissue wasting due to the breakdown of tissue protein stores. The degree of malnutrition is hidden until the excess fluid is removed.

Nephrosclerosis

A hardening of the renal arteries, known as **nephrosclerosis,** is caused by arteriosclerosis and results in a decreased blood supply to the kidneys. The condition is **hypertensive kidney disease** and can eventually destroy the kidney.

Progressive Nature of Kidney Failure

Kidney disease can be acute or chronic. The earliest clinical evidence of nephropathy is the appearance of low levels (30 mg/day or 20 g/min) of albumin in the urine, referred to as **microalbuminuria.**

In acute renal failure, referred to as **acute kidney injury (AKI),** the kidneys stop working entirely or almost entirely. Acute kidney injury occurs suddenly and is usually temporary. It can last for a few days or weeks.

Chronic kidney disease (CKD) occurs when progressively more nephrons are destroyed until the kidneys simply cannot perform vital functions. CKD occurs over time and is usually irreversible.

As individual nephrons are damaged, the remaining nephrons work harder to maintain metabolic homeostasis. As each functional nephron's workload is increased, the nephron becomes more susceptible to work overload and damage. The normal composition of the blood becomes altered when the remaining functional nephrons cannot assume any additional workload.

At such time, serum levels of **blood urea nitrogen (BUN), creatinine,** and uric acid become elevated. In some clients, even though the underlying condition (e.g., diabetes mellitus, hypertension) is treated, chronic renal disease may lead to **end-stage renal disease (ESRD).** During ESRD, most or all of the kidneys' ability to produce urine and regulate blood chemistries is severely compromised; dialysis or kidney transplant is required for survival.

Sodium Depletion

Often, the first sign of CKD is sodium depletion. This occurs when the kidneys lose their ability to reabsorb sodium in the tubule. Symptoms associated with sodium depletion include:

- A reduction of renal blood flow
- Dehydration
- Lethargy
- Decreased glomerular filtration rate (GFR)
- Uremia (see next section)
- Deterioration in neurological symptoms, including headaches, disorientation, and, in severe cases, seizures and coma

The client's blood pressure and body weight drop. Urine volume may be increased initially in CKD. A loss of body fat and protein content is responsible for the weight loss. The client's serum albumin level may fall as protein is lost in the urine.

Sodium Retention

As kidney function further deteriorates, some of these symptoms reverse. The kidneys lose the ability to excrete sodium. When this occurs, symptoms include:

- Sodium retention
- Overhydration

- Edema
- Hypertension
- Congestive heart failure (CHF)

The body can excrete little or no urine. The GFR gradually declines in CKD. CKD has been formally classified into five stages based on the GFR. Table 19-1 lists the stages of CKD and describes each stage along with the corresponding GFR. Most clients with a GFR below 25 milliliters per minute will eventually require either dialysis or transplantation, regardless of the original cause of failure. Nutrition therapy for CKD is to maintain good nutritional status (preventing malnutrition), slowing progression of the disease, and treating complications (NIH, 2014).

Progression to Uremia

If the client progresses to stage 5 CKD, **uremia** develops. Uremia is the name given to the toxic condition associated with renal failure. Uremia is produced by retention in the blood of nitrogenous substances normally excreted by the kidneys. The uremic client manifests many symptoms in virtually every body system as toxic waste products build up in the blood. The client may complain of:

- Fatigue
- Weakness
- Decreased mental ability
- Twitching and cramping muscles
- Anorexia
- Nausea
- Vomiting
- **Stomatitis,** an inflammation of the mouth
- Taste changes, especially for meats

To complicate matters further, gastrointestinal ulcers and bleeding are common. All of these symptoms have a direct effect on the client's willingness to eat.

Halting the Progression

Health-care professionals have known for many decades that clients with CKD who have sustained a loss of GFR may

continue to lose renal function until they develop terminal renal failure. The National Kidney Disease Education Program recommends diet therapy to slow the progression of CKD by:

- Controlling blood pressure
- Reducing excessive protein intake
- Managing diabetes

Aggressive antihypertensive treatment includes reducing sodium intake to no more than 1,500 mg per day and the use of angiotensin-converting enzyme (ACE) inhibitors or angiotensin receptor blockers (ARB) to slow the rate of progression of nephropathy (NIH, 2014).

Treatment of Kidney Disease

Kidney functions cannot be assumed by another organ. There is no cure for CKD. However, many clients can be treated with dialysis (an artificial kidney) or a kidney transplant. Artificial kidneys have been widely used since the 1960s to treat clients with severe kidney failure.

Dialysis

Dialysis means the passage of solutes through a membrane. Two functions of the kidneys are:

1. The removal of waste products
2. The regulation of fluid and electrolyte balance

By removing waste products from the blood and assisting in the maintenance of fluid balance, dialysis reduces the symptoms of:

- Uremia
- Hypertension
- Edema
- The risk of CHF

Dialysis is usually started when GFR is less than 15 mL/minute and the client develops symptoms of severe fluid overload, high potassium levels, acidosis, or uremia. Dialysis cannot restore the lost hormonal functions of the kidney. In addition, dialysis cannot correct the anemia that occurs because of a lack of erythropoietin. Some dialysis clients still need treatment for hypertension.

Hemodialysis

During **hemodialysis,** blood is removed from the client's artery through a tube, is forced to flow over a semipermeable membrane where waste is removed, and then is rerouted back into the client's body through a vein. Before dialysis can be initiated, an access site that allows blood to be removed from the body and returned back to the body at the time of dialysis must be surgically created. Ideally, this access will be a **fistula** created several months before dialysis is anticipated.

Figure 19-3 illustrates a client undergoing a hemodialysis treatment. A solution called the **dialysate** is placed on one

TABLE 19-1	Stages of Chronic Kidney Disease and Glomerular Filtration Rate (GFR)	
STAGE	**GFR**
1. Some kidney damage with normal or elevated GFR	≥90
2. Kidney damage with mildly decreased GFR	60–89
3. Mild to severe loss of kidney function with decreased GFR	30–59
4. Severe loss of kidney function with decreased GFR	15–29
5. Kidney failure	<15 Dialysis, transplant, hospice, or palliative care

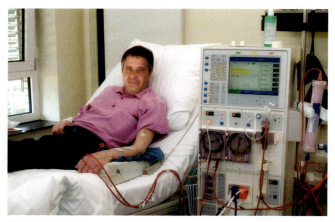

FIGURE 19-3 Client undergoing hemodialysis at dialysis center.

side of the semipermeable membrane, and the client's blood flows on the other side. The dialysate is similar in composition to normal blood plasma but may be manipulated to remove varying amounts of waste products. The client's blood has a higher concentration of urea and electrolytes than the dialysate has, so these substances diffuse from the blood into the dialysate. Sodium modeling may be used during dialysis. Modeling involves changing the concentration of sodium in the dialysate, which can improve the amount of fluid removed during the treatment. The composition of the dialysate varies according to the client's requirements.

Dialysis staff members usually administer in-center hemodialysis treatments for 3 to 4 hours, three times per week. Home hemodialysis is becoming more widely used in the United States. The client and a care partner learn to do the procedure in their own home. In-home treatment regimens vary from 3 to 6 days per week for 2 to 4 hours per treatment. Nocturnal hemodialysis may be done at home or in a center. These treatments are long, slow, daily, or every other day for 6 to 8 hours while the client sleeps. Dialysis is not as effective as normal kidney function because blood cleansing occurs only when clients are attached to artificial kidneys. Normal kidneys clear the blood 24 hours a day, 7 days a week.

Peritoneal Dialysis

The **peritoneum** is the lining of the abdominal cavity. During **peritoneal dialysis,** the dialysate is placed directly into the client's abdomen by means of a soft permanent catheter implanted between the abdominal wall and the peritoneum. The dialysate enters the body through a permanent catheter placed in the abdominal cavity. The peritoneum functions as the semipermeable membrane, allowing waste products and excess fluid to pass from blood into the dialysate. Various glucose concentrations are used in the dialysate to manipulate the amount of fluid removed.

The most common types of peritoneal dialysis are **continuous ambulatory peritoneal dialysis (CAPD)** and **automated peritoneal dialysis (APD).** The advantage of

peritoneal dialysis is that the client's blood levels of sodium, potassium, creatinine, and nitrogen stay within a more stable range and allow for a more liberal diet than in hemodialysis. Large shifts in fluid balance are also avoided. However, part of the glucose in the dialysate is available to the client as calories. The higher the glucose concentration used, the more calories are absorbed. The decision about which treatment is best is based on the client's medical condition, lifestyle, and personal preference. For example, a client with poor personal hygiene would not be a good candidate for peritoneal dialysis because of a high risk for infection.

CONTINUOUS AMBULATORY PERITONEAL DIALYSIS

Clients choosing CAPD are dialyzing constantly. With this method, the client instills 1.5 to 3 liters of dialysate into the abdominal cavity via a catheter. The fluid remains in the cavity for 4 to 6 hours while the client continues with activities of daily living. During this time, waste products and excess fluids diffuse through the peritoneal membrane into the dialysate. The dialysate is then drained and discarded, and then replaced with fresh solution in a process called an **exchange.** Each exchange takes 30 to 40 minutes, and clients perform four to five exchanges daily to achieve good dialysis.

AUTOMATED PERITONEAL DIALYSIS (APD)

APD is a process in which the "exchanges" just described are done during the night by means of a machine, called a cycler. The machine automatically fills and drains the dialysate. This process is done during sleeping hours, each cycle lasts $1\frac{1}{2}$ hours (NKF, 2015).

Kidney Transplant

Although kidney transplant can restore full renal function, it is considered a treatment, not a cure. Immunosuppressants to prevent rejection of the transplanted kidney are necessary. Some commonly used immunosuppressants are azathioprine, corticosteroids, and cyclosporine. These medications have many side effects, including diarrhea, nausea, and vomiting, which influence nutrient intake and absorption. A heart-healthy diet should be followed after a transplant, and other nutritional changes may be needed in an individual with diabetes or other health conditions.

Nutritional Care

The nutritional needs of clients with kidney diseases are changing constantly. The reason for the change is that the disease state and treatment approach are not static. Clients with kidney disease require constant assessment, monitoring, and counseling. In addition, providing quality nutritional care to these clients, who frequently must be coaxed to eat, is challenging. Anorexia, nausea, and vomiting are frequent complaints, particularly in the hospital.

Client–nurse interactions are important because nurses can influence and enhance client adherence to prescribed diets. Close communication among all members of the health-care team is vital to meeting the dynamic nutritional needs of these clients. The Academy of Nutrition and Dietetics (2013) and NKF (2015) consider coordination of care imperative in the practice guidelines for medical nutrition therapy for CKD. These two organizations are working together to develop new nutritional guidelines for CKD, anticipated to be published in 2018 (Academy of Nutrition and Dietetics, 2016).

Malnutrition

Malnutrition in hemodialysis clients is associated with increased mortality and morbidity. Moderate to severe malnutrition is estimated to occur in approximately 34% of clients on hemodialysis. Among the reasons for the malnutrition are:

- Increased catabolism
- Metabolic changes caused by excretion changes in different nutrients
- Decreased food intake because of restrictions and/or poor appetite
- Low economic status

Goals of Nutrition Therapy

Well-planned nutritional management is a fundamental part of any treatment plan for renal disease. Every client with renal disease requires an individualized diet based on the following goals:

- Attain and maintain optimal nutritional status.
- Prevent net protein catabolism.
- Minimize uremic toxicity.
- Maintain adequate hydration status.
- Maintain normal serum potassium levels.
- Control the progression of renal osteodystrophy (discussed later).
- Modify the diet to meet other nutrition-related concerns, such as diabetes, heart disease, gastrointestinal tract ulcers, and constipation.

- Retard the progression of kidney failure and postpone the initiation of dialysis.

No single diet is appropriate for all renal clients. Every client requires individual assessment, and every client's diet will likely change over time.

Dietary Components

Several basic components need to be monitored and, if possible, controlled in diets for kidney disease:

- Kilocalories
- Protein
- Sodium
- Potassium
- Phosphorus, vitamin D, and calcium
- Fluid
- Saturated fat and cholesterol
- Iron, vitamins, and minerals

The need to restrict or encourage the consumption of any of these nutrients changes according to the client's medical status and treatment approach. For example, at one time, client control of his or her potassium intake may not be necessary, but at another time, control may be vital. See Table 19-2, which displays nutrient modification required at the different disease stages.

Kilocalories

Clients with renal disease need additional kilocalories. In the absence of diabetes, clients on high-kilocalorie diets are usually given all the simple carbohydrates and monounsaturated and polyunsaturated fats they will eat. *Trans*-fats are minimized. The end products of fat and carbohydrate catabolism are carbon dioxide and water. Neither of these dietary constituents imposes a burden on the client's compromised excretory ability.

Inadequate nonprotein kilocalories, however, will encourage tissue breakdown and aggravate uremia. Clients with renal insufficiency need 35 to 40 kcal/kg per day. The use of a specialized oral supplement such as Suplena®, a

TABLE 19-2 **Stages of Chronic Kidney Disease, Nutrient Modification, and Rationale**

STAGE	NUTRIENT MODIFICATION	RATIONALE
1	CHO control if indicated	Control blood glucose levels.
2	Sodium Evaluate lipid levels and need to modify diet Potassium	Control blood pressure. CVD risk reduction Begin to monitor to minimize cardiac complications.
3	Phosphorus	Continue modifications of stages 1 and 2.
4	RDA for protein Potassium	Begin to monitor and treat as indicated to maximize bone health. Promote adequate and not excessive protein intake. Monitor monthly to avoid cardiac complications. All the above may slow the progression of kidney disease.
5	Highly individualized	As indicated by treatment approach, usual food intake, and laboratory values.

CHO, carbohydrate; CVD, cardiovascular disease; RDA, recommended dietary allowance.

low-protein, high-calorie product by Abbott Laboratories, is one example of an appropriate oral supplement for clients who are unwilling or unable to eat enough food. An adequate intake of kilocalories is crucial to the success of the dietary treatment.

In addition, individuals with diabetes and renal diseases need good control of blood sugar levels. Diets for renal disease can be high in simple sugars, and clients must learn how best to distribute the sugars through the day for optimal blood glucose control. In some cases, the primary nutritional goal is to decrease uremia, and blood glucose control may become less important. Consuming enough kilocalories while adhering to the other nutrient restrictions can be difficult for clients with CKD. See the Dollars & Sense 19-1 for a recipe for a fruit smoothie that is less costly and more palatable than most commercial oral supplements.

Protein

In renal clients, a primary goal of nutritional therapy is controlling nitrogen intake. Control may mean increasing or decreasing dietary protein as the client's medical condition and treatment approach change.

Because animal products contain all the essential amino acids, examples of foods containing protein of high biologic value include:

- Eggs
- Meat
- Dairy products

A vegetarian diet has been proven beneficial for clients with renal failure. Human and animal models suggest that vegetarian diets that are plentiful in some plant proteins may increase survival rates and decrease proteinuria, glomerular filtration rate, renal blood flow, and histological renal damage compared with nonvegetarian diets.

Vegetarian diets by nature are high in potassium and phosphorus because of all the vegetables, whole grains, and

fruits they contain. The client's goal is to eat the right combination of plant proteins while keeping potassium and phosphorus under control. A referral to a renal dietitian is important for these clients.

Protein restrictions are effective only if the client also consumes adequate kilocalories. Beginning renal insufficiency is usually called a predialysis and requires a restriction or modification of protein intake. Individuals with diabetes who have early stages of CKD should eat no more than 0.8 to 1 gram protein per kilogram of body weight. For nondiabetics with CKD, 0.8 grams protein per kilogram of body weight should be consumed. (Further lowering protein to 0.6 gram in nondiabetics could be beneficial but is a difficult regimen to follow.) This reduction may actually improve measures of renal function. For this reason, dietary intervention is now instituted when microalbumin appears in the urine (National Kidney Disease Education Program [NKDEP], 2015).

The treatment approach influences protein requirements. Hemodialysis clients need increased protein because hemodialysis results in a loss of 1 to 2 grams of amino acids per hour of dialysis. A client on CAPD has an even higher protein need because he or she dialyzes continuously. During dialysis, protein passes out of the blood with the waste products and into the dialysate fluid. When the dialysate fluid is discarded, a significant amount of protein is lost. A high-protein diet is necessary to replenish the losses.

Sodium

The desirable sodium intake for clients with kidney disease depends on individual circumstances. Serum sodium is not a reliable indicator of sodium intake in CKD. Dietary levels of sodium are based on blood pressure and fluid balance. The sodium intake of many clients with kidney failure must be restricted to prevent sodium retention with consequent generalized edema. Clients need to know that high sodium intake influences thirst and therefore fluid intake. Water softeners can be a significant source of sodium, and clients may be instructed to avoid them. The National Kidney Disease Education Program recommends a sodium intake of 1,500 mg per day or less (NIH, 2014).

The disease that precipitated renal failure plays a role in determining the need for sodium restriction. Because glomerulonephritis, for example, is more likely to produce hypertension and fluid retention, sodium restriction is often necessary. Low levels of sodium, absence of edema, and normal or low blood pressure commonly characterize other renal diseases, such as pyelonephritis. **Pyelonephritis** is an inflammation of the central portion of the kidney. In this situation, sodium intake may be higher than in the other groups of diseases but is individualized according to needs.

Potassium

Dietary potassium, like sodium, must be individually evaluated. **Hypokalemia** (low blood potassium level) must be avoided because it may introduce cardiac arrhythmias and eventually cardiac arrest. Boxes 19-1 and 19-2, respectively,

---

Dollars & Sense 19-1

Berry Smoothie

2 cups blueberries (fresh or frozen)
2 cups strawberries (fresh or frozen)
9 ounces silken tofu, extra firm
1/2 teaspoon ground ginger
2 pinches of red pepper flakes (optional)
1/4 teaspoon rum extract or vanilla extract
1 tablespoon honey or agave nectar
1 teaspoon lemon juice
1/2 cup ice

Use a blender to mix all ingredients thoroughly. Makes four servings.

1 cup serving contains 125 kilocalories, 1.8 grams fat, 44 mg calcium, 42 mg sodium, 100 mg phosphorus, 339 mg potassium, 22 grams carbohydrates, 15.5 grams of sugar, 6 grams fiber, and 6 grams protein (NKF, 2017).

BOX 19-1 ■ High-Potassium Foods

Clients should avoid these high-potassium foods in excess of ½ cups per day* or in the amount calculated by a dietitian.

Dairy Products
As calculated*

Meats
As calculated*

Starches
Bran cereals and bran products

Fruits
Orange, fresh
Mango, fresh
Nectarines
Papayas
Dried prunes
Avocado
Bananas

Vegetables
Bamboo shoots, fresh
Beet greens
Baked potato, with skin
Sweet potato fresh
Spinach, cooked
All others if eaten in excess of allowance*

Others
Chocolate, cocoa
Molasses
Salt substitute
Low-sodium broth
Low-sodium baking powder
Low-sodium baking soda
Nuts

*Dairy foods and meat products contain not only considerable potassium but also phosphorus and protein that need to be carefully planned in the diets of many clients.

BOX 19-2 ■ Low-Potassium Foods and Beverages*

Low-Potassium Foods
Bean sprouts, canned
Gum drops
Hard, clear candy
Nondairy topping
Honey
Jams and jellies
Jellybeans
Lollipops
Marshmallows
Suckers
Sugar
Lifesavers
Chewing gum
Poly-Rich (nondairy creamer)
Cornstarch

Low-Potassium Beverages
Carbonated beverages
Lemonade
Limeade
Cranberry juice
Popsicles (1 stick—60 mL of fluid)
Hawaiian Punch†
Kool-Aid†

Low-Potassium Unsweetened Beverages
Diet carbonated beverages
Diet lemonade
Diet Kool-Aid†

*Individuals with diabetes should not freely eat foods with sugar.
†These beverages are low in potassium but are often high in phosphorus and need to be restricted in many renal clients with a phosphorus dietary restriction.

list foods high and low in potassium. Salt substitutes are very high in potassium and should be avoided by renal clients. Water softeners may be a source of dietary potassium, and clients may be instructed to avoid water treated in such a manner. The need to restrict potassium generally increases in clients with decreased urinary output.

ACE inhibitors have been shown to reduce the level of albuminuria and the rate of progression of renal disease to a greater degree than other hypertensive agents that lower blood pressure (NKDEP, 2015). Use of ACE inhibitors may exacerbate hyperkalemia in clients with advanced renal insufficiency; therefore, when used, serum potassium levels should be monitored.

The recommended intake of potassium is 2.0 to 3.0 grams per day for most clients. If a client's potassium level is elevated (5 to 6.5 mEq/L), dietary potassium intake should be minimized to less than 2.4 grams per day. When urinary output is 100 to 500 mL and serum potassium is 5.5 to 6.5, a 40- to 60-mEq (about 1,563 to 2,345 mg K) intake is suggested.

In cases of anuria or when serum potassium exceeds 6.5 mEq/L, a dietary intake of 20 to 25 mEq/L (about 780 to 975 mg K) is suggested. This suggestion is for the acute, critical-care client because of its poor palatability. Fundamental to understanding medical nutritional therapy for clients with renal disease is that overrestricting a client's diet is never appropriate because of the danger of tissue catabolism and malnutrition. Before reducing diet, check the client's medications to be sure that he or she is not on potassium supplements. If the client is undergoing hemodialysis, also check the potassium level of the dialysate to see that all potassium that can be safely removed is being removed.

The potassium content of fruits and vegetables varies according to the form and the preparation method. For example, ½ cup of canned pears in heavy syrup has about 80 milligrams of potassium, and one fresh pear has about 210 milligrams. Potassium is water-soluble. For this reason, some renal clients on low-potassium diets are taught to use large amounts of water to prepare vegetables and to discard the water after cooking to decrease the vegetable's potassium content. Unfortunately, the process also decreases water-soluble vitamins. Most renal clients need renal vitamin supplements. Clients should eat fruits or vegetables in the form given on the list.

Phosphorus, Vitamin D, and Calcium

In the body, phosphorus, vitamin D, and calcium are all normally balanced. In clients with kidney disease, vitamin D cannot be activated, a situation leading to a low serum calcium level. At the same time, the kidneys cannot excrete phosphorus, a situation leading to an elevated serum phosphorus level.

When serum calcium level drops, calcium is released from the bones because of the increased secretion of **parathyroid hormone (PTH)**. PTH is secreted in an effort to correct the calcium imbalance. This chain of events may lead to renal **osteodystrophy** and **vascular calcification**, which are complications of chronic renal disease. **Renal osteodystrophy** leads to faulty bone formation. **Vascular calcification** contributes to the high incidence of cardiovascular disease seen in clients with CKD.

Control of blood levels of calcium and phosphorus involves several treatment approaches. First, clients with hypocalcemia and secondary hyperparathyroidism are given activated vitamin D orally or, if they are on hemodialysis, intravenously during their treatment. Activated vitamin D cannot be given when serum calcium or phosphorus levels are very high or vascular calcification may result.

Phosphorus is a mineral found in the bones and is needed along with calcium to build strong bones. When there is extra phosphorus in the body that the kidneys cannot excrete, calcium is pulled from the bones, which can make them brittle. High phosphorus levels must be controlled with the initiation of dietary phosphorus restriction. Phosphorus is found mainly in (see Box 19-3):

- Dairy products
- High-protein foods
- Whole-grain products
- Inorganic phosphate additives

Clients must learn how to read the ingredient label to avoid as many phosphate additives as possible. Although the amount added to a given food is small, these additives are 100% absorbed, while organic phosphates found naturally in foods have a much lower absorption rate. Phosphate additives are found in fast foods, processed foods, and canned and bottled beverages. Clients with CKD, especially in stages 3 through 5, need to watch their phosphorus intake. By limiting protein in the diet, phosphorus is also limited. If further reductions are needed, the dietitian should meet with the client to determine how a further reduction in phosphorus-containing foods can be managed (NKDEP, 2015).

Phosphate binders may be added to a client's regimen if dietary modification does not produce desired results. This is especially true for clients in stage 3 through 5 of CKD. Phosphate binders are medications that bind phosphorus in the GI tract, allowing the resulting complex to be eliminated in the stools. These medications *must* be taken while a client eats his or her meals (Academy of Nutrition and Dietetics, 2013; NKF, 2017). A **calcimimetic** may also be added to the treatment regimen. This medication acts directly on the parathyroid gland to reduce the release of PTH.

Fluid

Some predialysis (renal insufficiency) and most dialysis clients generally must restrict fluid intake because their kidneys can no longer excrete excess fluid. Table 19-3 lists guidelines for distributing fluids between meals and medications. Clients on hemodialysis are restricted to 500 to 1,000 milliliters plus 24-hour urinary output. This fluid restriction allows for fluid gain of 2 to 2½ kilograms between dialysis treatments. Predialysis clients do not generally have fluid restrictions unless their clinical condition indicates a need. For clients on CAPD, fluid restriction is "as tolerated" according to their daily weight fluctuations and blood pressure.

Saturated Fat and Cholesterol

Clients with renal disease frequently have hyperlipidemia. High serum lipid levels increase the progression of renal

---

BOX 19-3 ■ Foods High in Phosphorus

Dairy Foods	Raisin bran	**Dried Beans**	Pumpkin seeds
Milk	Whole wheat	Navy beans	Sunflower seeds
Cheese	Biscuits	Kidney beans	
Cocoa	Waffles	Lima beans	**Other**
Condensed milk	Pancakes	Pinto beans	Cola drinks
Evaporated milk	Cereals with nuts	Lentils	Chocolate
Cottage cheese	Cheese crackers	Black-eyed peas	Toffee
Yogurt	Cheese curls	Soybeans	Caramel
Custard			Fudge
Ice cream	**Meats**	**Nuts and Seeds**	Mushrooms
Pudding	Sardines	Almonds	Molasses
Cream soups	Herring	Cashews	Raisins and dates
	Smelt	Coconut	Other dried fruits
Grains	Liver	Pecans	Casseroles with cheese or cream
Bran	Sweetbreads	Walnuts	soup
Bran flakes	Tripe/menudo	Peanuts	
Bran muffins	Egg yolk (more than 2 per day)	Peanut butter	
Brown rice			

TABLE 19-3   Guidelines for Fluid-Restricted Clients

IF THE FLUID RESTRICTION IS	USE THIS AMOUNT OF FLUIDS WITH MEALS	USE THIS AMOUNT OF FLUIDS WITH MEDICATIONS
1,000 mL (4 cups)*	600 mL (2½ cups)	400 mL (1½ cups)
1,200 mL (5 cups)	700 mL (3 cups)	500 mL (2 cups)
1,500 mL (6 cups)	1,000 mL (4 cups)	500 mL (2 cups)
2,000 mL (8 cups)	1,000 mL (4 cups)	1,000 mL (4 cups)

All foods contain some fluids, but it is especially important to count the following as part of the fluid allowance:

Milliliters of Fluid per ½ Cup

Water	120	All juices	120	Watermelon	100
Coffee	120	Soda-pop	120	Sherbet	65
Tea	120	Ice	60	Ice cream	40
Decaf Coffee	120	Gelatin	100	Ice milk	40
Milk	120	Soup	120	Popsicle	80

All cup measures are approximations.

disease, which contributes to an increased risk of cardiovascular disease. The NKF recommends clients follow a healthy lifestyle to help lower cholesterol, which includes a diet low in saturated fat and cholesterol, regular physical exercise (30 minutes per day), healthy weight maintenance, no smoking, no more than 1 alcoholic beverage per day (with physician approval), and low-fat cooking methods (bake, broil, steam).

Significant hypertriglyceridemia is commonly present in clients with a history of kidney disease. The nutritional care of clients with elevated triglycerides includes a modified fat diet, modification of carbohydrate intake, and encouragement to increase exercise—as tolerated and with their physician's knowledge. Clients are counseled to avoid saturated fat and *trans* fat and to increase their intake of monounsaturated fat.

Iron

Anemias in clients with kidney disease may be due to:

- A lack of the kidney's production of erythropoietin
- A decreased oral iron intake, which commonly occurs as a result of dietary restriction
- Blood loss

Epoetin alfa, a pharmaceutical form of erythropoietin, may be used to increase red blood cell production and thereby correct the anemia. The treatment for iron-deficiency anemia is oral or IV iron and an increase in dietary sources of iron.

A diagnosis of iron-deficiency anemia can be made by a laboratory measure of ferritin. **Ferritin** is the storage form of iron found primarily in the liver. A small amount of ferritin circulates in the blood and reflects the amount of iron in body stores. A laboratory value of >100 micrograms per mL is recommended for CKD clients, ensuring adequate iron for erythropoietin-stimulated production of red blood cells (NKDEP, 2015).

Vitamin and Mineral Supplementation

Unless supplements are given, chronically uremic clients are prone to deficiencies of water-soluble vitamins. Losses are most notable with pyridoxine, ascorbic acid, and folic acid. Supplementation of these nutrients is recommended for clients on dialysis. Fat-soluble vitamins are not lost in the dialysate, and supplementation is not indicated except with vitamin D for another reason (see previous discussion). Because the body's ability to excrete excess fat-soluble vitamins is compromised, toxicity is a potential problem.

Teaching Diet for Kidney Disease

In 1993, the American Dietetic Association and the National Kidney Foundation introduced the National Renal Diet, a uniform diet that could be used across the country. The second edition, introduced in 2002, included more simple lists with more emphasis on clients' involvement in determining and managing their own diets. The edition starts with survival information and allows the dietitian to introduce new topics as client interest and blood chemistries indicate the need for further diet modification and teaching.

The importance of individualizing medical nutrition therapy for the client with CKD cannot be overemphasized. Regular contact with a renal dietitian increases the client's ability to change established behaviors and also allows for the most liberal diet possible. Table 19-4 shows the guidelines for medical nutrition therapy of clients with kidney disease by treatment approach.

Renal Disease in Children

Growth failure is commonly seen in children with chronic renal failure treated with dialysis, but it is not an inevitable complication. Inadequate caloric consumption and metabolic acidosis are reasons for the poor growth. These children usually need to have their sodium, potassium, and

TABLE 19-4 Selected Nutritional Parameters for Varying Levels of Kidney Failure

NUTRITIONAL PARAMETER	NORMAL KIDNEY FUNCTION	STAGES 1–4 CHRONIC KIDNEY DISEASE	STAGE 5 HEMODIALYSIS	STAGE 5 PERITONEAL DIALYSIS	TRANSPLANT
Calories (kcal/kg per day)	30–37	<60 years: 35 >60 years: 30–35	<60 years: 35 >60 years: 30–35	<60 years: 35 including calories from dialysis	Initial: 30–35 Maintenance: 25–30
Protein (grams/kg per day)	0.8	0.6–0.75 50% HBV	1.2 50% HBV	1.2–1.3 50% HBV	Initial: 1.3–1.5
Fat (percent total kcal)	30%–35% Clients considered at highest risk for cardiovascular disease: emphasis on <10% saturated fat, PUFA, MUFA, 250–300 mg cholesterol/day				
Sodium (mg/day)	<2,300 mg/day*	≤1,500 mg/day†	≤1,500 mg/day†	≤1,500 mg/day†	<2,300 mg/day*; monitor medication effect
Potassium (mg/day)	Unrestricted	Correlated to laboratory values	2,000–3,000 (8–17 mg/kg per day)	3,000–4,000 (8–17 mg/kg per day)	Unrestricted; monitor medication effect
Calcium (mg/day)	Unrestricted	1,200	<2,000 from diet and medications	<2,000 from diet and medications	1,200
Phosphorus (mg/day)	Unrestricted	Correlated to laboratory values	800–1,000, adjusted for protein	800–1,000, adjusted for protein	Unrestricted unless indicated
Fluid (mL/day)	Unrestricted	Unrestricted with normal urine output	1,000 + urine output	Monitored; 1,500–2,000	Unrestricted unless indicated

Meant as guidelines only for initial assessment; individualization to client's own metabolic status and coexisting metabolic conditions is essential for optimal care. HBV, high biological value; MUFA, monounsaturated fatty acids; PUFA, polyunsaturated fatty acids.
*Source: Reprinted from Beto, JA, and Bansal, VK: Medical nutrition therapy in chronic kidney failure: integrating clinical practice guidelines. J Am Diet Assoc 104:407, 2004. Copyright 2004, with permission from the American Dietetic Association. Updated sodium values based upon *2010 Dietary Guidelines for Americans and †National Institutes of Health, 2011.*

protein intake rigidly controlled, and this control may contribute to poor food intake. Anorexia and emotional disturbances are also contributing factors. Continually reinforcing the rationale for medical nutrition therapy and providing meal and snack ideas and emotional support can help to improve adherence.

Suggestions for improving children's intake include:

- Involving the children in selecting and preparing foods (insofar as possible)
- Serving meals in an appealing, attractive manner (e.g., serving contrasting colors and textures of foods, using decorative tableware and dishes)
- Serving small, frequent meals
- Ensuring that the child has someone with him or her at mealtime
- Planning special mealtime events such as picnics (even if they are held in the hospital playroom)

Kidney Stones

Kidney stones may be found in the bladder, kidney, ureter, or urethra. During urine formation, the urine moves from the collecting tubules into the renal pelvis. From the **renal pelvis,** the urine moves down the **ureter** and into the

urinary bladder. Finally, urine passes from the bladder down the urethra and exits the body.

A stone, also called a **urinary calculus,** is a deposit of mineral salts held together by a thick, syrupy substance. A urinary calculus can block the movement of urine from the body. Symptoms of a blockage include:

- Sudden severe pain
- Loss of kidney function
- **Hematuria** (blood in the urine)
- Urinary tract infections, including kidney infections

A kidney stone can also pass out of the body with the urine.

Causes

The cause of most kidney stones is unknown. Some possible causes include:

- An abnormal function of the parathyroid gland
- Disordered uric acid metabolism (as in gout)
- An excessive intake of animal protein and sodium
- Immobility, being overweight
- Kidney infections (forming struvite stones)
- Genetic disorder causing cystine to leak through kidneys into the urine (cystine stones)

At higher risk for kidney stones are men, people with a sedentary lifestyle, Asians, and whites. Typically, kidney stones occur in clients who are between 30 and 50 years of age. A determination of the stone's composition may lead to a restriction of dietary substrates (the substance acted on). Frequent dietary substrates of kidney stones are oxalic acid and purines. Decreased fluid intake and strongly concentrated urine or low urine volume are risk factors.

Treatment

All clients with kidney stones should drink sufficient water, 6 to 8 cups of water per day are recommended. The primary reason for increasing fluid intake is to prevent formation of concentrated urine, in which crystals are more likely to combine and precipitate.

Oxalates

Calcium oxalate is the most common constituent of kidney stones. Some individuals are genetically susceptible to stone formation. A diet excluding foods high in oxalates (see Table 19-5) is frequently prescribed for clients with kidney stones if laboratory analysis shows that removed or passed stone is high in oxalates. Additionally, reducing sodium to 2,300 mg and limiting animal protein in the diet are recommended because excess sodium and protein cause the kidneys to excrete calcium in the urine. Having enough calcium in the diet, 800 mg per day (through food or supplements taken with food), helps prevent calcium oxalate stones (NIH, 2017).

Calcium

Historically, if laboratory analysis of a surgically removed or passed stone found it to be high in calcium, a low-calcium diet was prescribed (600 milligrams per day). Today, it is known that kidney stones are not caused by dietary calcium. Kidney stones are of less concern with an increased calcium intake than with a decreased intake. Calcium in the digestive track binds with oxalates from foods and keeps it from entering the blood and then the urinary tract where stones can form. Consuming 800 mg of calcium per day helps prevent kidney stones and also helps maintain bone density (NIH, 2017).

Uric Acid Stones

Stones composed of uric acid form when the urine is persistently acidic. Animal protein is rich in purines, which may increase uric acid in the urine. If uric acid is concentrated in the urine, it can form a stone by itself or with calcium. Meat consumption should be limited to 6 ounces per day in individuals who form uric acid stones (NIH, 2017). Purines are sometimes a complication of **gout,** a hereditary metabolic disease that is a form of arthritis. One symptom of gout is inflammation of the joints. The metabolism of uric acid is related to dietary **purines,** a product of protein digestion. A purine-restricted diet is commonly prescribed for gout. Table 19-6 shows purines

TABLE 19-5   Foods High in Oxalates

MG/100 GRAMS	
Beverages	
Coffee, instant dry	143.0
Tea, brewed	12.5
Fruits	
Blackberries, raw	12.4
Gooseberries, raw	19.3
Plums, raw	11.9
Grains	
Bread, whole-wheat	20.9
Vegetables	
Beets, raw	72.2
Beets, boiled	109.0
Carrots, boiled	14.5
Green beans, raw	43.7
Green beans, boiled	29.7
Rhubarb, raw	537.0
Rhubarb, stewed	447.0
Spinach, boiled	571.0
Miscellaneous	
Cocoa, dry	623.0
Ovaltine, powder	45.9
Peanuts	95.3
Mixed Nuts	137.7

Source: Values taken from Pennington, JA, and Douglass, JA: Bowes and Church food values of portions commonly used, ed 18. Lippincott Williams & Wilkins, Philadelphia, 2004, and oxalate.org, 2017.

TABLE 19-6   Purines in Food

GROUP A: HIGH CONCENTRATION (150–1,000 MG/100 GRAMS)	
Liver	Sardines (in oil)
Kidney	Meat extracts
Sweetbreads	Consommé
Brains	Gravies
Heart	Fish roes
Anchovies	Herring

GROUP B: MODERATE AMOUNTS (50–150 MG/100 GRAMS)	
Meat, game, and fish other than those mentioned in Group A	Asparagus
	Cauliflower
Fowl	Mushrooms
Lentils	Spinach
Whole-grain cereals	
Beans	
Peas	

GROUP C: VERY SMALL AMOUNTS: NEED NOT BE RESTRICTED IN DIET OF PEOPLE WITH GOUT	
Vegetables other than those mentioned above	Coffee
Fruits of all kinds	Tea
Milk	Chocolate
Cheese	Carbonated beverages
Eggs	Tapioca
Refined cereals, spaghetti, macaroni	
Butter, fats, nuts, peanut butter*	
Sugars and sweets	
Vegetable soups	

Fats interfere with the urinary excretion of urates and should be limited if the objective is to promote excretion of uric acid.
Source: From Taber's Online, FA Davis, Philadelphia, 2017. Used with permission.

in foods. Many physicians do not prescribe a low-purine diet for gout because the condition can be more effectively controlled by medications.

Clinical Application 19-2 summarizes the recommendations for medical nutrition therapy for kidney stones.

Surgery

Surgery is sometimes necessary to remove large kidney stones. Surgical removal of the stones prevents infection, reduces pain, and prevents a loss of kidney function.

Urinary Tract Infections

One form of **urinary tract infection (UTI)** is **cystitis,** an inflammation of the bladder. This condition is prevalent in young women. Recurrent UTI means that the individual has three or more bouts of infection per year. Conclusive evidence-based research does not exist to demonstrate a benefit in consuming high levels of vitamin C or cranberry juice in the diet as a way to prevent or treat UTIs. Clients with UTIs should be encouraged to drink ample fluids, 6 to 8 glasses per day (NIH, 2017).

CLINICAL APPLICATION   19-2

Dietary Approaches to Prevent Kidney Stones

TYPE	DRINK 2–3 L OF FLUID/DAY	REDUCE SODIUM TO ≤2,300 MG/DAY	LIMIT PROTEIN TO 6 OZ/DAY	CONSUME ≤800 MG OF CALCIUM/DAY	LIMIT OXALATE INTAKE FROM FOOD	DRINK CITRUS DRINKS*
Calcium oxalate	X	X	X	X	X	X
Calcium phosphate	X	X	X	X		X
Uric acid	X		X			X
Struvite	X					X
Cystine	X (or more)					X

*Studies suggest that citrus drinks such as lemonade and orange juice protect against kidney stones because the citrate stops crystals from growing into stones.
Source: Adapted from National Institutes of Health, 2013 (NIH Publication No. 13-6425).

KEYSTONES

- The basic functional unit of the kidney is the nephron.

- Millions of nephrons work together to form urine and remove unnecessary substances from the blood.

- Glomerular filtration rate (GFR) is a measure of kidney function.

- The kidneys are also the site where vitamin D_3 (calcitriol) and erythropoietin are activated.

- Kidney failure can be acute or chronic. Chronic renal disease is progressive. Treatment for kidney failure is dialysis or a kidney transplant.

- Nutritional management of clients with renal disease is a fundamental part of treatment.

- Clients with kidney disease require constant assessment, monitoring, and counseling.

- The dietary components that may need modification are kilocalories, protein, sodium, potassium, phosphorus, fluid, cholesterol, and saturated fat.

- Vitamin and mineral supplements are often prescribed for clients with renal disease.

- Frequently, the diet these clients follow must be modified as their medical condition and treatment changes.

- Some nutritional intervention is necessary for clients with kidney stones and urinary tract infections. The fluid intake of these clients should be high.

CASE STUDY 19-1

Mr. U is a 55-year-old man who works full time and has a sedentary lifestyle. He is 5 ft 10 in. tall, has a medium frame, and weighs 68 kg. His ideal and usual weight is 76 kg. During the past 6–9 months, he has been anorectic and has had intermittent nausea and episodes of vomiting. He receives 4 hours of hemodialysis 3 times per week. His predialysis blood chemistry values were as follows:

- Blood urea nitrogen, 63 mg/dL
- Sodium, 135 mmol/L (135 mEq/L)
- Potassium, 4.0 mmol/L (4.0 mEq/L)
- Phosphorus, 2.0 mg/dL
- Calcium, 9.0 mg/dL
- Albumin, 3.3 g/dL
- Urine output ranges between 800 and 1,000 mL per day.

On arrival in the hemodialysis unit today, the client complained of hopelessness and a fear of dying. He complained that he cannot meet the nutritional goals set by the dietitian because he just keeps getting "sick and sicker and is afraid of dying."

The client's medical record lists religious preference as Catholic.

CARE PLAN

Subjective Data
Client complains of anorexia, nausea, and vomiting; a lack of hope; and a fear of dying.

Objective Data
Client tearful today. ■ Documented history of anorexia, emesis, and nausea. ■ His body weight is stable.

Analysis
Anorexia, nausea, and vomiting likely related to fear as evidenced by statement, "I have given up hope and am afraid of dying."

Plan

DESIRED OUTCOMES EVALUATION CRITERIA	ACTIONS/ INTERVENTIONS	RATIONALE
The client will maintain a sense of purpose despite fear.	Assist the client/family to identify areas of hope in life.	Clients and family members who can list foods and fluids that are better tolerated will provide hope.
Involve the client actively in his own care.	Explain to the client that despite his uncomfortable symptoms, his body weight is stable.	It is more effective to begin every counseling session with a review of the client's positive behaviors.
Seeks information to reduce fear.	As client has an ongoing relationship with the dietitian, he or she may be able to expand client's repertoire of food- and fluid-related coping mechanisms.	Dietitians in hemodialysis centers visit clients at least monthly and frequently more often.
Help client expand spiritual self.	Ask the client if he would like you to arrange a visit from a Catholic priest or his designee.	Helping a client connect to his spiritual self helps maintain a sense of purpose despite fear.

TEAMWORK 19-1

DIETITIAN'S NOTES

The following Dietitian's Notes are representative of the documentation found in a client's medical record.

Subjective: *Visited client per nursing request today. Client asked for specific information to decrease vomiting and nausea and increase food intake. He describes his food intake as sporadic. Lately food intake has been less than he would like. He states that he has not missed any days of work due to illness. Client states that his wife has been especially helpful with meal preparation and grocery shopping, but nothing sounds good to him. Usually eats/drinks a half cup dairy, four starches, two vegetables, five meats, three fruits, and six fats. However, he is discouraged when he cannot rigidly follow this pattern every day.*

Objective: *Weight stable at 76 kg; Compazine (for nausea) 2 times per day as needed; albumin 3.3 g/L; blood urea nitrogen 63 mg/dL; phosphorus 2.0 mg*

Analysis: *Client is eating about 66 grams of protein on days he does not experience nausea and vomiting. Phosphorus of 2.0 may be related to too many phosphate binders and not eating enough. Recommend that client try eating an extra egg or two each day on the days he is not nauseated. Also, recommended that he sip four cans of Nepro® (Abbott) on days he cannot eat and just to try a few sips every hour on the hour. Four cans of Nepro would provide 960 mL and 1,700 kcal, and 76.2 grams of protein. Client was reminded that this would use 960 mL of his fluid allowance. Client appeared relieved to have a plan he could follow on days when he was not "up to eating."*

Plan:
- *Recommended that client take one less phosphate binder per day until his next treatment*
- *Will speak again with client during his next hemodialysis treatment and provide positive reinforcement*
- *Client needs to consume more kcal*

Daily Renal Diet Plan Goals

NUTRIENT	LEVEL	RATIONALE
Energy (kcal)	2,300–2,700	30–35 kcal/kg HBW
Protein (grams)	91	1.2 grams/kg HBW
Sodium (mg)	2,000	Control fluid weight gain
Potassium (mg)	3,000	≤40 mg/kg HBW
Phosphorus (mg)	1,080 mg	10–12 mg/kg of protein
Fluid (mL)	1,500–1,750	750 mL plus urine output

HBW, Healthy body weight (may be called standard body weight or ideal body weight).

CRITICAL THINKING QUESTIONS

1. Explain the relationship of the dietary protein modification to the signs and symptoms Mr. U is experiencing.

2. Mr. U eats only about half his needed kilocalories. What should you do?

3. Mr. U decides he would like to try continuous ambulatory peritoneal dialysis (CAPD). How would his diet probably change?

CHAPTER REVIEW

1. Which of the following is a nutritional goal for a child with renal failure?
   1. Maintain current hydration status
   2. Promote normal growth and development
   3. Maximize uremia
   4. Stimulate client well-being

2. Kidney disease cannot be caused by:
   1. Consumption of toxic metals
   2. Consumption of 1 to 3 L a day of water
   3. Infection
   4. Trauma

3. Kilocalories usually need to be increased in protein-restricted diets because an adequate kilocalorie intake:
   1. Assists in the control of serum potassium
   2. Is necessary to prevent renal anemia
   3. Controls and prevents osteodystrophy
   4. Spares protein

4. The _____ intake from food is not monitored in renal clients.
   1. Vitamin D
   2. Fluid
   3. Protein
   4. Sodium

5. The most important nutritional consideration in treating clients with kidney stones is to:
   1. Limit calcium intake
   2. Restrict all end products of protein metabolism
   3. Restrict all food sources of calcium, oxalic acid, and purines
   4. Increase fluid intake

6. In a diet for CKD, stages 1–4 without dialysis, the following may commonly be restricted:
   1. Protein, iron, vitamin C
   2. Protein, kilocalorie, iron, phosphorus
   3. Protein, fluid, phosphorus, sodium, potassium
   4. Protein, fluid, potassium, vitamin C

CLINICAL ANALYSIS

1. Bill, age 10, has acute glomerulonephritis. His mother explains that Bill had a streptococcal infection 1 week before the illness. When planning Bill's care, the nurse recognizes that he needs help in understanding his diet. Bill's restrictions will include:
   a. A low-fat diet
   b. A calcium restriction
   c. A daily measurement of urine output (if any) and plan for his fluid intake
   d. A high-protein diet

2. Mr. Jones, a 49-year-old mechanic, has been admitted to the hospital with diagnosis of renal failure. Mr. Jones has been following a 40-gram protein, 2-gram sodium, 2-gram potassium, 1,000-mL fluid restriction for the past 5 years. Mr. Jones is scheduled for surgery tomorrow to have a permanent fistula implanted for hemodialysis. Mr. Jones's nutritional needs will change after he is maintained on hemodialysis to:
   a. More oranges, bananas, and baked potatoes
   b. More lean meat, eggs, fish, low-fat dairy products, and peanut butter
   c. Less starches, breads, and cereals
   d. Less margarine, oil, and salad dressings

3. Mr. Jones is found to have an elevated serum phosphorus level after 6 months on hemodialysis. He should:
   a. Restrict his intake of dairy products and peanut butter
   b. Restrict his intake of red meats
   c. Increase his intake of sugar, honey, jam, jelly, and other simple sugars
   d. Discontinue his phosphate binders

CHAPTER 20

Diet in Digestive Diseases

After completing this chapter, the student should be able to:

- Describe the preoperative limitations of specific fluids recommended by the American Society of Anesthesiologists.
- Distinguish between the dietary preparation for gastrointestinal surgery and the dietary preparation for surgery on other body systems.
- Compare the diet-related interventions for postprandial hypotension and dumping syndrome.
- Identify the mealtime treatment of gastroesophageal reflux disease and hiatal hernia.

- Explain the dietary treatment of celiac disease related to its pathophysiology.
- Differentiate nutritional care for clients with Crohn disease from that for ulcerative colitis.
- Relate the nutritional care for clients with hepatitis to that for cirrhosis.
- Describe the nutritional aspects of medical treatment for cholecystitis.
- Discuss cystic fibrosis as to impact on digestion and dietary treatment.

The gastrointestinal (GI) tract functions both as a barrier to substances from the environment and as an entry point for nutrients and other substances. Many disorders that affect the GI tract and its accessory organs (liver, gallbladder, and pancreas) influence the nutritional status of clients. Most surgical procedures have an impact on GI tract function and require special dietary measures, both preoperatively and postoperatively. This chapter covers dietary modifications for surgical clients and for clients with common disorders and diseases of the digestive system.

Dietary Considerations With Surgical Clients

Because of its role in tissue building and healing, protein is crucial in surgical clients. Protein depletion increases the risk of:

- Infection because the body cannot manufacture enough white blood cells
- Shock because low serum albumin prevents the return of interstitial fluid to the blood vessels
- Wound **dehiscence** because local edema persists and interferes with healing

Individuals with diseases affecting the GI tract are at special risk when facing surgery because such diseases interfere with nutrition. In cases involving GI surgery, the GI tract is incised and sutured, so postoperative feeding may be postponed to allow for healing. If the GI tract is permanently

modified, specialty nutritional care is needed to optimize use of the remaining organs. Surgical clients with liver disease also need special attention. The liver has many functions, some of which are listed in Table 20-1. Because of the liver's role in metabolizing and detoxifying drugs, clients with liver disease must be carefully managed when surgery is necessary. Moreover, some anesthetics, analgesics, and anti-infectives are toxic to the liver.

Preoperative Nutrition

Before elective surgery is undertaken, nutritional deficiencies should be identified and corrected. Preoperative undernutrition is linked to increased postoperative complications. Nutritional status should be assessed using client history, physical examination, and laboratory tests. Those most at risk are those who have had a 5% or more weight loss in the previous 1 to 3 months, have a BMI <18.5, and/or have had a 25% to 75% reduction in oral intake; take steroids; and have cancer or immunosuppression (as a result of disease or medication) (Mohabir & Gurney, 2015; Webb, 2015). Many overweight or obese clients are instructed to lose weight to reduce the risks of surgery. If the client is anemic, an iron preparation may be prescribed. Other nutrients can be provided as needed. At least 2 to 3 weeks are required for objective evidence of the effectiveness of nutritional therapy. Clinical Application 20-1 relates one possible cause of malnutrition in surgical clients.

Preventive nutritional support is effective for malnourished surgical clients or those whose oral intake will be

TABLE 20-1 Examples of Liver Functions

RELATED TO	PRODUCES/PROCESSES	STORES	BREAKS DOWN
Carbohydrate	Glucose from galactose and fructose Glucose from glycogen Glucose from glycerol and protein	Glycogen	
Fat	Fat from glucose Cholesterol Fatty acids and glycerol from cholesterol, phospholipids, and lipoproteins Lipoproteins Water-soluble bilirubin (from fat-soluble) Bile	Fat	
Protein	Albumin Some globulins Prothrombin Fibrinogen Transferrin Enzymes to convert ammonia to urea		
Vitamins	Retinol-binding protein Other transport proteins Activates thiamin Activates vitamin B_6 Processes vitamin D	A, D, E, K Thiamin Riboflavin B_6 Folic acid B_{12} Biotin	
Minerals		Iron	Worn-out red blood cells
Other			*Acetaminophen* Alcohol *Aldosterone* Bacteria Barbiturates Estrogen Glucocorticoids *Morphine* *Progesterone* Some anesthetics

CLINICAL APPLICATION 20-1

Surgical Clients with Rampant Dental Caries

Within a period of weeks, three clients on a gynecological surgical unit suffered postoperative wound disruptions. Each disruption was a **dehiscence,** a separation of the wound edges. Dehiscence occurs most frequently between the 5th and 12th postoperative days. Risk factors for dehiscence include:

- Obesity
- Malnutrition
- Dehydration
- Abdominal distention
- Infection
- Increased abdominal pressure from improper deep breathing and coughing

All three clients had at least one of the risk factors. One client ran a postoperative fever, which could have been caused by infection or dehydration. The other two clients had such severely carious teeth that it would have been difficult for them to chew in the months before surgery. They probably were malnourished. Marked dental caries suggest a need for a thorough nutritional assessment. Carious teeth can cause and be caused by poor eating habits.

compromised after surgery. In clients undergoing elective major GI surgery, perioperative nutrition therapy for 7 days before surgery (>10 kcal/kg/day) is associated with a 50% reduction in nosocomial infection and total complications. Individuals who were determined to be of low nutritional risk before surgery had no change in outcomes even if receiving presurgical nutrition therapy (McClave, DiBaise, Mullin, & Martindale, 2016). Preoperative fasting protocols have been liberalized based on research showing slight risk of pulmonary aspiration with modern anesthetics. Guidelines for anesthesia administration to healthy individuals scheduled for elective procedures permit greater oral intake than in the past (Table 20-2). The guidelines do not supplant the need for individual assessment. Nor do they apply to individuals with GI motility or metabolic disorders, individuals with potential airway problems, or women in labor.

For the next step modifying preoperative fasting protocols, see Clinical Application 20-2. Whatever the prescribed fast, a client's compliance with it should be assessed at the time of the procedure (American Society of Anesthesiologists, 2017).

TABLE 20-2   Preoperative Fasting Recommendations to Minimize Aspiration Risk

ORAL INTAKE	MINIMUM FASTING TIME	COMMENT
Clear liquids	2 hours	Examples: water, fruit juices without pulp, carbonated beverages, clear tea, black coffee No alcohol
Breast milk	4 hours	For otherwise healthy neonates and infants
Infant formula and nonhuman milk	6 hours	Nonhuman milk is similar to solids in gastric emptying time.
Light meal	6 hours	Example: toast and clear liquids
Regular meal including fat or meat	8 hours	Fat and meat delay gastric emptying
Fried or fatty foods	May require >8 hours	Amount and type of food should be considered. Fasting for >8 hours may be associated with hypoglycemia in children.

Adapted from American Society of Anesthesiologists, 2017.

CLINICAL APPLICATION   20-2

Preoperative Clear Liquids

There is some evidence that the use of preoperative carbohydrate loading through consumption of clear liquid carbohydrate beverages in individuals without diabetes may decrease insulin resistance seen after surgery and in starvation. Carbohydrate loading may also reduce hospital length-of-stay (LOS) post-surgery. However, in some studies there was no difference in LOS when carbohydrate beverages were consumed versus water or placebo. When compared with fasting versus carbohydrate beverages, there was improvement in LOS. Therefore, the recommendation is that clear liquids may be consumed up to 2 hours before elective surgery (Carmichael et al, 2017).

Postoperative Nutrition

Intravenous (IV) fluids are continued after surgery. The usual minimum replacement is 2 liters of 5% glucose in water in 24 hours. This amount contains 100 grams of glucose and delivers 340 kilocalories. Although this will not meet a person's resting energy expenditure, it will prevent ketosis. Guidelines recommend the early discontinuation of IV fluids in the postoperative period, after recovery room discharge, and the encouragement of clear fluids as tolerated.

Peristalsis is the passage of **flatus** (gas) via the rectum. This used to be an indication that the individual was ready to begin oral nutrition; however, there was a lack of evidence to support this. Early enteral nutrition therapy after elective surgery, in the surgical ICU and for individuals undergoing surgery for complications of pancreatitis, has been shown to be associated with significant reductions in infection, hospital length-of-stay (LOS), and mortality (McClave, DiBaise, Mullin, & Martindale, 2016). The clinical practice guidelines for "Enhanced Recovery After Colon and Rectal Surgery" recommends that individuals who undergo elective colorectal surgery be offered a regular diet immediately after surgery. Early feeding (<24 hours) accelerates GI recovery and decreases LOS, complications, and mortality. "Sham feeding" (chewing sugar-free gum for ≥10 minutes 3 to 4 times per day) after colorectal surgery also demonstrates small improvements in GI recovery and may be associated with a decreased LOS, possibly due to an increase in bowel motility (Carmichael et al, 2017).

Clients may progress from clear liquids to full liquids, a soft diet, and then a regular diet as soon as possible (see Chapter 14). The progression time varies with the client and surgical procedure. It may be hours or days. If "diet as tolerated" is ordered, the client should be asked what foods sound appealing. Sometimes a full dinner tray when the client does not feel well "turns off" the small appetite he or she has.

For clients undergoing elective major upper GI surgery requiring postoperative nutritional support, enteral feeding is considered as the most desirable form of postoperative feeding. In well-nourished clients, early parenteral nutrition provides no benefit and may cause harm. However, in malnourished clients who cannot be fed enterally, providing parenteral nutrition may reduce complications and mortality (McClave, DiBaise, Mullin, & Martindale, 2016).

Surgical removal of a part of the GI tract, such as the stomach, duodenum, jejunum, or ileum, may result in malabsorption of specific nutrients. Similarly, realignment of parts of the tract can interfere with the digestive processes (Fig. 20-1).

Note that bile salts are absorbed in the ileum. Although the loss of bile salts in the feces may seem harmless, the body ordinarily recycles these salts over and over in the management of fats. Prolonged impaired absorption of bile salts can result in failure to absorb fat and fat-soluble vitamins.

Disorders of the Mouth and Throat

Varied conditions such as dental caries, oral surgery, surgery of the head and neck, fractured jaw, cancer chemotherapy, or radiation therapy can cause difficulty with chewing and swallowing. Special feeding techniques and scrupulous oral hygiene may be required. Often the client requires a feeding tube, as covered in Chapter 14. Suggestions to manage **dysphagia** are described in Chapter 9 and interventions for

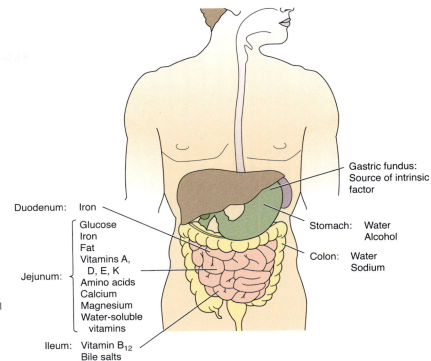

FIGURE 20-1 The chief sites of absorption for various nutrients. Disease or resection of an area will increase the risk of deficiency of specific nutrients. *(Adapted from Scanlon, VC, and Sanders, T: Student Workbook for Essentials of Anatomy and Physiology, ed 6. FA Davis, Philadelphia, 2011, p. 283, with permission.)*

anorexia appear in Chapter 21. Box 24-2 summarizes the dietary management of many symptoms.

Disorders of the Esophagus

Its sole purpose is to conduct food to the stomach, but the esophagus sometimes malfunctions. Achalasia, gastroesophageal reflux, and hiatal hernia are types of esophageal disorders.

Achalasia

Failure of the GI muscle fibers to relax where one part joins another is called **achalasia.** When it occurs in the **cardiac sphincter,** which separates the stomach from the esophagus, the condition is termed *cardiospasm.* The cause is believed to be damage to the nerves of the esophagus, inherited, and/or an autoimmune disorder (National Institutes of Health [NIH], 2016).

Very hot or cold foods may trigger esophageal spasm, and anxiety seems to aggravate the condition. Symptoms are described as "something sticking in my throat" and a feeling of fullness behind the sternum (breastbone). Vomiting may occur with achalasia, and aspiration of vomitus can cause pneumonia.

In mild cases, avoiding spicy foods and minimizing dietary bulk may be effective. Diets for these clients require much individual attention. Rarely does one achalasia client have intolerances for the same foods as another client. Plenty of liquids with small, frequent meals may help. Treatment of severe cases involves stretching the cardiac sphincter or surgically incising it to enlarge the passage.

Gastroesophageal Reflux Disease

Some regurgitation of stomach contents into the esophagus occurs in normal individuals. Usually the presence of stomach contents in the esophagus stimulates esophageal contractions that return the refluxed material to the stomach. If excessive reflux occurs, either in frequency or volume, or if the esophagus fails to contract in response to stomach contents, the individual has **gastroesophageal reflux disease (GERD).** Approximately 20% of the U.S. population is affected by GERD (Vaez et al, 2017).

Approximately 50% of infants have regurgitation (gastroesophageal reflux [GER]) within the first 3 months of life, which resolves by age 12 to 14 months. If an infant's symptoms do not resolve or cause an inability to feed, the infant may have GERD. Symptoms may include arching of the back during or immediately after feeding; colic without medical cause; coughing, gagging, wheezing; poor feeding, growth, or weight grain; vomiting; weight loss; and malnutrition. Treatment may include:

- Small, frequent feedings thickened with cereal
- Upright positioning 30 minutes after feeding
- Burp after 1-2 ounces of formula or after nursing from each breast (NIH, 2015)

In adults, risk factors for gastroesophageal reflux are:

- Hiatal hernia with incompetent lower esophageal sphincter (Fig. 20-2)
- Medications or foods that reduce the effectiveness of the lower esophageal sphincter

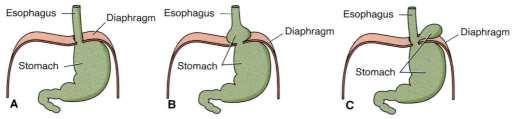

FIGURE 20-2 In hiatal hernia, the upper part of the stomach squeezes into the chest cavity through the esophageal opening in the diaphragm. *A, Normal anatomy. B, Sliding hiatal hernia. C, Rolling hiatal hernia. (Reprinted from Williams, LS, and Hopper, PD: Understanding Medical-Surgical Nursing, ed 4. FA Davis, Philadelphia, 2011, p. 727, with permission.)*

- History of nasogastric intubation with a duration of more than 4 days
- Surgery on the pyloric sphincter
- Smoking
- Conditions that raise intra-abdominal pressure such as pregnancy and obesity

The stomach is normally protected from hydrochloric acid by a thick layer of mucus. Because the esophagus is not so protected, repeated bouts of gastroesophageal reflux can lead to esophagitis and ulcer formation that, when healed, may cause a stricture at the site of the scar tissue. See Peptic Ulcers section in this chapter.

The prominent symptom of gastroesophageal reflux is heartburn with pain occurring behind the breastbone. Sometimes the pain radiates to the neck and the back of the throat. Lying down or bending over may increase reflux and aggravate the pain. If the passage becomes narrowed, **dysphagia** may become bothersome, resulting in anorexia, malnutrition, and weight loss and possibly leading to aspiration pneumonia.

Treatment may include medications (proton-pump inhibitors such as *omeprazole* and histamine H_2 antagonists such as *ranitidine*) as well as diet modification.

Dietary treatment involves several principles:

- Decreasing gastric pressure on the lower esophageal sphincter (small, frequent meals)
- Normal amounts of dietary protein (associated with tightening the cardiac sphincter)
- Avoidance of foods and behaviors that relax the sphincter:
  - Fat and chocolate
  - Peppermint and spearmint
  - Caffeine, alcohol, tobacco

Timing of intake is an important self-care strategy. Avoidance of meals less than 3 hours before bedtime plays a role in prevention of nighttime reflux (NIH, 2014). Table 20-3 details diet and lifestyle strategies for gastroesophageal reflux. It may not be necessary to implement every element. One client with severe nighttime heartburn found that elevating the head of the bed on blocks and eliminating a predinner cocktail was enough to significantly reduce his heartburn and improve his sleep. Similarly, an expectant mother may easily identify foods that cause heartburn (increasingly uncomfortable later in pregnancy with expanding pressure on the stomach) and eliminate those for its duration. If GERD persists, it may cause abnormal cells to develop in the esophagus, which increases the chances of

TABLE 20-3　Diet for Gastroesophageal Reflux and Hiatal Hernia

DESCRIPTION	INDICATIONS	ADEQUACY
The diet is designed to minimize reflux through timing of intake, limiting fat, and exclusion of sphincter relaxants. Adjunctive treatment involves lifestyle changes.	Esophageal reflux, hiatal hernia, esophageal ulcers, esophagitis, esophageal strictures, heartburn	The diet may not meet the Recommended Dietary Allowance for vitamin C and iron in the premenopausal woman.

LIFESTYLE CHANGES	CHOOSE	DECREASE
Meal pattern	Six small meals Chew thoroughly. Limit liquids with meals if causing distention or early satiety.	Eating within 3 hours of bedtime
Adjunctive therapy	Remain upright 3 hours after meals. Relax at mealtime—sit down. Use blocks to elevate head of bed 6 inches. Consider weight loss if needed. Implement appropriate regular physical activity.	Lying down in the hour after eating

Adapted from NIH, 2014.

cancer. Invasive testing using an endoscope and ultimately a surgical procedure may be necessary.

Hiatal Hernia

The *esophageal hiatus* is the opening in the diaphragm through which the esophagus is attached to the stomach. A **hiatal hernia** is a protrusion of the stomach through the esophageal hiatus into the chest cavity (see Fig. 20-2). The symptoms of hiatal hernia are similar to those of gastroesophageal reflux, and its medical treatment is the same. Persistent symptoms despite conservative treatment might lead the client to elect surgical repair of the hernia.

Disorders of the Stomach

Disorders of the stomach often require diet modification and, in some cases, surgery. The following sections concern two common disorders, gastritis and peptic ulcers, and one disorder mainly associated with diabetes mellitus, delayed gastric emptying. Also included is an exaggerated physiological response that can cause problems for older adults, postprandial hypotension.

Gastritis

Inflammation of the stomach is **gastritis** that can be acute or chronic. Worldwide, the most common cause is infection with *Helicobacter pylori* (*H. pylori*), usually causing nonerosive gastritis, which may be acute or chronic (see Peptic Ulcer Pathophysiology section in this chapter).

Reactive gastritis may be acute or chronic, caused by damage to the stomach lining due to (NIH, 2015):

- Reflux of bile from the small intestine into the stomach (especially after partial gastrectomy)

- Chemical injury from alcohol, cocaine, aspirin, other nonsteroidal anti-inflammatory drugs (**NSAIDs**), bile reflux, or acid
- Underperfusion of the gastric mucosa following trauma or sepsis
- Infection usually from *H. pylori*
- Autoimmune response targeting cells in the stomach lining, typically nonerosive

Symptoms of gastritis are:

- Nausea
- Vomiting
- Epigastric pain

Signs of erosive gastritis are red blood in vomit; red blood or black tarry stools; feeling dizzy or faint; shortness of breath; and paleness.

Figure 20-3 illustrates the abdominal quadrants and regions used to record signs and symptoms revealed during the assessment process. The illustration also shows the underlying soft structures contained in the quadrants and the bony structures in the regions.

There is no evidence that eating, diet, or nutrition play a role in causing or preventing gastritis (NIH, 2015). More often than not, discovering which foods aggravate an individual's pain and discomfort with gastritis is a trial-and-error process. Tolerances vary from person to person. Prolonged or recurrent gastritis deserves medical attention to diagnose and treat the underlying problem.

Delayed Gastric Emptying

Gastroparesis is a disorder that produces symptoms of gastric retention without physical obstruction. Peristalsis is weak, resulting in large particles of food poorly prepared for digestion and in retained liquids whose exit from the

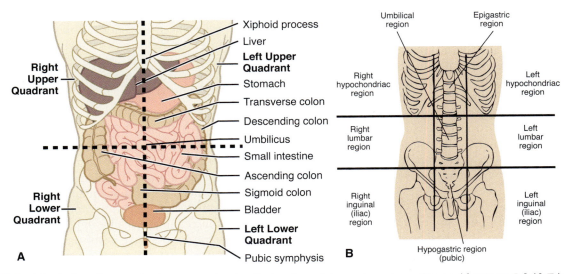

FIGURE 20-3 Abdominal quadrants and regions are used to describe locations of signs and symptoms. *(Reprinted from Venes, D [ed.]: Taber's Cyclopedic Medical Dictionary, ed 22. FA Davis, Philadelphia, 2013, pp. 4 and 2009, with permission.)*

stomach depends on gravity. Ingested food may remain in the stomach for a prolonged period. Gastroparesis does not have a clear etiology, but it is believed to be caused by damage to the vagus nerve, which signals stomach muscles as a part of normal digestion. Gastroparesis is seen in diabetes; nervous system disorders, such as multiple sclerosis and Parkinson disease; abdominal or esophageal surgery; infection; hypothyroidism; and as a side effect of some medications, such as narcotic pain relievers (Mayo Clinic, 2017). Signs and symptoms include:

- Abdominal pain, bloating, and acid reflux
- Nausea and vomiting
- Erratic changes in blood glucose levels
- Anorexia, weight loss, and malnutrition

Individuals with diabetes are significantly impacted by erratic blood glucose levels. The individual's health-care provider may require changes in blood glucose checks (increased frequency and timing to after meals) and changes in medications, administration timing, and doses.

Treatment of delayed gastric emptying focuses on (Mayo Clinic, 2017; American Diabetes Association, 2017):

- Eating small, frequent meals
- Eating slowly, chewing food thoroughly, sitting upright after meals
- Reducing the fat ingested (which remains in the stomach longer than carbohydrate or protein)
- Decreasing fiber intake
- Drinking plenty of water (1 to 1.5 liters/day), avoiding carbonated beverages and alcohol
- Avoiding smoking and tobacco smoke
- Gentle exercise (walking) after meals

If adequate nutrition cannot be provided orally, jejunal feeding may be necessary. In severe cases of gastroparesis, medications may be prescribed and stimulatory techniques may be implemented.

Peptic Ulcers

Peptic ulcer disease is a common illness that affects individuals aged above 65 years. Approximately 1.6 million cases are diagnosed annually, with 10% of men and 5% of women affected during their lifetimes (Taber's, 2017).

Esophageal, gastric (stomach), and duodenal ulcers are called *peptic ulcers* and form when the mucosa is insufficiently resistant to stomach acids. If just the superficial cells are involved, the lesion is an **erosion.** If the muscular layer is involved, the person has an **ulcer.**

Pathophysiology

More than half of the world's population is infected with *H. pylori*, a bacterium that has been associated with chronic gastritis, peptic ulcer, and gastric cancer. The United States has a 35.6% overall prevalence of *H. pylori*; however, indigenous Alaskans have a 74.8% prevalence (Bjorkman, 2017).

Peptic ulcers are caused by factors that increase gastric acid production or impair mucosal barrier protection. *H. pylori* and NSAIDs disrupt normal mucosal defense and repair, making the mucosa more susceptible to acid. NSAID use and resulting mucosal damage may provide an opening for opportunistic infection by *H. pylori*. Contributing risk factors are caffeine consumption, use of tobacco products, and severe physiological stress. There is no clear understanding of the relationship between peptic ulcer and emotional stress (Taber's, 2017).

Signs and Symptoms

Both gastric and duodenal ulcers cause epigastric pain. The pain from gastric ulcer is a burning, gnawing pain occurring 1 to 2 hours after meals and may be relieved by ingesting food. Heartburn, nausea, vomiting, **hematemesis**, **melena**, and unexplained weight loss may also be experienced (Taber's, 2017).

Complications

Hemorrhage is the most common complication of peptic ulcer disease and may lead to anemia. If the blood is vomited immediately after bleeding begins, it is bright red. If it stays in contact with digestive juices for a time, the vomitus is brown-black and granular, resembling coffee grounds. The medical term for this is *coffee-ground emesis*. Other complications of peptic ulcer are infection, if there is a perforation in the stomach or intestine, making the individual vulnerable to *H. pylori*, and obstruction of the GI tract due to inflammation and scarring (Mayo Clinic, 2017; Taber's, 2017).

Scar tissue from a healed ulcer can restrict the gastric outlet, causing pyloric obstruction. If the ulcer continues to erode through the entire stomach or intestinal wall, the result is a **perforated ulcer.** Leakage of GI contents into the sterile abdominal cavity causes **peritonitis,** an inflammation of the peritoneum (the lining of the abdominal cavity).

Treatment

Medical treatment for *H. pylori* infection includes combinations of antibiotics and other drugs. Only if such treatment proves ineffective is surgery considered. No specific dietary causes or diet-based treatments have been rigorously studied in gastritis or gastric ulceration and avoidance of foods and practices that cause symptoms is recommended (NIH, 2015).

MEDICAL

Before the advent of antiulcer medications, clients with peptic ulcers were usually advised to take antacids every 2 hours, alternating with milk and cream. Later research demonstrated that milk is a potent *inducer* of gastric acid secretion.

Current guidelines suggest the use of triple-antibiotic therapy as first-choice treatment of *H. pylori* infection. Because of increasing resistance of pathogenic bacteria to antibiotics, probiotics have been suggested as adjunctive therapy in treatment of peptic ulcers. More research is needed before definitive strategies in the use of probiotics can be recommended for client use (Khoder, Al-Menhali, Al-Yassir, & Karam, 2016).

For more information on probiotics and prebiotics, see Box 20-1.

New medications have revolutionized the treatment and are almost always effective without a drastic change in diet. In addition to antibiotics to eradicate *H. pylori*, commonly prescribed medications are:

- *Cimetidine, famotidine,* and *ranitidine,* which block histamine-stimulated gastric acid secretion
- *Omeprazole,* which suppresses gastric acid production

Smoking should be stopped, and alcohol consumption ceased or limited. There is no evidence that changing the diet speeds ulcer healing or prevents recurrence (Mayo Clinic, 2017).

SURGICAL

When surgery is necessary, the ulcer is removed, and the remaining GI tract is sutured together. Surgical procedures designed to eliminate the diseased area include gastroduodenostomy (stomach and duodenum anastomosed) and gastrojejunostomy (stomach and jejunum anastomosed). **Anastomosis** is the surgical connection between tubular structures. Figure 20-4 illustrates these two procedures.

After gastric surgery, parenteral and enteral feedings are used singly or in combination. If enteral feeding is used, the tube must be inserted beyond the area that was resected

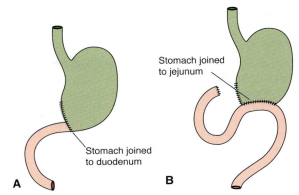

FIGURE 20-4 Common gastric resection procedures. *A,* Gastroduodenostomy or Billroth I procedure. *B,* Gastrojejunostomy or Billroth II procedure. *(Reprinted from Williams, LS, and Hopper, PD: Understanding Medical-Surgical Nursing, ed 4. FA Davis, Philadelphia, 2011, p. 738, with permission.)*

(removed). Nutritional care includes delivering nutrients to ensure maximal use of the remaining functions of the GI tract. After a client is advanced to an oral diet, he or she may experience **dumping syndrome,** a complication of a surgical procedure that removes, disrupts, or bypasses the pyloric sphincter. Dumping syndrome occurs in 20% to 50% of clients after gastric surgery (Kanth & Roy, 2016). Clinical Application 20-3 describes the dumping syndrome in more detail.

Postprandial Hypotension

Postprandial hypotension is a drop in systolic blood pressure of 20 mm Hg or more within 2 hours after beginning a meal. Postprandial hypotension occurs in up to one-third of older people but virtually never occurs in younger people. It is more likely to occur in people who have high blood pressure or disorders that impair the brain centers controlling the autonomic nervous system (Higginson, 2017).

Symptoms and complications include:

- Dizziness
- Light-headedness
- Falls

Normally the body compensates for the increased blood flow to the digestive tract after meals, but in the elderly, the mechanisms maintaining adequate circulation to the rest of the body become less effective. Greater effects are seen when the stomach empties more rapidly.

To prevent postprandial hypotension, a person should:

- Limit carbohydrate intake
- Take frequent small meals
- Lie in a semirecumbent position for 90 minutes after eating
- Schedule antihypertensive medications between rather than just before meals (Higginson, 2017).

Special dietary additives or medications to delay gastric emptying are sometimes prescribed.

BOX 20-1 ■ Probiotics and Prebiotics

Probiotics are food products or oral supplements containing a sufficient number of viable microorganisms to improve the intestinal microbial balance of the host to potentially confer health benefits. They are similar to the intestinal bacteria found in the gut and are thought to help repopulate and balance the gut flora (Wolfram, 2016). Illness and antibiotic therapy can cause a disruption in the gut flora, which commonly causes diarrhea (ConsumerLab, 2017).

The number of microorganisms that must be ingested to obtain a beneficial effect varies depending on the reason for its use; however, a probiotic should typically contain several billion microorganisms. The exact effect probiotics have on the GI tract is still under study, but it is thought that they may inhibit bacterial growth and may boost the immune system (ConsumerLab, 2017).

The traditional delivery method for probiotics is in dairy products, but new technologies using spray or freeze-drying extend shelf life and permit the use of tablets and capsules. Those dietary supplements are not routinely tested by government agencies (see Chapter 15) but ConsumerLab's (2017) voluntary certification program tests for viability of the organisms, lack of potentially harmful organisms, and appropriate disintegration. Probiotics are found in fermented or aged milk and milk products, such as yogurt, kefir, and aged cheeses (Wolfram, 2016). The most reliable food source is yogurt labeled "live and active culture." To earn this seal, the product must contain at least 100 million bacteria per gram of yogurt at the time it is made and must not have been heat treated because heat kills the bacteria. Nondairy sources of probiotics include kimchi, sauerkraut, miso, tempeh, and cultured nondairy yogurts (Wolfram, 2016). **Prebiotics** are nondigestible food ingredients that are linked to the favorable growth of positive gut bacteria and may enhance calcium absorption. Good prebiotic food sources are artichokes, asparagus, bananas, soybeans, garlic, leeks, onions, and whole-wheat foods (Wolfram, 2016).

CLINICAL APPLICATION   20-3

Dumping Syndrome

The pyloric sphincter normally allows only small amounts of gastric contents into the duodenum at a time. Altered gastric emptying is seen after gastric surgeries (due to cancer and for weight loss) and esophageal surgery (Mayo Clinic, 2015). In dumping syndrome, concentrated liquid is suddenly "dumped" into the intestine. Depending on the time elapsed after a meal dumping syndrome is characterized as

- Early (30–60 minutes **postprandial**)
  - Abdominal pain and cramping, bloating, diarrhea due to large osmolar load in small intestine
  - Hypotension, tachycardia, dizziness due to compensatory fluid shifts
- Late (longer than 60 minutes postprandial)
  - Carbohydrate load increases blood glucose
  - Hypersecretion of insulin produces rapid decrease in blood glucose resulting in hypoglycemia
- Sweating, shakiness, difficulty concentrating (Kanth & Roy, 2016)

Dumping syndrome is most often associated with a total or partial gastrectomy involving resection of two-thirds of the stomach. The same signs and symptoms can occur in a client after **vagotomy** or one receiving enteral feeding if the nasogastric tube is accidentally carried down into the duodenum.

Treatment includes medications, dietary modification, and surgical reconstruction.

Medications that may be helpful are:

- *Acarbose,* which delays and reduces glucose absorption
- *Octreotide,* which can delay gastric emptying and small bowel transit and inhibit insulin production and postprandial vasodilation (Kanth & Roy, 2016)

Dietary treatment of the dumping syndrome attempts to delay gastric emptying and to distribute the increased osmolality to the bowel over time. Table 20-4 depicts diet principles, which prevent or treat dumping syndrome.

Disorders of the Intestines

To obtain satisfactory diagnostic radiographic or endoscopic studies of the bowel, it must be emptied. This is usually accomplished by a clear liquid diet followed by laxatives. Explaining the procedures and the necessity for them helps to gain the client's cooperation. For inpatients, the nurse should ensure that the client receives maximum nourishment when tests are completed for the day. Frequently, another series of tests is scheduled for the next day.

Problems with Elimination

Several problems with frequency and consistency of bowel movements are common. These include irritable bowel syndrome, diarrhea, and constipation.

Irritable Bowel Syndrome

Irritable bowel syndrome (IBS) is estimated to affect 10% to 15% of the population, about twice as many women as men, usually in people younger than 45 years. It is a chronic **functional** GI disorder characterized by a combination of abdominal pain or discomfort and altered bowel habits. A diagnosis of IBS is made if symptoms have lasted more than 6 months; at least three times a month for at least 3 months for which other GI causes have been excluded; pain or discomfort is relieved after having a bowel movement; and there is a change in the frequency or appearance of bowel movements (NIH, 2015).

The most common signs and symptoms of irritable bowel syndrome are:

- Bloating, abdominal distention
- Abdominal pain, often relieved by passage of stool
- Constipation or diarrhea or alternating episodes of both
- Mucus in stools

The causes of IBS are not well understood. Motility problems, bacterial overgrowth in intestines, infections, genetics,

TABLE 20-4   Diet for Dumping Syndrome

DESCRIPTION	INDICATIONS	ADEQUACY
This diet consists of six small feedings, high in protein and fat and low in simple sugars.	This diet and adjunct therapy, used after surgical removal of the pyloric sphincter or other treatments that speed gastric emptying, is designed to prevent rapid emptying of hypertonic gastric contents into the small intestine. Examples of such operative procedures include vagotomy, pyloroplasty, hemigastrectomy, total gastrectomy, esophagogastrectomy, Whipple procedure, gastroenterostomy, and gastrojejunostomy. As the body adapts to its new condition, specific foods may be tolerated later in convalescence.	Deficiencies secondary to surgery or malabsorption may require supplementation. Among the nutrients likely to be needed are the vitamins B_{12}, D, and folic acid and the minerals calcium and iron.
LIFESTYLE CHANGES	CHOOSE	DECREASE
Meal pattern	Six small servings. Eat slowly and chew thoroughly.	Fluids with meals Very hot or cold foods that stimulate peristalsis
Adjunctive therapy	Lie down for $1/2$ to 1 hour after meals. Fiber supplements (pectin, guar gum) that form gels with carbohydrates are effective for hypoglycemia by decreasing glucose absorption and increasing intestinal transit time (Mayo Clinic, 2015).	

food sensitivities, and mental health issues are thought to contribute to IBS (NIH, 2015). Treatment for IBS is symptomatic. Medications to treat the symptoms of diarrhea and constipation, probiotics, and treatment for mental health issues may help. Implementation of a Low FODMAP Diet is recommended (see Clinical Application 20-4).

Diarrhea

Passage of liquid or unformed feces, diarrhea, is an important cause of morbidity and mortality in the elderly and in children (see Chapter 11). Most instances of diarrhea in adults are self-limiting and resolve without treatment or the need for extensive medical work-up. In many cases, the cause of diarrhea cannot be found. If an adult is in little jeopardy from an electrolyte imbalance, self-treatment for diarrhea following the conservative regimen listed in Table 20-5 is appropriate. Oral rehydration solutions can be used (see Chapter 8 for Pedialyte). A low-fiber/residue diet (Table 20-6) may be required to slow intestinal motility.

CLINICAL APPLICATION   20-4

Low FODMAP Diet

The Low FODMAP (**f**ermentable **o**ligosaccharides, **d**isaccharides, **m**onosaccharides, **a**nd **p**olyols) diet, accepted as an effective strategy for managing symptoms of irritable bowel syndrome (IBS) in Australia, has sparked interest worldwide. The targets of restriction are short-chain carbohydrates that have been shown to induce IBS symptoms of abdominal pain, bloating, flatus, and diarrhea due to their poor absorption, osmotic activity, and rapid fermentation.

The richest sources of the FODMAPs are:

- Fructooligosaccharides (fructans)—wheat, rye, onions, garlic, artichokes
- Galactoligosaccharides (GOS)—legumes (soy, beans, chickpeas, lentils), cabbage, Brussels sprouts
- Lactose—milk, dairy products, beer, prepared soups and sauces
- Fructose—honey, apples, dates, mangoes, papaya, pears, prunes, watermelon, high-fructose corn syrup
- Sorbitol—apples, pears, stone fruits, sugar-free mints/gums
- Mannitol—mushrooms, cauliflower, sugar-free mints/gums

Not all FODMAPs will trigger symptoms for all clients. Only those that are malabsorbed are likely to be clinically significant:

- Fructans and GOS are always malabsorbed and fermented by intestinal **microflora.** This process results in gas production and associated flatulence in healthy people. With the altered gut flora, motility disorders, and hypersensitivity in IBS, the symptoms may be that much more evident.

- The remaining FODMAP carbohydrates will induce symptoms only in the proportion of clients with IBS that malabsorb them.
- A trial of a full Low FODMAP Diet can be conducted for 4–6 weeks, after which structured rechallenges with the potentially well-absorbed carbohydrates (lactose, fructose, sorbitol, and mannitol) can begin.

The Low FODMAP Diet is not simple to implement correctly. Lactose is only a FODMAP in individuals with lactase insufficiency (see Chapter 9). Individualizing the diet is particularly important for vegetarians, who may depend on legumes for protein intake, but may also highlight to clients that they can cope with garlic as a minor ingredient or wheat products occasionally, which would expand the nutritional composition of the diet long-term. The key issue is the total FODMAPs ingested at a meal, not the individual items. Additionally, FODMAPs have prebiotic effects due to the production of short-chain fatty acids after fermentation. Therefore, all clients should be encouraged to try to reintroduce FODMAPs to a level that they can comfortably tolerate.

The low-FODMAP diet requires a registered dietitian's expertise both to maximize compliance with instigating the complete list of FODMAP sources and to avoid an overly restricted approach. The latter is of great import in the event the diet is successful and likely to be followed long-term. The low-FODMAP diet is recommended for IBS, suggesting that this should be the first dietary strategy tried (NIH, 2015).

TABLE 20-5 Self-Treatment for Diarrhea*

TIME	ORAL INTAKE	COMMENTS
First 12 hours	Water or oral hydration solutions at room temperature	Easily absorbed fluids to maintain hydration
Second 12 hours	Clear liquids, no caffeine or extremes of temperature	If up to 5% body weight lost; if more than 5% lost, seek medical attention
		Very hot, very cold, or caffeinated beverages stimulate peristalsis.
Third 12 hours	Full liquids	Experiment with milk in case lactose intolerance has developed.
Fourth 12 hours	Soft diet	Include applesauce or banana for pectin; rice, pasta, and bread without fat (digested by enzymes usually unaffected by gastroenteritis).
By 48th hour	Regular diet	Seek medical treatment if diarrhea has not resolved and regular diet is not tolerated. Other reasons for medical attention: dehydration, abdominal distension, fever, bloody stools.

*Appropriate for healthy adults.

TABLE 20-6   Low-Fiber/Residue Diet

DESCRIPTION	INDICATIONS	ADEQUACY
The low-fiber diet limits milk and milk products and excludes any food made with seeds, nuts, and raw or dried fruits and vegetables. Digestibility of fiber is not appreciably altered by pureeing. The purpose of the diet is to decrease colonic contents by limiting fiber intake to 10–15 grams per day.	The diet can be used for severe diarrhea, partial bowel obstruction, and acute phases of inflammatory bowel diseases, ulcerative colitis and Crohn disease. Postoperatively the diet may be used in the progression to a general diet. Long-term use of the diet is not recommended because it may aggravate symptoms during nonacute phases of disease.	Strict reduction in milk and milk products, vegetables, and fruits may necessitate supplementation of calcium, vitamin C, folate, and other nutrients. If used long-term, a registered dietitian should be consulted regarding nutritional adequacy.

Adapted from NIH, 2014; NIH, 2016.

Medical consultation becomes important if diarrhea:

- Lasts for more than 4 days
- Causes severe pain in the abdomen or rectum
- Provokes a fever of 102°F or higher
- Produces blood in the stool or black, tarry stools
- Is accompanied by signs of dehydration

In addition to these concerns, if a client has medical conditions for which fasting, dehydration, or infectious disease is a hazard, a physician should be consulted.

TRAVELER'S DIARRHEA

The classic definition of traveler's diarrhea is passage of at least three unformed stools per day plus one or more signs or symptoms of an enteric infection (nausea, vomiting, fever, abdominal pain, cramps, fecal urgency). Traveler's diarrhea is a self-limited infection that affects approximately 40% of travelers to developing countries (Taber's, 2017).

The most common causes of traveler's diarrhea cases are a variety of bacterial enteropathogens, but noroviruses are also an important cause of morbidity among travelers. Destination is the most significant risk factor for developing traveler's diarrhea (Mayo Clinic, 2016):

- High-risk areas of Asia, Africa, Central and South America, Mexico, and the Middle East
- Areas that pose some risk, Eastern Europe and the Caribbean

Other risk factors are (Mayo Clinic, 2016):

- Immunocompromised states
- Lowered gastric acidity
- Individuals with diabetes, inflammatory bowel disease, or cirrhosis of the liver, making them more prone to infections

Traveler's diarrhea is commonly experienced in underdeveloped countries with substandard sanitation infrastructure. To minimize risk, people should avoid (Taber's, 2017):

- Drinking tap water and ice made from it
- Foods washed in water and served raw
- Uncooked seafood
- Raw or poorly cooked meats

OTHER CAUSES

Diarrhea may be iatrogenic (produced by treatment) accompanying antibiotic therapy or tube feeding. In the acute hospital setting, especially critical care units, diarrhea is a common complication of enteral feeding due to either bacterial growth in the feeding, if mishandled, or the osmotic effect of the formula.

Probiotics may accelerate recovery from acute infectious diarrhea and prevent antibiotic-associated diarrhea (see Box 20-1). Another possible cause of diarrhea is celiac disease (see Genomic Gem 20-1 and Clinical Application 20-5).

GENOMIC GEM 20-1

Celiac Disease

The National Institutes of Health (NIH) estimates that 1 in 141 Americans has celiac disease and most don't know it. **First-degree relatives** (parent, sibling, child) of those with the disease have a 4%–15% chance of developing celiac disease (NIH, 2017). Genetic predisposition to celiac disease is strongly linked to genes that encode inherited human leukocyte antigen (HLA), specifically alleles HLA-DQ2 and HLA-DQ8. These alleles are found in 30% of the general population. Only 1% of individuals in the general population with the gene variants develop celiac disease; however, those who have a first-degree relative with celiac disease have a 3% chance of developing the disease (Celiac.org; NIH, 2017).

Because only a few genetically susceptible individuals develop celiac disease, its etiology is considered to be multifactorial involving a combination of:

- Genetic predisposition
- Ingestion of gluten (see Chapter 9)
- An autoimmune response that produces chronic inflammation of the small intestine

At present, a strict gluten-restricted diet is the only treatment. Selecting such a diet should become easier because in 2013, the FDA published the first regulation defining "gluten-free" for voluntary food labeling that covers other terms such as "no gluten," "without gluten," and "free of gluten." Such foods must contain less than 20 parts per million of gluten.

Constipation

Each person develops a usual bowel pattern, and so a bowel movement every day or every second or third day may be perfectly normal for a given individual. **Constipation** refers to a decrease in a person's normal frequency of defecation, especially if the stool is hard, dry, or difficult to expel. Female sex, older age, low-fiber diet, a sedentary lifestyle, malnutrition, **polypharmacy**, recent surgery, and a lower socioeconomic status have all been identified as risk factors for constipation. Between 1/6 to 1/3 of the U.S. population reports having constipation (NIH, 2015; Taber's, 2017).

Symptoms of constipation include fewer than normal (for an individual) bowel movements, stool that is difficult or painful to pass, and abdominal pain or bloating. The following factors may contribute to constipation (NIH, 2015):

- Diets low in fiber
- Lack of physical activity
- Medications (opiates, anticonvulsants, diuretics, antidepressants, antacids, anticholinergics)
- Travel
- Health conditions (pregnancy, neurological conditions such as Parkinson disease, diabetes, hypothyroidism, GI diseases/disorders)
- Older age

After disease conditions causing constipation have been diagnosed and treated or ruled out, recommended lifestyle changes to treat constipation include (NIH, 2015):

- Gradually increase dietary fiber (see Clinical Calculation 20-1).
- Drink adequate water.
- Exercise regularly.
- Evacuate at a regular time (usually after a meal to take advantage of the body's programming), or without delay when feeling the urge.

In some cases of fecal impaction, the client may experience diarrhea. Clinical Application 20-6 explains this paradox.

CLINICAL APPLICATION 20-5

Celiac Disease

Celiac disease is a digestive disorder triggered by consuming gluten in the diet, causing damage to the small intestine. Gluten is found in wheat, barley, and rye commonly found in foods (bread, pasta, cookies, convenience foods, and cakes) and also may be found in some cosmetics, vitamins, supplements, and medications.

Celiac disease is more common in Caucasians, women, those with other autoimmune diseases, and those with a relative diagnosed with celiac disease. Common GI symptoms include:

- Children can have abdominal pain and bloating, chronic diarrhea, constipation, gas, nausea, pale foul-smelling stools, steatorrhea, and vomiting.
- Adults who have digestive symptoms may have abdominal pain and bloating, intestinal blockages, and intestinal or gastric ulcers.

Other symptoms include:

- Infants may present with failure to thrive. Older children are seen with short stature, delayed puberty, dental enamel defects, and weight loss.
- Adults present with anemia, weak and brittle bones, bone or joint pain, depression, dermatitis, infertility, miscarriage, and fatigue.

Source: NIH, 2016.

CLINICAL CALCULATION 20-1

Constipation and Fiber Intake

Achieving the recommended fiber intake of 21–38 grams per day is a matter of prudent choices at every meal. Listed below are examples of high-fiber foods on the left and foods in the same category on the right with less fiber.

HIGHER-FIBER FOODS	GRAMS OF FIBER	LOWER-FIBER FOODS	GRAMS OF FIBER
Breakfast			
All-bran buds, 1/3 cup	13	Corn flakes, 1 cup	1
Orange sections, 1 cup	4	Orange juice from frozen concentrate, 1 cup	0
Lunch			
Wendy's chili, small	5	Campbell's microwavable chicken noodle soup, 1 cup	2
Raw apple with skin, 2¾" diameter	4	Raw apple peeled, 2¾" diameter	2
Dinner			
Whole-wheat spaghetti, 1 cup cooked	6	White spaghetti, 1 cup cooked	3
Banana, 1 cup sliced	4	Watermelon 1 cup diced	1
Total	36		9

Many other foods also contribute to fiber intake and can be evaluated via labels or at http://ndb.nal.usda.gov or http://nutritiondata.self.com. Individuals who wish to correct constipation without medications should determine their present fiber intake and increase it gradually to the Recommended Dietary Allowance while also drinking *sufficient water.*

CLINICAL APPLICATION 20-6

Distinguishing Diarrhea From Fecal Impaction

If a client usually is constipated and then has diarrhea, the nurse should check the rectum for impacted stool. The stool will be dry and hard and the client will not be able to pass it unassisted. The diarrheal stool is passed around the impaction.

As in many cases, prevention is preferable to diagnosis and treatment. Institutionalized clients should be monitored for elimination problems. Frequency and consistency of bowel movements should be charted and appropriate interventions implemented before impaction results.

Inflammatory Bowel Diseases (IBDs)

The Centers for Disease Control and Prevention (CDC) estimated that in 2015, three million adults in the United States had IBD, an increase in 1 million from 1999. The peak age at onset is 20 to 30 years, although IBD may occur at any age (Centers for Disease Control and Prevention [CDC], 2017). The exact etiology of IBDs are unknown, and it is believed that the interactions among genetics, environment, intestinal **microbiota,** and immune system are involved in the pathogenesis of IBDs (Loddo & Romano, 2015). Normally, the immune cells protect the body from infection. In people with IBD, however, the immune system attacks the cells of the intestines. In the process, the body sends white blood cells into the lining of the intestines where they produce chronic inflammation.

The two most common IBDs are **Crohn disease (CD)** and **ulcerative colitis (UC).** The two diseases share some similar characteristics but also have major differences (see Tables 20-7 and 20-8 and Genomic Gem 20-2).

Clients are advised to eat a healthy diet, making necessary diet changes to help alleviate IBD symptoms. General goals for nutritional care of IBD clients include the following (NIH, 2016):

- The prevention and correction of malnutrition through screening and monitoring
- The prevention of osteoporosis
- In children, the promotion of optimal growth and development

Specific actions to achieve those goals include the following:

- Keep a food diary to help avoid foods that clearly worsen symptoms
- Take small, frequent meals
- Drink adequate fluids
- Limit excess fat
- Take vitamin/mineral supplements only as ordered by health-care provider
- Eliminate dairy foods if lactose intolerant

Table 20-9 lists general uses of nutritional modalities for IBD.

Nutritional Therapy

Beyond general goals, the nutritional care of clients with IBD must be individualized according to the nutritional status of the individual, the location and extent of the disease, and the surgical and medical treatments. Although certain food choices enhance risk of IBD, elimination of individual food items will not likely alter the course of the disease (Forbes et al, 2017). To maintain nutritional status, foods should not be eliminated from the diet without a fair trial. Restrictions should be limited to foods that produce gas or loose stools. Suspected foods

TABLE 20-7 Similarities Between Crohn Disease (CD) and Ulcerative Colitis (UC)	
Etiology	Loss of tolerance to intestinal bacteria
Theories	Autoimmune interaction of genetic susceptibility and environment
Familial links	Clients who have a **first-degree relative** with inflammatory bowel disease (IBD) have up to a 7% increased risk of developing IBD (Walfish & Companioni, 2016). See Genomic Gem 20-2.
Contributing dietary factors	A diet rich in fruit and vegetables, rich in omega-3 fatty acids, and low in omega-6 fatty acids is associated with a decreased risk of developing CD or UC, but there is no IBD diet that can promote remission in clients with active disease. Active monitoring and treatment for malnutrition is recommended (Forbes et al, 2017).
Geographic/ethnic factors	Higher frequency in people of Northern European and Anglo-Saxon origin. Two to 4 times more common among people of Ashkenazi Jewish descent than non-Jewish individuals from the same geographic location. Decreased incidence in Central and Southern Europe and South America, Asia, and Africa. Increasing incidence among blacks and Latin Americans living in North America (Walfish & Companioni, 2016).
Signs and symptoms	Diarrhea, abdominal pain Weight loss Decreased bone mineral density
Associated conditions	Arthritis, joint pain Eye irritation Kidney stones Liver disease

TABLE 20-8   Differences Between Crohn Disease (CD) and Ulcerative Colitis (UC)

	CD	UC
Location	Anywhere in GI tract, 80% of the cases are in the small bowel	Large intestine
Distribution	Diseased areas alternate with healthy tissue	Usually starts in rectum and spreads upward in continuous pattern
Lesions	Involves all layers of intestinal wall	Confined to mucosal and submucosal layers
Associated conditions*	Problems with skin Gallstones	Osteoporosis Colon cancer if entire colon affected over 8–10 years
Environmental factors	Associated with smoking	A possible increase in the United States in clients who use NSAIDs, antibiotics, oral contraceptives; there may be some decrease with smokers.
Complications	Blockage of the intestine due to swelling and scar tissue (most common) Fistulas, abscesses	Toxic megacolon

*Uncertain pathophysiology; may be result of inflammation.
Source: Forbes et al, 2017.

GENOMIC GEM 20-2

Inflammatory Bowel Disease

Having a relative with inflammatory bowel disease (IBD) accounts for an 8–10-fold increased risk of developing Crohn disease (CD) or ulcerative colitis (UC). If a disease is entirely due to genes, its concordance in identical (*monozygotic*) twins would approach 100% and that in nonidentical (*dizygotic*) twins 50%. Identical twins more often have CD, than do fraternal twins. The concordance rate in monozygotic twins is 50% in CD compared with 10% in dizygotic twins. Twin studies provide evidence for a genetic link to IBD, which is stronger for CD than for UC. A child has a 26-fold increase for developing CD and a 9-fold increase for UC when another sibling already has it. Factors influencing development of IBD:

1. Genetic mutation encodes susceptibility. More than 200 loci have been identified.
2. A trigger initiates inflammation, such as environment (see Table 20-8).
3. Intolerance to normal gut microorganisms develops.

One gene involved in CD encodes for a bacterial defense peptide expressed in ileal mucosa, the site most affected in CD (Dryden & Seidner, 2014). Another identified inherited defect found in clients with CD is a mutation of a gene on chromosome 16, which results in abnormal chronic inflammation in response to bacteria such as *Escherichia coli* in the digestive tract (Thomas & Greer, 2010).

One suggested trigger is dietary change, specifically adoption of the Western diet. IBD cases in Japan have increased significantly over the past 3 decades with total kilocalories from fat and animal protein displacing those from rice. Refined sugars, fatty foods, and fast foods all enhance development of CD and ulcerative colitis (Dryden & Seidner, 2014).

Sources: Loddo & Romano, 2015; Forbes et al, 2017.

TABLE 20-9   Nutritional Care in Inflammatory Bowel Disease

	CROHN DISEASE (CD)	ULCERATIVE COLITIS (UC)
Oral intake	After exacerbation: low-fat, low-fiber, high-protein, high-kilocalorie in small frequent feedings Progress to normal diet as tolerated Avoid foods high in **oxalate** (see Table 19-5) Omega-3 fatty acid supplements should not be used	As unrestricted and balanced as possible Omega-3 fatty acid supplements should not be used
Enteral feeding by mouth or feeding tube	Used when needed as supportive therapy to undernutrition in addition to regular food, or in clients with intestinal strictures or stenosis	Can be used as supportive therapy in clients with severe UC
Parenteral nutrition (PN) Evidence-based guidelines do not recommend as primary treatment	In chronic disease, for clients with a very short gut, prolonged ileus or obstruction, or anastomotic fistulas	PN should only be used if intestinal failure occurs
Probiotics/prebiotics	Should not be used	Certain probiotic strains may be beneficial/ Prebiotics may be useful in the maintenance of remission in some clients

Source: Forbes et al, 2017.

should be tried in small amounts to determine tolerance levels.

Surgical Treatment

Surgery may be recommended when IBD becomes medically unmanageable. The portion of the bowel that is inflamed can be surgically resected but may cause major nutritional complications.

ILEOSTOMY

In an **ileostomy,** the end of the remaining portion of the small intestine (the **ileum**) is attached to a surgically established opening in the abdominal wall called a **stoma,** from which the intestinal contents are discharged. This results in a shorter gut that may create additional nutritional hazards for the client.

An ileostomy produces liquid drainage containing active enzymes that irritate the skin. In addition, nutrient losses are great. A loss of as much as 2 liters of fluid per day immediately after surgery is possible. Over time, the bowel adapts to some extent, and drainage decreases to 300 to 500 milliliters. This amount, however, is more than the 100 to 200 milliliters of water lost in the normal stool. In addition to fluid and electrolyte losses, ileostomy clients have decreased fat, bile acid, and vitamin B_{12} absorption. Clinical Application 20-7 describes innovations for controlling ileostomy drainage.

COLOSTOMY

A **colectomy** is the surgical removal of part or all of the colon. Depending on the pathology, the surgeon may connect the remaining bowel to allow evacuation through the anus or make an artificial opening in the abdominal wall to allow the passage of waste. In a **colostomy,** a part of the large intestine is resected, and a stoma is created in the abdominal wall. Clients who have surgery to divert intestinal contents through the abdominal wall often suffer psychological trauma in addition to the physical change.

CLINICAL APPLICATION   20-7

Continent Ileostomies (Abdominal Pouch)

Ordinarily if an ileostomy is performed, the client must wear an appliance to contain the drainage. Other procedures afford a measure of control of the drainage.

Continent ileostomies sometimes can be constructed from the remaining intestine, creating an intestinal reservoir or pouch just inside the abdominal wall. The pouch is emptied by inserting a catheter into the stoma several times a day.

Sometimes an ileoanal anastomosis is done so that the anal sphincter can be used to control elimination. Even after the bowel adapts to its shorter length, the client has 7–10 bowel movements per day.

It is important for all health-care providers to know which procedure has been performed so that the surgeon's and client's expectations can be reinforced when teaching the client.

In contrast to an ileostomy, a colostomy after the convalescent period may be so continent that a dry dressing is all that is necessary to cover the stoma. The client may do daily irrigations or not, as the surgeon suggests. Sometimes, after the initial learning process, the client knows best.

DIETARY GUIDELINES FOR OSTOMY CLIENTS

A soft or general diet is usually served to ostomy clients after recovery from surgery with restrictions based on individual tolerance. Stringy, high-fiber foods are initially avoided until a definite tolerance has been demonstrated and then are best tried in small amounts one at a time. Stringy, high-fiber foods include:

- Celery, corn, cabbage, coleslaw, peas, sauerkraut, spinach
- Coconut, dried fruit, membranes on citrus fruits, pineapple
- Popcorn, nuts, seeds, and skins of fruits and vegetables

In addition, some clients avoid **cruciferous** vegetables, beans, fish, eggs, beer, and carbonated beverages because they produce excessive odor or gas. Certain foods may be therapeutic because they thicken the stool: applesauce, banana, cheese, creamy peanut butter, pasta, white bread, and white rice.

Clients with ostomies should be encouraged to:

- Eat at regular intervals, 5 to 6 times a day.
- Chew food well to avoid blockage at the stoma site.
- Drink adequate amounts of fluid.
- Avoid foods that produce excessive gas, loose stools, offensive odors, or undesirable bulk.
- Avoid excessive weight gain that will affect the stoma.

Diverticular Disease

A **diverticulum** (plural: diverticula) is an outpouching of intestinal membrane through a weakness in the intestine's muscular layer, chiefly in the colon (Fig. 20-5). Once thought to be a condition nearly confined to the elderly, 35% of U.S. adults <50 years of age and 58% of those aged above 60 have diverticular disease. In the United States, approximately 200,000 people are hospitalized annually (NIH, 2016).

Of environmental factors contributing to diverticular disease, dietary fiber deficiency has received the most attention, although data are limited and conflicting. Whether a deficiency is causative or not, fiber may improve symptoms and decrease complications. Other factors that may increase risk of diverticular disease are:

- Genetics
- Obesity and lack of exercise
- Medications (NSAIDs and steroids) and smoking

Contrary to a long-standing belief, avoidance of seeds and nuts to reduce risk is not supported by the literature (NIH, 2016). Individual clients, however, may dispute the reports in the literature, steadfastly maintaining those foods increase symptoms and choosing to avoid them.

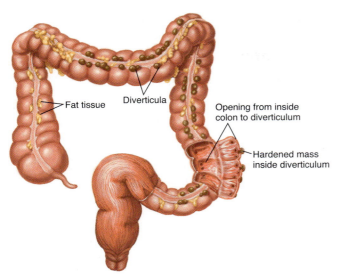

FIGURE 20-5 Diverticula of the colon. (*Reprinted from Venes, D [ed.]: Taber's Cyclopedic Medical Dictionary, ed 22. FA Davis, Philadelphia, 2013, p. 715, with permission.*)

Diverticulosis

The presence of diverticula is called **diverticulosis.** A common location is the point at which a blood vessel enters the intestinal muscle. A proposed causative factor in diverticulosis is the increased force needed to propel insufficient intestinal contents through the lumen.

Frequently a person with diverticulosis has no signs or symptoms. After a diagnosis of diverticulosis, a high-fiber diet of 14 grams per 1,000 calories consumed per day is advised. An individual consuming 2,000 kilocalories would therefore ingest 28 grams of fiber. This should be accompanied by an adequate fluid intake (NIH, 2016).

Diverticulitis

When diverticula become inflamed, the condition is termed *diverticulitis.* An endoscopic view is shown in Figure 20-6. These clients typically present with left lower quadrant pain,

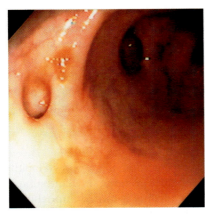

FIGURE 20-6 Diverticulitis, seen endoscopically. (*Reprinted from Venes, D [ed.]: Taber's Cyclopedic Medical Dictionary, ed 22. FA Davis, Philadelphia, 2013, p. 715, with permission.*)

fever, and elevated white blood count. The diagnosis may be confirmed using a computed tomography (CT) scan (NIH, 2016).

Initial therapy for uncomplicated diverticulitis is supportive, including monitoring, bowel rest, and antibiotics. Diet is advanced through clear liquids, low-fiber/residue (see Table 20-6), and general menus as the client's condition improves. After that, a high-fiber diet as for diverticulosis is prescribed. Clients should receive detailed instructions on the incorporation of fiber into the diet after they have followed a low-fiber diet. Fiber should be reintroduced gradually to avoid the abdominal cramping, bloating, and gas pains that can occur with drastic changes in fiber intake.

Diseases of the Liver

Some of the many functions of the liver are listed in Table 20-1. Major liver diseases, hepatitis and cirrhosis, often require careful nutritional management as part of a complex treatment regimen.

Hepatitis

Inflammation of the liver, or **hepatitis,** can result from viral infections, alcohol, drugs, or toxins. Acetaminophen poisoning is the most common cause of acute liver failure, accounting for approximately 48% of cases in the United States, leading to 29% of these individuals requiring a liver transplant, which has a 28% rate of mortality. Other hepatotoxic substances, including alcohol, contribute additively to the risk of acetaminophen toxicity (Yoon et al, 2016).

Viral hepatitis is caused by infection with any of at least five distinct viruses: hepatitis A virus (HAV), hepatitis B virus (HBV), hepatitis C virus (HCV), hepatitis D virus (HDV), and hepatitis E virus (HEV). Most viral hepatitis infections in the United States are attributable to HAV, HBV, and HCV (CDC, 2015). Table 20-10 compares those three types by mode of transmission, high-risk populations, and vaccine availability.

Signs and Symptoms

Regardless of type or cause, symptoms are:

- Anorexia
- Nausea
- Epigastric discomfort
- Fatigue
- Weakness

Signs of hepatitis are vomiting, diarrhea, and jaundice caused by the inability of the liver to convert fat-soluble bilirubin to a water-soluble (conjugated) form. The degree of jaundice gives a rough estimate of the severity of the disease. Physical examination shows an enlarged and tender liver and an enlarged spleen.

Treatment

Only HCV can be cured with direct-acting antiviral medications. The course of treatment normally lasts 12 to 24 months.

TABLE 20-10 Common Types of Viral Hepatitis

	HEPATITIS A	HEPATITIS B	HEPATITIS C*
Cases of chronic disease	Uncommon in the United States, 2,500 cases in 2014	About 2.2 million Americans have chronic hepatitis B	About 3.3 million Americans have chronic hepatitis C
Usual mode of transmission	Fecal–oral: contaminated food and water	Body fluids Rare—transplanted organs Inanimate objects contaminated with body fluids, including medical equipment, razors, toothbrushes, acupuncture and tattoo needles Virus is stable on environmental surfaces at least 7 days	Parenteral equipment: medical, religious, recreational, sexual contact Rarely: perinatal transmission, transplanted organs
High-risk populations	Household and sexual contacts of acute cases Travelers to developing countries Individuals having unprotected sex Injecting drug users	Household and sexual contacts of infected persons, including perinatal Injecting drug users Individuals having unprotected sex Health-care and public-safety workers exposed to blood and body fluids in their work Accidental needle sticks of health-care workers and caregivers working with infected individuals	Individuals who share injecting equipment Health-care workers using parenteral equipment (needle-stick accidents) HIV-infected individuals
Vaccine	Yes, if at least 12 months of age Routine vaccination recommended before traveling to developing countries	Yes, universal vaccination of infants beginning at birth Screening of pregnant women; immunoprophylaxis to infants born to infected women; those of unknown infection status Vaccination of previously unvaccinated children, adolescents, organ transplant recipients Vaccination of high-risk adults	No; the 6 genotypes and approximately 100 subtypes of the virus impede development of effective vaccines

*Most common bloodborne infection in the United States.
Adapted from NIH, 2017.

Treatment for other forms of viral hepatitis involves combinations of interferon and antiviral drugs to modify the course of the disease. The medications have significant side effects that require careful monitoring (NIH, 2017). The cornerstones of treatment are:

- Bed rest
- Abstinence from alcohol and other substances toxic to the liver
- Optimum nutrition to permit the liver to heal

Convalescence may take from 3 weeks to 3 months. Clients on bed rest, especially debilitated clients with hepatitis, are more susceptible to pressure injuries than the average client because of decreased synthesis of albumin and the globulins. If the client abstains from alcohol, the hepatitis is often reversible. Full recovery is measured by the return of liver function tests to normal and may take more than a year.

Nutritional Care

A healthy eating pattern, such as those outlined in the *2015-2020 Dietary Guidelines for Americans*, is recommended for clients with hepatitis. Alcohol is hepatotoxic and should not be ingested (NIH, 2017). Clients who experience extreme fatigue and may have a diminished appetite should be encouraged to eat up to 6 small meals per day.

Cirrhosis of the Liver

Cirrhosis of the liver is the 12th leading cause of death in the United States, responsible for more than 32,000 deaths each year. The most common causes of cirrhosis are alcoholism and chronic viral hepatitis. The only treatment for end-stage liver disease that affects survival is liver transplantation (NIH, 2014).

In **cirrhosis,** the liver becomes scarred and ineffective at regeneration. The major nutritional effects of alcoholism are summarized in Clinical Application 20-8, and its connection to mortality is described in Clinical Application 20-9.

Several barriers interfere with alcoholism case–finding:

- Alcoholism's multiple and varied manifestations
- The health-care provider's personal definition of alcoholism
- Denial by the client and family

Clinical Application 20-10 shows an example of a brief, effective screening tool to identify possible alcohol misusers. Such specific information might be useful in counseling clients. Regardless of the tool or free-form used, health-care providers should assess lifestyle factors that contribute to illness and a note should be made of the client's definition of a drink that may not match that of a **standard drink.**

Pathophysiology

Alcohol needs no digestion. It is absorbed rapidly, 20% from the stomach and 80% from the small intestine. Immediately after absorption, alcohol is carried throughout the body. In the liver, which is subjected to higher concentrations than other organs, it is metabolized at the rate of $1/2$ ounce of alcohol per hour. This refers to the alcohol content, not the whole beverage. This rate cannot be rushed, and giving coffee

CLINICAL APPLICATION 20-8

Nutritional Effects of Alcoholism

Alcoholism is a disease of alcohol consumption that leads to alcoholic liver disease (ALD), which includes a range of liver injury, including alcoholic hepatitis and cirrhosis. Muscle wasting, weight loss, and nutritional deficiencies are common in ALD. In addition to complete alcohol withdrawal, the following nutritional interventions are recommended to counteract commonly seen deficiencies:

- Nutritional assessment to evaluate for malnutrition—typically seen in 20%-60% of clients with alcoholic cirrhosis and 100% of hospitalized clients with alcoholic hepatitis.
- Caloric needs should be determined by indirect calorimetry—provide frequent meals, nighttime snack, a daily protein intake of 1.0-1.5 g/kg/day, and avoidance of unnecessary restrictions (e.g., sodium unless edema or ascites present).

Enteral nutrition therapy is preferred over parenteral nutrition therapy and is associated with improvement in nutritional status in individuals unable to meet their nutritional needs through food alone. Screen for and treat micronutrient deficiencies of water-soluble and fat-soluble vitamins and minerals. Deficiencies commonly seen in ALD:

- Folate—due to reduced dietary intake, malabsorption, reduced liver uptake and storage, and increased urinary excretion. It has been estimated that 80% of individuals hospitalized who have alcoholism have low serum folate, with 44% of them severely depleted.
- Thiamin (vitamin B1)—due to reduced dietary intake, malabsorption, and reduced liver uptake and storage. Deficiency causes confusion and hypoactivity.
- Cyanocobalamin (vitamin B12)—due to reduced dietary intake. Deficiency may cause extremity weakness and anemia.
- Vitamin D—due to decreased dietary intake, possibly less sun exposure, abnormal metabolism related to hepatic damage. May cause muscle weakness. Low vitamin D levels may be a biomarker of the severity of liver damage.
- Glucose—IV glucose should be administered to cirrhotic clients fasting for more than 12 hours.
- **Branch chain amino acids** (BCAA)—supplements should be administered to ALD clients with hepatic encephalopathy.

Sources: Rossi, Conte, & Massironi, 2015; MerckManuals.com, 2017.

CLINICAL APPLICATION 20-9

Alcohol Contributes to Mortality

The World Health Organization (WHO) estimates that in 2012 alcohol was responsible for 3.3 million deaths, representing 5.9% of all deaths. Alcohol abuse is a factor in more than 200 disease and injury conditions. The global burden of disease and injury attributable to alcohol is 5.1% (WHO, 2015).

In the United States, it is estimated that excessive alcohol use leads to approximately 88,000 deaths annually. The shortening of lives for those who die because of excessive alcohol use is estimated to average 30 years. Excessive drinking is responsible for 1 in 10 deaths among adults aged 20-64 years (CDC, 2016).

CLINICAL APPLICATION 20-10

Questionnaire for Identifying Alcohol Misuse (NIH, 2015)

The **AUDIT-C Questionnaire** focuses on the amount and frequency of alcohol consumption. It asks, all within the past year:

1. How often did you have a drink* containing alcohol?
   a. Never = 0
   b. 2 to 4 times per month = 2
   c. 2 to 3 times a week = 3
   d. 4 or more times a week = 4
2. How many drinks did you have on a typical day when you were drinking?
   a. None, I do not drink = 0
   b. 1 or 2 = 0
   c. 3 or 4 = 1
   d. 5 or 6 = 2
   e. 7 to 9 = 3
   f. 10 or more = 4
3. How often did you have six or more drinks on one occasion?
   a. Never = 0
   b. Less than monthly = 1
   c. Monthly = 2
   d. Weekly = 3
   e. Daily or almost daily = 4

The AUDIT-C is scored on a scale of 0-12 (scores of 0 reflect no alcohol use). In men, a score of 4 or more is considered positive; in women, a score of 3 or more is considered positive. Generally, the higher the AUDIT-C score, the more likely it is that the patient's drinking is affecting his/her health and safety.

*A standard drink is 0.5 oz of alcohol found in 12 oz of beer, 5 oz of wine, or 1.5 oz distilled spirits.

or other stimulants to an inebriated person induces not sobriety but merely alert intoxication.

If the liver is not able to repair the damage caused by alcohol, dying liver cells are replaced by scar tissue. Figure 20-7 traces the path from cell death to several cardinal signs of cirrhosis. Because the liver has multiple functions, one pathological change reinforces another. Common complications include portal hypertension; esophageal varices; gallbladder and bile duct stones; edema and ascites; liver cancer; and hepatic encephalopathy (NIH, 2014). The signs and symptoms of cirrhosis appear in Box 20-2.

The end result of cirrhosis is liver failure, which can lead to hepatic coma. See hepatic encephalopathy in Clinical Application 20-11.

Dietary Treatment for Cirrhosis

Malnutrition is commonly seen in cirrhosis.

In general, nutrition in clients with stable cirrhosis features these key components:

- Avoidance of alcohol
- Ingestion of four to six meals per day
- Late evening snack to avoid fasting-associated catabolism

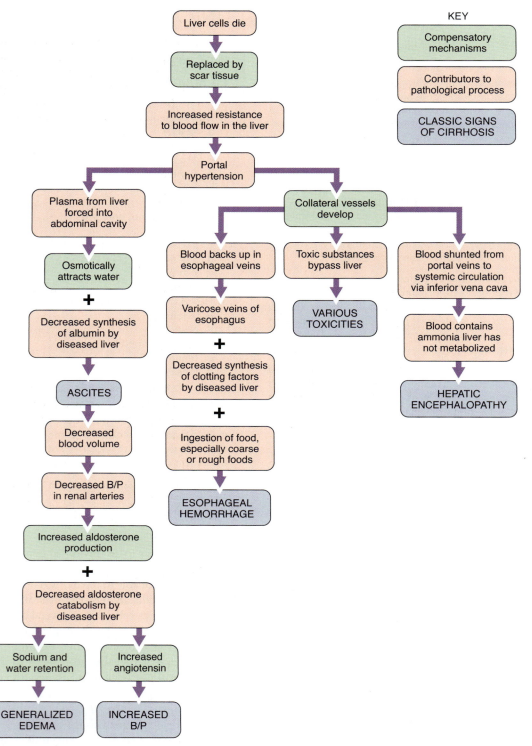

KEY

Compensatory mechanisms

Contributors to pathological process

CLASSIC SIGNS OF CIRRHOSIS

FIGURE 20-7 Progression of pathology leading to the classic signs and symptoms of cirrhosis of the liver. Many other manifestations appear given the multiple functions of the liver.

- Protein intake of 1.0 to 1.5 grams per kilogram of body weight
- Sufficient kilocalories to avoid muscle catabolism, and provision of a liquid supplement if client has diagnosed malnutrition or is unable to consume enough kilocalories from foods

- Monitored vitamin status and appropriate supplementation
- Sodium restriction based on **ascites** level

The dietary management of these clients, particularly those with end-stage liver disease, is complex and constantly changing, requiring the continuing services of an expert dietitian.

BOX 20-2 ■ Signs and Symptoms of Cirrhosis	
Symptoms	**Signs**
■ Anorexia	■ Abdominal distention
■ Epigastric pain	■ Vomiting
■ Nausea that worsens as the day goes on	■ **Steatorrhea**
	■ Jaundice
	■ Ascites
	■ Edema
	■ GI bleeding

CLINICAL APPLICATION 20-11

Hepatic Encephalopathy

This liver-caused brain disease accounts for 22,931 hospitalizations, with an average length-of-stay of 8.5 days. The cause is thought to be multifactorial, but excessive ammonia retained in the body causes neurocognitive manifestations.

Ammonia is produced by intestinal bacteria and by digestive enzymes breaking down protein. Even if the person consumes no protein foods, the bacteria work on the castoff cells of the GI tract and on the blood from GI bleeding, which is common in alcoholic cirrhosis. Ordinarily, the liver degrades ammonia to urea, which is excreted in urine by the kidneys, but in liver failure, blood ammonia levels rise. Ammonia is toxic to all cells, including those of the liver and the brain.

Some signs and symptoms of hepatic encephalopathy include:

■ Personality changes
■ Irritability
■ Weakness
■ Apathy
■ Confusion
■ Sleepiness

Primary treatment of hepatic encephalopathy is administration of a nonabsorbable disaccharide, *lactulose*. This drug, given orally or by enema, acidifies the large intestine. The change in pH causes ammonia to be converted to ammonium ions, which are not absorbed but eliminated in the feces. If *lactulose* is not sufficient, the antibiotic *rifaximin* (which remains in the lumen of the intestine) may be added to decrease the bacteria present.

The goal of nutritional management of clients with hepatic encephalopathy should be to promote good nutrition because malnutrition is commonly found in individuals who have hepatic encephalopathy. Nutritional recommendations include an energy intake of 35–40 kcal/kg ideal body weight (IBW), a 1.2–1.5 g/kg IBW protein intake, and 25–45 g of fiber daily.

Branched-chain amino acids (BCAA) may be selected as therapy because clients with liver cirrhosis often lack BCAA, which is thought to contribute to hepatic encephalopathy. Oral BCAA improve manifestations of hepatic encephalopathy, but have no effect on mortality or nutritional status. Mild hepatic encephalopathy may respond positively to probiotics, but they should not replace other therapies.

Source: Suraweera, Sundaram, & Sab, 2016.

Gallbladder Disease

On the underside of the liver is a small pouchlike organ called the **gallbladder.** Its function is to concentrate and store bile until needed for digestion. The liver secretes 600 to 800 milliliters of bile per day that the gallbladder, by eliminating the water content, reduces to 60 to 160 milliliters. Bile functions to emulsify large fat droplets into smaller droplets, exposing greater surface area to the action of lipase.

Causative Factors

The presence of gallstones is called **cholelithiasis** (Fig. 20-8). Risk factors for gallstones include (Marcason, 2015):

■ Female sex—especially pregnant, on hormone therapy, or using birth control pills
■ Age above 60
■ Weight loss using a very low-calorie diet
■ Increased fat and sugar intake
■ Sedentary lifestyle
■ Hispanic or Native American heritage
■ Type 2 diabetes and/or hyperinsulinemia
■ Dyslipidemia

When the gallbladder becomes inflamed from irritation by stones (90% of the cases), parasitic infection, or prolonged fasting associated with parenteral nutrition, the condition is labeled **cholecystitis.**

Symptoms and Treatment

The cardinal symptom of gallbladder disease is pain after ingestion of fat caused by spasms of the gallbladder. The pain is located in the right upper quadrant and often radiates to the right shoulder.

Dietary Modifications

For chronic gallbladder disease, the client should follow a healthy eating pattern, limiting fat. Obese clients should

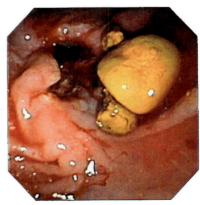

FIGURE 20-8 Gallstones seen endoscopically (original magnification × 3). *(Reprinted from Venes, D [ed.]: Taber's Cyclopedic Medical Dictionary, ed 22. FA Davis, Philadelphia, 2013, p. 987, with permission.)*

lose weight. Some clients obtain relief with the restriction of dietary fat; others do not. A reasonable approach to fat restriction is to:

- Select skim milk dairy products
- Limit fats or oils to 3 teaspoons per day
- Consume no more than 6 ounces of very lean meat per day

Another approach is to eliminate foods that cause symptoms. Clients usually can identify foods that cause them pain. Fried foods are the worst offenders. Gas-forming foods also are often poorly tolerated. Table 20-11 identifies some foods that are low in fat and some that are high in fat.

Medical and Surgical Treatments

Asymptomatic gallstones are usually just monitored. Surgery is the preferred option to treat symptomatic gallbladder disease, but medical management may be recommended to allow inflammation to subside, for individuals who are poor surgical risks, or for individuals who wish to delay surgery to accommodate their priorities.

The usual surgical procedure in the United States is laparoscopic **cholecystectomy.** Clients and physicians still may opt for removal of the gallbladder through the traditional open incision if the stones are large or the gallbladder is infected. The removal of the stones without the gallbladder is a *cholecystotomy.*

After traditional cholecystectomy, the client may initially receive nothing by mouth or clear liquids. Then the diet is progressed as tolerated. After laparoscopic cholecystectomy, clients may receive a general diet immediately. Postsurgery, 5% to 40% of people have nausea, vomiting, gas, bloating, diarrhea, and abdominal pain.

Later in convalescence, balanced meals should be well tolerated because bile enters the duodenum continuously. Clients who become nauseated and suffered pain after eating certain foods preoperatively, however, may continue to avoid them postoperatively because of the association.

Two alternate, less invasive treatments have been devised to treat gallstones. One technique involves an oral agent to dissolve the stones, *ursodiol.* This is indicated for cholesterol stones only, not pigment stones; only those less than 1.5 centimeters in diameter; and in cases where reformation of stones is not expected—for instance, when caused by rapid weight loss (Drugs.com, 2017).

Another method is to break up the stones using shock waves through a procedure called *lithotripsy.* It is used infrequently because it is labor-intensive, requires expensive

TABLE 20-11 Comparison of Fat Content of Selected Foods

LOW-FAT FOODS	FAT (GRAMS)	HIGH-FAT FOODS	FAT (GRAMS)
Starch/breads			
Angel food cake, $1/12$	<1	Pecan pie, $1/6$ of pie	24
Italian bread, 1 slice	<1	Bread stuffing, $1/2$ cup	13
English muffin, 1	1	Danish pastry	12
Raisin toast, 1 slice	1	Croissant, 1	12
Pancake, 4-inch, 1	2	Glazed raised doughnut, 1	13
Meats, fish, and poultry			
Beef round, 3 oz lean roasted	9	Beef prime rib, 3 oz lean only	24
Chicken breast, 3 oz roasted, without skin	9	Chicken, deep-fried thigh, 1	14
Boiled ham, 3 oz	9	Spare ribs, 3 oz	24
Tuna, $1/2$ cup water-packed	6	Tuna, $1/2$ cup oil-packed, drained	24
Fruits and vegetables			
Banana, $8^3/4$ inch long, 1	1	Avocado, 1	30
Raisins, 1 cup	1	Coconut, dried, 1 cup	50
Potato, baked, 1	<1	French fried potato, $2 \times 3^1/2$ inches, 15 pieces	12
Onion, raw, sliced, 1 cup	<1	French fried onion rings, 4	10
Milk products			
Cottage cheese, 1%, $1/2$ cup	1	Cottage cheese, 4%, $1/2$ cup	5
Mozzarella, part skim, 1 oz	5	Cheddar, 1 oz	9
Skim milk, with added milk solids, 1 cup	1	Whole milk, 1 cup	8
Frozen yogurt, low-fat, 1 cup	4	Ice cream, regular, hard, vanilla, 1 cup	14
Fast foods*			
Arby's		Beef 'n Cheddar sandwich	20
Junior Roast Beef sandwich	8	Quarter Pounder with cheese	26
McDonald's		6-inch tuna	25
Hamburger	9	Spicy Chicken sandwich	22
Subway			
6-inch roast beef	5		
Wendy's			
Ultimate Chicken Grill sandwich	10		

*Check with the restaurant. Recipes may be revised.

equipment, and, compared with laparoscopic procedures, less universally effective.

Diseases of the Pancreas

In addition to the endocrine secretions, insulin, glucagon, and somatostatin, the **pancreas** secretes at least 10 digestive enzymes, including amylase, lipase, trypsin, and chymotrypsin. It also secretes bicarbonate to aid electrolyte balance. Because of those many secretions, diseases of the pancreas create major nutritional consequences. Two important disorders of the pancreas affecting nutrition are pancreatitis and cystic fibrosis.

Pancreatitis

Pancreatitis, the inflammation of the pancreas, is the most common disease that affects the pancreas (Baumler, 2016). Normally, the pancreatic enzymes necessary for digestion are inactive in the pancreas and become activated only on entering the duodenum. Otherwise, the active enzymes would digest the pancreas itself. In **pancreatitis,** the retained pancreatic enzymes become activated and do digest the pancreatic tissue. In severe cases, the enzymes escape into the general circulation causing inflammation in distant organs.

Acute Pancreatitis

In the United States, common causes of acute pancreatitis cases are attributed to alcohol abuse, gallstones, and high triglycerides. Each year there are more than 300,000 admissions to hospitals due to acute pancreatitis.

The characteristic symptom of acute pancreatitis is excruciating pain in the left upper quadrant. Pain may start out mild, but worsens after eating. Pain may last for several days. Nausea and vomiting accompany an attack (Pancreas Foundation, 2017). Laboratory tests reveal elevated levels of serum amylase and lipase (Basnayake, 2015).

Nutritionally, mild pancreatitis may be treated with (Pancreas Foundation, 2017):

- Nothing by mouth for 24 to 48 hours to avoid stimulating the pancreas
- Aggressive hydration with IV fluids
- After 48 hours, the client should be able to consume food to support the increased kilocalories required for healing the inflammation
- A client unable to eat should be started on EN therapy, via a feeding tube

Chronic Pancreatitis

In chronic pancreatitis, persistent inflammation results in permanent structural damage with fibrosis and ductal strictures. Repeated injury to the tissue is thought to cause chronic pancreatitis. The most common cause of chronic pancreatitis in the United States is alcoholism; however, less than 10% of alcoholics develop pancreatitis. Other environmental factors, such as tobacco smoke, are potent additional risk factors, doubling the risk for chronic pancreatitis over nonsmokers. There is some evidence that individuals who consume a high-fat diet develop chronic pancreatitis at a younger age, but more studies are necessary before clear conclusions may be made. The genetic component of pancreatitis may be triggered by excessive alcohol intake (Baumler, 2016).

In the United States, fewer than half the cases of chronic pancreatitis result from alcoholism, and 10% to 30% are **idiopathic.** Other known causes include hereditary pancreatitis, autoimmune pancreatitis, hyperparathyroidism, and obstruction of the main pancreatic duct (Baumler, 2016).

Most often, these clients present with severe abdominal pain that may last many hours or several days. Episodes typically subside spontaneously after 6 to 10 years as the cells that secrete digestive enzymes are destroyed. General dietary management principles depend on the stage of disease but progressively are likely to include:

- Total abstinence from alcohol (and, although not dietary, from smoking)
- Small, frequent nutritionally balanced meals, keeping fat to no more than 30% of the diet
- Vitamin–mineral supplements if prescribed by healthcare provider
- If underweight
  - 35 kilocalories per kilogram of body weight daily
  - 1.0 to 1.5 grams of protein per kilogram of body weight per day
- Pancreatic enzyme supplements, which help but do not substitute for normal function
- Oral nutritional supplements may be required to boost the total caloric intake
- Rarely, short-term parenteral nutrition to replace nutrient stores
- Monitoring for and treating diabetes resulting from loss of **endogenous** insulin and glucagon secretions. Diabetes develops in 90% of clients with chronic pancreatitis (Baumler, 2016).

Cystic Fibrosis

Originally considered a disease of childhood because of limited life expectancy, **cystic fibrosis (CF)** is increasingly seen in adults, currently affecting 30,000 children and adults in the United States (70,000 worldwide). More than 50% of the CF client population is aged 18 or older, but more than 75% of clients are diagnosed by age 2 (Cystic Fibrosis Foundation, 2017).

Pathophysiology

The chief cause of morbidity and mortality in cystic fibrosis is obstruction of exocrine glands with thick mucus, affecting multiple organ systems. GI manifestations of cystic fibrosis is characterized by:

- Pulmonary dysfunction and infection, resulting in increased caloric requirements and decreased appetite

- Pancreatic impairment, causing insufficient production of pancreatic enzymes contributing to malabsorption of fat, protein, and fat-soluble vitamins often resulting in malnutrition
- Cystic fibrosis-related diabetes
- Altered motility of the GI tract and small bowel bacterial overgrowth

Obstruction by viscid material in the lumen of the glands interferes with the digestive secretions of the pancreas. Fat malabsorption may result in the passage of bulky, fatty, foul-smelling feces and protein malabsorption, which leads to stunted growth (deficit in height for age).

Treatment

- Supportive care is the foundation of CF treatment with the overall goal that every client should achieve normal growth. Children under the age of 2 who are not growing well should receive a trial zinc supplement.
- With appropriate pancreatic enzyme replacement, most clients can maintain a reasonable nutritional

status with a normal diet. Advanced pulmonary manifestations may require enteral feeding not only to maintain weight and growth but also because better nutritional status improves muscle strength and lung function.

CF clients have specific nutritional requirements:

- Energy needs that may be 110% to 200% of those normally recommended, with unlimited fat in meals
- Oral nutritional supplements or enteral tube feeding to meet estimated daily energy requirements
- Supplemental pancreatic enzyme therapy to control symptoms and permit adequate food intake for normal growth and weight gain despite not completely correcting nutrient malabsorption
- Yearly monitoring of serum vitamin A, E, and D levels and supplementation as needed; hypervitaminosis A has been reported
- Adequate salt intake and monitoring of electrolytes (Sabharwal, 2016)

KEYSTONES

- Recommended preoperative intake allows clear fluids up to 2 hours before anesthesia, breast milk 4 hours, infant formula and nonhuman milk 6 hours.
- Dumping syndrome and postprandial hypotension require similar dietary interventions. Meals should be dry, frequent, and low in simple sugars. Lying down after eating helps retain stomach contents for a longer time.
- For gastroesophageal reflux (GERD) and hiatal hernia, meals should be small and frequent with normal protein and limited fat. Remaining upright after eating encourages movement of stomach contents into the duodenum.
- Celiac disease develops in a genetically predisposed individual in whom exposure to dietary gluten leads to

damage to the small intestine. The treatment is a gluten-free diet for life.
- Medical nutrition therapy for inflammatory bowel disease includes good nutrition and adequate fluid and caloric intake with more frequent feedings, as necessary. A food diary may help identify a client's food intolerances, if any.
- Keys to nutritional treatment of hepatitis and cirrhosis of the liver are abstinence from alcohol and optimum nutrition.
- Cholecystitis is treated medically with a low-fat diet. To prevent cholelithiasis, eating breakfast or drinking two glasses of water on arising empties the gallbladder of concentrated bile that results from a long overnight fast.

CASE STUDY 20-1

An outpatient, Ms. C, a 40-year-old woman, has just been evaluated for right upper quadrant pain. The pain occurs after meals and radiates to the right shoulder. Ms. C has noticed that her stools have become pale gray in the past 2 months.

Ultrasound examination of the gallbladder showed the presence of numerous stones. None is obstructing the duct system yet.

Ms. C is a single parent of four children, aged 4 to 17 years, and is employed as a secretary. If surgery does become necessary, she would like to delay it until the youngest child is in school. For that reason, she is electing medical management.

Usual food intake: no breakfast; coffee and doughnut mid-morning; "this week's special" lunch-meat sandwich and chips at noon; casseroles for dinner.

Stated she does not know much about nutrition, that she shops as her mother did, and that she cooks food her children will eat. Rarely buys fresh fruits or vegetables because of the cost.

CARE PLAN

Subjective Data

Pain in right upper quadrant immediately after eating ■ Pale stools for 2 months by history ■ Usual intake: high fat, low fiber
■ Admitted lack of knowledge about nutrition

Objective Data

Gallstones per ultrasound ■ Measured height 5 ft 4 in. ■ Measured weight 165 lb ■ BMI 28.3. ■ BP 139/89

Analysis

Need for diet instruction related to prescribed low-fat diet for cholecystitis as evidenced by self-report
■ Potential increased risk for surgical complications related to overweight and prehypertension

Plan

DESIRED OUTCOMES EVALUATION CRITERIA	ACTIONS/ INTERVENTIONS	RATIONALE
Client will verbalize foods to avoid on low-fat diet by end of teaching session.	Explain low-fat diet, adapting to client's lifestyle. Provide written instructions for client to take home.	Having written instructions available as a teaching tool structures the session and may stimulate questions the client would not think of otherwise. Taking the material home will reinforce the instruction.
Client will state means to modify meals to accommodate prescribed diet by end of teaching session.	Explore Ms. C's preferences for adding fiber to her diet.	Soluble fiber will combine with cholesterol, which comprises most gallstones, and carry it out of the body. Building on the client's choices increases the chances of compliance.
Client will think through her ability to implement the diet and voice hesitations by the end of this visit.	Obtain client's reaction to diet and offer alternatives to her present meal pattern.	Considering the client's wishes affirms her status as an individual. Personalizing the diet for her circumstances will increase the chances of success.
Client will accept referral to social worker to maximize nutrition for self and family.	Make appointment with social worker for Ms. C before she leaves today.	Completing arrangements before the client leaves avoids the possibility of procrastination.

TEAMWORK 20-1

SOCIAL WORKER'S NOTES

The following Social Worker's Notes are representative of the documentation found in a client's medical record.

Referred by nurse instructing client on low-fat diet for cholecystitis

Subjective: *Head of household of five; divorced 6 months; ex-husband unemployed and behind on child support*

Objective: *Earning slightly more than minimum wage per paycheck stub*

Analysis: *Eligible for Head Start and Supplemental Nutrition Assistance Program (SNAP)*

Plan: *Identify barriers to participation; assist with applications; encourage attendance at nutrition education sessions provided by Head Start*

CRITICAL THINKING QUESTIONS

1. How will dietary modification affect the children?

2. If Ms. C were not in such a dire financial situation and ineligible for assistance, what other approaches to improving the family's nutritional intake could be tried?

3. How would you follow up on Ms. C's implementation of the low-fat diet as well as her overweight and hypertension (assuming other measurements confirm the readings)?

CHAPTER REVIEW

1. Which of the following foods are recommended for a client with diverticulosis?
   1. Bologna sandwich with white bread and mayonnaise
   2. Corn on the cob with a veggie burger, whole-wheat bun, lettuce and tomato
   3. Canned peaches with cottage cheese
   4. Banana-nut waffles with butter and syrup

2. The American Society of Anesthesiologists' guidelines suggest which of the following intakes is permissible for healthy individuals undergoing elective procedures?
   1. Water and apple juice until 1 hour before the procedure
   2. Plain tea and unbuttered toast with clear jelly 6 hours before scheduled surgery
   3. Infant formula or breast milk 4 hours before an elective procedure begins
   4. Light meal containing meat at 5 a.m. before a procedure scheduled for noon

3. Clients who have had resection of the ileum should be monitored for:
   1. Iron-deficiency anemia
   2. Fat-soluble vitamin deficiency
   3. Calcium and phosphorus deficiency
   4. Vitamin B_{12} deficiency

4. A client with cirrhosis of the liver should be asked if he or she experienced _____ before ordering a diet.
   1. A headache
   2. Vomiting of blood
   3. A recent course of antibiotic therapy
   4. Hives

5. Which of the following meal components is likely to lessen symptoms of the dumping syndrome?
   1. Mashed fresh strawberries
   2. Orange sherbet
   3. Salt-free tomato juice
   4. Whole-wheat toast with dietetic jelly

6. Chronic pancreatitis is:
   1. Curable, requires pancreatic enzymes, affects digestion
   2. Caused by diabetes, chronic renal insufficiency, requires a low-sodium diet
   3. Requires pancreatic enzymes, causes diabetes, causes dumping syndrome
   4. Causes diabetes, requires long-term pancreatic enzyme therapy, is the most common disease of the pancreas

CLINICAL ANALYSIS

1. Mr. W is a 55-year-old man admitted to the acute care unit for jaundice and ascites secondary to cirrhosis of the liver. He has gained 15 pounds in the past 3 weeks, and his serum sodium is 125 mEq/L. He is a diagnosed alcoholic who has been through a detoxification program several times in the past 5 years. The dietitian has instructed Mr. W on a 1,500-mg sodium diet with a fluid restriction of 1,000 mL per day.
   When the nurse does the beginning of shift assessment, Mr. W says that he tried "cutting down on salt" when he started gaining weight, but it didn't work. Which of the following statements best reflects a good understanding of Mr. W's pathology and treatment?
   a. Just cutting out added salt is not enough, because many foods are naturally high in sodium.
   b. Fluids are always restricted with a low-sodium diet.
   c. The ascites is caused by the inability of the liver to produce water-soluble bilirubin.
   d. Besides retaining sodium, Mr. W has ascites due to decreased blood pressure in the liver.

2. Mr. W vomits immediately after his next meal. The physician then orders a hydrating solution of 5% dextrose in water intravenously. If thiamin is not included in that order, the nurse should inquire about it because:
   a. Thiamin is necessary to predigest the dextrose for immediate absorption.
   b. Deficiency of thiamin causes delirium tremens.
   c. Intravenous glucose without thiamin in the cirrhosis client can lead to symptoms of confusion and decreased activity.
   d. Thiamin prevents folic acid stores from being diluted by the hydrating solution.

3. Ms. M has been diagnosed with gastroesophageal reflux disease. Dietary instructions should include taking:
   a. Normal amounts of protein to help tighten the cardiac sphincter.
   b. Mint teas to counteract the bitter taste caused by reflux of gastric contents into the esophagus.
   c. Small amounts of wine with dinner to aid in relaxation and enjoyment of the meal.
   d. Whole milk products to increase the kilocalorie density of the diet.

CHAPTER 21

Diet and Cancer

After completing this chapter, the student should be able to:

- Relate nutritional factors to the incidence of cancers at the most common sites.
- Summarize dietary guidelines for the prevention of cancer.
- Compare the New American Plate® to MyPlate (Chapter 1) as to its potential value as a teaching tool.
- Interpret the lack of validation of population correlations of fruit and vegetable intake with cancer occurrence in more focused research.
- Describe examples of the associations that have been found between diet and cancer.

- Explain the difficulty of generalizing dietary behaviors to adopt or to avoid with the goal of preventing cancer.
- Identify measures to increase oral intake for anorexic clients with cancer.
- Discuss strategies to prevent infections in the immunosuppressed client.
- List four classes of drugs that may be used to affect food intake and weight in clients with cancer.
- Describe three approaches to increase oral intake for a cancer client with mouth ulcerations.
- Define *cachexia* and correlate its characteristics with the challenges of managing the condition.

Definitions and Statistics

According to Hippocrates's definition, cancer means "crab," for the creeping way in which it spreads. *Cancer* is a general term for more than 200 types of malignant neoplasms.

Terminology

A **neoplasm** is a new and abnormal formation of tissue (tumor) that grows at the expense of the healthy organism.

- **Benign** tumors are localized but potentially dangerous if situated in vital organs.
- **Malignant** (cancerous) tumors infiltrate surrounding tissue and spread to distant parts of the body.
- **Sarcomas** arise from connective tissue, such as muscle or bone and are more common in young people.
- **Carcinomas** occur in epithelial tissue, including cancers of the lung, breast, prostate, and colon, and are more common in older people.

Characteristics common to all types of cancer are uncontrolled growth and the ability to spread to distant sites (**metastasize**). To determine the severity of a client's disease, both microscopic and macroscopic measures are used. Although particular cancers have specific systems, in general, the scales for both run from one (least severe) to four (most severe).

- **Grade** of malignancy refers to the extent to which the cells under the microscope resemble normal cells, with grade 1 most like normal cells and grade 4 least like them.

- **Stage** of disease refers to the physical location of the tumor, with stage I localized and stage IV involving distant metastases.

Incidence and Mortality

In the United States, more than 20% of cancer deaths are attributed to body fatness, physical inactivity, excess alcohol consumption, and/or poor nutrition (American Cancer Society [ACS], 2017). Cancer is the second most common cause of death in the United States after heart disease.

The incidence of the three most common cancers for men (prostate, lung/bronchus, colorectal) and women (breast, lung/bronchus, colorectal) of different ethnicities is illustrated in Figure 21-1. The factors that drive these disparities as well as the causes of cancer are complex and often incompletely understood. Certain cancers appear in great numbers in particular countries. Clinical Application 21-1 summarizes some of these findings. For all groups, cancer of lung is the chief cause of cancer deaths (World Health Organization [WHO], February, 2017).

Diet and Cancer Development

New insights into the benefits obtained from foods show that:

- Food can provide benefits beyond its intrinsic nutrient content (see Functional Foods in Chapter 1)

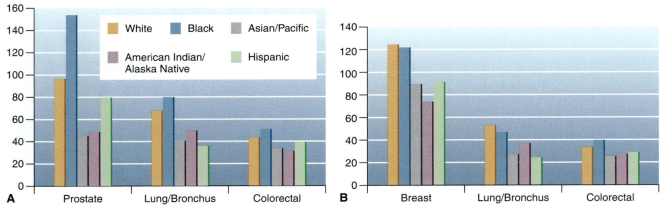

FIGURE 21-1 The three most common cancers for men *(A)* and women *(B)* in the United States, 2014. Rates are per 100,000 persons and are age-adjusted to the 2000 U.S. standard population. The ethnic groups are white, black, Asian/Pacific, American Indian/Alaska Native, and Hispanic. *(Data from U.S. Cancer Statistics Working Group. United States Cancer Statistics: 1999-2014 Incidence and Mortality Web-based Report. Atlanta: U.S. Department of Health and Human Services, Centers for Disease Control and Prevention and National Cancer Institute; 2017. Available at www.cdc.gov/uscs.)*

CLINICAL APPLICATION 21-1

Diet–Cancer Links in Various Populations

Residents of a given country experience similar environmental factors, including diet. They also may have **genes** that are similar compared with those found in people elsewhere.

- Stomach cancer is common where nitrates and nitrites are prevalent in food and water and where cured and pickled foods are popular. These areas include Korea, Japan, and China. Gastric cancer is the third leading cause of cancer-related deaths in China (Pan et al, 2017).
- Gastric cancer is the second cause of cancer-related deaths in Mexico, with a positive correlation being made to diets high in salt, processed meats, chili peppers, and alcoholic drinks (Denova-Gutierrez, Hernandez-Ramirez, & Lopez-Carrillo, 2014).

Studies of immigrants are especially enlightening. In Japan, the incidence of stomach cancer is higher and the incidence of prostate and colon cancer is lower than those in the United States. In second-generation Japanese immigrants to the United States, however, the distribution of cancers becomes similar to that of other Americans. One study compared gastric cancer prevalence between Asian immigrant and native Asians and found a decreased incidence of gastric cancer in Asian immigrants, which suggests that lifestyle plays a part in the development of gastric cancer (Kim, Park, Nam, & Ki, 2015).

Foods contain thousands of bioactive molecules that have the potential to alter gene and protein expression. Developing personalized nutrition for cancer prevention and therapy will require:

- Understanding **genotypes** and **phenotypes**
- Identifying bioactive food components that can favorably intervene in cellular processes

Bioactive food components with anticancer potential can affect the expression of genes involved in cell proliferation, differentiation, and death that are frequently altered in cancer. More studies will be required to fully understand how diet plays a role in cancer prevention. Until the era of personalized nutrition arrives, the American Cancer Society has issued general recommendations to decrease cancer risk (Box 21-1). The American Institute of Cancer Research developed the New American Plate® (Fig. 21-2), which exemplifies the guidelines. The image is a tool, not a specialized diet, for Americans to use in order to evaluate what they are eating to reduce cancer risk by addressing the following components:

- Eat plant-based meals that are $\frac{2}{3}$ or greater of vegetables, fruits, whole grains, or beans and $\frac{1}{3}$ or less of animal proteins.
- Control portion sizes.
- Maintain a healthy BMI by using the above guidelines (The American Institute of Cancer Research, 2017).

Dietary Habits Linked to Cancer

Table 21-1 shows four dietary conditions that are convincingly related to cancers arising in specific organs. Many other items have been studied that may be related to particular cancers, but the evidence is not as strong as for the ones listed. Numerous factors can impede certainty in nutrition research:

- Inconsistent results from small studies or varying designs
- Isolated nutrients or foods studied, thus oversimplifying the nutritive process
- Interventions too small, durations too short to produce an effect

Obesity

Excess adipose tissue has been found to produce cytokines, which contribute to chronic inflammation in the body. Environments of chronic inflammation can contribute to the development of abnormal malignant cells.

BOX 21-1 ■ Recommendations to Decrease Cancer Risk

For Community Action
- Increase access to healthful foods in schools, worksites, and communities.
- Decrease access to and marketing of foods and drinks of low nutritional value, particularly to youth.
- Provide safe, enjoyable, and accessible environments for physical activity in schools and workplaces, and for transportation and recreation in communities.

For Individual Choices
- Maintain a healthy weight throughout life. Be as lean as possible without being underweight.
  - Avoid excess weight gain at all ages. For the overweight person, even a small amount of weight loss has health benefits.
  - Limit intake of high-calorie foods and drinks.
- Adopt a physically active lifestyle. Some activity above one's usual level can produce health benefits.
  - Adults: 150 minutes of moderate-intensity or 75 minutes of vigorous-intensity activity per week, preferably distributed throughout the week.

- Children and teens: 1 hour of moderate or vigorous physical activity daily with vigorous activity 3 days per week.
- Limit sedentary behavior: sitting, lying down, screen-based entertainment.
- Consume a healthy diet, emphasizing plant food sources.
  - Choose amounts to maintain a healthy weight.
  - Limit intake of processed meat and red meat.
  - Consume at least 2½ cups of vegetables and fruits daily.
  - Select whole grains in preference to refined grain products.
- If alcohol is chosen, limit consumption to one **standard drink** per day for women and two for men.

Adapted from American Cancer Society, 2017. ACS Guidelines for Nutrition and Physical Activity. Available at https://www.cancer.org/healthy/eat-healthy-get-active/acs-guidelines-nutrition-physical-activity-cancer-prevention/guidelines.html.

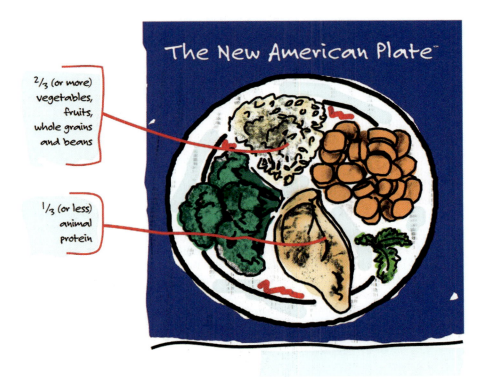

FIGURE 21-2 Vegetables, fruits, whole grains, and beans cover two-thirds (or more) of the New American Plate® with the remaining one-third (or less) of the plate reserved for fish, poultry, meat, and low-fat dairy foods. *(The New American Plate® is a registered trademark of the American Institute for Cancer Research, 2000. Reprinted with permission.)*

Systemic inflammation can worsen when clients are obese and consume diets high in fat and refined sugars (Donohoe, Doyle, & Reynolds, 2015).

Accumulation of body fat contributes to cancers of the colon, kidney, pancreas, endometrium, gallbladder, and adenocarcinoma of the esophagus. Regarding breast cancer, premenopausal women with greater body fat have reduced risk, whereas in postmenopausal women, there is a positive but weak association between adiposity and breast cancer. For colon cancer, increasing weight, hip circumference, waist circumference, BMI, and waist-to-hip ratio is associated with increased risk and risk of developing a more advanced stage of the disease (Neumann et al, 2015).

Therefore, some of the associations between dietary fat intake and cancer may be explained by excess energy intake, leading to overweight and obesity. Strong evidence remains to support the link between animal fat consumption and

TABLE 21-1   Dietary Habits Convincingly Linked to Particular Cancers

CANCER SITE	OVERWEIGHT-OBESITY	RED OR PROCESSED MEAT	ALCOHOL	SALT-PRESERVED FOODS
Breast	X		X	
Colorectal	X	X	X	
Endometrium	X			
Esophagus	X		X	
Gallbladder	X			
Kidney	X			
Larynx			X	
Liver	X		X	
Oral cavity			X	
Pancreatic	X	X		
Pharynx			X	X
Prostate		X		
Ovarian	X			
Stomach		X		X

Data from American Cancer Society (2015, October 26). World Health Organization Says Processed Meat Causes Cancer, available at https://www.cancer.org/latest-news/world-health-organization-says-processed-meat-causes-cancer.html; National Cancer Institute (2017, January 17). Obesity and Cancer, available at https://www.cancer.gov/about-cancer/causes-prevention/risk/obesity/obesity-fact-sheet; National Cancer Institute (2013, June 24). Alcohol and Cancer Risk, available at https://www.cancer.gov/about-cancer/causes-prevention/risk/alcohol/alcohol-fact-sheet; Denova-Gutierrez et al (2014); Neumann et al (2015).

risk of aggressive or advanced prostate cancer (Xu et al, 2015). An important consideration in carcinogenesis is abnormal glucose and insulin metabolism especially in obese sedentary persons. High-**glycemic-index** diets have been associated with insulin resistance, and insulin resistance has been associated with pancreatic cancer. This association requires further investigation.

Red or Processed Meat

Red meat intake has been linked with risk of cancers of the colon, rectum, and prostate. Evidence has demonstrated that increased consumption of animal fats from red meat increases premenopausal breast cancer risks (Aupperlee et al, 2015). The Nurses' Health Study (NHS) has demonstrated that women who consumed red meat daily, including pork, lamb, and beef, had a 2.5 higher risk of developing colorectal cancer than women who consumed red meat less than once per month, and other sources of fat, chicken, dairy, and vegetables did not have the same correlation (Dong-Hoon, NaNa, & Giovannucci, 2016).

Heterocyclic aromatic amines (HCAs) and polycyclic aromatic hydrocarbons (PAHs), formed by high-temperature cooking of muscle meats, have been identified as risk factors for colorectal cancer. There have been inconsistent results on the effect of HCA and colorectal cancer, but limiting consumption is still recommended (Potera, 2016). The amount of HCAs in a meal can be reduced by:

- Marinating meat for at least 30 minutes before cooking with a mixture of vinegar, lemon juice, or wine with herbs and spices
- Precooking larger cuts of meat to decrease time exposed to flames

- Choosing lean cuts of meat to avoid flare-ups to reduce risk of charring (American Institute for Cancer Research, 2017).

For someone interested in reducing meat intake, Dollars & Sense 21-1 offers an alternative burger.

Dollars & Sense 21-1

Easy and Inexpensive Veggie Burger

This recipe uses spices liberally. Other choices might be just as tasty or more so if fresh herbs are used. Salt is absent. Frying until crispy is necessary to hold the shape.

1 cup cooked unsalted beans well drained (black are good, others worth trying)
½ cup chopped raw onion (compensates for lack of salt)
⅛ tsp. powdered garlic
½ tsp. dried thyme
½ tsp. dried rosemary
½ tsp. dried parsley
½ tsp. Mrs. Dash Caribbean Citrus Salt-free Seasoning (or other flavor)
¼ tsp. black pepper
½ slice sour dough bread torn into ¼ inch crumbs
1 egg, beaten
2 tbsp. canola or olive oil for frying

Mash beans with potato masher or fork. Stir in rest of ingredients except egg and oil. If desired, taste at this point (before raw egg is added) and adjust seasoning. Add egg and mix well. Heat oil in skillet. Shape mixture into two patties. Fry in skillet over medium heat with adequate space between. Try to turn just once to keep intact. Cooking aromas suggest when first side is browned.

Slide out of skillet onto whole-wheat buns. Serve with usual burger condiments.

Assuming that other ingredients or substitutes are on hand, the cost for beans, onion, egg, breadcrumbs, and buns was $2.14 for two bean burgers.

Alcohol

Risk for the cancers associated with alcohol (see Table 21-1) increases significantly with the consumption of more than two drinks per day. The risks are equal whether the drink is 12 ounces of beer, 5 ounces of wine, or 1.5 ounces of liquor. Substantial evidence indicates that alcohol is the most consistent dietary risk factor that increases the risk of breast cancer (Rice et al, 2015). Women at high risk of breast cancer might reasonably consider abstaining from alcohol.

In cases of upper gastrointestinal cancer, the carcinogenic effects of alcohol may be caused by direct contact; in cancer of the liver, by toxicity.

Salt-Preserved Foods

Dietary salt intake was directly associated with risk of gastric cancer (see Clinical Application 21-1). A systemic review concluded that dietary salt intake is positively associated with the risk of gastric cancer but noted that some salty foods are also high in nitrites, also related to gastric cancer. In addition, most studies assessed salt intake by questionnaire rather than 24-hour urinary sodium excretion, which is recommended by the World Cancer Research Fund as the best measurement of salt intake.

A Diet to Prevent Cancer

The campaign to improve fruit and vegetable intake for general health continues (Fig. 21-3), but behavior change comes slowly. Studies looking at fruit and vegetable intake in 2013 demonstrated that most adults in the United States consumed under the recommended amount (Moore &

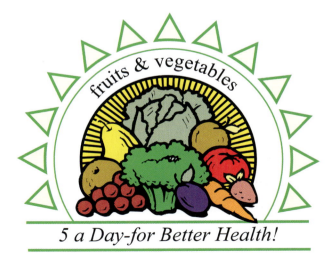

FIGURE 21-3 National 5 a Day program logo. The program logo and slogan are registered service marks. To use them, food industry and state health authority partners sign a license agreement to follow guidelines that maintain the scientific integrity of all messages and other communications to the public. (Reprinted from Foerster, SB, et al: California's "5 a Day—for Better Health" campaign: an innovative population-based effort to effect large-scale dietary change. Am J Prev Med 11:124, 1995, with permission.)

Thompson, 2015). Isolating the effects of vegetables and fruits from lifestyle is also problematic. People who eat large amounts of vegetables and fruits also tend to eat less meat and to be physically active. The WHO (June 17, 2017) recommends a diet low in fat, sodium, and sugar and consuming greater than 400 grams, or at least 5 servings, of fruits and vegetables per day to reduce the risk of noncommunicable disease including cancer.

Changing Emphasis on Fruits and Vegetables

Still included in the ACS recommendations (see Box 21-1) is consumption of 2½ cups of fruits and vegetables daily. Scientific emphasis on overall fruit and vegetable intake to prevent cancer has been moderated because large prospective studies showed weak or absent effects on cancer risk, perhaps because all fruits and vegetables were lumped together for analysis. In addition, potatoes and some fruit juices have high glycemic indexes and increase insulin secretion (see Obesity section earlier in this chapter).

Although blanket protection against cancer by fruits and vegetables is unlikely, as sources of beneficial phytochemicals, certain fruits and vegetables may bolster defenses against the development of cancer (Table 21-2).

Complicating the interpretation of the evidence is the concept that dietary patterns can result in synergistic and antagonistic interactions among bioactive components that likely contribute to the inconsistencies in observed biologic responses to functional foods. Additionally, the focus on identifying bioactive components in fruits and vegetables with the goal of developing single agents using a pharmacologic approach has been criticized on the basis that no chemopreventive strategies that are standard of care in medical practice have resulted from that approach.

Although there is little research regarding the ability for specific fruits and vegetables to prevent or reduce the risk of cancer, we do recognize the benefits of diets high in fruits and vegetables. When eaten in whole form, fruits and vegetables offer additional fiber and phytochemicals that offer protective benefits. A diet high in fruits and vegetables helps to maintain a lower BMI, which is associated with decreased cancer risk.

Balance, Moderation, and Variety—Again

Unfortunately, there is no nutritional bulletproof vest against cancer. Population studies that found links between vegetable and fruit intakes and decreased cancer cases investigated whole foods. Whether the specific components can be proven to prevent cancer remains to be seen. For most people, including generous amounts of plant products in the diet is a healthful strategy.

Consumption of vegetables and fruits is especially important if they replace other more kilocaloric-dense foods. On the other hand, if the produce is fried or served with rich sauces, or the fruit is converted to high-kilocaloric beverages, the goal of reaching and maintaining a healthy weight will be thwarted.

TABLE 21-2   Potential Cancer Risk Reduction From Phytochemicals

PHYTOCHEMICAL	SOURCE	BENEFIT
Carotenoids	Red, orange, and green fruits and vegetables	May inhibit cancer cell growth, antioxidant
Flavonoids	Apples, citrus fruit, onion, soy products, coffee, and tea	May inhibit inflammation and tumor growth
Indoles	Cruciferous vegetables, including broccoli, cauliflower, Brussels sprouts	May induce detoxification of carcinogens
Isoflavone	Cruciferous vegetables	May limit production of cancer-related hormones, works as antioxidant
Polyphenols	Cherries, rosemary	Prevent cancer formation and prevent inflammation

Adapted from: American Institute of Cancer Research (2017). Phytochemicals: the cancer fighters in your food. Available at http://www.aicr.org/reduce-your-cancer-risk/diet/elements_phytochemicals.html.

Nutrition for Cancer Clients

A cancer survivor is anyone who has been diagnosed with cancer, from the time of diagnosis through the rest of his or her life. The 5-year survival rate is the percentage of persons still living 5 years after diagnosis. The 5-year relative survival rate for all cancers combined is now approximately 69%. Among whites, it is about 67.5%; among blacks, about 61%. For the five cancers most commonly diagnosed in adults, the 5-year survival rates were as follows:

- Breast, 89.7%
- Bladder, 77.5%
- Prostate, 98.9%
- Colorectal, 65.1%
- Lung, 17.7% (National Institutes of Health, National Cancer Institute; September 12, 2016)

Given advances in early detection and treatment, the number of cancer survivors in the United States is estimated to exceed 12 million. Approximately 1 in every 25 Americans is a cancer survivor, and about 68% of Americans diagnosed with cancer now live more than 5 years. The trajectory of cancer survivorship is marked by three general stages:

1. Acute stage—diagnosis through recovery.
2. Extended—cancer-free, maintaining remission, or living with cancer; feelings of anxiety or fear often remain.
3. Permanent—Longer-term survival client may have long-term effects from diagnosis or treatment.

Good nutrition can have a role across each stage. Malnutrition in cancer clients affects prognosis and choices of treatment. Malnutrition is present in 15% to 40% of clients at diagnosis with an increased percentage to 80% in advanced stages of disease (Vidal-Casariego, Pintor-de la Maza, Calleia-Fernandez, & Villar-Taibo, 2015). For any given type of tumor, survival is shorter in clients with significant pretreatment weight loss (more than 10% of usual body weight).

Nutrition and Physical Activity During Active Treatment and Recovery

All of the major modalities of cancer treatment, including surgery, radiation, and chemotherapy, can significantly affect nutritional needs by:

- Altering usual eating habits
- Adversely affecting digestion, absorption, and metabolism of food

A complete nutritional assessment should begin as soon after diagnosis as possible to identify any nutritional deficiencies. The physical changes evoked by treatments are only part of the difficulty encountered in adequately nourishing cancer clients. Likely to also affect food intake are psychological factors, such as pain, anxiety, depression, xerostomia, and early satiety.

During active cancer treatment, the overall goals of nutritional care should be to:

- Prevent or resolve nutrient deficiencies
- Achieve or maintain a healthy weight
- Preserve lean body mass
- Minimize nutrition-related side effects

Randomized controlled trials have demonstrated that aerobic exercise significantly reduced cancer-related fatigue during and postcancer therapy. In relation to diagnosis, exercise decreased fatigue in clients with breast or prostate cancer but not in those with hematological malignancies. Aerobic exercise and/or physical activity significantly reduced fatigue but further studies need to be done on type, intensity, and duration that is needed for benefit (Mitchell et al, 2014).

Concerns that the estrogenic activity of isoflavones may have adverse effects on breast cancer recurrence have been assuaged. One study demonstrated risk reductions of 29% for breast cancer in Asian women who consumed a high-soy diet, greater than 20 grams per day, compared to a low-soy diet, less than 5 grams per day (Watson, Stalker, Jones, & Moorehead, 2015). A moderate amount of soy is 1 to 2 standard servings of whole-soy foods, such as tofu, soy milk, and edamame (American Institute for Cancer Research, 2017).

Living After Recovery

Determining exactly when a cancer's aberrant cell division began is difficult because of:

- Cancer's long development time
- The complex interaction between cancer cells and the body's defenses

Equating the beginning of the cancer with the date of diagnosis is measurable but misleading. Consequently, it may be too much to expect that lifestyle changes after diagnosis would make a major difference in the client's outcome.

Nevertheless, during this posttreatment phase, setting and achieving lifelong goals for weight management, a physically active lifestyle, and a healthy diet are important to promote overall health, quality of life, and longevity.

Weight Management

The ACS advises cancer survivors to achieve and maintain a healthy weight. The ACS advocates that individuals use My-Plate Supertracker tools to help manage weight, and ensure that physical activity recommendations are being met, and dietary guidelines are being followed.

Physical Activity

The ACS advises cancer survivors to engage in regular physical activity, to avoid inactivity, and return to normal daily activities as soon as possible after diagnosis. Specifically, the ACS recommends 150 minutes of exercise per week, including strength training at least 2 days per week (ACS, 2017).

The American College of Sports Medicine concurs with the ACS with the caveat to consult with the medical staff to assess tumor site–specific issues. Receiving particular mention are clients with breast cancer, prostate cancer, intestinal stomas, and morbid obesity. The National Comprehensive Cancer Network [NCCN], which produces evidence-based standards of care guidelines, recommends that survivors obtain referral to physical therapy to facilitate exercise during fatigue (NCCN, April 10, 2017).

In short, individual assessment underlies safe implementation of an exercise program in cancer survivors. Many survivors can safely begin a low- to moderate-intensity exercise program, such as walking, without supervision or exercise specialist evaluation.

Dietary Patterns

The ACS advises cancer survivors to consume a diet that is high in vegetables, fruits, and whole grains and to follow the Guidelines on Nutrition and Physical Activity for Cancer Prevention summarized in Box 21-1. Despite efforts to find a "magic bullet" among micronutrients, none has been demonstrated to be effective in humans with an established cancer. Studies have concluded that Western diets high in animal fats and sugars and low in fiber increase the risk of colon cancer and breast cancer (Microbiota Key to Diet-Associated Risk for Colon Cancer, 2015; Gtahani et al, 2017).

Advanced Cancer and End of Life

A diagnosis of cancer does not necessarily mean that the person will die of cancer. For instance, women with low-grade localized endometrial cancer were most likely to die of cardiovascular disease, whereas women with high-grade advanced cancer were most likely to die of endometrial cancer.

That is not to minimize the fact that it is estimated that there will be 600,920 deaths from cancer in the United States in 2017 (ACS Facts and Figures, 2017). Those clients should receive the best care available with emphasis on maximizing the quality of their remaining life.

Diet and Exercise

Recommendations for nutrition and physical activity in those who are living with advanced cancer are best based on individual nutrition needs and physical abilities. To the extent possible, physical activity should be encouraged.

Although advanced cancer is sometimes accompanied by substantial weight loss, it is not inevitable that individuals with cancer lose weight or experience malnutrition. In general, the goal should be to optimize nutritional state and encourage repair of tissues not only during cancer surgery or procedures but throughout the course of cancer therapy to decrease morbidity and increase quality of life.

Many clients with advanced cancer choose to adapt their food choices and meal patterns to meet nutritional needs and to manage cancer symptoms or treatment side effects. Additional nutritional supplementation such as nutrient-dense beverages and foods can be consumed by those who cannot eat or drink enough to maintain sufficient energy intake. The use of enteral nutrition and parenteral nutrition support should be individualized with recognition of overall treatment goals (control or palliation) and the associated risks of medical complications and/or ethical dilemmas. Modalities of nutritional support for cancer clients are shown in Table 21-3. The goal of nutrition intervention is to support anabolism, body composition, functional status, and quality of life. When designed in a structured, formal nutrition care process, nutrition support can be effective in clients with cancer and all clients should have a nutritional assessment at diagnosis.

Enteral and parenteral nutrition are covered in detail in Chapter 14. Care of the client with terminal illness is the subject of Chapter 24.

TABLE 21-3   **Nutritional Therapies for Cancer Clients**

	INDICATIONS	CLINICAL RESULTS	PRECAUTIONS
Oral	Clients with decreased kilocaloric or nutrient intake	Enhanced long-term oral intake Weight maintenance Preservation of lean body mass Improved quality of life	Dietitian's conversion of prescribed diet to acceptable meal plan is critical to success
Enteral	Head and neck or thoracic cancer with obstructive masses If oral food intake is insufficient despite dietary counseling and supplements Severe mucositis	Weight gain Decreased infectious complications than with PN Prevents dehydration and interference with treatment due to inflammation of the mouth	Monitor swallowing ability to discontinue artificial feeding when appropriate Pulmonary aspiration is the most concerning complication
Parenteral	Negative side effects of treatment, including radiation enteritis or chemotherapy/radiation diarrhea Malnourished clients before chemotherapy or surgery	Improved nutrient laboratory values	Prolonged survival if nutritional goals are met In most cases, inappropriate if diagnosis is terminal Increased risk of infection compared to enteral nutrition
Pharmacotherapy			
Appetite stimulants	*Megestrol* *Cyproheptadine* *Prednisolone* *Dexamethasone*	Weight gain, much of it fat Improved quality of life	Decreased proinflammatory cytokines Decreased nausea Increased caloric intake
Antidepressant drugs	*Sertraline* *Citalopram*	Relief of anorexia Possible weight gain	Major depression occurs in about 6.4%–17.8% of advanced-cancer clients 50% of advanced-cancer clients met diagnostic criteria for psychiatric conditions
Antiemetic drugs	*Fosaprepitant* *Ondansetron* *Dexamethasone* *Methylphenidate*	Reduce incidence of electrolyte imbalance, dehydration, malnutrition Combination therapy typically is most effective	Up to 80% of clients receiving chemotherapy will experience nausea
Stimulant		Relief of anorexia Relief of depression	Causes anorexia in clients without cancer

Adapted from Cotogni (2016); Mondello et al (2015); Bausewein et al (2015); Thomas, Randolph, & Pruemer (2015); Koth & Kolesar (2017).

Common Nutritional Problems

Some nutritional problems in cancer clients are due to the disease, and others are due to treatment modalities. Common problems affecting the consumption of meals and nourishment of cancer clients are early satiety and anorexia, taste alterations, local effects in the mouth, nausea, vomiting, diarrhea, and altered immune response. Cachexia is a wasting condition seen in cancer and other diseases.

EARLY SATIETY AND ANOREXIA

Although they may look starved, cancer clients may take a few bites of food and declare that they are full. They may say that they have no appetite at all. The main source of this symptom is the cancer itself, by mechanisms that are beginning to be understood. Control of the disease improves the appetite.

Sometimes, however, the physical pressure from the tumor or **third-space** fluid accumulation may give a feeling of fullness. Relieving that problem may improve food intake.

Some additional factors may interfere with appetite. The psychological stress of dealing with cancer may produce anxiety or depression. The person may be grappling with a body image change or may be going through the grieving process for the loss of a body function or the potential loss of life itself.

Interventions

- Encourage eating whether hungry or not.
- Exercise appropriately before meals.
- Serve small, frequent, attractive meals.
- For inpatients, serve favorite foods from home or a family-shared meal.
- For children, serve food in shapes or decorated with the child's name.
- Vary supplement flavors to prevent taste fatigue.
- Offer 1 ounce of a complete supplement every hour.
- Add nutrients to regular foods.
  - $1\frac{1}{3}$ cups (or whatever amount satisfies) of instant dry skim milk powder in 1 quart of liquid milk increases

the nutrient density, with little or no change in palatability.

- 1 tablespoon of dry skim milk powder in mashed potatoes or puddings.

TASTE ALTERATIONS

Cancer clients may have changes in taste perceptions, particularly a decreased threshold for bitterness. Accordingly, they will often say that beef and pork taste bitter or metallic. Some clients report a decreased sensation of sweet, salty, and sour tastes, and they desire increased seasonings. These taste changes are caused by the cancer and the various modes of therapy. In some cases, taste acuity returns 2 to 3 months after cessation of treatment. Unfortunately, clients who have undergone treatment for head and neck cancers may have permanent changes in taste (McLaughlin & Mahon, 2014).

Interventions

- Provide oral hygiene before meals to freshen the mouth.
- Offer lemon-flavored beverages to improve taste sensations.
- Cook in a microwave oven or in glass utensils to minimize the metallic taste.
- Offer plastic table service if metal utensils are a problem.
- Serve eggs, fish, poultry, and dairy products that may be better received than beef or pork.
- Serve meat cold or at room temperature to lessen the bitter taste.
- Add sweet sauces and marinades to the meat to improve its palatability.

LOCAL EFFECTS IN THE MOUTH

Because of the rapid cellular turnover in the oral mucosa, a common adverse reaction to chemotherapy and radiotherapy is **stomatitis**. Also, clients being treated with radiation for head and neck cancers often experience inflammation or ulcers in the mouth, decreased and thick saliva, and swallowing difficulty. Any of these conditions may interfere with nutritional intake.

Interventions

- For all: provide oral hygiene, before and after meals.
- For mouth ulcerations, try the following strategies:
  - Serve soft, mild foods.
  - Top foods with sauces, gravies, and dressings, which may make foods easier to eat.
  - Serve cream soups and milk, which provide much nutrition for the volume ingested.
  - Serve cold foods, which have a somewhat numbing effect and may be better tolerated than hot food.
  - Include liquids with meals to help wash down the food.
  - Introduce drinking straws, which may detour liquids around mouth ulcerations.
  - Avoid these irritants (a highly recommended strategy): hot items, salty or spicy foods, acidic juices, and alcohol (even in mouthwash).

- If necessary, seek an anesthetic mouthwash, which can be prescribed. If the mouth is anesthetized, clients should be instructed to chew slowly and carefully to avoid biting their lips, tongue, or cheeks.
- For dry mouth, try the following strategies:
  - Include adequate hydration to help keep the mouth moist.
  - Present food with lubricants such as gravy, butter, margarine, milk, beer, or bouillon to aid intake.
  - Offer sugarless hard candy, chewing gum, or popsicles to stimulate saliva production.
- For swallowing difficulty, try the following strategies (see also the box on dysphagia in Chapter 9):
  - Advise the client to make swallowing a conscious act (inhaling, swallowing, and exhaling) to lessen the risk of choking.
  - Suggest experimenting with head position, which may ease the dysphagia. Tilting the head backward or forward may help.
  - Serve foods that are nonsticky and of even consistency to minimize swallowing difficulty. Lumpy gravy and mixed vegetables, for example, are hard to manage.
  - Suggest dunking bread products in beverages to help lubricate the passage.
  - Refer to a speech therapist as necessary.

NAUSEA, VOMITING, AND DIARRHEA

This triad of symptoms often accompanies radiation treatment or chemotherapy, as well as certain types of tumors. Because the gastrointestinal tract cells are normally replaced every few days, these rapidly dividing cells are more vulnerable to cancer treatments than other body cells. Not all clients suffer these side effects to the same extent, and the effects generally cease when the treatment is completed. See also Table 21-3 for antiemetic therapy.

Some clients are disabled by diarrhea but reluctant to seek help, perhaps believing that their situation is normal. Both during and after treatment ends, questions about specific symptoms could bring to light a condition amenable to correction.

Radiation enteritis involves injury to the intestine. Clients at greater risk of radiation enteritis are those:

- Who receive radiation to abdomen or pelvis
- Who have had previous abdominal surgery
- Who have hypertension, diabetes mellitus, or pelvic inflammatory disease
- Who receive chemotherapy along with the radiation
- Who are older in age

Interventions

For nausea and vomiting, try the following strategies:

- Offer the client dry crackers before rising.
- Schedule meals at times of the day when nausea is least.
- Serve liquids 30 to 60 minutes after solid food.

- Limit fats in the diet to promote gastric emptying.
- Teach the client to eat slowly and chew thoroughly.
- Suggest the client rest after eating.
- Recommend that the client save favorite foods for times of feeling well to avoid food aversion.
- Instruct the client to take antiemetics and analgesics as prescribed. Pain also causes nausea.
- Advise the client or caregiver to minimize strong cooking odors by
  - Selecting milder foods
  - Ventilating the kitchen
  - Preparing food in a microwave oven or by boil-in-bag methods

For diarrhea, try the following strategies:

- Add pectin-containing (apple, banana) foods to the client's intake.
- Implement a low-fiber diet (see Chapter 20).
- Test for and treat lactose intolerance.
- Consult with a dietitian about special feedings.

ALTERED IMMUNE RESPONSE

Sometimes antineoplastic agents suppress the client's immune system. Clients receiving them are at risk for overwhelming infections from organisms that would not affect other persons. Clients receiving radiation therapy or radiation as part of bone marrow transplantation also are at high risk for infections and need to be protected from all organisms, even those that are harmless to most healthy people. Clinical Application 21-2 relates the role of the aging immune system to cancer.

Interventions

Depending on the client's condition, the following strategies may be used.

- Institute protective isolation to minimize exposure to microorganisms.
- Observe strict procedures for food safety and sanitation (see Chapter 13).

CACHEXIA

A state of malnutrition and wasting is called **cachexia**, but muscle wasting due to cancer differs from that which occurs in starvation and aging. Also seen in other advanced diseases, a degree of cancer-induced cachexia is experienced by up to 80% of advanced-stage cancer clients (Camargo et al, 2015).

Cancer cachexic results from a complex cascade of physiologic and metabolic derangements involving synthesis, storage, and degradation of all three macronutrients, including fat, carbohydrate, and protein. Cachexia is characterized by:

- Systemic inflammation
- Negative protein and energy balance
- Involuntary loss of lean body mass (Aoyagi et al, 2015)

The cause of cancer-cachexia is complex and research believes that it is a combination of secretion of tumor-derived factors, changes in cytokine levels, and treatment-induced anorexia that contribute to impaired pathways that regulate normal eating (Mondello et al, 2015). Diagnostic components

CLINICAL APPLICATION   21-2

Role of the Immune System in Cancer

Age is the most important risk factor for tumorigenesis. More than 60% of new cancers and more than 70% of cancer deaths occur in persons older than 65 years. Many lines of evidence point to the most important factor simply being the passage of time allowing for prolonged exposure to environmental carcinogens. Immune competence tends to decrease with age, a phenomenon termed *immunosenescence*. Immunosenescence has been associated with negative outcomes such as disposition for new infections and pathologic conditions with a suspected role in the development of cancer (Onyema et al, 2015). Further research is necessary in this area.

The immune system can recognize and eliminate tumor cells, but the tumors also can interfere with and evade immune responses through multiple mechanisms. The increased incidence of cancer in AIDS clients and organ transplant clients on immunosuppressive drugs demonstrates the consequence of a weakened immune system.

Part of the body's immune defense is provided by certain white blood cells called **T-lymphocytes.** These cells have the task of recognizing foreign materials, including cancer cells, as "nonself" and acting to destroy the invaders. Some of the T-lymphocytes develop into killer cells, which bind to the foreign cell membrane and release lysosomal enzymes into the foreign cell to destroy it.

The T-lymphocytes mature in the **thymus** gland in the chest, hence the name *thymic lymphocytes*. Possibly contributing to the development of cancer in the elderly is the deterioration of the immune system, because the thymus gland begins to shrink at sexual maturity, and by age 50 only 10% of the original gland remains.

Present knowledge only suggests that the age-related immune alterations are likely to favor the development of tumors.

include unintentional weight loss of >5% over 6 months, loss of skeletal muscle mass, and low kilocaloric intake.

Cachexia can result in:

- Impaired physical function
- Increased psychosocial distress
- Reduced tolerance to treatment
- Decreased quality of life
- Increased mortality (Sun, Quan, & Yu, 2015)

The result is inefficient use of whatever nutrients are supplied to the client. Treatment of cachexia is complex and often not possible in end-stage disease. Treatment should include a combination of modalities. Figure 21-4 shows a woman with cachexia.

Interventions

Depending on the cachectic client's condition and wishes and the provider's judgment, the following strategies to improve nutrition may be implemented.

- Best choice—aggressive treatment of the cancer.
- Appropriately treat symptoms interfering with nutritional intake (see Chapter 24).
- Reassure client that poor appetite is caused by the cancer not by his or her lack of effort.

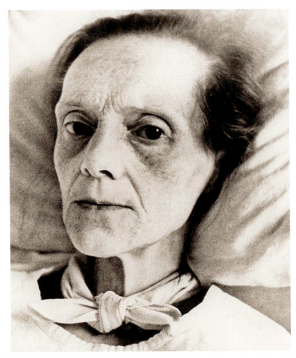

FIGURE 21-4 This woman is cachectic, showing signs of malnutrition and wasting. *(Reproduced from* Nutrition Today, *16(3), cover, © Williams & Wilkins, 1981, with permission.)*

- Encourage available medications (see Table 21-3) to improve the quality of life.
- In selected clients, supplementation with omega-3 fatty acids (fish oil) or protein may be advised (Gullett et al, 2011).

The Charting Tip in Box 21-2 advocates forethought when documenting cancer clients' at-home treatments and diet plans.

One should not expect identical disease outcomes in different people. Just as human beings vary in characteristics, so do cancers differ from one another. Much of the difference in treatment outcomes for clients with cancer stems from variations in tumor biology.

BOX 21-2 ■ Charting Tip

When admitting a client who provides much of his or her own care at home, try to learn all about treatments and dietary preferences and document them. It is essential for these clients to have complete nutritional assessments upon admission. If the client becomes less self-sufficient after surgery or after beginning cancer therapy, the staff will not have to ask multiple questions before providing care. Recording this information in the electronic medical record ensures that others besides the nurse who obtained it will be able to meet the client's needs.

KEYSTONES

- Alcohol intake plus overweight and obesity, caused by poor diet and inactivity, are related to breast and colon cancer occurrence. Red or processed meat intake is related to prostate cancer occurrence.
- The best dietary advice to prevent cancer: avoid obesity, stay physically active, consume a healthy plant-based diet with limited red and processed meats, and drink minimal amounts of alcohol if at all.
- The New American Plate® includes amounts and sample foods in the graphic but omits specific reference to dairy foods. MyPlate includes online resources to assist in implementation. Depending on the learner's motivation and abilities, either could serve as a starting point for instruction.
- Studying fruits and vegetables in general may not contain sufficient items that really might be of benefit. In more focused studies, the selected study components are likely an infinitesimal part of the whole food from which it comes. A study may be too short to account for the long lead-time in cancer development.
- The anorexic client with cancer could benefit from appropriate exercise before meals, small amounts of complete nutritional supplements hourly, added dry milk powder to appropriate foods, and efforts to make mealtime special and pleasurable.

- Protective isolation is common for clients with altered immune responses. Dietary strategies to protect the immunosuppressed client are directed at strict adherence to food safety and sanitation procedures. Some providers may wish to limit the client's access to unpasteurized, uncooked, and unwashed foods.
- Appetite stimulants may succeed in increasing a cancer client's weight (mostly fat) and are credited with increasing the quality of life. An anabolic steroid has been approved to increase lean body mass in cancer clients. Antidepressants and a stimulant may also relieve anorexia.
- Nutrient intake in clients with mouth ulcerations may be enhanced by using straws to bypass the sores; by serving cool, smooth, bland nutrient-dense foods; and by avoiding acidic, salty, and spicy foods.
- Cachexia is a wasting condition thought to be caused by an inflammatory response to the tumor. The result is a complex cascade of physiologic and metabolic derangements involving synthesis, storage, and degradation of all three macronutrients: fat, carbohydrate, and protein. Weight loss in cachexic clients cannot be reversed by increased nutrient intake alone. Controlling the cancer is the best method of reversing cachexia.

CASE STUDY 21-1

Mrs. Z is a 67-year-old widow who had a lumpectomy for breast cancer yesterday. If no complications arise, she is scheduled for discharge tomorrow. The nurse providing her morning care asked how she felt.

"Terrible."

"Do you need something for pain?"

"No, I had something a little while ago. I'm just overwhelmed. This happened so fast. I don't know how I'm going to manage all I have to do. The doctor said I was a good candidate for lumpectomy but I don't know how I will get to radiation therapy. He also said I should lose weight. What good will that do—I've already got cancer!"

"Had cancer. It's gone, remember?"

The nurse continued to explore Mrs. Z's risk factors conversationally. She eats the typical Western diet, red meat about every other day, a glass of wine, maybe two, daily with dinner. It was a habit she and her husband had until his death from colon cancer 9 months ago shortly after they retired and moved south. Mrs. Z is 5 ft 4 in. tall and weighs 175 lb. She has no children, no relatives in the area, and no church affiliation.

CARE PLAN

Subjective Data
Uncertain of ability to obtain radiation treatment ■ Lacks information about risk factors for breast cancer ■ Feeling overwhelmed; widowed <1 year

Objective Data
Admission weight 175 pounds, height 5 ft 4 in. ■ BMI 30.1

Analysis
Lack of resources related to procuring cancer treatment; lack of information related to breast cancer prevention

Plan

DESIRED OUTCOMES EVALUATION CRITERIA	ACTIONS/ INTERVENTIONS	RATIONALE
Client will formulate plan to attend radiation therapy by discharge.	Refer to social worker to be seen today.	Ensuring that client has a bridge to continuing therapy will increase likelihood of completing the regimen.
Client will acknowledge three risk factors for breast cancer pertinent to her situation.	Teach that obesity and alcohol are recognized risk factors for breast cancer.	Acknowledging personal risk factors for breast cancer is the first step to changing behavior.
	Point out that · Diet is only one of many possible factors leading to cancer. · Physical activity has been linked to decreases in recurrence of breast cancer. · Lifestyle changes may prevent a second primary cancer in her unaffected breast that has been subjected to the same risk factors as the operated breast.	Recognizing the many factors that play a role in developing cancer should alleviate regrets and guilt about the cause of her cancer.
	Present or review information on a healthy diet according to the American Cancer Society.	Focusing on what can be done now and in the future to change her risk factors offers a measure of control to the client and encourages a positive outlook.

TEAMWORK 21-1

SOCIAL WORKER'S NOTES

The following Social Worker's Notes are representative of the documentation found in a client's medical record.

The social worker, after interviewing Mrs. Z, wrote the following:

Subjective: *Lacks transportation to radiation therapy.*

Widowed, without social support system in place.

States that the doctor recommended weight reduction.

Objective: *Coherent. Ready to accept advice.*

Analysis: *Immediate need is transportation to and from radiation therapy.*

Secondary need is social support system to cope with diagnosis and lifestyle changes.

Plan: *Set up transportation with American Cancer Society (ACS).*

Recommend follow-up with support group at ACS.

CRITICAL THINKING QUESTIONS

1. What additional assessment data might impact the design of Mrs. Z's nutritional care plan?

2. Was the nurse's statement, "Had cancer. It's gone …," a wise reply? Why or why not?

3. Do you think that there is a relationship between Mrs. Z's cancer and that of Mr. Z's illness and death? Why or why not?

CHAPTER REVIEW

1. A client with a strong family history of colon cancer asks the nurse for dietary advice to decrease cancer risk. Which of the following statements would be best?
   1. "There are no dietary modifications that will decrease your cancer risk."
   2. "You should consume a diet high in fruits and vegetables."
   3. "You should eat red meat only once daily."
   4. "Fruit juice is an acceptable substitution for whole fruits to reduce colon cancer risk."

2. Cruciferous vegetables that are thought to protect against cancer are:
   1. Corn, lima beans, and peas
   2. Carrots, green beans, and tomatoes
   3. Brussels sprouts, bean sprouts, and water chestnuts
   4. Broccoli, cauliflower, and cabbage

3. Which of the following foods is likely to be well received by a cancer client with mouth ulcerations?
   1. Hot chicken noodle soup
   2. Orange juice with orange sherbet
   3. Vanilla milkshake
   4. Bagel with cream cheese

4. Which of the following interventions except one are likely to assist a client with cancer who suffers from anorexia. Select all that apply.
   1. Confining the diet to full liquids
   2. Sipping complete nutritional supplements hourly between meals
   3. Serving meals attractively
   4. Exercising as possible before meals
   5. Serve small, frequent meals

5. Heterocyclic aromatic amines (HCAs), formed by high-temperature cooking of muscle meats, are risk factors for
   1. Breast cancer
   2. Colorectal cancer
   3. Lung cancer
   4. Prostate cancer

CLINICAL ANALYSIS

1. Mrs. R is a 70-year-old widow under treatment for breast cancer. She is being cared for by her daughter, Ms. S, with assistance from a home health-care service. Despite fairly good oral intake at the daughter's urging, Mrs. R continues to lose weight and now carries 95 lb on her 5-ft 4-in. frame. Her main complaint regarding food is its bitter taste.

   Ms. S asks why her mother continues to lose weight when she is taking half the meals and more than half the supplements offered. Which of the following replies by the nurse would be most appropriate?
   a. "Your mother must be too active and using more calories than she is taking in."
   b. "Probably the medications are dehydrating her. We should increase her fluid intake."
   c. "Frequently the tumor short-circuits the body's metabolism so that nutrients cannot be used normally."
   d. "She doesn't take in enough protein to prevent loss of muscle. We should try supplements of amino acid powders."

2. Ms. S expressed interest in learning what she could do to lessen her own chances of developing a malignancy of the breast. Which of the following suggestions have the best evidence for preventing breast cancer?
   a. Limit intake of red, processed, or charbroiled meats.
   b. Maintain a normal weight and minimize or avoid alcohol intake.
   c. Gradually increase fiber intake to 25 grams per day, accompanied by adequate fluid intake.
   d. Eat a variety of colorful fruits and vegetables every day.

3. Which of the following interventions could alleviate the metallic tastes Ms. R is experiencing?
   a. Cooking meats in the microwave oven in glass dishes
   b. Limiting the intake of dairy products
   c. Selecting only very tender cuts or ground beef
   d. Cooking fish outside on the grill to eliminate odors

CHAPTER 22

Nutrition in Critical Care

LEARNING OBJECTIVES

After completing this chapter, the student should be able to:
- List four hypermetabolic conditions that increase resting energy expenditure and hence kilocaloric requirements.
- Describe how metabolism differs in starvation and hypermetabolism.
- Discuss the effects of impaired respiratory function on nutritional status and appropriate nutritional therapy.
- List six recommendations for the safe refeeding of malnourished clients.

Clients admitted to critical care units have life-threatening injuries and illnesses. Acute conditions may include severe burns, trauma, and infections. The most likely chronic conditions related to admission to critical care units are respiratory and cardiac problems. This chapter focuses on clients admitted with respiratory problems. Chapter 18 focused on cardiac care. The body responds to life-threatening injuries and illnesses with a hypermetabolic response. The provision of nutritional care for these clients is a challenge. Under- or overfeeding these clients may result in a loss of lean body mass and death, respectively.

Stress and Critical Care

Metabolically the body responds to starvation by decreasing energy expenditure and to hypermetabolism by increasing energy expenditure. Some of the major complications seen in critical care include:

- Inflammation
- Sepsis (blood infection)
- Gastrointestinal (GI) effects
- Wounds
- Fluid imbalances
- Multisystem organ failure

The Stress of Starvation

The physical stress of starvation alters nutrient needs. Biologically, our bodies evolved to cope with periods of feast or famine. Our response to the stress of starvation evolved slowly over the course of millions of years. The human body's response to food deprivation allowed a person to survive despite inadequate food for longer periods than after other physical assaults.

Uncomplicated starvation means that the client is experiencing food deprivation without an underlying disease state. During uncomplicated starvation, clients expend about 70% of the kilocalories they normally need to maintain body weight. Because of the biochemical adaptation to starvation, these clients require fewer kilocalories than is normal for their height and weight.

The breakdown or catabolism of nutrient stores to meet energy needs characterizes our initial response to starvation. Every cell within the human body needs a constant supply of energy to function. During starvation, a series of four chemical reactions occurs to meet each cell's energy needs:

1. **Glycogenolysis** is the breakdown of glycogen (the liver's carbohydrate stores). This breakdown releases glucose into the bloodstream. However, the body's limited glycogen stores last only a few hours.
2. **Gluconeogenesis** is the production of glucose from noncarbohydrate stores (only the glycerol portion of triglycerides and amino acids derived from proteins in muscle and organ mass). The primary source of glucose in early starvation is the increased rate of gluconeogenesis, which causes a reduction of lean body mass.
3. **Lipolysis** is the breakdown of adipose tissue for energy. This breakdown releases free fatty acids into the bloodstream. In prolonged starvation, adaptive mechanisms conserve body protein stores by enabling a greater proportion of energy needs to be met by increased fatty acids, with a decreased requirement for glucose.
4. **Ketosis** is the accumulation of ketone bodies: acetone, beta-hydroxybutyric acid, and acetoacetic acid. Ketosis results from the incomplete metabolism of fatty acids, generally from carbohydrate deficiency, and occurs commonly in starvation. The body uses some ketone bodies for energy during prolonged starvation to meet the central nervous system's need for glucose. This use of ketones reduces, but does not eliminate, the need for glucose.

These chemical reactions are summarized in Figure 22-1.

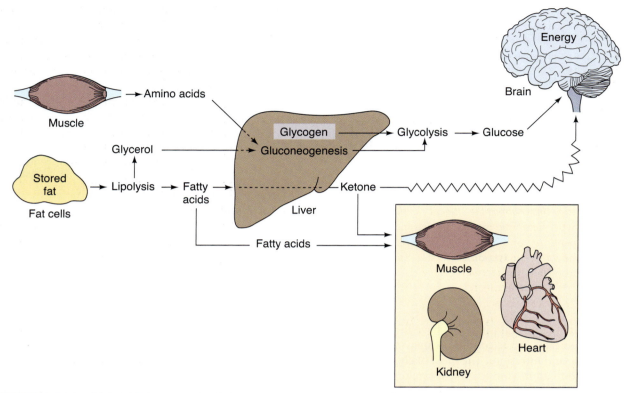

FIGURE 22-1 Origin of fuel and fuel consumption during starvation. The primary source of glucose in early starvation (after the depletion of glycogen stores) is the increased rate of gluconeogenesis. In prolonged starvation, adaptive mechanisms conserve protein by enabling a greater proportion of energy needs to be met by ketone bodies, with a decreased requirement for glucose.

Each body cell needs glucose, fatty acids, or the end products of fatty acids and amino acids for energy. Body cells need fuel constantly. Amino acids can be used for energy, but only after the liver converts them into glucose or fat. Specific organs have a preference for glucose as a fuel source. The brain, for example, prefers glucose for energy. Some cells can also use ketone bodies for energy. The brain will use ketone bodies but prefers glucose. For the most part, the human body can use only a small part of the fat molecule, the glycerol portion, to manufacture glucose. Therefore, after the liver's glycogen stores are depleted, body protein stores must be continually broken down to supply the brain with glucose during starvation.

The heart, kidney, and skeletal muscle tissues prefer fatty acids and ketone bodies for their fuel sources. As a result, even if a starving person is fed glucose (as in intravenous feeding), some fat is still needed to prevent the breakdown of adipose tissue. A balance of the end products of fat and carbohydrate metabolism is necessary for survival.

In prolonged starvation, most body organs switch to a less-preferred fuel source. Even the brain increasingly uses more ketone bodies for energy after adaptation to starvation than before. The breakdown of muscle tissue continues in prolonged starvation but at a much lower rate. The human body also becomes more efficient in reusing amino acids for protein synthesis. Thus, urea nitrogen excretion decreases during prolonged starvation.

The rate of tissue breakdown in prolonged starvation also decreases because the metabolic rate and total energy expenditure decrease to conserve energy and prolong life. The catabolic or starved individual spontaneously decreases physical activity, increases sleep, and has a lower body temperature. All of these adaptations during prolonged starvation serve one purpose—to prolong life. The human body gets "more miles per gallon" as a result of individual body organs switching to a less-preferred fuel source.

Hypermetabolism

An abnormal increase in the rate at which fuel or kilocalories are burned is called **hypermetabolism.** Characteristics of this condition are:

- Increased metabolic rate
- Negative nitrogen balance
- Hyperglycemia
- Increased oxygen consumption

Box 22-1 discusses the benefits of intensive insulin therapy in critical care clients. The body increasingly uses protein obtained from internal body stores (lean body mass) to meet energy needs and depletes lean body mass.

Hormonal Response

The stress response in hypermetabolism is also mediated by hormones. The catecholamines, glucagon, and cortisol oppose insulin and are typically referred to as counter-regulatory hormones. Collectively these hormones influence glucose and fat metabolism by causing the breakdown of glycogen and amino acids to produce glucose and triglycerides from body fat stores. The body produces glucose so that it has the fuel to respond to stress. Two other hormones, aldosterone and antidiuretic hormone, also respond to stress, and the result is the retention of both water and sodium.

Metabolic Response

The metabolic response of the immune system to infection or injury is called the **inflammatory response.** The signs and symptoms of inflammation include:

- Swelling
- Redness
- Heat
- Pain

C-reactive protein (CRP) is released by the liver during acute phase of the inflammatory response and alters:

- Metabolism
- Heart rate
- Blood pressure
- Body temperature
- Immune cell function

CRP is frequently measured in critical care clients. One practical application of this metabolic response is that an individual's kilocalorie and protein intake may be sufficient, but their pre-albumin level remains depressed. The negative nitrogen balance seen cannot be prevented because metabolic processes during stress promote protein breakdown. The inflammatory response needs to run its course before anabolism begins again.

Early Feeding

When to start nutritional rehabilitation of the critical client is under debate. For example, when treating clients with burn injuries some physicians keep clients NPO (non per os) for the first 24 to 72 hours after admission, and others initiate tube feedings within 4 hours. Here, an important consideration is that **peristalsis,** the wavelike motion that propels food through the GI tract, ceases in some burn clients. Until peristalsis returns, the client's stomach should not be the site of choice for a tube feeding.

In addition, other critically ill clients may have an ileus caused by muscle paralysis or an obstruction. Physicians who do feed clients early insert the feeding tube into the client's intestines past the ileus and deliver a very slow, continuous-drip feeding. The slow, continuous drip minimizes the likelihood of the feeding collecting in the intestines.

Most institutions have a policy of measuring **gastric residual volume (GRV)** in clients with gastric tube feedings. To measure stomach contents that have not been absorbed, the nurse will periodically suction the stomach's gastric contents using a large bore syringe. Institutions will have varying policies regarding nursing intervention if GRV is 250 mL or greater. Research is supporting that tube feedings should not be stopped or reduced in clients with an isolate GRV of 250 mL when the client demonstrates no other signs of feeding intolerance (Heydari & Zeydi, 2014). Overestimating feeding intolerances by nurses can result in undernourishment in clients. There is a movement in institutional policy increasing GRV to 500 mL or greater before withholding feedings and recommending the use of monitor GRV be eliminated as an assessment tool in the critically ill client receiving enteral nutrition (McClave et al, 2016). If the critically ill client is adequately fluid resuscitated, then enteral nutrition should be started within 24 to 48 hours after surgery or admission to the critical care unit. Enteral nutrition is associated with a reduction in infectious complications and may reduce length of stay as opposed to parenteral nutrition.

Although early enteral feeding offers many advantages, in many cases it is not medically feasible. A functioning GI tract is a prerequisite to enteral feeding. These conditions preclude the use of enteral feedings:

- Low mesenteric blood (ischemic bowel)
- Severe hypotension
- Perforate bowel
- Peritonitis
- Chemotherapy- or radiation-induced mucositis
- Multisystem organ failure

For these clients, intravenous nutrition is obligatory. Clinical Calculation 22-1 demonstrates the calculation of a sample central parenteral solution. See Dollars & Sense 22-1 for information regarding the cost of intensive care treatment.

Examples of Hypermetabolism

Cancer, major surgery, burns, infections, and trauma are the physical stressors that have the greatest impact on metabolism. The needs of clients with cancer are described in Chapter 21. This section of this chapter focuses on the

CLINICAL CALCULATION   22-1

Calculating a Sample Central Parenteral Nutrition (CPN) Solution

These are the steps for calculating the total kilocalories and grams of protein in the following CPN solution: 500 mL D_{50}, 500 mL amino acids 10%, 250 mL lipid 10%.

DEXTROSE

D_{50} = 0.50 × 500 mL = 250 grams of dextrose
250 grams × 3.4 kcal/gram = 850 kcal

AMINO ACIDS

500 mL × 0.10 = 50 grams of protein
50 grams of protein × 4 kcal/gram = 200 kcal

LIPIDS

250 mL × 1.1 kcal/mL = 275 kcal

TOTAL KCALORIES

850 from dextrose + 200 from protein + 275 from lipid = 1,325 kcal

---

Dollars & Sense 22-1

Cost of Intensive Care Stay

Admissions to intensive care units result in burdening expense for hospitals as well as for the client. The mean cost of a terminal intensive care stay is estimated to be $39,300 ± $45,100, with day one charges of the stay being the most expensive (Khandelwal et al, 2016). Providing nutrition to the critically ill contributes to the cost of admission. Clients who require central parenteral nutrition will require placement of a central venous access device, specialized IV formula, and specialized equipment to deliver the solution, which all have associated costs. The Academy of Nutrition and Dietetics (2013) has confirmed that the use of enteral tube feeding reduces the cost of medical care in the critically ill client when compared to the use of CPN.

---

nutritional needs of clients experiencing surgery, burns, infections and fevers, and trauma. Nutritional support during extreme stress is needed to decrease the length of the stress, prevent complications, and minimize suffering.

SURGERY

Uncomplicated minor surgery increases the surgical client's kilocaloric requirement by only 5%. Surgery needed to repair soft tissue trauma requires a 14% to 37% increase in kilocalories. A surgical client with complications may require a large increase in kilocalories.

BURNS

Major burns are the most extreme state of stress a client can sustain and produce a hypermetabolic state that raises kilocaloric needs higher than those of most other stresses. Kilocaloric requirements may be as high as 8,000 calories per day. Even a client who was well nourished before becoming burned may rapidly develop protein–calorie malnutrition. The degree to which the metabolic rate increases

is directly related to the body surface area burned. The percentage of body surface area burned is determined by totaling the percentages in Figure 22-2A. Figure 22-2B illustrates first-degree (superficial), second-degree (partial thickness), and third-degree (full-thickness) burns. Studies

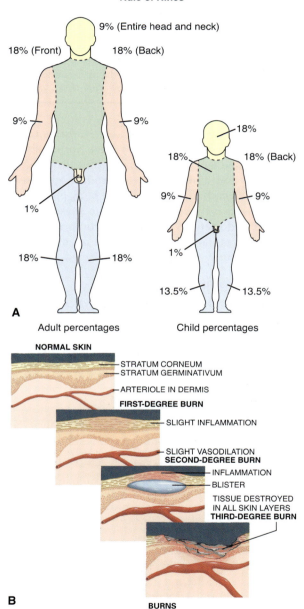

FIGURE 22-2 *A,* The percentage of body surface area burned is determined by comparing the body surface area of the client's burns to the percentages given in the chart. For example, if a client has extensive burns over both legs, the total body surface area burned would be 36% (18% for the first leg plus 18% for the second leg). *(Reprinted from Venes, D [ed]: Taber's Cyclopedic Medical Dictionary, ed 21. FA Davis, Philadelphia, 2010, by Beth Anne Willert, MS, Illustrator, with permission.)* *B,* Burns are classified as first degree, second degree, and third degree. *(Reprinted from Thomas, CL [ed]: Taber's Cyclopedic Medical Dictionary, ed 18. FA Davis, Philadelphia, 1997, p. 278, by Beth Anne Willert, MS, Illustrator, with permission.)*

show that the hypermetabolic state may remain elevated for 1 to 2 years after a severe thermal injury (Lunawat, Vishwani, Datey, & Singh, 2015).

An increase in waste products in some clients with burns requires an increase in fluids. Extra fluids help the kidneys eliminate waste products. Capillary permeability is increased in burn clients; thus, plasma proteins, fluids, and electrolytes escape into the burn area and interstitial space. This shift reduces the volume of plasma, and so fluid volume needs to be replaced. Fluid resuscitation in smaller burns, less than 20% total body surface area for adults, can be accomplished through a combination of oral and intravenous fluids. Adults and children with burns greater than 20% of total body surface area will require intravenous fluids resuscitation. The formula that is used to calculate fluid resuscitation needs in adults within the first 24 hours is called the Parkland Formula. It is important for the nurse to realize that the formula is only a guide to fluid resuscitation. The nurse is still responsible for assessing the client for adequate perfusion and circulation by monitoring vital signs, capillary refill, urine output, and laboratory values. The volume may need to be adjusted to a higher or lower rate based on the client's response to the fluid (see Clinical Calculation 22-2).

Burn clients are particularly susceptible to **sepsis,** the state in which disease-producing organisms are present in the blood. Sepsis is a medical emergency that causes an overwhelming, uncontrolled, systemic inflammatory response leading to tissue and organ failure and death. Major sepsis further increases a client's metabolic rate. Clients with indwelling catheters and central venous access devices are at risk for sepsis. Sepsis, of course, is not limited to burn clients; clients with surgical trauma or infections such as pneumonia or urinary tract infections may also suffer from sepsis.

For all burn clients, a nutritional assessment is essential to minimize complications and allow nutritional therapy to be evaluated effectively. The food intake of these clients should be monitored and documented. The kilocalories and grams of protein consumed or taken intravenously should be monitored per the facility's policy.

A high-protein, high-kilocalorie diet is ordered for most burn clients as soon as oral intake is medically feasible. Often the diet is initially offered in six small meals. Complete nutritional oral supplements are commonly used to increase the client's kilocaloric and protein intake. The protein content of the diet can be increased by providing a between-meal feeding high in protein, a serving of 2 eggs at breakfast, and a 4-ounce serving of meat at both lunch and supper. If the client drinks a full 8 ounces of milk with each meal, this further increases the protein content of the diet.

TRAUMA

Trauma is a physical injury or wound caused by an external violence. Stab and gunshot wounds, multiple fractures, and injuries acquired in motor vehicle accidents are examples of trauma. Victims of traumas may become hypermetabolic, depending on the severity of the injury, and vitamin and mineral supplements may be necessary.

Vitamin C plays a role in wound healing, and its administration restores healing. Vitamin C functions as a cofactor in the hydroxylation of proline into collagen and enhances cellular and humoral response to stress. Vitamin A, calcium, and zinc are also important in wound healing. Vitamin A enhances fibroplasia and collagen accumulation in wounds. Calcium is needed for calcium-dependent collagenases, iron for the formation of collagen, and zinc as a cofactor for enzymes responsible for cellular proliferation.

INFECTIONS AND FEVER

Malnutrition decreases resistance to infection, and infection aggravates malnutrition by depleting body nutrient stores. Fever characteristically accompanies infection but can also result from a variety of causes. The body needs extra kilocalories and fluids during fever because it takes more energy to support the higher metabolic rate. Infection may result in:

- Decreased food intake and absorption of nutrients
- Altered metabolism
- Increased excretion of nutrients

Extra protein is also needed to produce antibodies and white blood cells to fight the infection. Perspiration entails a loss of fluids from the body, and many clients with fever have increased perspiration. Fluid may also be lost in vomiting and diarrhea and needs to be replaced.

Protein and Kilocalorie Needs

The client with hypermetabolism has an increased need for protein. Kilocalorie intake should maintain energy balance

---

CLINICAL CALCULATION 22-2

Parkland Formula

4 × client's weight in kilograms × percentage of burn = total fluid volume to be infused over the first 24 hours. Half of the volume is infused over the first 8 hours and the rest of the volume is infused over the next 16 hours.

A 186-pound man sustained second- and third-degree burns over 20% of his body after pouring gasoline on burning leaves and tree limbs.

STEP ONE: CALCULATE WEIGHT IN KILOGRAMS

186 pounds ÷ 2.2 = 85 kilograms in body weight

STEP TWO: CALCULATE FLUID NEEDS FOR THE FIRST 24 HOURS

4 × 85 kilograms × 20 BSA = 6,800 mL/24 hours

STEP THREE: CALCULATE FLUID VOLUME TO BE INFUSED OVER FIRST 8 HOURS

Half the volume is infused over the first 8 hours
[6,800 mL ÷ 2 = 3,400 mL]
3,400 mL ÷ 8 hours = 425 mL/hour × 8 hours then the remaining volume
3,400 mL ÷ 16 hours = 213 mL/hour × 16 hours

without overfeeding. Many critical care clients have GI problems and poor food intake.

PROTEIN

Injury or illness requires active protein formation. These states all require a constant supply of protein:

- Surgical wound healing
- Tissue repair
- Replacement of red blood cells and plasma protein lost in hemorrhage
- Immune response to infection

The extent of hypermetabolism and catabolism depends on the degree of injury and client response to the injury.

Protein Needs

The protocol for calculating a client's protein requirement varies from institution to institution. For non–critical care clients, 0.8 to 1.2 grams of protein per kg of ideal body weight (IBW) or actual body weight (ABW) formula is often used. For critical care clients, 1.2 to 2 grams of protein per kilogram per day, or higher, in burns or multitrauma clients is used (McClave, Taylor, Martindale, & Warren, 2016).

Urine Assessment of Protein Status

Total urinary excretion of nitrogen increases with the client's stress level. Urinary creatinine measurements may be used to estimate muscle protein reserves. One problem common to the use of all urinary measurements is the completion of an accurate 24-hour urine collection. Nurses are typically responsible for collecting a 24-hour urine specimen from the client. If even one voiding is discarded, the measurement will be inaccurate.

KILOCALORIES

Clients who are hypermetabolic have an increased need for kilocalories. Clients lose weight because an increased need for energy coupled with a possibly inadequate energy intake and/or protein intake promotes weight loss.

Kilocalorie Needs

Energy expenditure is the number of kilocalories that an individual uses to meet the body's demand for fuel. The most accurate method for measuring energy expenditure is indirect calorimetry (see Chapter 5). However, many facilities lack the equipment and trained personnel to complete this procedure. Each organization usually has a protocol to follow to calculate the number of kilocalories to be initially delivered via nutritional support. The client is then monitored closely to determine metabolic response to the initial kilocalorie estimate.

The number of required kilocalories is typically calculated by either kcal/kg or one of several different predictive formulas. Research has found that predictive formulas often are only 37% to 65% accurate in estimating caloric needs of critically ill clients. Three of these formulas are discussed here. Propofol is a commonly used medication to sedate mechanically ventilated clients. This medication is administered parenterally in a 10% fat emulsion. It is important to consider the number of calories derived from fat in this medication and include them when assessing the total overall kilocalories the client received.

Equations

Three different equations to predict kilocaloric need are discussed.

HARRIS–BENEDICT EQUATION. Although the Harris–Benedict equation is still widely used to estimate resting energy expenditure (REE) for critically ill clients, there is conflicting evidence on the formula's accuracy of predicting kilocalorie needs. Research has found that predictive formulas often are only 37% to 65% accurate when compared to calculation with indirect calorimetry of critically ill clients (Ferreira-Picolo, Fabiane-Lago, & Fabiane-Menegueti, 2016). A brief explanation of the equation is presented in Clinical Calculation 22-3.

STRESS FACTORS. When using the Harris–Benedict equation, the use of stress factors is common. Research has shown that different types of stress increase kilocaloric needs differently. A stress factor is a number assigned to a given pathological state to predict how much a client's kilocaloric need has increased as a result of the type of stress the client is experiencing.

Table 22-1 lists various types of physical stress and the stress factor used for each disease state. Stress factors are used most often with the Harris–Benedict equation. The Ireton–Jones (1992 version) equation considers stress factors in the equation.

As the table shows, a client with burns on more than 50% of the body has a stress factor of 2.0. This means that kilocaloric need is twice (200%) his or her REE. In contrast, the stress factor after minor surgery is 1.05. This means that a client who has had minor surgery needs only 5% more kilocalories than his or her REE. Depending on the physical activity of the client, a factor for this is sometimes used. Stress factors are convenient to use in estimating kilocaloric needs when using predictive equations for clients with multiple stressors.

IRETON–JONES, 1992. Another equation is the Ireton–Jones, 1992 version. Clinical Calculation 22-4 provides the formula used to estimate energy expenditure with this equation. This equation includes stressors for the ventilator dependent, burned, and trauma client.

MIFFLIN–ST. JEOR. Yet another equation is the Mifflin–St. Jeor. Clinical Calculation 22-5 provides the formula used to estimate energy expenditure with this equation. The Mifflin–St. Jeor formula takes into account activity factors (Table 22-2).

Predictive equations are used to initially determine a client's kilocaloric goal rate. Without indirect calorimetry, the best method to determine if too much or too little energy is being given to a client is to closely monitor body weight, laboratory values, nutritional intake, and sometimes blood gases at predetermined intervals.

It is important to recognize that calculating nutritional needs for intensive care clients requires specialized training and the calculations will be performed by registered

CLINICAL CALCULATION 22-3

Calculating Kilocaloric Needs Using the Harris–Benedict Predictive Equation

MALE CLIENT

Energy Need = Resting Energy Expenditure (REE) × Activity Factor × Stress Factor

Step 1: Use the following **Harris–Benedict equation** to calculate the male client's resting energy expenditure:

$$REE = 66 + (13.7 \times weight\ in\ kg) + (5 \times height\ in\ cm) - (6.8 \times age)$$

Step 2: Multiply an activity factor by the client's REE (see Table 22-2).

$$REE \times Activity\ Factor$$

Step 3: Multiply the answer obtained in step 2 by the appropriate stress factor (Table 22-1).

$$REE \times Activity\ Factor \times Stress\ Factor$$

FEMALE CLIENT

Energy Need = REE × Activity Factor × Stress Factor

Step 1: Use the following Harris–Benedict equation to calculate the female client's resting energy expenditure:

$$REE = 655 + (9.6 \times weight\ in\ kg) + (1.8 \times height\ in\ cm) - (4.7 \times age)$$

Step 2: Multiply an activity factor by the client's REE (see Table 22-2).

$$REE \times Activity\ Factor$$

Step 3: Multiply the answer obtained in step 2 by the appropriate stress factor (see Table 22-1).

$$REE \times Activity\ Factor \times Stress\ Factor$$

EXAMPLE CALCULATION

Assume that you need to estimate the kilocaloric need of a 154-lb (70-kg) man who is 5 ft 5 in. (165 cm) tall and 25 years old. Assume that he is confined to bed and has a fractured long bone.

Sample calculation for step 1:
70-kg man who is 165 cm tall and 25 years old

$$REE = 66 + (13.7 \times 70) + (5 \times 165) - (6.8 \times 25)$$
$$REE = 66 + 959 + 825 - 170$$
$$REE = 1,680$$

Sample calculation for step 2:

$$REE \times Activity\ Factor$$
$$1,680 \times 1.2$$
$$2,016$$

Sample calculation for step 3:

$$Answer\ from\ step\ 2 \times Stress\ Factor$$
$$2,016 \times 1.35$$
$$2,721.6 = client's\ estimated\ energy\ need$$

TABLE 22-1 Stress Factors Used to Determine Kilocalories With Harris–Benedict Equation

STRESSOR	FACTOR
Surgery	1.1–1.3
Anabolism	1.5–1.75
For each degree F above 98.6°	1.07
Cancer	1.6
Soft tissue trauma	1.14–1.37
Long bone fracture	1.6
Burns (0%–20% of body surface area)	1.25
Burns (20%–40% of body surface area)	1.5
Burns (>40% of body surface area)	1.85
Peritonitis	1.2–1.5
Major sepsis	1.4–1.8

CLINICAL CALCULATION 22-4

Ireton–Jones (IJ), 1992 Equation

An explanation of the equation components is followed by example equations.

(A) = Age in years
(W) = Weight in kilograms
(S) = Sex; male = 1; female = 0

DIAGNOSIS OF TRAUMA

(T) = present = 1; absent = 0

DIAGNOSIS OF BURN

(B) = present = 1; absent = 0

BODY MASS INDEX (BMI) >27

(0) = present = 1; absent = 0

CLIENT WHO IS BREATHING SPONTANEOUSLY

$$IJ_{(s)} = 629 - 11(A) + 25(W) - 609(0)$$

CLIENT WHO IS VENTILATOR DEPENDENT

$$IJ_{(V)} = 1,925 - 10(A) + 5(W) + 281(S) + 292(T) + 851(B)$$

CLINICAL CALCULATION 22-5

Mifflin–St. Jeor

An explanation of the equation components is followed by example equations.

(A) = Age in years
(W) = Weight in kilograms
(H) = Height in centimeters

MEN

$$REE = (9.99 \times W) + (6.25 \times H) - (4.92 \times A) + 5$$

WOMEN

$$REE = (9.99 \times W) + (6.25 \times H) - (4.92 \times A) - 161$$

Once REE is calculated the result can be multiplied by the stress factors in Table 22-1 and the activity factors in Table 22-2.

TABLE 22-2	Activity Factors Commonly Used to Calculate a Client's Activity Kilocalories
Little or no activity	1.2
Light activity	1.375
Moderate activity	1.55
Very active	1.725
Exceedingly active	1.9

dietitians in collaboration with the physician and pharmacists. The nurse is responsible for accurate, timely, and safe administration, and as stress factors change the nurse can report these findings to the medical team.

The B vitamins help release the chemical energy stored in foods. Whenever a client requires increased kilocalories, the need for the B-vitamin complex automatically increases. When anabolism or the building of body tissue is indicated, vitamin C requirements are increased.

Hypermetabolic clients usually need to build up depleted tissue stores. Evidence demonstrates that there is significant lean muscle mass loss after 10 days in bed (Perry, 2016). Critically ill clients may have increased micronutrient needs, but research is lacking to make specific recommendations.

Gastrointestinal Complication

Ulcers and some intestinal diseases are aggravated by stress. A client may report that he or she has specific food intolerances when under stress but that the same food is easily tolerated at other times. This change is partially due to impairment of GI function during episodes of stress and the use of some medications. Decreased motility can cause the development of anorexia, abdominal distention, gas pains, and constipation. These symptoms may contribute to food intolerances or reduced food intake.

Food Intake

The volume of food a client consumes and the desire to prepare food are influenced by stress. The time at which food is eaten also may be important. The best approach is to offer small frequent meals or oral nutritional supplements between meals.

Nutrition and Respiration

The scientific literature addresses the relationship between good nutrition and respiration:

Respiration refers to the exchange of gases (oxygen and carbon dioxide) between a living organism and its environment. The air or oxygen inhaled and the carbon dioxide exhaled is the act of ventilation.
Ventilation means breathing.
Pulmonary means concerning or involving the lungs.

Chronic obstructive pulmonary disease (COPD) refers to a group of lung diseases with a common characteristic of chronic airflow obstruction. COPD has become the fourth leading cause of death in the United States.
Respiratory failure is an acute or chronic disease caused by an imbalance between the amount of gases entering the lungs and the demand of body cells for gases, resulting in tissue hypoxia.
Acute respiratory failure is an imbalance caused by a disease that affects ventilation in a client who has a healthy lung and normal alveoli.
Chronic respiratory failure results from a disease in the bronchial structures or functioning (alveoli) structures of the lung. Malnutrition is commonly seen in clients with respiratory diseases.
Acute respiratory distress syndrome (ARDS) is often caused by conditions such as pneumonia and is characterized by a rapid onset of dyspnea and severe deficits in gas exchange. O_2 saturation reflects the percentage of hemoglobin saturated with oxygen and is an indicator of inadequate oxygen delivery to tissues. Normal oxygen (O_2) saturation in adults is usually 95% to 100% in adults and 95% in the elderly. Critical O_2 saturation is equal or less than 90%.

Effects of Impaired Nutritional Status on Respiratory Function

Poor nutrition is related to inadequate pulmonary function in five important ways:

1. Clients with respiratory diseases or inadequate respiratory function frequently have an inadequate food intake, which is related to anorexia, shortness of breath (SOB), or GI distress. Shortness of breath during food preparation and consumption of meals may limit kilocaloric intake. Inadequate oxygen delivery to the cells causes fatigue. Impaired GI tract motility is common in clients with respiratory diseases (see point number three).

2. Kilocaloric requirements are often increased in clients with pulmonary disease. It has been estimated that clients with COPD used 10 times the amount of calories to breathe than those without pulmonary disease. As a result of the combined effects of decreased food intake and increased energy requirements, weight loss is commonly seen in these clients.

3. A client's catabolism can affect pulmonary function. When kilocaloric intake is decreased, the body begins to break down muscle stores, including those of the respiratory muscles. A loss in the lean mass of any muscle affects the muscle's function. The lung's structure itself is thus affected as a result of catabolism, often referred to as pulmonary cachexia. Malnutrition may also result in decreased lung tissue cell replacement or growth. GI distress is common in clients with pulmonary disease and is related to malnutrition. A loss of GI structure

including muscle mass may lead to hemorrhage and paralytic ileus. **Paralytic ileus** is the temporary cessation of peristalsis and contributes to decreased food intake and the feeling of anorexia. In addition, paralytic ileus may lead to a translocation of bacteria. Decreased peristalsis in the GI tract fosters the movement (translocation) of bacteria from the GI tract into the bloodstream. This translocation, in turn, leads to sepsis, or blood-borne infection, a sometimes fatal complication.

4. Malnutrition increases the risk of respiratory tract infections. Lung infection is frequently the cause of death in pulmonary clients. In severe malnutrition, the body decreases the production of antibodies, which are necessary to fight infection. Also, as a result of starvation, the lungs decrease production of pulmonary phospholipid (a fat-like substance). Phospholipids assist in keeping the lung tissue lubricated and help to protect the lungs from any inhaled disease-producing organisms.

5. Improved nutritional status has been shown to be associated with a better ability to wean clients from ventilators. A ventilator is a machine that provides gases under pressure to clients who are unable to breathe on their own because of an insufficient number of ventilations or inspired volume amounts for cellular respiration.

Clients on ventilators do not have to use their respiratory muscles to breathe. Active muscle movement stimulates muscle growth through protein stimulus. This is the same principle that applied to physical exercise increasing muscle size. To some extent, all the respiratory muscles **atrophy,** or waste away, due to inactivity while a client is artificially breathing.

Clients on ventilators are usually weaned slowly from these machines as their conditions improve. Some experts have attributed clients' ability to be successfully weaned from ventilators to an increase in protein synthesis. Good nutrition stimulates respiratory muscle growth.

In mechanically ventilated clients, there is good data to indicate that once a client is extubated, swallowing dysfunction and a real risk of aspiration is present in most clients and may last up to several days.

Nutritional Therapy

Respiratory disease can affect food intake and nutrient utilization. Many clients with respiratory diseases also have problems with water balance.

Energy Nutrient Utilization

Care must be taken not to overfeed clients with reduced respiratory function. Excess intake can raise the demand for oxygen and the production of carbon dioxide beyond the client's capacity. The total number of kilocalories fed to the pulmonary client should be closely monitored. A nutritional assessment helps estimate the client's kilocaloric need

and assists in therapy. Clients should be advised to consume full-fat, high-energy foods (Hodson, 2016).

Research has shown that in individuals with COPD, the presence of lower body mass index (BMI; <20 kg/m²) increases 1-year mortality 4-fold higher when compared to overweight or obese (BMI; >25 kg/m²) clients with COPD (Hodson, 2016). This means that these clients require close monitoring with appropriate follow-up. Too many kilocalories may increase carbon dioxide production and too few kilocalories may result in a weight loss and contribute to a decreased body mass with a subsequent poor outcome. Kilocalories are typically given on the low side of the 25 to 35 kcal/kg initially and increased slowly.

Vitamins and Minerals

Clients who have had a poor nutrient intake are at risk for nutrient deficits. Even if intake is adequate, nutritional depletion may occur in severe COPD clients, resulting in a need for supplementation of vitamins and minerals. Specific nutrients depleted in pulmonary disease include:

- Iron
- Vitamin A
- Vitamin C
- Vitamin D
- Vitamin E
- Selenium

Usually electrolyte levels are closely monitored in ICU clients because of fluid imbalances and the occurrence of **respiratory acidosis** and **respiratory alkalosis.** Some clients' intravenous solutions require daily manipulation to correct imbalances of electrolytes.

An adequate intake of vitamins A and C is essential for helping to prevent pulmonary infections and decrease the extent of lung tissue damage. The diet should include foods high in vitamin A, such as:

- Fortified milk
- Dark green or yellow fruits and vegetables
- Some breakfast cereals (check the label)
- Cheese
- Eggs

The diet should include foods high in vitamin C, such as:

- Citrus fruits and juices
- Strawberries
- Fortified breakfast cereals (check the label) should also be included.

Sources of vitamins A and C should be carefully chosen to ensure that they do not contribute to gas production.

Low bone density is problematic in many clients with COPD. Among the reasons for this are glucocorticosteroid therapy, reduced physical activity, a history of tobacco use, an inadequate calcium and vitamin D intake, and the pulmonary disease process itself.

Fat

The COPD client needs to be conscientious regarding fat intake. Fat metabolism generates less CO_2 than metabolism of carbohydrates, which is a benefit to the client. Clients with COPD tend to retain higher levels of CO_2, which can worsen respiratory distress. When choosing fats, the client needs to be advised to consume monounsaturated and polyunsaturated fats while avoiding *trans* fatty acids and saturated fats. Some studies have suggested that omega-3 fatty acids may have protective antioxidant effects on the lungs, but further studies need to be conducted (Lin, Lin, Wu, Cheng, & Yeh, 2016). Excess fat intake can lead to weight gain and increased adipose tissue around the midsection, which can increase respiratory effort in the COPD client.

Water, Phosphorus, and Magnesium

Water balance and serum phosphorus levels need to be closely monitored. Clients with COPD and acute respiratory failure often need fluid restriction. Fluid restriction assists in the control of **pulmonary edema** or a movement of fluid into interstitial lung tissue.

Low serum phosphorus levels or hypophosphatemia are often seen in clients who are respirator dependent. Phosphorus leaves the intracellular space and moves into the extracellular space during starvation. Serum phosphorus levels are in the normal or near-normal range at this point.

With refeeding, phosphate moves back into the intracellular space. At this point, the serum phosphorus level may drop below normal. If this occurs, it is crucial that the client receive phosphate replacement. Because acute hypophosphatemia has been reported to cause respiratory failure, serum phosphorus levels should be monitored in all clients receiving aggressive nutritional support. A magnesium deficiency appears to cause a loss of muscle strength and should, therefore, be monitored closely.

Feeding Techniques

Many of these clients lack the energy to eat. Complaints of fatigue are common. The GI distress experienced by these clients contributes to the anorexia. Box 22-2 lists interventions that can be used to improve nutrition in COPD clients.

Refeeding Syndrome

Refeeding is the reintroduction of kilocalories and nutrients by oral or other routes. **Refeeding syndrome** is a detrimental state that results when a previously severely malnourished person is reintroduced to food and nutrients improperly. Complications with refeeding can occur regardless of the

---

BOX 22-2 ■ **Interventions for Clients With COPD**

- Avoid gas-causing foods, such as carbonated beverages, cruciferous foods, and fried foods.
- Ensure adequate daily calcium intake.
- Encourage clients to eat little amounts frequently. Encourage six small energy-dense meals a day.
- Maintain adequate hydration to assist in thinning secretions.
- Choose foods that are easily prepared and chewed.
- Advise clients to clear their airways before eating.
- Limit sodium intake to prevent water retention.
- Chew slowly to avoid swallowing air.
- Drink fluid between meals.
- Sit upright at a table for all meals.
- Wear oxygen via nasal cannula during meals to increase oxygen level.

---

route by which nutrients are delivered, whether oral, enteral, or parenteral.

The term *refeeding syndrome* has been used to describe a series of metabolic and physiological reactions that occur in some malnourished clients when nutritional rehabilitation is begun. Improper refeeding of a chronically malnourished client can result in congestive heart failure (CHF) and respiratory failure. Clients at risk include those with:

- Alcoholism
- Chronic weight loss
- Hyperglycemia, or insulin-dependent diabetes mellitus
  Included also are clients on:
- Chronic antacid or
- Diuretic therapy

Elderly persons living alone who choose not to eat or are unable to eat because of progressive infirmity are likely candidates. Any incompetent mentally or physically challenged adult or abused child who has not been eating, either by choice or because of neglect, is also at risk of experiencing refeeding syndrome.

Starvation leads to both a loss of the lean body mass in the heart and respiratory muscles and decreased insulin secretion. When carbohydrate intake is low, the pancreas adapts by decreasing insulin secretion. With the reintroduction of carbohydrates into the diet, insulin secretion will increase. The increased insulin secretion is associated with increased sodium and water retention.

Other hormones are also activated with carbohydrate feeding. As a result of hormone action, increases in metabolic rate, oxygen consumption, and carbon dioxide production occur. The net effect of these metabolic changes is an increased workload for the cardiopulmonary system. Refeeding may increase the work of the cardiopulmonary system beyond its diminished capacity (due to the loss of lean body mass) and cause CHF and respiratory failure.

Starvation also leads to an increase in extracellular fluid and an increased loss of intracellular phosphorus, potassium, and magnesium. The degree of intracellular loss of these minerals reflects the degree of loss of lean body mass. Before refeeding, serum phosphorus and magnesium levels may remain in the lower range of normal, whereas the intracellular and total body stores of these minerals are depleted.

After refeeding, these minerals are redistributed from the extracellular to the intracellular compartments. Repeated laboratory measurements taken after refeeding is started may show low serum levels of phosphorus, magnesium, and potassium. Failure to correct for these mineral deficiencies may be fatal for the client.

Principles of Safe Refeeding

Health-care workers need to be aware of the dangers of refeeding a severely malnourished or starved client. Starved or severely malnourished clients may be seen in outpatient settings as well as in hospital intensive care units and long-term care facilities. The recommendations in Clinical Application 22-1 may help health-care workers avoid the refeeding syndrome.

Refeeding the malnourished client requires a team effort. A careful diet history taken by the dietitian can assist in the identification of clients likely to become victims of refeeding syndrome. Indications of a significantly altered status include changes in:

- Taste
- Appetite
- Intake
- Weight
- Consumption of a special diet

Correction of electrolyte abnormalities by the health-care provider before implementing nutritional support can prevent death. Careful observation and monitoring by the nutritional support service can identify early signs of this syndrome. Open and prompt communication among all health-care team members may be crucial to the client's survival.

CLINICAL APPLICATION   22-1

Recommendations for Refeeding the Malnourished Client

These seven points are broad guidelines for working with malnourished clients.

1. Health-care professionals need first to recognize clients at risk. Refeeding syndrome occurs in:
   - Clients with frank starvation, including war victims undergoing repletion
   - Chronically ill clients who are malnourished
   - Clients on prolonged intravenous dextrose solutions without other modes of nutritional support
   - Hypermetabolic clients who have not received nutritional support for 1–2 weeks
   - Clients who report prolonged fasting
   - Obese clients who report a recent loss of a considerable amount of weight
   - Chronic alcoholics
   - Clients with anorexia nervosa
2. Health-care workers practicing in outpatient settings not directly under the supervision of a physician need to develop a referral plan in the event they suspect that a client is a likely candidate for refeeding syndrome. These clients require the expertise of a physician.
3. A health-care provider needs to test for and correct all electrolyte abnormalities before initiating nutritional support, whether by the oral, enteral, or parenteral route. Many physicians depend on other health-care workers to assist in the monitoring of:
   - Serum phosphorus
   - Magnesium
   - Potassium values

For nurses practicing within hospitals, this means notifying the provider on receipt of laboratory test results showing low serum levels of these minerals. It is especially important to notify the physician before implementing changes in:
   - Tube feeding
   - Oral diets
   - The rate of intravenous nutrition
4. The health-care provider needs to restore circulatory volume and to monitor pulse rate and intake and output before initiating nutritional support. Again, many providers depend on nurses and other health-care workers to assist in monitoring these signs.
5. The kilocaloric delivery to a previously starved client should be slow. Tube-fed and parenterally fed clients who have been previously malnourished need to be closely monitored for the following items:
   - Rate
   - Total volume
   - Concentration of kilocalories delivered
     These items should be increased one at a time:
   - Concentration
   - Volume
   - Rate of kilocaloric intake
6. Stepwise advancement to a higher kilocaloric intake should not occur unless the client is metabolically and physiologically stable.
7. Electrolytes should be monitored before nutritional support is started and at designated intervals thereafter.

KEYSTONES

- Hypermetabolism differs from starvation in that resting energy expenditure (REE) increases during hypermetabolism and decreases during a prolonged state of starvation.

- Major surgery, severe infections, fever, major burns, and severe trauma are all examples of hypermetabolic states.

- Respiratory status profoundly affects nutrient need and utilization as well as food intake.

- Nutritional support can decrease catabolism of the respiratory muscles, improve immune function, minimize carbon dioxide production, and improve the likelihood of successfully weaning clients who are on mechanical respirators.

- Refeeding a previously starved client involves some risks. Refeeding may increase the work of the cardiopulmonary system beyond its diminished capacity and cause congestive heart failure and respiratory failure.

CASE STUDY 22-1

Mr. X is a 68-year-old man who was admitted to the intensive care unit (ICU) with a diagnosis of bilateral pneumonia that was resistant to a 10-day prior course of antibiotic therapy. On admission, the client presented in acute distress: clammy to touch; weak; and unable to sit on examination table without assistance and support. Recumbent vital signs revealed the following: blood pressure 110/65; pulse 120 and weak; respiratory rate 28 breaths per minute and shallow; and sublingual temperature of 102.5°F (39.17°C). Medical history obtained from client was unremarkable and, in particular, no history of respiratory distress, smoking, or exposure to inhalation of toxic substances such as asbestoses.

His O_2 saturation was 83 on admission and his PCO_2 53. Imaging studies showed diffuse bilateral pulmonary infiltrates and small to moderate bilateral plural effusions. His albumin level was 2.5. Based on these findings and the blood gases, mechanical ventilation was instituted.

Mr. X is 5 ft 11 in. tall and weighs 140 lb (63.6 kg). His body mass index is 19.5. He reported a 9-lb weight loss over the past 3 weeks. He admits to living a sedentary lifestyle and reports a poor food intake. He states that his wife died about 6 months ago, and since then he has quit eating much. Mr. X admits his personal hygiene has also been poor. The neighbor brought him to the hospital and stated Mr. X appeared to have lost "a lot of weight."

An orally placed feeding tube with the tip placed in the stomach was inserted and placement was confirmed by diagnostic imaging. His kilocaloric need was estimated to be 1,590–2,226 based on 25–35 kcal/kg and his actual body weight. His protein needs were estimated to be 1.2–1.5 grams/kg or 75.8–95.4 grams/day, also based on his actual body weight.

The dietitian recommended a formula with a 1.5 kcal/mL concentration. A 24-hour continuous feeding of 1,435 total milliliters at 59 mL per hour was recommended as a goal. An initial rate of 20 mL per hour with a gradual increase of 10 mL every 8 hours as tolerated was set until the goal rate was reached. In addition, 750 mL water would be needed to meet fluid needs and should be used to flush the tube, as tolerated by the client.

On the third day of his hospital stay, the client's phosphorus, potassium, and magnesium, which had been in the normal range on admission, dropped below normal. These electrolytes were replaced intravenously by physician's order. The client remained and tolerated the tube feeding without problems for the next 6 days.

The physician started to wean the client from the mechanical ventilator 24-hours ago as his pneumonia related-symptoms responded well to the intravenous antibiotic treatment. The client states that he does not know why he got so ill.

CARE PLAN

Subjective Data

Denies knowledge of the relationship among lifestyle behaviors and infection ■ Reported significant weight loss and very poor food intake and sedentary behaviors

Objective Data

BMI = 19.5 on admission ■ Mechanical ventilation for the past 8 days second to pneumonia ■ Tube feeding well tolerated since admission ■ On admission visually presented with dirty hands, soiled clothing, and body odor

Analysis

Client's condition related to poor personal hygiene as a result of grieving and knowledge deficit

Plan

DESIRED OUTCOMES EVALUATION CRITERIA	ACTIONS/ INTERVENTIONS	RATIONALE
Client expresses feelings about loss.	Actively listen to the client, particularly when he mentions his wife.	Client needs much assistance learning to ask for help.
Client seeks social support	Offer social services referral.	The social worker will be able to determine client's eligibility for treatment and match Mr. X's financial resources to specific doctors or programs.
Client states that good nutrition and moderate exercise, and proper hygiene are important for disease resistance.	Explain the relationship between lifestyle behaviors and resistance to infectious disease.	Knowledge is the first step to behavioral change.
	Offer client a referral to the dietitian to discuss healthful eating and easily prepared meals.	The dietitian has reliable educational materials suitable for most populations.

TEAMWORK 22-1

SOCIAL WORKER'S NOTES

The following Social Worker's Notes are representative of the documentation found in a client's medical record.

Met with client per physician and nursing request. Although we did discuss his wife's death, client did not express grief or sadness. Also, phoned client's next closest relative, a sister living out-of-state. She indicated concern with her brother's inability to move forward with his life. She claims that before her sister-in-law's death, her brother was a well-groomed, cheerful person. At first, she denied any family history of mental illness. After some discussion, she admitted that her mother had committed suicide when she and her brother were very young. Long-term counseling and possibly medication are indicated. Mr. X has mental health coverage. Recommend referral to psychiatrist and possibly discharge to outpatient mental health program per the psychiatrist's evaluation.

TEAMWORK 22-2

DIETITIAN'S FOLLOW-UP NOTES

The following Dietitian's Notes are representative of the documentation found in a client's medical record.

Spoke with client initially 1 day after his present hospital admission to assess his nutritional needs and write recommendations. At that time, client was tearful about his poor health habits. He did not mention much about his deceased spouse except to say that she died 6 months ago. Concur with social worker's note. Client does not currently appear able to meet his own nutritional needs on discharge. Will defer education until after psychiatrist's evaluation. In the meantime, client is consuming sips of clear liquids only as he is still in the process of being weaned from the ventilator. The client agreed to try a complete liquid supplement, a few sips every hour. The client needs much encouragement.

CRITICAL THINKING QUESTIONS

1. After 2 days of monitoring the client's kilocalorie and protein intake and despite encouragement to eat from the nurses and the dietitian, the client refuses to eat much food. His kilocalorie intake is less than 500, with only 12 grams of protein. What would you recommend?

2. The client has concerns regarding access and preparation of foods at home. What suggestions would you give the client? What referrals can be made?

3. You question the client's mental competence. What should you do?

CHAPTER REVIEW

1. Which of the following is true about clients who have a life-threatening injury or illness?
   1. Their resting energy expenditure is about 70% of the kilocalories normally needed to maintain body weight.
   2. They have a decreased need for fluids.
   3. Biologically, their organs do not adapt to their increased need for kilocalories by switching to a less preferred fuel source.
   4. They need 0.8–1.2 grams of protein per kilogram of actual body weight.

2. Which of the following conditions does not increase a client's resting energy expenditure?
   1. Infection
   2. Chronic obstructive pulmonary disease
   3. Starvation
   4. Burn

3. A burn client's need for kilocalories is related to:
    1. The amount of protein eaten
    2. The total body surface area burned
    3. The volume of food tolerated
    4. The amount of existing nutrient stores

4. Malnutrition is commonly seen in clients with pulmonary disease due to which of the following? Select all that apply.
    1. Many of these clients have a decreased food intake.
    2. Many of these clients expend more kilocalories to breathe.
    3. Many of these clients have impaired gastrointestinal tract function.
    4. Many of these clients have an extraordinary ability to fight infection.
    5. Many of these clients have difficulty breathing and chewing at the same time.

5. Experts advocate the following when refeeding a malnourished client:
    1. Immediately pushing kilocalories and protein to replenish lost stores
    2. Progressing the rate, volume, and concentration of a tube feeding as rapidly as possible
    3. Full participation of all members of the health-care team to manage commonly seen metabolic abnormalities
    4. Correction of the hyperphosphatemia seen during the refeeding of a malnourished client

CLINICAL ANALYSIS

1. Mr. L is suffering from second- and third-degree burns over 40% of his body. His physician has decided to use topical agents and leave the wound open to air. In the first 30–40 days postburn, the health-care team is planning nutritional support. The best supplemental feedings for the client would be:
    a. A high-fat feeding such as a milkshake made with ½ cup skim milk and 1 cup of ice cream
    b. A high-carbohydrate feeding such as soda with added honey
    c. A polymeric (complete nutritional) supplement that is acceptable to the client
    d. A high-kilocalorie dessert such as apple pie, cake, or ice cream

2. Mrs. J is an alcoholic who has previously reported that she has not eaten "food" for at least the past 3 months. She stated that her primary source of kilocalories has been alcohol. After her treatment for alcohol withdrawal on another unit, she was transferred to the unit where you work. The physician has ordered a high-kilocalorie, high-protein diet. So far, she has eaten 100% of the three high-kilocalorie, high-protein trays she has received while on your unit. While reviewing the client's laboratory values, you notice her serum phosphorus, magnesium, and potassium levels have just recently decreased. Mrs. J's depressed phosphorus values may be related to:
    a. A movement of phosphorus into the extracellular space
    b. A total compartmental depletion of phosphorus
    c. A lack of phosphorus in Mrs. J's present dietary intake
    d. A movement of phosphorus into the intracellular space

3. Mr. C is a heavy smoker. He was recently admitted to your unit with carbon dioxide retention and a diagnosis of chronic obstructive pulmonary disease. He complains of gas pains. The client will not derive benefit from:
    a. Caffeinated beverages
    b. Broccoli, onions, peas, melons, and cabbage
    c. Six small meals
    d. Custard, hot cooked cereals, bananas, ground meats, and mashed potatoes

CHAPTER 23

Diet in HIV and AIDS

LEARNING OBJECTIVES

After completing this chapter, the student should be able to:

- Define AIDS and HIV and list transmission routes for the virus.
- List nutrition-related complications seen in clients infected with HIV and, for each complication, describe interventions to improve nutritional status.
- Discuss why malnutrition is commonly seen in clients with HIV or AIDS.
- Describe why each client with AIDS needs an individualized nutritional assessment.

Acquired immune deficiency syndrome (AIDS) is a life-threatening disease and a major public health issue. The **human immunodeficiency virus (HIV)** causes AIDS. The impact of this virus on our society is and will continue to be a challenge. In 2015, 36.7 million people were living with HIV globally, with 2.1 million newly affected (HIV.gov, 2017). This chapter discusses the prevention, diagnosis, and treatment of HIV **infection.** HIV is complicated by the side effects of medications, coinfections with other infectious disease, wasting, and lipodystrophy. The course of AIDS is often complicated by malnutrition. For these reasons, a major portion of this chapter is devoted to the nutritional care of clients infected with HIV.

Human Immunodeficiency Virus

The human immunodeficiency virus attacks both the immune system and the nervous system. **Immunity** refers to resistance to or protection against a specified disease.

When the HIV virus enters the bloodstream, it begins to attack cells with a specific protein called CD_4 on their surfaces. CD_4 is present on lymphocytes. Health-care providers may also refer to T cells when discussing HIV/AIDS. The terms *T cells* and CD_4 are often used interchangeably. Lymphocytes are the main source of the body's immune capability, which involves humoral immunity produced by B cells and cell-mediated immunity produced by T cells. CD_4 levels decrease as the HIV disease progresses.

A healthy, uninfected person usually has 500 to 1,000 CD_4 cells/mm³. The HIV virus enters the cell, conscripts its DNA, and reprograms it to reproduce the virus. Loss of CD_4 function leaves an individual susceptible to infections and certain cancers. Evidence shows that the AIDS virus may also attack the nervous system, causing damage to the brain. See Box 23-1 for route of HIV transmission and prevention strategies.

Acquired Immune Deficiency Syndrome

AIDS is defined by the presence of HIV infection and a low level of white blood cells or T cells of less than 200 cells in every microliter of blood. It is a disease complex characterized by a collapse of the body's natural immunity against disease. Every part of the human body may be affected.

On average, HIV takes about 10 to 12 years, without treatment, to progress to AIDS. The survival rate for newly diagnosed clients initiating therapy is now estimated to be decades (see Box 23-2). There are a multitude of factors that influence the progression of the disease, including nutritional status, virulence of the strain of the virus, and the presence of other infection. The inability to adhere to, or lack of access to, antiretroviral (medication) therapy may also contribute to progression of the disease.

No Known Cure

Dramatic but expensive treatment advances have changed the health-care community's view of AIDS. The use of active antiretroviral therapy (ART) has decreased mortality rates. However, findings indicate that in the vast majority of clients receiving ART, who had undetectable levels of HIV-1 RNA in plasma, the virus has not been eradicated. Clients will require treatments continuously for the rest of their lives. Also, ART is not a treatment option for much of the world's population. Sadly, the medications are too costly (Dollars & Sense 23-1).

Primary Transmission
- Primarily transmitted through unprotected sexual contact with infected partner; anal sex increases risk
- Sharing needles or syringes

Less Common Route of Transmission
- Infants born to HIV-infected mothers
- Being accidently stuck with HIV-contaminated needle
- Receiving blood products or organ transplants
- Being bitten by an HIV-positive person
- Contact between broken skin, wounds, or mucous membranes with HIV-positive blood or body fluids

Ways HIV Is Not Transmitted
- Air or water
- Insect bites
- Saliva, tears, or sweat
- Casual contact such has hugs or handshakes

Prevention
- Be aware of HIV status
- Limit sexual partners
- Correct and consistent use of condoms if sexually active
- Don't share needles
- Health-care workers should use Universal Precaution when exposed to blood or bodily fluids (see Fig. 23-1)

BOX 23-2 ■ HIV in Aging Population

The Centers for Disease Control and Prevention (June 9, 2017) reports that of the percentage of people newly diagnosed with HIV in 2015, 12% were aged 50–59 years and 5% were 60 years old or older. Special considerations need to be made with the aging population who are living with HIV/AIDS. **Frailty** is a syndrome that is characterized by a progressive decline in system functions, including physical, social, and psychological attributes, which increases the risk of adverse outcomes (Feng et al, 2017). Frailty often results in loss of independence with increased nursing home admissions and an increase in illness and death. Clinical manifestations include low endurance, poor strength, impaired balance, unintentional weight loss, and low physical activity (Ngangbam, 2017). Older people will undergo natural age-related changes such as loss of muscle mass, and it is unknown how the virus will affect this progression. The older population with HIV may see an increase in complications related to both age and chronic inflammatory status that requires further investigation (Leng & Margolick, 2015).

Dollars & Sense 23-1

No Money for Medications

The cost of ART therapy can place a financial burden on clients, and their families, who are uninsured or underinsured. Studies have confirmed the correlation that lower income communities have greater prevalence of HIV in epidemic proportions (CDC, May 18, 2017). Below is the cost of the preferred first-line regimen utilizing generic medications that are not combined.

Medication	Dose	Monthly Cost	Annual Cost
Tenofovir	1 tablet daily	$1,197.32	$14,367.84
Lamivudine	1 tablet daily	$283.89	$3,406.68
Efavirenz	1 tablet daily	$1,010.13	$12,121.56
		Total annual cost	$29,896.08

Adapted from U.S. Department of Health and Human Services. AIDS*info*. Guidelines for the Use of Antiretroviral Agents in HIV-1-Infected Adults and Adolescents: Limits to Treatment Safety and Efficacy. Updated July 14, 2016. Available at: https://aidsinfo.nih.gov/guidelines/html/1/adult-and-adolescent-arv-guidelines/459/cost-considerations-and-antiretroviral-therapy

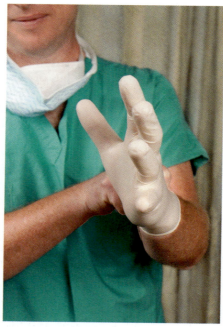

FIGURE 23-1 A health-care worker donning a pair of beige latex gloves to protect himself from body fluids. *(From CDC/Amanda Mills, 2011.)*

Signs and Symptoms

The natural history of HIV infection is divided into three stages:

1. Acute infection
2. Clinical latency
3. AIDS

Stage 1: Acute Infection

An HIV-infected individual may experience no symptoms or develop an acute flulike illness, with symptoms appearing from 2 to 4 weeks to up to 3 months after exposure to the virus. This is often referred to as acute retroviral syndrome (ARS) or primary HIV infection. Typically, the symptoms are not severe enough for the infected individual to seek medical attention. During this early phase, there are higher levels of the virus circulating in the blood, which can make the virus more easily transmittable. It is important to note that not every person infected with HIV will develop these symptoms.

Stage 2: Clinical Latency

This stage may also be referred to as *asymptomatic HIV* or the *chronic HIV* stage. The individual may be **asymptomatic** for years after becoming infected with the virus. This stage can last an average of 10 years. About 25% of HIV-infected people do not know that they are infected, and the danger lies in their ability to infect others unknowingly. Even though the person may be symptom-free, viral replication continues at a slower rate than in the acute infection stage. Clients may seek health care with minor infections and wasting syndrome, unaware of their HIV infection.

If the infection is untreated, CD_4 cells decline steadily during the latency stage.

Stage 3: AIDS

A diagnosis of AIDS is made whenever a person is HIV infected and has a CD_4 count of less than 200 cells/mm^3. Nutrition-related AIDS-defining illnesses include wasting, nutrient malabsorption, and oropharyngeal and esophageal *candidiasis* (thrush).

The Epidemic

The AIDS epidemic started in Africa, and the first cases of the syndrome were described in the United States in the early 1980s. Untreated case fatality rates initially approached 100%. With the introduction of ART, the HIV-related death rate has declined approximately 70% since 1995.

The epidemic increasingly affects persons infected through heterosexual contact, women, minorities, and people with low incomes. These affected groups are usually diagnosed at a later stage of infection when related disease is present and often delay care for themselves because they must care for others or have competing subsistence needs for their time and resources. Sub-Saharan Africa is the country most severely affected with 1 in every 25 adults living with HIV (World Health Organization [WHO], Global Health Observatory (GHO) Data, 2017). Genomic Gem 23-1 provides insight into why certain groups are more severely affected by this virus.

Complications of HIV Infection

The HIV-infection complications explained in this text include opportunistic infections such as thrush, tuberculosis (TB), and *Pneumocystis carinii* pneumonia; gastrointestinal dysfunction; AIDS dementia complex; organ dysfunction; wasting; and lipodystrophy. Boxes 23-3 and 23-4 discuss characteristics of AIDS and the common problems these clients experience.

Opportunistic Infections

Parasitic, bacterial, viral, and fungal organisms are everywhere in our environment. A healthy person's immune system keeps these organisms in check and under control. AIDS places the client at high risk for certain infections, called **opportunistic infections.** Following the guidelines for safe food handling is especially important for this population. Opportunistic infections commonly seen in clients with AIDS include thrush, TB, and *Pneumocystis* pneumonia.

GENOMIC GEM 23-1

HIV Infections by Race, Sexual Orientation, and Ethnicity

For some time, the continent of Africa has had the highest prevalence of HIV infection in the world, with 25.6 million people who live in Africa living with HIV and with more than two-thirds of the global total of new HIV diagnoses occurring on the continent (WHO, Global Health Observatory (GHO) Data, 2017).

Researchers have found a mutation in the Duffy antigen receptor expression (DARC). This mutation gives profound protection against some malaria species in West Africa (Horuk, 2015). Unfortunately, this mutation leads to significantly increased susceptibility to HIV-1 infection in those of African heritage and paradoxically to prolonged survival in HIV-1-infected individuals. This mutation may explain both the high incidence and prevalence of HIV in those of African heritage. Researchers think that the gene variant arose tens of thousands of years ago, in response to a deadly strain of malaria.

BOX 23-3 ■ Signs and Symptoms of AIDS

AIDS is characterized by:

- Fatigue
- Anorexia
- Diarrhea
- Weight loss
- Fever
- Decreased white blood cell count, or **leukopenia**
- Muscle wasting

BOX 23-4 ■ Conditions Seen in Clients with HIV/AIDS

Common problems associated with AIDS include:

- Opportunistic infections
- Gastrointestinal dysfunction
- Tumors
- AIDS dementia complex (ADC)
- Organ dysfunction

Thrush

A physical assessment may show signs of **thrush,** a thick whitish coating on the tongue or in the throat that may be accompanied by sore throat (see Fig. 23-2). Thrush is a fungal infection that can cause oral ulcers, frequent fevers, and gastrointestinal inflammation. Basic teaching for mouth care by the health educator should include the following information:

- Use a prescribed antifungal medication as directed.
- Use a cotton swab instead of a toothbrush if brushing is painful or causes bleeding. Commercial mouthwash may cause discomfort or pain.

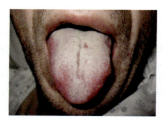

FIGURE 23-2 Thrush may cause mouth pain and interfere with nutritional intake. A soft diet may be helpful. *(Courtesy of Dr. William Gerstein; From Barankin, B, and Freiman, A: Derm Notes: Dermatology Clinical Pocket Guide. FA Davis, Philadelphia, 2006, p. 73.)*

- Avoid hot foods.
- Try soft foods, such as scrambled eggs, cottage cheese, mashed potatoes, mashed winter squash, puddings, custards, milk, juices (not citrus), and canned fruits such as peaches, pears, apricots, and bananas.
- Cut meat into small pieces or grind or blend it.
- Supplement the diet with a complete oral nutritional supplement.
- Use a straw.
- Application of anesthesia gel before eating.
- Tilt the head forward or backward to ease swallowing.
- Avoid any food that causes discomfort. Fried, spicy, sour, salty, and sticky foods may not be tolerated, such as chips, nuts, seeds, raw vegetables, peanut butter, pickles, citrus fruits and juices, and tomatoes.

Tuberculosis

TB is spread from person to person through tiny airborne particles. By sharing surroundings with a person who has active pulmonary TB, a susceptible person may inhale the disease-producing bacteria. Fortunately, most people who have inhaled these particles never become contagious or develop active TB; however, even a healthy immune system cannot kill all the particles. HIV infection weakens the body's immune system and makes it more likely that the individual who has inhaled TB-related particles will develop active TB. In 2015, out of 10.4 million new cases of TB, 1.2 million were HIV positive (WHO, HIV/AIDS: Tuberculosis & HIV, 2018).

Pneumocystis Pneumonia

Pneumonia, characterized by shortness of breath, fatigue, and anorexia, is also common in AIDS clients. About 60% of AIDS clients are infected with one type of pneumonia-causing organism, called *Pneumocystis jiroveci*, formerly called *Pneumocystis carinii*, hence the name **Pneumocystis pneumonia (PCP)**. PCP is the most common pulmonary opportunistic infection in clients with HIV. The organisms settle in the person's lungs, causing progressively worsening breathing problems and eventually leading to death. Many times clients with this infection are too tired to cook meals.

Gastrointestinal Dysfunction

The gastrointestinal tract is a common site for expression of HIV-related symptoms. The client may feel pain in the mouth or esophagus due to the growth of opportunistic infections.

The client may have difficulty swallowing because of open lesions or sores.

AIDS commonly affects both the small and large intestine. The enzymes necessary for digestion and absorption in the wall of the small intestine may be lacking or present in insufficient amounts. Malabsorption may occur with diarrhea. Gut failure may follow. Medications to control these infections also contribute to the gastrointestinal dysfunction.

AIDS Dementia Complex

AIDS dementia complex (ADC) is the most common HIV-caused central nervous system illness associated with AIDS. Early symptoms of ADC are difficulty concentrating, slowness in thinking and response, and memory impairment. Behavioral symptoms include social withdrawal, apathy, and personality changes. Motor symptoms include clumsiness of gait, difficulty with fine motor movements, and poor balance and coordination. Clients frequently become so mentally impaired that they cannot procure and prepare their own meals.

Organ Dysfunction

AIDS affects many organs in the body, leading to organ dysfunction. Diseases of the gallbladder, liver, and kidneys are seen in some AIDS clients:

Cholecystitis, inflammation of the gallbladder, can occur in conjunction with certain opportunistic infections seen in AIDS clients.

Hepatomegaly, an enlarged liver, is frequently seen, and symptoms include pain, fever, and abnormal liver function test results, especially of the alkaline phosphatase level. Liver disease is one of the leading causes of mortality in HIV-positive clients and over 60% of these deaths are attributed to being co-infected with the hepatitis C virus (HCV) (Jaquet et al, 2017).

Pancreatitis, inflammation of the pancreas, has also been noted in some infected clients.

AIDS can lead to **end-stage renal failure** within weeks.

Wasting

AIDS wasting syndrome is characterized primarily by involuntary weight loss, consisting of both lean and fat body mass. Despite treatment with medication, wasting remains a leading AIDS-defining event and is associated with high morbidity and mortality. Analysis of body composition, measurement of soft tissue volumes (muscle, fat, and organ), and diagnostic imaging of adipose tissue distribution make it possible to define wasting syndrome in terms of total weight loss and tissue compartment loss.

Wasting may be caused by undernutrition or nutrient malabsorption. The body does not compensate by decreasing resting energy expenditure as it does during starvation. Thus, kcalorie need remains elevated, and when accompanied by anorexia, the result is a high fatality rate.

AIDS-related wasting syndrome is described as a 10% weight loss from baseline with diarrhea or chronic weakness and fever for more than 30 days without a known cause.

Lipodystrophy

Lipodystrophy, an adverse effect of ART, is a syndrome causing peripheral fat wasting and fat accumulation centrally. Metabolic abnormalities in total cholesterol, increased low-density lipoprotein, and increased triglycerides may necessitate that clients modify their diets accordingly. Box 23-5 describes the signs and symptoms of lipodystrophy.

Treatment

A variety of new medications show some promise of killing or inhibiting the activity of the HIV virus. Clinical Application 23-1 discusses medication treatment for AIDS. Clients with HIV and AIDS take multiple prescribed medications, and almost all these clients need extensive counseling on food and medication interactions. Resistance training may be beneficial for these clients, especially those who are losing lean body mass. Realistically, health-care intervention can only suppress most infections for these clients, not cure them.

Other medications may be useful in reversing the nutritional decline and sequelae associated with AIDS: Marinol (dronabinol) and Megace (megestrol acetate) have both been shown to have significant efficacy in:

- Appetite stimulation
- Increased kilocalorie intake
- Reversing weight loss
- Improving a client's sense of well-being

Meal plans to support medication regimens include not only meal timing but also carbohydrate, fat, and protein distribution and symptom management strategies.

Prevention and Counseling

All states and the District of Columbia have specific laws regarding HIV testing. Screening for HIV should be part of routine medical screening with an option to decline. Current guidelines recommend that adolescents and adults aged 13 to 64 years be tested for HIV in all health-care settings (WHO, January 4, 2017). It is also recommended that clients who may be younger or older who are at high risk be tested. It is important that no client be tested without informed consent. Every client must be notified either verbally or in writing before the screening. Notification of a positive HIV test finding may create a crisis for the individual. A person who has had pretest counseling is more prepared and likely to cope better.

Counseling the individual on how best to fight the virus is important; for example, the HIV-positive individual needs to receive all current immunizations to boost his or her immunity. Behaviors that interfere with wellness and reduce immunity include:

- Drinking alcohol
- Smoking
- Illegal drug use
- Poor nutrition

These should be discouraged. Adequate rest and exercise can improve general good health and should be encouraged.

Nutrition and HIV Infection

Nutritional management is both a preventive and a therapeutic treatment in HIV infection. A malnourished client has a limited ability to fight infection. A well-nourished individual infected with the HIV virus is better able to resist opportunistic infections and tolerate the side effects of treatment. Good nutritional status may influence response to medications by:

- Decreasing the incidence of adverse drug reactions
- Providing nutrients for reactions evoked by medications
- Supporting organ functions

Worldwide, few people who have advanced disease are receiving antiretroviral treatment. Micronutrient supplements have been proposed as a low-cost intervention that may slow the progression of HIV disease. The impact of micronutrient supplementation may be less in the developed nations of the world because the general population is less likely to be malnourished.

Malnutrition in AIDS Clients

Malnutrition in clients with HIV/AIDS causes a number of physiological alterations that may lead to decreased resistance to infection and is an important predictor of morbidity and mortality. People who are malnourished are six times more likely to die than those who are adequately nourished. A well-balanced diet is essential to optimal immune function (see Box 23-6).

Malabsorption

Diarrhea and malabsorption are nutrition-related problems for AIDS clients. Diarrhea is also a side effect of antiretroviral medications.

BOX 23-5 ■ Signs and Symptoms of Lipodystrophy

Characteristics of lipodystrophy:

- Increasing abdominal girth
- Decreasing fat in the extremities and face
- Advent of a buffalo hump
- Breast enlargement
- Increased serum triglyceride levels
- Increased glucose levels
- Increased insulin levels
- Increased blood pressure

CLINICAL APPLICATION

Medications Used for HIV and AIDS

Drug therapy for clients with HIV has increased in complexity. There are currently three classes of antiretroviral medications used during the initial treatment of an HIV-positive client, including nucleoside reverse transcriptase inhibitors (NRTIs), nonnucleoside reverse transcriptase inhibitors (NNRTIs), and integrase inhibitors (IIs). Lifelong medication therapy with combinations of these medications may be required for management and presents challenges to nutritional status by introducing potential interactions with food, body metabolism, and side effects. The following table lists first-line ART medications used in adults with HIV/AIDS, typical dosing, and food tips.

Common Medications Used in HIV/AIDS

MEDICATION GENERIC NAME	DOSING	FOOD TIPS
IIS		
Dolutegravir		
NNRTIs		
Efavirenz	Daily at bedtime	Take on an empty stomach; 1 hour before or 2 hours after a meal Take with a full glass of water Hyperlipidemia
Nevirapine		
NRTIs		
Tenofovir	Daily	Take with or without food May decrease bone density May cause or worsen renal failure
Emtricitabine	Daily	Take with or without food Lactic acidosis Liver failure/jaundice
Zidovudine	Daily	Take with or without food Lactic acidosis Muscle weakness Anemia Neutropenia
Lamivudine	Daily	No interaction with or without meals May cause lactic acidosis May cause pancreatitis May worsen hepatitis

How are the drugs mentioned in the table combined? Typically the client will take a combination of antiretrovirals based on efficacy, toxicity, pill burden, dosing frequency, drug–drug interactions, and comorbidities.

Preferred first-line regimen: *Efavirenz plus tenofovir plus lamivudine (or emtricitabine)*

It is important to note that many of the medications now come as a combination tablet.

Adapted from U.S. Department of Health and Human Services. AIDSinfo: Drugs available at https://aidsinfo.nih.gov/drugs; WHO (2016, June) Consolidation Guidelines in the Use of Antiretrival Drugs for Treating and Preventing HIV Infections: Recommendations for a Public Health Approach—Second Edition. Available at http://www.who.int/hiv/pub/arv/arv-2016/en/.

BOX 23-6 ■ Effects of Malnutrition

Malnutrition causes numerous physiological alterations within the body. Some of the changes include:

- Increased gut permeability, which allows more alien material to be absorbed into the body
- Decreased intestinal secretions; some of these secretions are necessary for the proper digestion and absorption of food
- Changes in intestinal flora, which may affect the utilization of nutrients
- Hormonal imbalances
- Decreased ability to repair tissue; the body ceases to replace and repair tissue because it lacks the raw materials to do so

Mucosal atrophy and decreased digestive enzyme activity contribute to the malabsorption and diarrhea seen in persons with AIDS. Carbohydrate and fat malabsorption are frequently seen in AIDS clients with diarrhea. Gastrointestinal problems such as diarrhea may occur in children with HIV infection due to disaccharide intolerance rather than to enteric infection with known pathogens.

Malabsorption of fat, simple sugars, and vitamin B_{12} occurs in clients with intestinal infections. AIDS clients who have diarrhea or malabsorption clearly have additional vitamin and mineral needs. Clinicians should measure 25-hydroxy vitamin D levels as an indicator of fat-soluble vitamin absorption.

Studies have demonstrated that vitamin D deficiency is associated with increased risk of HIV disease progression and death (Manion et al, 2017). Initially, dietary treatment involves identification of the cause of the diarrhea and a determination of which nutrients the client cannot absorb. The concentration of hydrogen in the breath can be measured after oral lactose or sucrose administration to determine whether the client is intolerant to either of these sugars. An elevated breath hydrogen level implies intolerance because hydrogen is primarily a product of metabolism of these sugars by colon bacteria.

Fecal microbiological evaluations and intestinal biopsies are used to determine absorptive capability. In some clients infected with HIV, malabsorption of sucrose, maltose, lactose, and fat has been documented, even in the absence of diarrhea.

Clients with a form of carbohydrate intolerance may benefit from either a lactose-restricted or a disaccharide-free diet. A disaccharide-free diet is indicated for severe intolerance to sugar. Sucrose needs to be broken down into glucose and fructose (lactose into glucose and galactose; maltose into glucose and glucose) before absorption is possible.

A disaccharide-free diet excludes most fruits and vegetables and many starches and is nutritionally inadequate. Vitamin C is deficient, and daily supplementation is recommended. Some of these clients may tolerate a small amount of sugar, but they usually need assistance in understanding their tolerance level. A lactose-free diet may be sufficient for clients who are deficient only in lactase.

A low-fat diet may be necessary to control **steatorrhea.** Several additional meal-planning tips are suggested to promote the client's well-being and to control malabsorption:

- Fluids should be encouraged to maintain hydration when large fluid volume is lost in stools.
- Yogurt and other foods that contain the *Lactobacillus acidophilus* culture may be helpful if bacteria overgrowth is a problem secondary to long-term anti-infective use.
- Small, frequent meals make the best use of a limited absorptive capacity of the gut.
- A multivitamin supplement is indicated to increase the amount of vitamin available for absorption. Clients should always consult with their health-care providers before beginning supplements.
- Oral liquid nutritional supplements may be helpful.
- Aggressive nutritional support such as enteral and parenteral nutrition, if appropriate, should be considered.
- Pancreatic enzymes (Pancrecarb) may be prescribed as indicated.
- Sorbitol, which is used as a sweetening agent in both sugar-free candies and some medications, has been shown to cause diarrhea and should be avoided.
- Caffeine should be avoided because it stimulates peristalsis.
- Fiber-containing supplements may be useful.

In some situations, the malabsorption is highly resistant to treatment. Nutritional therapy goals should maximize client comfort. The benefits of overly restricting the client's diet may not suffice to offset the resulting loss in client comfort in an incurable situation.

Increased Nutritional Requirements

There is an increase in resting energy expenditure of approximately 10% in clients with HIV/AIDS. HIV wasting and secondary infections increase resting energy expenditure and increase kilocalorie, protein, and certain mineral and vitamin requirements.

Historically, dietitians have used the Harris–Benedict equation and multiplied the appropriate stress and activity factors to estimate kilocaloric requirements. Many software programs in use are still based on this equation. The Academy of Nutrition and Dietetics in its Evidence-Based Library recommends that kilocaloric needs be measured by indirect calorimetry. If this technology is not available, using formulas such as Harris–Benedict equation (see Clinical Calculation 22-3) or Mifflin–St. Jeor equation (see Clinical Calculation 22-5) is appropriate for estimating the client's energy needs.

Hypometabolism

Not all clients with AIDS become hypermetabolic. Hypometabolic clients need a gradual increase in kilocalories and a lower kilocalorie:nitrogen ratio. These clients should also be monitored for refeeding syndrome.

Decreased Food Intake

Anorexia can be a major problem for many clients with AIDS. A poor food intake may be the result of fever, respiratory infections, drug side effects, gastrointestinal complications, oral and esophageal pain, and emotional stress. Clients with ADC may experience mechanical problems with eating.

Nutritional Care in AIDS

Manifestations of the HIV virus vary greatly from one client to another. Therefore, nutritional care must be tailored to each client's unique set of symptoms. Quality nutritional care starts with screening.

Screening

Screening HIV-infected clients for nutritional problems is a crucial component of quality client care. Early indicators of decreased nutritional status include decreases in usual body weight, low weight for height, a low albumin level, and a body mass index (BMI) less than 20.

The following should be included in the assessment process:

- A baseline measure of percent body fat and lean body mass to monitor disease progression
- Recent food intake

- Comorbidities and opportunistic infection
- Oral or gastrointestinal symptoms
- Barriers the client may have to safe nutritious food
- Lack of food and poor food choices, which are linked to transmission of HIV infection and a poor response to treatment

Referral to a social worker is always indicated to address these challenging issues.

Planning Nutrient Delivery

In keeping with the general principle "if the gut works, use it," every effort should be made to feed the client orally. The following dietary modifications to oral intake may be helpful:

- Changing the meal plan, which may resolve the anorexia commonly seen in AIDS clients
- Offering small, frequent feedings
- Serving food cold or at room temperature, which may help some clients consume more kilocalories
- Modifying seasonings and kilocaloric density, which may improve intake
- Modifying texture, which may assist the client with poor chewing ability or oral lesions

If the client is unable to consume sufficient nutrients from table foods, supplemental feedings or other enteral feedings should be considered. The type of malnutrition should influence the food and supplements offered, which the dietitian usually determines.

If the client is unable to consume sufficient nutrients orally and the gut is working, a tube feeding may be considered. Percutaneous endoscopic gastrostomy (PEG) tubes are often used. If the gut is not functioning properly, peripheral parenteral nutrition (PPN) or central parenteral nutrition (CPN) may be considered. The goal should always be to prolong living, not to prolong dying. A client has the right to refuse any alternative-feeding route offered.

Monitoring

To ensure that adequate nutrients are being consumed, body weight, waist circumference, and nutritional intake should be monitored every few weeks along with BMI and percent body fat. The loss of lean tissue central to body metabolism may be present throughout the disease process, regardless of weight maintenance, suggesting that weight is not a good early indicator of declining nutritional status. Throughout this process, health-care workers should maintain a supportive, nonjudgmental approach, which is the key to establishing a trusting relationship.

Client Teaching

An assessment of the client's knowledge level and understanding of an individualized meal plan is appropriate. All AIDS clients need instruction on food safety because low

immune system functioning makes them much more susceptible to food-borne illnesses. Education will minimize the likelihood of opportunistic infection. Instructions on dietary modifications, including nutrient-dense meals and the use of supplemental feedings, are also indicated (see Box 23-7).

Food Faddism and Quackery

Some clients with AIDS are vulnerable to both food faddism and quackery because they become desperate to try anything that arouses hope.

Food faddism is an unusual pattern of food behavior enthusiastically adapted by its adherents.

Food quackery is the promotion for profit of a medical scheme or remedy that is unproved or known to be false.

Health-care educators need to carefully balance and consider the danger of unusual food behaviors versus taking away any hope the client may have. Clients may tune out educators if they perceive that their beliefs and feelings are discounted without sensitivity. Some unusual food behaviors are not harmful, and some food behaviors can result in negative health consequences.

Follow-Up Care

The nutritional status of a client may depend on appropriate follow-up care. A referral should be made to a community agency, a home health-care program, an outpatient clinic, or a dietitian to provide continuity of care.

BOX 23-7 ■ Counseling the Client With HIV and AIDS

These nutritional principles are important to discuss with HIV and AIDS clients soon after the initial diagnosis:

- Review the principles of safe food handling and storage with the client (see Chapter 13).
- Review MyPlate guidelines as a basis for dietary intake.
- Discuss considering multivitamin and mineral supplement.
- Discourage inappropriate weight loss; many HIV clients lose lean body mass first and fat second. Address prevention, restoration, and maintenance of optimal body composition with emphasis on lean tissue. Encourage physical activity.
- If indicated, encourage more and frequent meals to increase energy intake. Teach regarding consuming foods with high nutrient density. Snacks, complete nutritional supplements, and intravenous feedings may be necessary.
- Suggest increasing whole-grain and fiber intake, which may include soluble-fiber supplementation.
- Discuss potential medication–nutrition interactions.
- Review use of nutrient supplements and potential interactions with nonprescription and herbal supplements.
- Address food and nutrition security issues. Refer to the social worker if the client lacks enough food.
- During counseling, evaluate signs and symptoms and tailor counseling to the client's unique needs. In addition, closely monitor the client's blood lipids, triglyceride, glucose, and cholesterol levels and recommend modification of the diet as indicated.

KEYSTONES

- The AIDS epidemic is worldwide.
- Although ART treatment has reduced mortality rates, no cure has been found for AIDS.
- Transmittal routes include blood-to-blood, perinatal, and sexual contact.
- Health-care professionals can protect themselves from AIDS by using extreme care when handling blood and equipment that has been in contact with blood; practicing safe sexual behaviors can help to protect everyone from AIDS.
- HIV attacks the immune system and leaves its victims defenseless against opportunistic infections.
- AIDS is a disease with many clinical complications.
- Nutritional management is both a preventive and a therapeutic treatment in clients infected with HIV.
- Increased nutrient needs, decreased food intake, and impaired nutrient absorption contribute to the malnutrition seen in AIDS clients.

CASE STUDY 23-1

Mrs. S is a 30-year-old woman who acquired HIV from her drug-abusing husband and subsequently infected their son in utero. She could not believe the test results when she was first told. Now she is seeking nutritional information to allow her to increase her chance for a quality life and her son's chance to survive infancy. Her knowledge of basic nutrition is good. She expressed some concern about transportation and has already missed her 6-week postpartum visit because her husband sold their car for money to buy drugs. She is also unable to go to the grocery store easily. She is 5 ft 6 in. tall and weighs 120 lb. All her laboratory work was within normal limits. Percent body fat is 25%.

CARE PLAN

Subjective Data
Lack of information on relationship of nutrition to AIDS ▪ Concrete goals established

Objective Data
HIV-positive tests, both mother and infant ▪ Percent body fat, 25%

Analysis
Lack of information related to modifying AIDS progression and changing unhealthy home environment

Plan

DESIRED OUTCOMES EVALUATION CRITERIA	ACTIONS/ INTERVENTIONS	RATIONALE
Client will verbalize areas in which nutrition could affect AIDS development.	Reinforce need for regular, balanced meals. Emphasize adequate kcalories.	The stress of receiving this diagnosis may impede use of previously learned information.
	Instruct Mrs. S to keep home environment clean, especially kitchen, bathroom, and basements, where molds and fungi could thrive. Teach client to monitor herself and her son for changes in health related to food intake or digestion.	Organisms that are harmless to persons with normal immune systems can cause opportunistic infections in HIV-infected persons. Discovering beginning malabsorption problems would permit treatment before malnutrition becomes apparent.
Client will monitor her percent body fat.	Explain the relationships among percent body fat, percent lean body mass, and exercise.	Exercise can prevent a loss of lean body mass. Weight can be stable, but body fat content can increase.
Client will keep her medical appointments and obtain groceries as needed.	Refer to social worker for help with transportation and food assistance programs.	The social worker has knowledge of available local resources.

TEAMWORK 23-1

SOCIAL WORKER'S NOTE

If the client is an inpatient, the social worker typically writes in the discharge planning section of the medical record. If the client is an outpatient, the social worker typically phones the physician's office directly with a solution to the problem and writes a short note to be placed in the medical record.

I met with the client, who described a sad home situation. We discussed the need for her to remove herself and infant from her present environment. I arranged for client to move into a shelter for abused women. She agreed to do this immediately.

TEAMWORK 23-2

DIETITIAN'S NOTES

The following Dietitian's Notes are representative of the documentation found in a client's medical record.

Subjective: *Met with the client, who expressed an interest in making improvements to her diet. She currently eats three times each day and does not avoid any of the major food groups. She does not take a multivitamin/mineral supplement.*

Objective: *5 ft 6 in. Percent body fat 25%; 120 lb*

Analysis: *Ideal body weight range 117–143 lb. Weight in kg is 54.5 kg. Estimated kcal need at 25–35 kcal/kg and 54.5 kg equals 1,363–1,907. Estimated protein need at 1.0–1.5 grams/kg equals 54.4–82 grams. Client's reported food intake, based on a 24-hour dietary recall and cross-checked with a food frequency, showed a kcalorie intake between 1,400 and 1,600. Her usual protein intake is between 40 and 50 grams per day. We discussed options for the client to increase her protein intake.*

Plan: *Recommend the addition of one cup of low-fat yogurt or milk per day. Client agreed to do this.*

CRITICAL THINKING QUESTIONS

1. The client has developed mouth sores from thrush and would like you to arrange for her to have CPN. She claims that it is just too painful to eat. What would you recommend?

2. The client's child has been diagnosed HIV positive. During a home visit, you notice that the kitchen is filthy. You instruct the client on food safety and sanitation. On a return visit, despite prior instruction on food safety, you notice that the client's kitchen is still not clean. The client claims that she is too tired to clean. What do you do?

3. The client went to a health food store and purchased several bottles of vitamin pills and herbal supplements. She believes that she can take these in lieu of eating. What should you do?

CHAPTER REVIEW

1. The health-care worker's best insurance against HIV transmission on the job is:
   1. Frequent hand washing
   2. Universal precautions
   3. Body substance isolation
   4. Adherence to all food safety policies and procedures

2. A client on ART can partially compensate for fat redistribution syndrome by:
   1. Taking medications as prescribed
   2. Taking supplemental vitamins and minerals
   3. Consuming a low-fat diet
   4. Exercising

3. Compared with wasting, cachexia is:
   1. A slower process
   2. The result of both a protein and kilocalorie deficit
   3. Always the result of a poor food intake
   4. Best treated by the inclusion of 400 additional kilocalories per day

4. Clinicians measure ____ as an indicator of fat-soluble vitamin absorption.
   1. Folate
   2. Zinc
   3. 25-hydroxy vitamin D
   4. Glucose

5. Educating a client with AIDS about food safety is important:
   1. To minimize the risk of rare tumors
   2. To prevent body fat redistribution
   3. To enhance renal function
   4. To prevent opportunistic infections

CLINICAL ANALYSIS

1. Mr. Y, a 45-year-old man, was diagnosed as HIV-positive 1 month ago. His height is 6 ft 0 in., and his weight is 178 lb and stable. He reports no signs or symptoms and has not seen a physician yet. He wants to know what he should eat. As the nurse during this first visit, you might discuss:
   a. The many benefits of ART
   b. Food safety, exercise, good nutrition, and the importance of follow-up with a physician
   c. The expected outcome and potential complications
   d. Vitamin and mineral supplementation, increased kilocaloric needs, and the treatment for malabsorption

2. Carlos, a 25-year-old man, presents with severe diarrhea. He was diagnosed with HIV about 8 years ago. He has five to six watery stools each day that do not appear to be related to his medications. His height is 5 ft 10 in., and his weight is 140 lb (usual weight is 175 lb). He is an inpatient, and the physician has ordered a stool culture, but the results are not back. You recommend:
   a. Extra fluids with meals to prevent dehydration
   b. A clear-liquid, complete nutritional supplement
   c. A high-fat and high-fiber diet to provide both kilocalories and bulk to his diet
   d. Six small meals with a milkshake between meals to push kilocalories and protein

3. Dave, a 36-year-old man, complains of fatigue. He is often too tired to cook and has little interest in food. He lives alone and is on disability. His CD_4 cell count is 400, and his viral load is 100,000. You recommend:
   a. Tube feeding
   b. Referral to a social service agency
   c. Meals-on-Wheels
   d. Six small meals daily

CHAPTER 24

Nutritional Care of the Terminally Ill

LEARNING OBJECTIVES

After completing this chapter, the student should be able to:

- Differentiate between palliative and curative nutritional care.
- State-appropriate nutritional screening questions for the terminally ill client.
- List at least two appropriate dietary management techniques for symptom control for each of the following: anemia, anorexia, cachexia, constipation, cough, dehydration, diarrhea, dysgeusia, esophageal reflux, fever, fluid accumulation, hiccups, incontinence, jaundice and hepatic encephalopathy, migraine headache, nausea and vomiting, pruritus, stomatitis, weakness, wounds and pressure injuries, and **xerostomia.**
- State-appropriate assessment questions for a terminally ill client.
- Discuss the ethical and legal considerations for feeding a terminally ill client.

This chapter discusses clients who have been certified by physicians to be terminally ill. An individual is considered terminally ill if he or she has a medical prognosis of 6 months or less based on the usual disease progression. Although a physician can estimate life expectancy based on disease progression, this is not an exact science. A client diagnosed with a terminal disease may live longer than or not as long as predicted because the disease may not follow its usual progression. Individuals who have been certified by a physician as terminally ill can elect to use the hospice benefit under federal guidelines. Hospice is the major health-care program for the terminally ill in the United States.

Dealing With Death

Our culture emphasizes the enjoyment of life. At the beginning of the 20th century, most people died at home, and many died young. Death was a part of everyday life. Over the past 50 years, most people have died in hospitals or long-term care facilities. Often an ambulance is called if a person is dying.

Although health-care workers have received much training on how to reverse the effects of disease, we have received much less training on how to assist our clients with dying. With changes in the health-care system bringing decreased lengths of hospital stays, an increasing number of clients will again be cared for in their homes. Training health-care workers to provide home care for terminally ill clients is becoming essential.

Nutritional and dietary issues are at the center of some ethical questions concerning the care of these clients. Health-care professionals need to address clients' values, goals of care, and preferences with regard to treatment to truly become client advocates.

The Dying Process

Death is an unavoidable part of the life cycle. Both physiological and psychological changes occur as part of the dying process. The client's age, diagnosis, and physical condition influence physiological changes. Regardless of the underlying disease, cardiopulmonary failure is the final cause of death. Pulmonary and circulatory failure may be gradual or sudden. The major signs and symptoms in the final days and hours of life include:

- Cessation of eating and drinking
- Oliguria and incontinence
- Muscle weakness
- Difficulty in breathing
- Cyanosis
- Decreased mental alertness
- Changes in vital signs

Hospice team members may describe clients with a terminal diagnosis as actively dying. An actively dying client has a life expectancy of a few hours or a few days. The reason for the actively dying designation is to determine staff needs.

Cessation of Eating and Drinking

Life will soon cease when a client's eating and drinking diminishes critically. Oral intake dwindles because a client has no desire to eat or because disease prevents digestion. This greatly decreased oral intake is often worrisome to family members.

Health-care workers need to counsel family members that dehydration at this time is believed to have a euphoric effect and is not painful. Clinical Application 24-1 discusses the physiological responses to fluid restriction. Fluids and comfort care such as the following actions can reduce the thirst sensations from dehydration:

- Ice chips if alert
- Lubricating the lips with moistened gauze or a water-soluble product
- Small amounts of food and water if desired by the client

Withholding and minimizing hydration can have the desirable effect of reducing:

- Disturbing oral secretions
- Bronchial secretions
- Need for frequent urination
- Cough from diminished pulmonary congestion
- Edema

It is not compassionate to force food or fluids on a client who is actively dying.

Oliguria and Incontinence

Because oral intake is usually decreased for several days before death, urine output is often diminished and may cease. The color of the urine may become very dark. A period of incontinence often precedes the oliguria, and anuria occurs. General fatigue, muscle weakness, and decreased mental acuity are among the reasons for the incontinence. Bedding should be changed as quickly as possible to avoid skin irritation. Death usually occurs within 48 to 72 hours after urine output stops.

CLINICAL APPLICATION   24-1

Physiological Response to Fluid Restriction

Young, healthy, active individuals who are deprived of water develop thirst, dry mouth, and headache, followed by fatigue; cognitive impairment occurs as dehydration progresses and becomes severe with abnormal electrolytes, rising blood urea nitrogen, and hemoconcentration. If water is not taken, renal failure is likely.

In terminally ill clients, dehydration results in the same signs and symptoms. However, studies have shown that metabolic changes may produce a sedative effect on the brain just before death. In cases where the evidence strongly suggests that hydration or feeding does not provide benefit, the health-care team has a responsibility to explain this to the client and/or family.

One study demonstrated that hospice nurses had positive views of terminal dehydration while acute care nurses felt dying clients needed artificial hydration and nutrition (Lachman, 2015). This study highlights the need for better education of nurses as well as families.

Difficulty in Breathing

Most clients have some difficulty breathing before death. Caregivers may become alarmed when they hear a loud, hoarse, and bubbling sound. These sounds are caused by the passage of breath through pharyngeal and pulmonary secretions that lodge at the back of the client's throat. These sounds are known as **terminal respiratory secretions,** often referred to as the "death rattle" by the lay public. Most clients will die within 24 to 48 hours after the development of this symptom. It is believed that the client does not experience increased suffering, but the symptom can be distressing for loved ones. Interventions that can be used to reduce symptoms and maintain a clear airway include elevating the head of the bed, positioning the client on his or her side and frequent turning, avoiding overhydration, using a humidifier, opening a window or using a fan to circulate air in the room, and use of anticholinergic medication such as scopolamine in order to decrease the amount of secretions. Suctioning is not recommended because it can cause discomfort in the client. All terminally ill clients do not have these sounds with respiration. Some clients experience apnea (a temporary cessation of breathing). A change such as one of these in breathing is an indicator that life will soon cease.

Cyanosis

Slightly bluish, grayish, or dark purple discoloration of the skin caused by poor oxygenation is called **cyanosis.** The client's feet, legs, hands, and groin feel cold. Many health-care workers believe that this is one of the most useful indicators that the end of life is approaching. Slowed circulation and decreased tissue perfusion cause these signs.

Decreased Mental Alertness

The amount of blood reaching the brain, lungs, liver, and kidneys decreases as general circulation slows. Sleepiness, apathy, disorientation, confusion, restlessness, and finally a decreased level of consciousness that frequently progresses to a sleeplike state are among the signs that death is imminent.

Changes in Vital Signs

Signs of impeding death include:

- A decrease in body temperature
- A rise and then a decrease in pulse rate
- A rise and then a decrease in respirations
- A fall in blood pressure

Death occurs when there is no pulse and respiration ceases.

Family members and caregivers of terminally ill clients often express fear at the thought of being alone with an actively dying client. For this reason, health-care workers often remain with the client and their loved ones during this time. Some health-care workers resist working with the terminally ill because they think that they cannot cope with this experience. However, death is not always a painful experience. Health-care workers who share the death experience with a client and the client's family often describe the experience as rewarding and profound.

Palliative Versus Curative Care

Palliative care has been defined as the active total care of an individual when curative measures are no longer considered an option by either the medical team or the client. The goal of curative care is arresting the disease. The goal of palliative care is the relief of symptoms to alleviate or ease pain and discomfort. Emphasis in palliative care is placed on addressing:

- Pain and symptom control
- Spiritual and psychological support
- Improving quality of life

These concerns are common in dying clients. Palliative care is defined by the World Health Organization (2017) as "An approach that improves the quality of life of patients and their families facing the problems associated with life-threatening illness, through the prevention and relief of suffering by means of early identification and impeccable assessment and the treatment of pain and other problems physical, psychosocial and spiritual." Palliative care programs address and include the client and family members in the plan of care, and care can be provided at any time during the course of the disease, not just at the end of life.

Hospice dates back to medieval times. During the crusades, travelers needed a place to stop for comfort. The Knights of Hospitallers of the Order of St. John of Jerusalem in the 12th century sheltered the sick and religious pilgrims. They established hospices in England, Germany, Italy, Cyprus, and Rhodes. The soul, mind, and spirit were considered as much in need of help as the body.

Around the 15th century, anatomical and surgical practices developed. Physicians moved into hospitals that emphasized curative treatments. Monks and nuns remained in cloisters and cared for the people the physicians could not heal, including the disabled, the chronically ill, and the terminally ill.

During the 18th and 19th centuries, great advances in curative treatments occurred, and hospitals became highly specialized in acute life-threatening situations. Hospitals were less able to offer shelter to people nearing life's end. At the same time, caring for the terminally ill became less a private or religious function and more a public and governmental one.

The modern hospice has its roots in the late 19th century, when a place of shelter for the incurably ill was founded in Dublin. The British physician Dr. Cicely Saunders inspired the hospice movement in the United States. Dr. Saunders is noted for her work in pain control and for the founding of St. Christopher's Hospice in London in 1967. The first operational hospice program in the United States was established in New Haven, Connecticut, in the early 1970s.

Hospice philosophy includes the belief that death is a natural aspect of life. Hospice is committed to the philosophy that persons have the right to die in the setting of their choice and to be as comfortable as possible. Central to the hospice philosophy is the idea that palliative care is appropriate when treatment of the client's disease becomes ineffective and irrelevant.

In 2014, it was estimated that 1.6 to 1.7 million people received hospice services and 58.9% of those clients died at home with their family or loved ones providing their primary care (National Hospice and Palliative Care Organization, 2015).

Nutrition Screening

All palliative care begins with the establishment of the goals of care. Studies suggest that what terminally ill clients want is to:

- Have their pain and other symptoms relieved
- Improve their quality of life
- Avoid being a burden to their family
- Have a close relationship with loved ones
- Maintain a sense of control

The goal of palliative nutritional care is to assist the client and caregiver with any food-related concerns. These difficulties may be related to uncomfortable symptoms and attitudes and beliefs held about food. Screening the client with a terminal illness for food-related concerns is the first step. There are major differences between screening a client who is undergoing curative or preventive treatment and screening a terminally ill client who is receiving palliative care.

First, the health-care worker needs to ascertain if the client has any symptoms that may be diminished by nutritional intervention. Second, the attitudes and beliefs of the client or caregiver about food need to be examined. Some clients and their caregivers have difficulty accepting that the terminally ill client frequently eats much less than is needed to sustain life. Box 24-1 is an example of a nutrition screening form for the client with a terminal condition.

Health-care professionals, clients, and family members frequently want to discuss the use of an intravenous or tube feedings in a terminally ill client during the screening process. The use of any artificial feeding should always be considered but is often inconsistent with treatment goals. For example, in the case of a client with dementia who has dysphagia or stops eating, placement of a percutaneous endoscopic gastrostomy (PEG) tube may be considered but should not be routinely used if dysphagia is caused by end-stage disease (Brooke & Ojo, 2015). If the treatment goal of the client is to reduce suffering and enhance the quality of life, a PEG tube may not assist in meeting this goal. The position of the Academy of Nutrition and Dietetics is that individuals have the right to request or refuse nutrition and hydration as medical treatment. This refusal includes PEG tube placement.

BOX 24-1 ■ Sample Nutrition Screening Form

Name _____ Caregiver's Name _____
Date _____ Diagnosis _____

1. Have you had any concerns about weight changes or food intake?

No _____ Yes _____ Describe _____

2. For clients on tube feedings or parenteral feedings only: Have your feedings created or increased discomfort, diarrhea, distension, other?

Type: _____ Amount _____ Infusion rate _____

3. Do you feel your symptoms could be decreased or controlled through dietary change?

No _____ Yes _____ Describe _____

4. Do you feel diet or nutritional supplement would benefit you or your disease process?

No _____ Yes _____ Type _____

5. Do you believe that your diet caused your disease or will slow the progression of your disease?

No _____ Yes _____ Describe _____

6. Do you find eating enhances comfort?

No _____ Yes _____

7. What concerns do you have regarding your diet intake? _____

8. Would you (client or caregiver) like to discuss food-related concerns with the dietitian?

No _____ Yes _____

Assessment

During the nutritional assessment, every question posed to the client or caregiver should have a purpose. Health-care workers generally need to know the results of laboratory tests, diagnostic procedures, physical examinations, and anthropometric measures as well as the level of immune function and food intake information to determine a client's nutritional status; however, this may have no value in the provision of nutritional care for a terminally ill client.

For example, why ask if a client drinks milk? Is it to estimate if the client is meeting the calcium, riboflavin, and vitamin D allowances? If it is determined that the client's milk intake is suboptimal, would anything be done about the inadequacy? If the client has diarrhea with severe abdominal cramping after the ingestion of milk, however, a recommendation to drink lactose-free milk would be appropriate. Unless the client will experience relief from bothersome symptoms, it is best not to recommend behavioral changes that may be difficult for the client to make. On the other hand, if the client expresses concern about the nutritional adequacy of his or her diet, nutrition education is not contraindicated (see Box 24-1).

Intervention and Symptom Control

Box 24-2 describes appropriate dietary management for symptom control for a client with a terminal illness. If a health-care worker feels uncomfortable discussing these

BOX 24-2 ■ Dietary Management for Symptom Control

Anemia
- Recommend a vitamin C source with red meats and iron-fortified foods.
- Discourage use of coffee, tea, and chocolate if the client has gastrointestinal bleeding.
- Recommend a multivitamin supplement if the client desires and the primary care provider approves but avoid megadose vitamins.

Anorexia
- Discuss practical issues with the client or caregiver, such as food attitudes, social aspects of eating, food preferences, and beliefs about food.
- Encourage concentration on the sensual pleasures of eating, such as table setting, garnishes, smells, and socialization.
- Evaluate the client's desire for a sense of well-being.
- Suggest use of small, frequent feedings.
- Educate the caregiver to recognize early signs of malnutrition and provide protein supplements, make food accessible, and encourage eating as desired by the client and caregiver if the client's prognosis is more than a few weeks.
- Evaluate the client's acceptance of a liquid diet and recommend complete oral nutritional supplements.
- Teach the caregiver that the client has the right to self-determination and may refuse to eat or drink when actively dying. The caregiver should continue to offer nourishment as a sign of love and caring but not harass the client to eat or drink.

Cachexia
- Teach relaxation techniques and encourage use before mealtime.
- Encourage the client and the caregiver to concentrate on the sensual pleasures of eating, such as setting an attractive table and plate and using food garnishes and providing an appetizing eating environment by removing bedpans and emesis basin before serving the food.
- Evaluate client for dysgeusia and dysphagia and xerostomia.

Constipation
- Encourage high-fiber foods (bran, whole grains, fruits, vegetables, nuts, and legumes) if an adequate fluid intake can be maintained.
- Instruct the client to avoid high-fiber foods if dehydration or an obstruction is suspected or anticipated.
- Assess the client's fluid intake and recommend an increased intake if needed.
- Recommend taking 1–2 ounces of a special recipe with the evening meal: 2 cups applesauce, 2 cups unprocessed bran (All-Bran®), and 1 cup of 100% prune juice. Refrigerate this mixture between uses and discard after 5 days if not used.
- Suggest limiting cheese and high-fat, sugary foods (doughnuts, cakes, pies, cookies) that may be constipating.
- Discontinue calcium and iron supplements if they contribute to constipation.
- Review the client's medications. If the client is taking bulking agents (milk of magnesia, magnesium citrate, Metamucil®, or Golytely®),

(continued)

BOX 24-2 ■ **Dietary Management for Symptom Control—cont'd**

a large fluid intake is essential. Suggest the client or caregiver to mask the taste of these medications in applesauce, mashed potatoes, gravy, orange juice, and nectars.

Cough

- Encourage fluids and ice chips.
- Recommend hard candy, including sour balls.
- Have the client try tea and coffee to dilate pulmonary vessels.

Dehydration

- Encourage intake of fluids such as juices, ice cream, gelatin, custards, puddings, and soups if the client's life expectancy is more than a few days.
- Encourage the client to try creative beverages such as orange sherbet and milkshake.
- Consider a nasogastric tube feeding for fluid delivery only after a discussion with other team members, client, and caregivers. Plain water and foods high in electrolytes can be delivered via a tube feeding.
- Consider a parenteral line only after a tube feeding is considered and rejected and after an in-depth discussion with the team members, client, and family. Client goals, expectations, and quality-of-life issues should all be very carefully considered. Parenteral lines for the delivery of nutrients and water are rarely indicated in terminally ill clients.

Diarrhea

- Consider modification of the diet to omit lactose, gluten, or fat if related to diarrhea.
- Suggest a decrease in dietary fiber content.
- Consider the omission of gas-forming vegetables if an association between the consumption of these foods and diarrhea can be ascertained.
- Consider the use of a low-residue diet.
- Encourage consumption of high-potassium foods (bananas, tomato juice, orange juice, potatoes) if the client is dehydrated.
- Recommend dry feedings (drink fluids 1 hour before or 30–60 minutes after meals).
- Encourage intake of medium-chain triglycerides and a diet high in protein and carbohydrates for steatorrhea due to pancreatic insufficiency.
- Consider the use of a complete oral nutritional supplement to provide adequate nutrient composition while helping the client overcome mild-to-moderate malabsorption.
- For copious diarrhea or diarrhea combined with a coccyx decubitus, consider use of a clear-liquid complete nutritional supplement or a predigested oral nutritional supplement.

Dysgeusia (abnormal taste)

- Encourage oral care before mealtime.
- Evaluate whether the client experiences a bitter, sweet, or no taste after food consumption.
- If foods taste bitter, encourage consumption of poultry, fish, milk and milk products, and legumes. Recommend the use of marinated meats and poultry in juices or wine. Sour and salty foods are generally not liked when a client experiences a bitter taste. Cook food in a glass or porcelain container to improve taste. Recommend a decreased use of red meats, sour juices, coffee, tea, tomatoes, and chocolate. The use of a modular protein supplement may be helpful if the client's protein intake is suboptimal.
- If foods taste sweet, recommend sour juices, tart foods, lemon juice, vinegar, pickles, spices, herbs, and the use of a modular carbohydrate supplement.
- If food has no taste, recommend foods served at room temperature, highly seasoned foods, and sugary foods.
- Recommend the use of sugar-free mints or gum.

Dyspnea (difficulty breathing)

- Encourage intake of coffee, tea, and chocolate. These foods are bronchodilators that increase blood pressure, dilate pulmonary vessels, increase glomerular filtration rate, and thus break up and expel pulmonary secretions and fluids.
- Encourage use of a soft diet. Liquids are usually better tolerated than solids. Cold foods are often better accepted than hot foods.
- Recommend small, frequent feedings.
- Encourage ice chips, frozen fruit juices, and popsicles; these are often well accepted.
- Consider the use of a complete high-fat, low-carbohydrate nutritional supplement. This decreases carbon dioxide retention and assists in breathing.

Esophageal Reflux

- Recommend small feedings.
- Discourage consumption of foods that lower esophageal sphincter pressure, such as high-fat foods, chocolate, peppermint, spearmint, and alcohol.
- Encourage the client to sit up while eating and for 1 hour afterward.
- Recommend avoidance of food within 3 hours before bedtime.
- Teach relaxation techniques.

Fever

- Recommend a high fluid intake.
- Consider a tube feeding for severe dehydration to maintain hydration after a discussion with team members. This is not recommended if death is imminent (hours/days).
- Recommend high-protein, high-caloric foods.

Fluid Accumulation

- Recommend a mild sodium restriction (<2 grams/day). Recommend a lower sodium restriction only if this is the wish of the client.
- Discourage a fluid restriction unless the client has significant hyponatremia.
- Provide a list of foods high in protein and potassium.

Hiccups

- Recommend smaller meals and slow eating.
- Discourage the use of a straw.
- Recommend the client swallow a large teaspoon of granulated sugar.

Hypoglycemia

- Assess the client's and caregiver's knowledge about diabetes and hypoglycemia.
- Determine if the client is truly insulin dependent as part of the admission assessment process.
  The following suggest true insulin dependence:
  - Introduction of insulin soon after the diagnosis
  - A history of previous ketoacidosis
  - Use of more than one daily dose of insulin for years
- Evaluate the client's expressed desire for extent of medical care. The primary guide for determining the level of nutritional intervention is the wish of the client.
- Determine the last time the client experienced the signs of a hypoglycemic episode. Many of these clients have deficiencies in the counter-regulatory hormones, especially epinephrine, and may lapse into a coma without any warning signs. Caregivers need to be informed of this potential complication. Educate the client and/or caregiver on the treatment of hypoglycemia.
- Monitor the client's blood glucose level. A suitable range for blood sugars would be 108–200 mg/dL in the hospice population.
- Encourage consumption of 30–50 grams of carbohydrate every 3 hours to prevent starvation ketosis. Each of the following is equal to 30–50 grams of carbohydrate: ¾ cup of Carnation Instant

BOX 24-2 ■ Dietary Management for Symptom Control—cont'd

Breakfast®, 1 cup of regular gelatin, 1 cup of vanilla ice cream, 1½ cups of ginger ale, 1 cup of orange juice, and 1 cup of apple juice.

Incontinence
- Discourage intake of coffee, tea, and carbonated beverages containing caffeine, especially before bedtime.
- Continue to encourage adequate fluid intake during the day.

Jaundice and Hepatic Encephalopathy
- Encourage a high-carbohydrate diet.
- Encourage a protein-restricted diet only if the client desires.
- Specialized oral nutritional supplements for clients with liver disease are often ineffective for the terminally ill but may be beneficial when the client desires to "live long enough to _____."
- Evaluate for the presence of esophageal varices. If present, provide soft foods.

Nausea and Vomiting
- Discuss practical issues with the client and caregiver such as food attitudes, social aspects of eating, and unpredictable food preferences.
- Recommend the client restrict fluids to 1 hour before or after meals to prevent early satiety.
- Assess if sweet, fried, or fatty foods are poorly tolerated; recommend avoidance if necessary.
- Evaluate if starchy foods such as crackers, breads, potatoes, rice, and pasta are better tolerated. Encourage increased consumption if helpful.
- Encourage the client to eat slowly, chew food well, and rest after each meal because these behaviors may increase food intake.
- Recommend that the client is not subjected to offensive odors during food preparation.
- Recommend that the person who has recently experienced severe nausea and vomiting try one to two bites of food per hour.
- Emphasize the sensual aspects of food, including appearance (serve garnished food on attractive tableware), odor of environment (remove bedpans and emesis basins from room), taste (cater to the client's likes and dislikes), and the importance of companionship during mealtime.
- Recommend the avoidance of food if nausea and vomiting become severe and food makes the client feel worse. Feeding may not be desirable if death is expected within hours or a few days and the effects of partial dehydration or the withdrawal of nutrition support will not adversely alter client comfort.
- Use of ginger to reduce effects of nausea.

Migraine Headaches
- Recommend that the client eat at regular intervals. Hunger or missed meals can trigger a migraine headache.
- Recommend that the highly motivated client keep a food diary and record the onset of any headaches. Migraine headaches can be triggered by one or many foods. Common food offenders include many common food additives, processed meats, peanuts and peanut products, soybeans, yeast, chocolate, aged cheeses, seasonings, caffeine, some types of alcohol, and flavorings.

Pruritus (severe itching)
- Recommend avoidance of known allergy foods.
- Encourage adequate fluid intake.
- Encourage adequate consumption of protein and fatty acids.

Stomatitis (inflammation of the mouth)
- Consider a multivitamin supplement with folic acid and vitamin B_{12}.
- Recommend avoidance of spicy, acidic, rough, hot, and salty foods.
- Recommend a consistency modification, such as pureed, soft, or liquid.
- Consider the use of a complete nutritional supplement.
- Recommend creamy foods, white sauces, and gravies.
- Consider between-meal supplements, such as milkshakes, eggnogs, and puddings.
- Recommend meals be served when the client's pain is under control.
- Recommend good oral care before and after meals.

Weakness
- Recommend a multivitamin–mineral supplement with folic acid, vitamin B_{12}, and iron.
- Encourage high-potassium foods (bananas, cantaloupe, milk, baked winter squash, etc.) if the client vomits easily.
- Recommend a modification in the food's consistency (mechanical soft or full liquid) to decrease the energy cost of eating.

Wounds and Pressure Injury
- Recommend the caregiver cater to the client's food preferences.
- Use of aggressive nutritional support is rarely effective but may be appropriate if the client and family express a desire to maximize quantity of life. For example, "I want to live and see my _____."
- Correct elevated glucose levels to decrease risk of infection.
- Evaluate the use of a multivitamin and mineral supplement that contains zinc and vitamin C. Because excess dietary zinc impedes healing, do not routinely recommend a zinc supplement without assessment information.
- Encourage protein and caloric intake equal to estimated needs only if the client desires and is able.
- Encourage the client to dip foods in gravy, margarine, butter, and olive oil to increase calorie intake.

Xerostomia (dry mouth)
- Encourage frequent sips of water or ice chips.
- Recommend the use of sugar-free chewing gum.
- Consider a modification of food consistency such as soft, mechanical soft, or full liquids.
- Recommend avoidance of extremely hot or cold foods. Foods served at room temperature are generally better tolerated.
- Recommend creamy foods, white sauces, and gravies.
- Encourage the client to dip foods in gravy, margarine, butter, olive oil, coffee, and broth.
- Consider the need for a complete liquid nutritional supplement between meals.

---

issues with the client or lacks the time to counsel the client, a referral to the dietitian is indicated.

Ethical and Legal Considerations

Many of the legal and ethical issues concerning health-care delivery and health-care provider–client relations involve the provision of nutrition and hydration. In the past, before the development of tube feedings and intravenous feedings, the inability to eat and drink by mouth meant death from progressive body wasting.

Now a decision needs to be made whether to feed a client. A client may experience a more comfortable death if he or she is slightly dehydrated. On the other hand, efforts to hydrate some clients (not those actively dying) may offer a benefit. This is controversial. Sometimes a client, significant other, or physician thinks that artificial hydration may promote client comfort and prolong life in a given situation.

Perhaps a client's vital signs had been fluctuating and are now stable. Ethicists use rational processes for determining the most morally desirable course of action in the face of conflicting value choices. The process of choosing an ethical course of action involves:

- Medical goals and proportionality
- Client preferences
- Quality of life
- Contextual features

Contextual features are the characteristics of a given situation.

Medical Care Goals and Proportionality

The medical care goals that apply to the client with a terminal illness include:

- Relieving symptoms, pain, and suffering
- Preventing untimely death ("I want to live long enough to ... .")
- Improving functional status or maintaining compromised status
- Educating and counseling the client and his or her significant others regarding the client's condition and prognosis
- Avoiding harming the client in the course of care
- Promoting health and preventing disease not related to the terminal disease

The physician or advanced-practice provider is responsible for the initial education and counseling of clients regarding their condition and prognosis.

The principle of proportionality is an important ethical consideration in the treatment of terminally ill clients. **Proportionality** means that a medical treatment is ethically mandatory to the extent that it is likely to confer greater benefits than burdens to the client. For example, many experts believe that a client who is actively dying and is slightly dehydrated has a more comfortable death. Dehydration has been reported to reduce:

- Disturbing oral secretions
- Bronchial secretions
- Need for frequent urination
- Cough from diminished pulmonary congestion
- Edema

Dehydration can sedate the brain just before death. Greatly diminished oral intake or its cessation is one of the signs that death is imminent. In another context, a client who is terminally ill but whose condition is stable

and enjoys many activities of daily living may appreciate or request education on how to maintain hydration. A nutritional intervention is appropriate if the client would receive greater benefits than burdens.

Client Preference

The most important ethical principle to consider is the client's right to self-determination. Some individuals may perceive suffering as an important means of personal growth or a religious experience. Other individuals may hope that a miracle cure will be discovered for his or her disease. Others may be ready for and accepting of death. Health-care workers have a responsibility to provide a combination of emotional support and technical nutritional advice on how best to achieve each client's goals. The American Nurses Association (2017) position on voluntary cessation of eating and drinking to hasten death can be made only by clients with decision-making capacity, not by surrogates, and these wishes should be followed if the client loses decision-making capacity.

Quality of Life

The most fundamental goal of medical care is an improvement in the quality of life for those who seek care. If improvement is not possible, a goal of medical care is maintenance of the same quality of life or slowing a decline in quality of life. Oral feeding is part of being human and associated with human dignity. Some clients derive some pleasure from the sensual aspect of food and the socialization that accompanies meals. Food conveys emotional, spiritual, sociological, and biological meanings.

If food remains enjoyable for a client with a terminal illness, the health-care worker should encourage mealtimes to be shared with loved ones. If eating is not a pleasant experience, however, it should not be overemphasized. Families and loved ones need to be educated that the loss in desire to eat and drink is common during the dying phase (Gillespie & Raftery, 2014).

Contextual

Every terminally ill client has his or her own story, with both a history and a future. A client's decision to eat or not to eat is part of his or her narrative. Two examples can illustrate why eating issues should always be given consideration when formulating a care plan.

Client 1 lives in a rooming house without air-conditioning; his family does not want to get involved; he does not have cooking facilities; he refuses to eat the meals delivered to him from the Senior Nutrition Center; and he insists that he wants to die at home. Client 1 refuses to eat.

Client 2 lives with his male companion in a beach house; his friend carries him every day to the beach to watch the sunset; meals are prepared for him by his companion and many other neighbors and friends. Client 2 tries to eat a small amount at least six times a day.

The willingness to eat is part of each man's story. The contextual features in a client's situation often relate to food acceptance. In Client 1's situation, the health-care worker may offer a valuable service by reassuring the client that he will not be abandoned because he refuses to eat. The fear of abandonment is among the most frequently cited apprehensions of dying. Even if a client refuses to eat, health-care workers should remain supportive. The client may change his or her mind. The health-care worker should not consider the rejection of food as a sign of personal or professional failure.

A consideration of a client's medical goals, preferences, quality of life, and contextual features may provide a framework for resolution of ethical dietary issues. Hospice programs have interdisciplinary care teams, and the interdisciplinary team conference is the best arena in which to discuss ethical feeding conflicts.

Legal Issues

The issue of whether to discontinue food and fluid to a client with a terminal illness first emerged in the 1960s. Clients have the legal right to refuse treatment, including artificial feedings. This right is based on the Fourteenth Amendment to the Constitution, which refers to the right to liberty, including the right to be left alone and not invaded or treated against one's will. Courts have recognized that competent adults have the right to refuse treatment, including artificial feeding.

Each state may exert its authority to expand the individual's right to liberty, however, based on other concepts. The preservation of life, the prevention of suicide, the protection of innocent third parties (such as minor children), and the protection of the ethical integrity and professional discretion of the medical profession are among these concepts. Health-care workers need to be familiar with the laws in their individual states and the policies and procedures of the organization for which they work.

They should also know their professional organization's standards of practice. In some states, a charge of battery can be made if a client is fed artificially against his or her wishes. In some states, a charge of negligence can be made if clients are allowed to intentionally starve themselves to death. Situations such as these should be discussed at the interdisciplinary team meeting or brought to the risk manager's attention. (The risk manager is hired by a health-care organization to identify, evaluate, and correct potential risks of injuring clients, staff, visitors, or property.)

With incompetent adult clients, caretakers and family should try to ascertain the client's wishes from past written and oral statements and actions. State laws differ as to whether nutrition and hydration are medically obligatory or medically optional. Some clients may wish for the withdrawal of antibiotics and ventilators but wish to continue nutritional support. This situation may occur when an individual has a PEG tube in place because of an inability to swallow, such as may occur with cancer of the esophagus.

What can health-care workers legally do if the client is incompetent and the family wants the feeding tube removed? What can the health-care worker legally do if family members disagree about whether to have the feeding tube removed? When in doubt, the best advice is to continue to feed the client until the health-care team, the institution's ethics committee, or the facility's risk manager reviews the case. The artificial feeding can be stopped at a future time if the decision is changed, but a deceased person cannot be brought back to life.

Individuals may make their wishes known in writing through advance directives, such as a living will or durable power of attorney. An **advance directive** is a signed document in which the client has specified what type of medical care is desired should he or she lose the ability to make decisions. A **durable power of attorney** for health care is a document in which the client gives another person power to make medical treatment and related personal care decisions for him or her. It can be used as an addition to the advance directive. Health-care workers are responsible for becoming familiar with a client's advance directive, durable power of attorney, and living will. In the event that a client does not have a written directive, the next of kin or guardian should be consulted about a probable preference for the level of nutritional intervention.

General Considerations

Palliative care does not automatically preclude aggressive nutritional support. The client's informed preference for the level of nutrition intervention is important. If the client wants maximal nutrition support and the policy of the organization is not to provide parenteral nutrition or tube feedings for terminally ill clients, the client has the right to be informed of the name of a facility that will provide this service. Artificial feeding generally is not desirable if death is expected within hours or a few days.

The effects of partial dehydration and the withdrawal of nutritional support will not adversely alter the client's comfort. Enteral or parenteral feeding would probably worsen the client's condition, symptoms, or discomfort when shock, pulmonary edema, diarrhea, or aspiration is a potential or actual complication. The client or surrogate needs to be informed of these facts when he or she requests maximal support.

KEYSTONES

- Death is an aspect of life.
- If we want to help the dying, we must examine our own attitudes toward death.
- Treatment for terminally ill clients is palliative.
- The goal of care is symptomatic relief to reduce or alleviate pain.
- Nutritional intervention can frequently alleviate or reduce the pain and suffering of a terminally ill client.
- The use of oral feedings should always be given consideration over tube and parenteral feedings.
- Oral feeding is ordinary care, whereas tube feedings and parenteral nutrition are considered by some to be extraordinary care.

- In the United States, the client's expressed desire is the primary guide for determining the extent of nutritional and hydration therapy.
- The U.S. Constitution guarantees clients the right to self-determination.
- Ethical and legal dilemmas should be brought to the attention of the interdisciplinary team, the risk manager, or the facility's ethics committee promptly.
- Artificial feeding should never be stopped unless one of these parties has investigated the situation and made a legal and ethical determination that the feeding should cease.
- Each health-care worker has an obligation to know his or her client's advance directive, durable power of attorney, and living will documentation.

CASE STUDY 24-1

Ms. Z is a 60-year-old woman who has a diagnosis of amyotrophic lateral sclerosis (ALS), also called Lou Gehrig disease, with a prognosis of less than 6 months. The client has at least two swallowing impediments. She is unable to dislodge food that collects under her tongue, in cheeks, and on her hard palate. She does not have adequate swallow control (the bolus goes down before she wants it to). Because of these impediments, Ms. Z is unable to tolerate thin liquids, and the maintenance of hydration and aspiration are of concern to the caregiver. Ms. Z is alert, oriented, and highly educated. She saw a television program that led her to believe that a high-protein diet would delay the progression of ALS. She would like instruction on a high-protein diet.

CARE PLAN

Subjective Data

Client believes that a high-protein diet will delay the progression of her ALS. ■ Caregiver is concerned about the danger of aspiration and the maintenance of hydration.

Objective Data

Diagnosis: ALS with a prognosis of less than 6 months ■ Lack of swallowing control

Analysis

Related to lack of desired information about foods high in protein as evidenced by verbal statements. ■ Deficient knowledge related to a lack of understanding of how to increase and/or maintain hydration with the client's swallowing impediments as evidenced by the caregiver's verbal statements.

Plan

DESIRED OUTCOMES EVALUATION CRITERIA	ACTIONS/ INTERVENTIONS	RATIONALE
The client will indicate how she can incorporate foods high in protein and of semisolid or pureed consistency into her diet.	Refer to dietitian.	Because a 70- to 80-g protein diet would most likely not harm the client and would make her feel in control, instruction on the diet is appropriate.
The caregiver will verbalize how to reduce the likelihood of aspiration by following safety precautions for clients with dysphagia.	Discuss feeding issues with the caregiver such as the correct body positioning and eating conditions. Eliminate distractions.	The risk of aspiration is high in clients with dysphagia.

DESIRED OUTCOMES EVALUATION CRITERIA	ACTIONS/ INTERVENTIONS	RATIONALE
	Position individual in an upright position (90 degrees at the hip) with feet flat on floor. Have client stay upright 30–40 minutes after a meal. Teach swallowing techniques such as tucking the chin and holding the breath while swallowing. Feed the client very small bites; $\frac{1}{2}$ to 1 teaspoon at a time. Encourage several dry swallows between bites of food. A wet-sounding voice with a gurgle may mean that food is resting on the vocal cords. Evaluate the cheeks after a meal to ensure pocketing did not occur.	

TEAMWORK 24-1

DIETITIAN'S NOTES

The following Dietitian's Notes are representative of the documentation found in a client's medical record.

Subjective: *The client requested a high-protein diet because she believes that it may delay the progression of her ALS. Client reports an intake of one poached egg, thickened whole milk, one slice of bread softened with gelatin, and one cup of thickened orange juice at breakfast. For lunch, client has a half banana, or half a tuna or chicken salad sandwich (bread softened with gelatin the night before). For dinner, the client has $\frac{1}{2}$ cup of pureed casserole (beef stew or macaroni and cheese with $\frac{1}{2}$ cup of added pureed vegetables), and a glass of thickened whole milk. She drinks at least three glasses of thickened water each day. She believes that she is 5 ft tall and weighs 90 lb. She denies a declining body weight.*

Objective: *Hospice client*

Analysis: *Ideal body weight 90–100 lb. Estimated kcalorie needs at actual body weight of 41 kg and 20–30 kcal/kg equal 820–1,230 kcal. Estimated protein needs at 1.2 grams/kg equal 49 grams. Client's reported protein intake is about 55 grams per day and her kcalorie intake is about 1,251 kcal per day. Client is currently eating about 1.1 grams of protein/kg of body weight. Reassured client and her daughter that her current intake is already high in protein and that both her stable body weight and reported food intake are within current guidelines. Both were reassured with the assessment.*

Plan: *No further action is necessary; however, my phone number was provided, and both parties were encouraged to call with any further food-related issues.*

CRITICAL THINKING QUESTIONS

1. The client's swallowing disorders are becoming more severe. Ms. Z is capable of eating only very small bites of food very slowly. The client's daughter is her caregiver, and she states, "It has been taking me 2 hours to feed my mother each meal. If I go any faster, she chokes. My husband is becoming very resentful and has asked me to make a decision. He says I can't continue to spend all day with my mother and ignore him." What would you say to this caregiver?

2. The caregiver believes that the client is still mentally alert and oriented, although the client cannot communicate. The client has progressed to the point where she has lost all motor function. She cannot talk or walk and has lost the use of her hands. The client's physician now believes that Ms. Z has an ileus (paralysis of the bowel). Why does this mean that the client cannot be fed orally? What are the treatment options? Who needs to be informed of the treatment options?

CHAPTER REVIEW

1. A diet prescription consistent with palliative care goals is:
   1. Forty grams of protein for liver failure
   2. Low-cholesterol, low-saturated-fat diet for hyperlipidemia
   3. Gluten-free diet for diarrhea and celiac disease
   4. High-calorie, high-protein diet for anorexia in an actively dying client

2. An appropriate nutritional screening question for a client with a terminal illness is:
   1. "How many times a day do you eat?"
   2. "How much weight have you lost in the past month?"
   3. "Do you look forward to meals?"
   4. "Do you include a green or yellow vegetable in your diet each day?"

3. The most important ethical principle to consider when a decision must be made about whether or not to feed a client is:
   1. The client's right to self-determination
   2. The principle of proportionality
   3. The client's medical goals
   4. The client's quality of life

4. Which recommendation would be appropriate for a client with end-stage congestive heart failure who requests dietary advice?
   1. Recommend a low-potassium diet
   2. Recommend a 1,000-mL fluid restriction
   3. Monitor the client's fluid intake and output
   4. Recommend a 1- or 1.5-gram sodium diet

5. The intervention appropriate for a terminally ill client with dyspnea who requests dietary treatment is:
   1. Encourage a high-fiber diet
   2. Consider a high-fat, low-carbohydrate complete nutritional supplement
   3. Recommend fresh fruits, whole grains, and vegetables
   4. Encourage avoidance of caffeine

CLINICAL ANALYSIS

1. Mr. O is actively dying. Mr. O's wife is concerned because her husband adamantly refuses all food and fluids. The nurse should:
   a. Call the doctor and request an order for a tube feeding
   b. Call the doctor and request an order for an intravenous feeding
   c. Instruct the caregiver to be more creative in the type of food and fluids she gives the client
   d. Counsel the caregiver that oral intake often ceases near the end of life

2. Mrs. P has terminal brain cancer and insulin-dependent diabetes mellitus; her life expectancy is a few days. She and her caregiver have been self-monitoring her blood glucose levels. The caregiver is quite concerned because Mrs. P's blood glucose levels are running between 80 and 120 mg/dL. Historically, the client claims to have followed her 1,200-kcalorie diet faithfully. Recently, her appetite is markedly reduced, and her blood glucose levels are elevated. The physician has been contacted and refuses to decrease the client's insulin further but recommends to Mrs. P's caregiver to stop monitoring the client's blood glucose levels. The nurse should:
   a. Encourage the caregiver to offer Mrs. P frequent sips of clear liquid fruit juices (about 30 grams of carbohydrate every 3 hours)
   b. Encourage the caregiver to continue to offer the client the 1,200-kcalorie diet to avoid a hypoglycemic episode
   c. Recommend the caregiver look for a new doctor because obviously the doctor does not know how to treat clients with insulin-dependent diabetes
   d. Contact the hospice medical director and ask for an order to decrease the client's insulin

3. Mr. J has a partial bowel obstruction and shows signs of dehydration. He has an order for Metamucil® as needed (prn). The nurse should immediately recommend:
   a. Eating high-fiber foods such as bran, whole grains, fruits, and vegetables
   b. Discontinuing the use of Metamucil
   c. Increasing the dose of Metamucil
   d. Eating cheese, cakes, pies, cookies, and doughnuts

Dietary Reference Intakes for Individuals: Recommended Dietary Allowances, Adequate Intakes, Acceptable Macronutrient Distribution Ranges, and Tolerable Upper Intake Levels

Dietary Reference Intakes (DRIs): Recommended Dietary Allowances (RDAs) and Adequate Intakes (AIs)—Vitamins (Food and Nutrition Board, Institute of Medicine, National Academies)

LIFE STAGE GROUP	VITAMIN A (mcg/d)[a]	VITAMIN C (mg/d)	VITAMIN D (mcg/d)[b,c]	VITAMIN E (mg/d)[d]	VITAMIN K (mcg/d)	THIAMIN (mg/d)
Infants						
0–6 mo	400*	40*	10*	4*	2.0*	0.2*
7–12 mo	500*	50*	10*	5*	2.5*	0.3*
Children						
1–3 y	300	15	15	6	30*	0.5
4–8 y	400	25	15	7	55*	0.6
Males						
9–13 y	600	45	15	11	60*	0.9
14–18 y	900	75	15	15	75*	1.2
19–30 y	900	90	15	15	120*	1.2
31–50 y	900	90	15	15	120*	1.2
51–70 y	900	90	15	15	120*	1.2
>70 y	900	90	20	15	120*	1.2
Females						
9–13 y	600	45	15	11	60*	0.9
14–18 y	700	65	15	15	75*	1.0
19–30 y	700	75	15	15	90*	1.1
31–50 y	700	75	15	15	90*	1.1
51–70 y	700	75	15	15	90*	1.1
>70 y	700	75	20	15	90*	1.1
Pregnancy						
14–18 y	750	80	15	15	75*	1.4
19–30 y	770	85	15	15	90*	1.4
31–50 y	770	85	15	15	90*	1.4
Lactation						
14–18 y	1200	115	15	19	75*	1.4
19–30 y	1300	120	15	19	90*	1.4
31–50 y	1300	120	15	19	90*	1.4

This table (adapted from the DRI reports, see www.nap.edu) presents Recommended Dietary Allowances (RDAs) in **bold type** and Adequate Intakes (AIs) in ordinary type followed by an asterisk (*). An RDA is the average daily dietary intake level—sufficient to meet the nutrient requirements of nearly all (97%–98%) healthy individuals in a group. It is calculated from an Estimated Average Requirement (EAR). If sufficient scientific evidence is not available to establish an EAR, and thus calculate an RDA, an AI is usually developed. For healthy breastfed infants, an AI is the mean intake. The AI for other life stage and gender groups is believed to cover the needs of all healthy individuals in the groups, but lack of data or uncertainty in the data prevents being able to specify with confidence the percentage of individuals covered by this intake.

[a]As retinol activity equivalents (RAEs). 1 RAE = 1 mcg retinol, 12 mcg β-carotene, 24 mcg α-carotene, or 24 mcg β-cryptoxanthin. The RAE for dietary provitamin A carotenoids is twofold greater than retinol equivalents (RE), whereas the RAE for preformed vitamin A is the same as RE.

[b]As cholecalciferol. 1 mcg cholecalciferol = 40 IU vitamin D.

[c]Under the assumption of minimal sunlight.

[d]As α-tocopherol. α-Tocopherol includes *RRR*-α-tocopherol, the only form of α-tocopherol that occurs naturally in foods, and the *2R*-stereoisomeric forms of α-tocopherol (*RRR*-, *RSR*-, *RRS*-, and *RSS*-α-tocopherol) that occur in fortified foods and supplements. It does not include the *2S*-stereoisomeric forms of α-tocopherol (*SRR*-, *SSR*-, *SRS*-, and *SSS*-α-tocopherol), also found in fortified foods and supplements.

[e]As niacin equivalents (NE). 1 mg of niacin = 60 mg of tryptophan; 0–6 months = preformed niacin (not NE).

[f]As dietary folate equivalents (DFE). 1 DFE = 1 mcg food folate = 0.6 mcg of folic acid from fortified food or as a supplement consumed with food = 0.5 mcg of a supplement taken on an empty stomach.

[g]Although AIs have been set for choline, there are few data to assess whether a dietary supply of choline is needed at all stages of the life cycle, and it may be that the choline requirement can be met by endogenous synthesis at some of these stages.

[h]Because 10% to 30% of older people may malabsorb food-bound B_{12}, it is advisable for those older than 50 years to meet their RDA mainly by consuming foods fortified with B_{12} or a supplement containing B_{12}.

[i]In view of evidence linking folate intake with neural tube defects in the fetus, it is recommended that all women capable of becoming pregnant consume 400 mcg from supplements or fortified foods in addition to intake of food folate from a varied diet.

[j]It is assumed that women will continue consuming 400 mcg from supplements or fortified food until their pregnancy is confirmed and they enter prenatal care, which ordinarily occurs after the end of the periconceptional period—the critical time for formation of the neural tube.

Sources: Dietary Reference Intakes for Calcium, Phosphorous, Magnesium, Vitamin D, and Fluoride (1997); *Dietary Reference Intakes for Thiamin, Riboflavin, Niacin, Vitamin B₆, Folate, Vitamin B₁₂, Pantothenic Acid, Biotin, and Choline* (1998); *Dietary Reference Intakes for Vitamin C, Vitamin E, Selenium, and Carotenoids* (2000); *Dietary Reference Intakes for Vitamin A, Vitamin K, Arsenic, Boron, Chromium, Copper, Iodine, Iron, Manganese, Molybdenum, Nickel, Silicon, Vanadium, and Zinc* (2001); *Dietary Reference Intakes for Water, Potassium, Sodium, Chloride, and Sulfate* (2005); *and Dietary Reference Intakes for Calcium and Vitamin D* (2011). *These reports may be accessed at* www.nap.edu.

RIBOFLAVIN (mg/d)	NIACIN (mg/d)[e]	VITAMIN B_6 (mg/d)	FOLATE (mcg/d)[f]	VITAMIN B_{12} (mcg/d)	PANTOTHENIC ACID (mg/d)	BIOTIN (mcg/d)	CHOLINE (mg/d)[g]
0.3*	2*	0.1*	65*	0.4*	1.7*	5*	125*
0.4*	4*	0.3*	80*	0.5*	1.8*	6*	150*
0.5	6	0.5	150	0.9	2*	8*	200*
0.6	8	0.6	200	1.2	3*	12*	250*
0.9	12	1.0	300	1.8	4*	20*	375*
1.3	16	1.3	400	2.4	5*	25*	550*
1.3	16	1.3	400	2.4	5*	30*	550*
1.3	16	1.3	400	2.4	5*	30*	550*
1.3	16	1.7	400	2.4[h]	5*	30*	550*
1.3	16	1.7	400	2.4[h]	5*	30*	550*
0.9	12	1.0	300	1.8	4*	20*	375*
1.0	14	1.2	400[i]	2.4	5*	25*	400*
1.1	14	1.3	400[i]	2.4	5*	30*	425*
1.1	14	1.3	400[i]	2.4	5*	30*	425*
1.1	14	1.5	400	2.4[h]	5*	30*	425*
1.1	14	1.5	400	2.4[h]	5*	30*	425*
1.4	18	1.9	600[j]	2.6	6*	30*	450*
1.4	18	1.9	600[j]	2.6	6*	30*	450*
1.4	18	1.9	600[j]	2.6	6*	30*	450*
1.6	17	2.0	500	2.8	7*	35*	550*
1.6	17	2.0	500	2.8	7*	35*	550*
1.6	17	2.0	500	2.8	7*	35*	550*

Dietary Reference Intakes (DRIs): Recommended Dietary Allowances (RDAs) and Adequate Intakes (AIs)—Elements (Food and Nutrition Board, Institute of Medicine, National Academies)

LIFE STAGE GROUP	CALCIUM (mg/d)	CHROMIUM (mcg/d)	COPPER (mcg/d)	FLUORIDE (mg/d)	IODINE (mcg/d)	IRON (mg/d)	MAGNESIUM (mg/d)
Infants							
0–6 mo	200*	0.2*	200*	0.01*	110*	0.27*	30*
7–12 mo	260*	5.5*	220*	0.5*	130*	11	75*
Children							
1–3 y	700	11*	340	0.7*	90	7	80
4–8 y	1000	15*	440	1*	90	10	130
Males							
9–13 y	1300	25*	700	2*	120	8	240
14–18 y	1300	35*	890	3*	150	11	410
19–30 y	1000	35*	900	4*	150	8	400
31–50 y	1000	35*	900	4*	150	8	420
51–70 y	1000	30*	900	4*	150	8	420
>70 y	1200	30*	900	4*	150	8	420
Females							
9–13 y	1300	21*	700	2*	120	8	240
14–18 y	1300	24*	890	3*	150	15	360
19–30 y	1000	25*	900	3*	150	18	310
31–50 y	1000	25*	900	3*	150	18	320
51–70 y	1200	20*	900	3*	150	8	320
>70 y	1200	20*	900	3*	150	8	320
Pregnancy							
14–18 y	1300	29*	1000	3*	220	27	400
19–30 y	1000	30*	1000	3*	220	27	350
31–50 y	1000	30*	1000	3*	220	27	360
Lactation							
14–18 y	1300	44*	1300	3*	290	10	360
19–30 y	1000	45*	1300	3*	290	9	310
31–50 y	1000	45*	1300	3*	290	9	320

This table (adapted from the DRI reports, see www.nap.edu) presents Recommended Dietary Allowances (RDAs) in bold type and Adequate Intakes (AIs) in ordinary type followed by an asterisk (*). An RDA is the average daily dietary intake level—sufficient to meet the nutrient requirements of nearly all (97%–98%) healthy individuals in a group. It is calculated from an Estimated Average Requirement (EAR). If sufficient scientific evidence is not available to establish an EAR, and thus calculate an RDA, an AI is usually developed. For healthy breastfed infants, an AI is the mean intake. The AI for other life stage and gender groups is believed to cover the needs of all healthy individuals in the groups, but lack of data or uncertainty in the data prevents being able to specify with confidence the percentage of individuals covered by this intake.

Sources: Dietary Reference Intakes for Calcium, Phosphorous, Magnesium, Vitamin D, and Fluoride (1997); Dietary Reference Intakes for Thiamin, Riboflavin, Niacin, Vitamin B6, Folate, Vitamin B12, Pantothenic Acid, Biotin, and Choline (1998); Dietary Reference Intakes for Vitamin C, Vitamin E, Selenium, and Carotenoids (2000); and Dietary Reference Intakes for Vitamin A, Vitamin K, Arsenic, Boron, Chromium, Copper, Iodine, Iron, Manganese, Molybdenum, Nickel, Silicon, Vanadium, and Zinc (2001); Dietary Reference Intakes for Water, Potassium, Sodium, Chloride, and Sulfate (2005); and Dietary Reference Intakes for Calcium and Vitamin D (2011). These reports may be accessed at www.nap.edu.

Copyrighted by the National Academy of Sciences, used with permission.

MANGANESE (mg/d)	MOLYBDENUM (mcg/d)	PHOSPHORUS (mg/d)	SELENIUM (mcg/d)	ZINC (mg/d)	POTASSIUM (g/d)	SODIUM (lcg/d)	CHLORIDE (g/d)
0.003*	2*	100*	15*	2*	0.4*	0.12*	0.18*
0.6*	3*	275*	20*	3	0.7*	0.37*	0.57*
1.2*	17	460	20	3	3.0*	1.0*	1.5*
1.5*	22	500	30	5	3.8*	1.2*	1.9*
1.9*	34	1250	40	8	4.5*	1.5*	2.3*
2.2*	43	1250	55	11	4.7*	1.5*	2.3*
2.3*	45	700	55	11	4.7*	1.5*	2.3*
2.3*	45	700	55	11	4.7*	1.5*	2.3*
2.3*	45	700	55	11	4.7*	1.3*	2.0*
2.3*	45	700	55	11	4.7*	1.2*	1.8*
1.6*	34	1250	40	8	4.5*	1.5*	2.3*
1.6*	43	1250	55	9	4.7*	1.5*	2.3*
1.8*	45	700	55	8	4.7*	1.5*	2.3*
1.8*	45	700	55	8	4.7*	1.5*	2.3*
1.8*	45	700	55	8	4.7*	1.3*	2.0*
1.8*	45	700	55	8	4.7*	1.2*	1.8*
2.0*	50	1250	60	12	4.7*	1.5*	2.3*
2.0*	50	700	60	11	4.7*	1.5*	2.3*
2.0*	50	700	60	11	4.7*	1.5*	2.3*
2.6*	50	1250	70	13	5.1*	1.5*	2.3*
2.6*	50	700	70	12	5.1*	1.5*	2.3*
2.6*	50	700	70	12	5.1*	1.5*	2.3*

Dietary Reference Intakes (DRIs): Recommended Dietary Allowances (RDAs) and Adequate Intakes (AIs)—Total Water and Macronutrients (Food and Nutrition Board, Institute of Medicine, National Academies)

LIFE STAGE GROUP	TOTAL WATER[a] (L/d)	CARBOHYDRATE (g/d)	TOTAL FIBER (g/d)	FAT (g/d)	LINOLEIC ACID (g/d)	α-LINOLENIC ACID (g/d)	PROTEIN[b] (g/d)
Infants							
0–6 mo	0.7*	60*	ND	31*	4.4*	0.5*	9.1*
7–12 mo	0.8*	95*	ND	30*	4.6*	0.5*	11.0
Children							
1–3 y	1.3*	130	19*	ND[c]	7*	0.7*	13
4–8 y	1.7*	130	25*	ND	10*	0.9*	19
Males							
9–13 y	2.4*	130	31*	ND	12*	1.2*	34
14–18 y	3.3*	130	38*	ND	16*	1.6*	52
19–30 y	3.7*	130	38*	ND	17*	1.6*	56
31–50 y	3.7*	130	38*	ND	17*	1.6*	56
51–70 y	3.7*	130	30*	ND	14*	1.6*	56
>70 y	3.7*	130	30*	ND	14*	1.6*	56
Females							
9–13 y	2.1*	130	26*	ND	10*	1.0*	34
14–18 y	2.3*	130	26*	ND	11*	1.1*	46
19–30 y	2.7*	130	25*	ND	12*	1.1*	46
31–50 y	2.7*	130	25*	ND	12*	1.1*	46
51–70 y	2.7*	130	21*	ND	11*	1.1*	46
>70 y	2.7*	130	21*	ND	11*	1.1*	46
Pregnancy							
14–18 y	3.0*	175	28*	ND	13*	1.4*	71
19–30 y	3.0*	175	28*	ND	13*	1.4*	71
31–50 y	3.0*	175	28*	ND	13*	1.4*	71
Lactation							
14–18 y	3.8*	210	29*	ND	13*	1.3*	71
19–30 y	3.8*	210	29*	ND	13*	1.3*	71
31–50 y	3.8*	210	29*	ND	13*	1.3*	71

This table (taken from the DRI reports, see www.nap.edu) presents Recommended Dietary Allowances in bold type and Adequate Intakes (AI) in ordinary type followed by an asterisk (*). An RDA is the average daily dietary intake level—sufficient to meet the nutrient requirements of nearly all (97%–98%) healthy individuals in a group. It is calculated from an Estimated Average Requirement (EAR). If sufficient scientific evidence is not available to establish an EAR, and thus calculate an RDA, an AI is usually developed. For healthy breastfed infants, an AI is the mean intake. The AI for other life stage and gender groups is believed to cover the needs of all healthy individuals in the groups, but lack of data or uncertainty in the data prevents being able to specify with confidence the percentage of individuals covered by this intake.
[a]Total water includes all water contained in food, beverages, and drinking water.
[b]Based on grams of protein per kilogram of body weight for the reference body weight, e.g., for adults 0.8 g/kg body weight for the reference body weight.
[c]Not determined.
Source: Dietary Reference Intakes for Energy, Carbohydrate, Fiber, Fat, Fatty Acids, Cholesterol, Protein, and Amino Acids (2002/2005) and Dietary Reference Intakes for Water, Potassium, Sodium, Chloride, and Sulfate (2005). The reports may be accessed at www.nap.edu.
Copyrighted by the National Academy of Sciences, used with permission.

Dietary Reference Intakes (DRIs): Acceptable Macronutrient Distribution Ranges (Food and Nutrition Board, Institute of Medicine, National Academies)

MACRONUTRIENT	RANGE (% OF ENERGY)		
	Children, 1–3 y	Children, 4–18 y	Adults
Fat	30–40	25–35	20–35
n-6 polyunsaturated fatty acids[a] (linoleic acid)	5–10	5–10	5–10
n-3 polyunsaturated fatty acids[a] (α-linolenic acid)	0.6–1.2	0.6–1.2	0.6–1.2
Carbohydrate	45–65	45–65	45–65
Protein	5–20	10–30	10–35

[a]Approximately 10% of the total can come from longer-chain n-3 or n-6 fatty acids.
Source: Dietary Reference Intakes for Energy, Carbohydrate, Fiber, Fat, Fatty Acids, Cholesterol, Protein, and Amino Acids (2002/2005). The report may be accessed at www.nap.edu.
Copyrighted by the National Academy of Sciences, used with permission.

Dietary Reference Intakes (DRIs): Acceptable Macronutrient Distribution Ranges (Food and Nutrition Board, Institute of Medicine, National Academies)

MACRONUTRIENT	RECOMMENDATION
Dietary cholesterol	As low as possible while consuming a nutritionally adequate diet
Trans fatty acids	As low as possible while consuming a nutritionally adequate diet
Saturated fatty acids	As low as possible while consuming a nutritionally adequate diet
Added sugars[a]	Limit to no more than 25% of total energy

[a]Not a recommended intake. A daily intake of added sugars that individuals should aim for to achieve a healthful diet was not set.
Source: Dietary Reference Intakes for Energy, Carbohydrate, Fiber, Fat, Fatty Acids, Cholesterol, Protein, and Amino Acids (2002/2005). The report may be accessed at www.nap.edu.
Copyrighted by the National Academy of Sciences, used with permission.

This glossary contains commonly used terms as well as terms that appear in **boldface** in the book.

Abdominal circumference (girth)—Distance around the trunk at the umbilicus.

Abdominal obesity—Excess body fat located between the chest and pelvis.

Abortifacient—Anything used to cause or induce an abortion.

Absorption—The movement of the end products of digestion from the gastrointestinal tract into the blood and/or lymphatic system.

Accreditation—Process by which a nongovernmental agency recognizes an institution for meeting established criteria of quality.

Acculturation—Process of adopting the values, attitudes, and behaviors of another culture.

Acetone—A ketone body found in urine, which can be due to the excessive breakdown of stored body fat.

Acetyl CoA—Important intermediate byproduct in metabolism formed from the breakdown of glucose, fatty acids, and certain amino acids.

Acetylcholine—A chemical necessary for the transmission of nervous impulses.

Achalasia—Failure of the gastrointestinal muscle fibers to relax where one part joins another.

Achlorhydria—Absence of free hydrochloric acid in the stomach.

Acidosis—Condition that results when the pH of the blood falls below 7.35; may be caused by diarrhea, uremia, diabetes mellitus, respiratory depression, and certain drug therapies.

Acquired immune deficiency syndrome (AIDS)—A disease complex caused by a virus that attacks the immune system and causes neurological disease and permits opportunistic infections and malignancies.

Acrodermatitis enteropathica—Rare autosomal recessive disease that causes zinc deficiency through an unknown mechanism of absorptive failure; fatal if untreated.

Acute illness—A sickness characterized by rapid onset, severe symptoms, and a short course.

Acute kidney injury (AKI)—Condition that occurs suddenly, in which the kidneys are unable to perform essential functions; usually temporary.

Adaptive thermogenesis—The adjustment in energy expenditure the body makes to a large increase or decrease in kilocalorie intake of several days' duration.

Additive—A substance added to food to increase its flavor, shelf life, and/or characteristics such as texture, color, and aroma.

Adequate Intake (AI)—The average observed or experimentally defined intake by a defined population or subgroup that appears to sustain a defined nutritional state; incorporates information on the reduction of disease risk; may be used as a goal for an individual's nutrient intake if an Estimated Average Requirement (EAR) or Recommended Dietary Allowance (RDA) cannot be set.

Adipose cells—Cells in the human body that store fat.

Adipose tissue—Tissue containing masses of fat cells.

Adolescence—Time from the onset of puberty until full growth is reached.

ADP (adenosine diphosphate)—A substance present in all cells involved in energy metabolism. Energy is released when molecules of ATP, another compound in cells, release a phosphoric acid chain and become ADP. The opposite chemical reaction of adding the third phosphoric acid group to ADP requires much energy.

Adrenal glands—Small organs on the superior surface of the kidneys that secrete many hormones, including epinephrine (adrenalin) and aldosterone.

Advanced directive—A signed document in which the client has specified what type of medical care is desired should he or she lose the ability to make decisions.

Aerobic exercise—Training methods such as running or swimming that require continuous inspired oxygen.

Afferent—Proceeding toward a center, as arteries, veins, lymphatic vessels, and nerves.

Afferent arteriole—Small blood vessel through which blood enters the glomerulus (functional unit of the kidney).

Aflatoxin—A naturally occurring food contaminant produced by some strains of *Aspergillus* molds; found especially on peanuts and peanut products.

AIDS dementia complex (ADC)—A central nervous system disorder caused by the human immunodeficiency virus.

ALA—*See* Alpha-linolenic acid.

Albumin—A plasma protein responsible for much of the colloidal osmotic pressure of the blood.

Aldosterone—An adrenocorticoid hormone that increases sodium and water retention by the kidneys.

Alimentary canal—The digestive tube extending from the mouth to the anus.

Alkaline phosphatase—An enzyme found in highest concentration in the liver, biliary tract epithelium, and bones; enzyme levels are elevated in liver, bone, and biliary disease.

Alkalosis—Condition that results when the pH of the blood rises above 7.45; may be caused by vomiting, nasogastric suctioning, or hyperventilation.

Allele—One of two or more different genes containing specific inheritable characteristics that occupy corresponding positions (loci) on paired chromosomes; an individual possessing a pair of identical alleles, either dominant or recessive, is homozygous for this gene.

Allergen—Substance that provokes an abnormal, individual hypersensitivity.

Allergy—State of abnormal, individual hypersensitivity to a substance.

Alopecia—Hair loss, especially of the head; baldness.

Alpha-linolenic acid (ALA)—A polyunsaturated omega-3 fatty acid found in some plants.

Alpha-tocopherol equivalent (*a*-TE)—The measure of vitamin E; 1 milligram of alpha-tocopherol equivalent equals 1.5 international units (IU) of natural alpha-tocopherol or 2.2 IU of synthetic vitamin.

Amenorrhea—Absence of menstruation; normally occurs before puberty, after menopause, and during pregnancy and lactation.

Amino acids—Organic compounds that are the building blocks of protein; also the end products of protein digestion.

Amniotic fluid—Albuminous liquid that surrounds and protects the fetus throughout pregnancy.

Amylase—A class of enzymes that splits starches—for example, salivary amylase, pancreatic amylase.

Anabolic phase—The third and last phase of stress; characterized by the building up of body tissue and nutrient stores; also called recovery phase.

Anabolism—The building up of body compounds or tissues by the synthesis of more complex substances from simpler ones; the constructive phase of metabolism.

Anaerobic exercise—A form of physical activity such as weight lifting or sprinting that does not rely on continuous inspired oxygen.

Anaphylaxis—Exaggerated, life-threatening hypersensitivity response to a previously encountered antigen; in severe cases, produces bronchospasm, vascular collapse, and shock.

Anastomosis—The surgical connection between tubular structures.

Anemia—Condition of less-than-normal values for red blood cells or hemoglobin, or both; result is decreased effectiveness in oxygen transport; causes may include inadequate iron intake, malabsorption, and chronic or acute blood loss.

Anencephaly—Congenital absence of the brain; cerebral hemispheres missing or reduced to small masses; fatal within a few weeks.

Angina pectoris—Severe pain and a sense of constriction about the heart caused by lack of oxygen to the heart muscle.

Angiotensin II—End product of complex reaction in response to low blood pressure; effect is vasoconstriction and aldosterone secretion.

Anion—An ion with a negative charge.

Anorexia—Loss of appetite.

Anorexia nervosa—A mental disorder characterized by a 25% loss of usual body weight, an intense fear of becoming obese, and self-starvation.

Anorexia of aging—Loss of appetite in an elderly individual related to physiologic, social, psychological, or medical causes.

Anorexigenic—Causing loss of appetite.

Antagonist—A substance that counteracts the action of another substance.

Anthropometric measurements—Physical measurements of the human body such as height, weight, and skinfold thickness; used to determine body composition and growth.

Anthropometry—The science of measuring the human body.

Antibody—A specific protein developed in the body in response to a substance that the body senses to be foreign.

Anticholinergic—An agent that blocks parasympathetic nerve impulses, thereby causing dry mouth, blurred vision due to dilated pupils, and decreased gastrointestinal and bronchial secretions.

Antidiuretic hormone (ADH)—Hormone formed in the hypothalamus and released from the posterior pituitary in response to blood that is too concentrated; effect is return of water to the bloodstream by the kidney.

Antigen—Protein or oligosaccharide marker on surface of cells; body can detect foreign antigens on organisms, foods, and transplanted tissues.

Anti-insulin antibodies (AIAs)—A protein found to be elevated in persons with insulin-dependent diabetes mellitus.

Antineoplastic drug—A drug that combats tumors.

Antioxidant—A substance that prevents or inhibits the uptake of oxygen; in the body, antioxidants prevent tissue damage; in foods, antioxidants prevent deterioration.

Antiretroviral—Substance or drug that stops or suppresses the activity of retroviruses such as human immunodeficiency virus (HIV).

Anuria—A total lack of urine output.

Apoferritin—A protein found in intestinal mucosal cells that combines with iron to form ferritin; it is always found attached to iron in the body.

Apolipoproteins—Protein components of lipoproteins that assist in regulating lipid metabolism; apo A, the primary high-density lipoprotein apoprotein, is inversely related to the risk for developing coronary artery disease.

Appetite—A strong desire for food or for a pleasant sensation, based on previous experience, that causes one to seek food for the purpose of tasting and enjoying.

Aquaporin—Water transport proteins, found in many cell membranes, that serve as water-selective channels and explain the speed at which water moves across cell membranes.

Arachidonic acid—An omega-6 polyunsaturated fatty acid present in peanuts; precursor of prostaglandins.

Ariboflavinosis—Condition arising from a deficiency of riboflavin in the diet.

Aromatic amino acids—Phenylalanine, tryptophan, tyrosine; ratio to branched-chain amino acids altered in liver failure.

Arrhythmia—Irregular heartbeat.

Arteriosclerosis—Common arterial disorder characterized by thickening, hardening, and loss of elasticity of the arterial walls; also called "hardening of the arteries."

Arthritis—Inflammatory condition of the joints, usually accompanied by pain and swelling.

Ascites—Accumulation of serous fluid in the peritoneal (abdominal) cavity.

Ascorbic acid—Vitamin C; *ascorbic* literally means "without scurvy."

Ash—The residue that remains after an item is burned; usually refers to the mineral content of the human body.

Aspartame—Artificial sweetener composed of aspartic acid and phenylalanine; 180 times sweeter than sucrose; brand names: Equal®, Nutrasweet®.

Aspergillus—Genus of molds that produce aflatoxins.

Aspiration—The state in which a substance has been drawn into the nose, throat, or lungs.

Assessment—An organized procedure to gather pertinent facts.

Astrocyte—A supporting cell of the central nervous system that contributes to the blood–brain barrier.

Asymptomatic—Without symptoms.

Ataxia—Defective muscular coordination, especially seen in voluntary movement attempts.

Atherosclerosis—A form of arteriosclerosis characterized by the deposit of fatty material inside the arteries; major factor contributing to heart disease.

Atom—Smallest particle of an element that has all the properties of the element. An atom consists of the nucleus, which contains protons (positively charged particles), neutrons (particles with no electrical charge), and surrounding electrons (negatively charged particles).

Atopy—Genetic predisposition to develop allergy primarily involving immunoglobulin E (IgE) antibodies; a child with two atopic parents has a 75% chance of similar symptoms; a child with one atopic parent has a 50% chance.

ATP (adenosine triphosphate)—Compound in cells, especially muscle cells, that stores energy; when needed, enzymes break off one phosphoric acid group, which releases energy for muscle contraction.

Atrophy—Decrease in size of a normally developed organ or tissue.

Autoimmune disease—A disorder in which the body produces an immunologic response against itself.

Automated peritoneal dialysis (APD)—A form of overnight, self-dialysis utilizing a cycler machine. The dialysate is allowed to remain in the abdominal cavity for 1½ hours before replacement.

Autonomy—Achieving independence; the psychosocial developmental task of the toddler.

Autosomal dominant gene—Dominant gene on any chromosome except X or Y; autosomal dominant inheritance: trait or disease transmitted from one parent even if the matching gene from the other parent is normal; example: familial hypercholesterolemia.

Autosomal recessive inheritance—Non–sex-linked pattern of inheritance in which an affected gene must be received from both parents for the individual to be affected; examples: **cystic fibrosis, phenylketonuria (PKU), galactosemia**, sickle cell disease. Note that the chance of normal, carrier, or affected children is the same with every pregnancy. Having had an affected child does not mean that the offspring of next three pregnancies will be normal or carriers.

Avidin—Protein in raw egg white that inhibits the B vitamin biotin.

Bacteria—Single-celled microorganisms that lack a true nucleus; may be either harmless to humans or disease producing.

Bacteriostat—Agent that prevents bacteria from growing and multiplying but does not necessarily kill them.

Balanced diet—A diet including sufficient foods from each of the major food groups daily; one containing all the essential nutrients in required amounts.

Bariatric surgery—Surgery performed to treat and control obesity.

Barium enema—Series of x-ray studies of the colon used to demonstrate the presence and location of polyps, tumors, diverticula, or positional abnormalities. The client is first administered an enema containing a radio-opaque substance (barium) that enhances visualization when the film is exposed.

Barium swallow—The primary diagnostic tool for direct visualization of the swallowing mechanism is called the *cookie swallow* or *modified barium swallow*. During this procedure, the client consumes three items of different viscosities. Each item contains a contrast medium that allows all phases of the swallowing mechanism to be visualized in x-rays. A physician is always present during this procedure.

Basal ganglia—Four masses of gray matter located in the cerebrum; contribute to the subconscious aspects of voluntary movement; inhibit tremors.

Benign—Not recurrent or progressive; nonmalignant; benign tumor may be life-threatening in crucial tissue such as the brain.

Beriberi—Disease caused by deficiency of vitamin B_1 (thiamin).

Beta-carotene—Carotenoid with the greatest provitamin A activity.

Beta-endorphin—Chemical released in the brain during exercise that produces a state of relaxation.

Bicarbonate—Any salt containing the $HCO_3{}^2$ anion; blood bicarbonate is a measure of alkali (base) reserve of the body; bicarbonate of soda is sodium bicarbonate ($NaHCO_3$).

Bile—Yellow secretion of the liver that alkalinizes the intestine and breaks large fat globules into smaller ones to facilitate enzyme digestive action.

Binge-eating disorder—Eating disorder in which the patient eats excess amounts of food and calories and does not purge.

Binging—Eating to excess; eating from 5,000 to 20,000 kilocalories per day.

Bioavailability—The rate and extent to which an active drug or nutrient or metabolite enters the general circulation, permitting access to the site of action; measured by concentration of the drug in body fluids or by the magnitude of the pharmacologic response.

Bioelectric impedance—Indirect measure of body fatness based on differences in electrical conductivity of fat, muscle, and bone.

Biological value—Scoring system of how well food proteins can be converted into body protein; eggs are norm of 100% of nitrogen being retained.

Biotin—B-complex vitamin widely available in foods.

Bladder—A body organ, also called the urinary bladder, which receives urine from the kidneys and discharges it through the urethra.

Blood–brain barrier—Specialized cells lining the brain capillaries that separate the brain from the circulatory system, thus protecting it from harmful substances.

Blood pressure—Force exerted against the walls of blood vessels by the pumping action of the heart.

Blood urea nitrogen (BUN)—The amount of nitrogen present in the blood as urea, often elevated in renal disorders; may be referred to as serum urea nitrogen (SUN).

B-lymphocytes (B-cells)—White blood cells that protect against infection by inducing antibody production; *see* Humoral immunity.

Body frame size—Designation of a person's skeletal structure as small, medium, or large; used to determine healthy body weight (HBW).

Body image—The mental image a person has of himself or herself.

Body mass index (BMI)—Weight in kilograms divided by the square of height in meters; BMIs of 19 to 24 are considered normal.

Body substance isolation—A situation in which all body fluids should be considered contaminated and treated as such by all health-care workers.

Bolus—A mass of food that is ready to be swallowed or a single dose of feeding or medication.

Bolus feeding—Giving a 4- to 6-hour volume of a tube feeding within a few minutes.

Bomb calorimeter—A device used to measure the energy content of food.

Botulism—An often fatal form of food intoxication caused by the ingestion of food containing poisonous toxins produced by the microorganism *Clostridium botulinum*.

Bowman capsule—The cuplike top of an individual nephron; functions as a filter in the formation of urine.

Branched-chain amino acids—Leucine, isoleucine, lysine, valine; sometimes used as therapy for hepatic coma.

Buffer—A substance that can react to offset excess acid or excess alkali (base) in a solution; blood buffers include carbonic acid, bicarbonate, phosphates, and proteins, including hemoglobin.

Bulimia—Excessive food intake followed by extreme methods, such as self-induced vomiting and the use of laxatives, to rid the body of the foods eaten.

C-reactive protein (CRP)—An abnormal protein produced by the liver in response to acute inflammation that is strongly associated with future vascular events.

Cachexia—State of malnutrition and wasting seen in chronic conditions such as cancer, AIDS, malaria, tuberculosis, and pituitary disease.

Calcidiol—25-hydroxyvitamin D [25(OH)D]; inactive form of vitamin D produced in the liver; circulating half-life of 15 days; serum level is best indicator of vitamin D status, reflecting vitamin D (from sun, food, and dietary supplements but not vitamin D stored in body tissues).

Calcification—Process in which tissue becomes hardened with calcium deposits; necessary for bone anabolism; pathological in vitamin D toxicity.

Calcitonin—Hormone produced by the thyroid gland that slows the release of calcium from the bone when serum calcium levels are high.

Calcitriol—1,25-dihydroxyvitamin D [1,25(OH)$_2$D]; physiologically active form of vitamin D produced primarily in the kidney; circulating half-life of 15 hours; serum levels typically not decreased until severe deficiency because of regulation by parathyroid hormone.

Calorie—A measurement unit of energy; unit equaling the amount of heat required to raise or lower the temperature of 1 gram of water 1.8°F (1°C).

Campylobacter—Flagellated, gramnegative bacteria; important cause of diarrheal illnesses.

Candida albicans—Microscopic fungal organism normally present on skin and mucous membranes of healthy people; cause of thrush, vaginitis, and opportunistic infections.

Capillary—Minute vessel connecting arteriole and venule; vessel wall acts as semipermeable membrane to exchange substances between blood and lymph and interstitial fluid.

Carbohydrate—Any of a group of organic compounds, including sugar, starch, and cellulose, which contains only carbon, oxygen, and hydrogen.

Carbonic acid—Aqueous solution of carbon dioxide; carbon dioxide in solution or in blood is carbonic acid.

Carcinogen—Any substance or agent that causes the development of or increases the risk of cancer.

Carcinoma—A malignant neoplasm that occurs in epithelial tissue.

Cardia—Upper orifice of the stomach connecting with the esophagus.

Cardiac arrhythmia—Irregular heartbeat.

Cardiac sphincter—Smooth muscle band at the lower end of the esophagus; prevents reflux of stomach contents.

Cardiomyopathy—Disease of heart muscle; may be primary due to unknown cause or secondary to another cardiac disorder or systemic disease.

Carotene—One of several yellow to red antioxidant pigments that are precursors to vitamin A.

Carotenemia—Excess carotene in the blood, producing yellow skin but not discoloring the whites of the eyes.

Carotenoid—Group of more than 500 red, orange, or yellow pigments found in fruits and vegetables, about 50 of which are precursors of vitamin A; includes carotene, which is such a precursor, and lycopene, which is not.

Casein—Principal protein in cow's milk.

Catabolic—The breakdown of molecules.

Catabolism—The breaking down of body compounds or tissues into simpler substances; the destructive phase of metabolism.

Catalyst—A substance that speeds up a chemical reaction without entering into or being changed by the reaction.

Cataract—Clouding of the lens of the eye.

Cation—An ion with a positive charge.

Cecum—The first portion of the large intestine between the ileum and the ascending colon.

Celiac disease (gluten-sensitive enteropathy)—An intolerance to dietary gluten, which damages the intestine and produces diarrhea and malabsorption.

Cell—The smallest functional unit of structure in all plants and animals.

Cellular immunity—Delayed immune response produced by T-lymphocytes, which mature in the thymus gland; examples of this type of response are rejection of transplanted organs and some autoimmune diseases.

Central parenteral nutrition (CPN)—Parenteral nutrition delivered into a large-diameter vein, usually the superior vena cava adjacent to the right atrium.

Cerebrovascular accident (CVA)—An abnormal condition in which the brain's blood vessels are occluded by a thrombus, an embolus, or hemorrhage, resulting in damaged brain tissue; stroke.

Cesarean delivery—Delivery of a baby through a surgical incision made into the mother's abdomen and uterus.

Chelating agent—A chemical compound that binds metallic ions into a ring structure, inactivating them; used to remove poisonous metals from the body.

Chemical digestion—Digestive process that involves the splitting of complex molecules into simpler forms.

Chemical reaction—The process of combining or breaking down substances to obtain different substances.

Chlorophyll—The green plant pigment necessary for the manufacture of carbohydrates.

Cholecalciferol—Vitamin D$_3$, formed when the skin is exposed to sunlight; further processed by the liver and kidneys; may be reported as serum 25-hydroxy-cholecalciferol.

Cholecystitis—Inflammation of the gallbladder.

Cholecystokinin—A hormone secreted by the duodenum; stimulates contraction of the gallbladder (releases bile) and the secretion of pancreatic juice.

Cholelithiasis—The presence of gallstones.

Cholestasis—Blockage of the flow of bile due to liver disease or obstructions in the duct system.

Cholesterol—A fatlike substance made in the human body and found in foods of animal origin; associated with an increased risk of heart disease.

Choline—Vitamin-like organic compound recognized as an essential nutrient; required for normal carbohydrate and fat metabolism and involved in protein metabolism.

Chromosomes—thread-like structure found in the nucleus of cells that contain DNA

Chronic illness—A sickness persisting for a long period that shows little change or a slow progression over time.

Chronic obstructive pulmonary disease (COPD)—A group of chronic diseases with a common characteristic of chronic airflow obstruction.

Chronic kidney disease (CKD)—An irreversible condition in which the kidneys cannot perform vital functions.

Chvostek's sign—Spasm of facial muscles following a tap over the facial nerve in front of the ear; indication of tetany.

Chylomicron—A lipoprotein that carries triglycerides in the bloodstream after meals.

Chyme—The mixture of partly digested food and digestive secretions found in the stomach and small intestine during digestion of a meal.

Chymotrypsin—A protein-splitting enzyme produced by the pancreas; active in the intestine.

Cirrhosis—Chronic disease of the liver in which functioning cells degenerate and are replaced by fibrosed connective tissue.

Client-care conference—A meeting that includes all health-care team members and may include the client or a significant other to review and update the client's nursing care plan.

Clostridium botulinum—An anaerobic (grows without air) organism that produces a poisonous toxin; the cause of botulism.

Clostridium perfringens—A bacterium that produces a poisonous toxin that causes a food intoxication; the symptoms are generally mild and of short duration and include intestinal disorders.

Cobalamin—Vitamin B_{12}; essential for proper blood formation.

Coenzyme—A substance that combines with an enzyme to activate it.

Cognitive—Of, relating to, or involving conscious mental activities such as thinking, understanding, learning, and remembering.

Colectomy—Surgical removal of part or all of the colon.

Collagen—Fibrous insoluble protein found in connective tissue.

Collecting tubule—The last segment of the renal tubule; follows the distal convoluted tubule. Several nephrons usually share a single collecting tubule.

Colloidal osmotic pressure (COP)—Pressure produced by plasma and cellular proteins.

Colon—The large intestine from the end of the small intestine to the rectum.

Colonic residue—Total solid material in the large intestine after digestion, including insoluble fiber, secretions, shed cells, and microorganisms. Fiber is the chief contributor to colonic residue and residual substance manageable by diet.

Colostomy—Surgical procedure in which an opening to the large intestine is constructed on the abdomen.

Comorbidity—A disease coexisting with the primary disease.

Complementation—Principle of meal planning advocating combining plant foods within a meal so that it contains all the essential amino acids; now applied to daily intake rather than to single meals.

Complement system—Series of about 25 proteins that work to "complement" the activity of antibodies in destroying bacteria; also helps to rid the body of antigen–antibody complexes; in carrying out these tasks, it induces an inflammatory response.

Complete protein—A protein containing all essential amino acids that humans need; usually found in animal sources such as milk, meat, eggs, and fish.

Complex carbohydrate—A carbohydrate composed of many molecules of $C_6H_{12}O_6$ joined together; polysaccharide; includes starch, glycogen, and fiber.

Compound—Two or more elements united chemically in specific proportions.

Compound fat—Substance obtained when one of the fatty acids joined to the glycerol molecule is replaced by another molecule, such as a protein.

Conditionally essential nutrient—Substance normally manufactured by the body; in certain situations, the body cannot manufacture an optimal amount.

Consanguinous union—Marriage of blood relatives; usually meaning second cousins or closer; genetic influence in unions between more distant relatives likely to differ only slightly from that in the general population.

Constipation—Decrease in a person's normal frequency of defecation; stool is often hard, dry, or difficult to expel.

Contamination iron—Iron that leaches from cookware into the food; in special circumstances, can become hazardous.

Continuous ambulatory peritoneal dialysis (CAPD)—A form of self-dialysis in which the dialysate is allowed to remain in the abdominal cavity for 4 to 6 hours before replacement.

Continuous feeding—Enteral feeding in which the formula drips slowly throughout the prescribed time span.

Contraindication—Any circumstance under which treatment should not be given.

Coronary heart disease (CHD)—Disease resulting from the decreased flow of blood through the coronary arteries to the heart muscle.

Coronary occlusion—Blockage of one or more branches of the coronary arteries, which supply the heart muscle with oxygen and nutrients.

Creatine—Nonprotein substance synthesized in the body from arginine, glycine, and methionine; combines with phosphate to form creatine phosphate, which is stored in muscle tissue as an energy source.

Creatinine—Nonprotein nitrogenous end product of creatine metabolism; because creatinine is excreted by the kidneys, serum creatinine levels are used to detect and monitor renal disease and to estimate muscle protein reserves.

Cretinism—A congenital condition resulting from a lack of thyroid secretions; characterized by a stunted and malformed body and arrested mental development.

Crohn disease—Inflammatory disease appearing in any area of the bowel in which diseased areas can be found alternating with healthy tissue.

Cross-contamination—The spreading of a disease-producing organism from one food, person, or object to another food, person, or object.

Cruciferous—Belonging to a botanical mustard family; includes broccoli, Brussels sprouts, cabbage, cauliflower, kale, kohlrabi, and Swiss chard.

Crystalluria—The presence of crystals in the urine; may be caused by the administration of sulfonamides.

Culture—The learned, shared, and transmitted values, beliefs, and norms of a particular group that guide its thinking, decisions, and actions in patterned ways.

Cyclical variation—A recurring series of events during a specified period.

Cystic fibrosis—Hereditary disease often affecting the lungs and pancreas in which glandular secretions are abnormally thick.

Cysteine—Sulfur-containing amino acid often lacking in legumes.

Cystitis—Inflammation of the bladder.

Cytochrome P450 enzymes—Group of genetically determined enzymes that help to metabolize fat-soluble vitamins, steroids, fatty acids, and other substances and to detoxify drugs and environmental pollutants; examples: CYP3A4 depicts family (3), subfamily (A), number (4).

Cytokine—One of more than 100 proteins mainly produced by white blood cells that function in inflammatory and specific immune responses.

Deamination—Metabolic process whereby nitrogen is removed from an amino acid.

Deciliter (dL)—100 milliliters or $\frac{1}{10}$ liter.

Decubitus ulcer—A pressure sore on the lower back, such as a bedsore.

Dehiscence—Separation of the edges of a surgical incision.

Delusion—False belief that is firmly maintained despite obvious proof to the contrary.

Dementia—The impairment of intellectual function that usually is progressive and interferes with normal social and occupational activities.

Dental caries—The gradual decay and disintegration of the teeth; a dental cavity is a hole in a tooth caused by dental caries.

Dental plaque—Colorless and transparent gummy mass of microorganisms that grows on the teeth, predisposing them to decay.

Deoxyribonucleic acid (DNA)—The hereditary material in humans and almost all other organisms; protein substance in the cell nucleus that directs all the cell's activities, including reproduction.

Desired outcome—The behavioral or physical change in a client that indicates the achievement of a nursing goal.

Development—Gradual process of changing from a simple to a more complex organism; involves psychosocial and physical changes, not only an increase in size.

Dextrose—Another name for the simple sugar glucose.

DHA—*See* Docosahexaenoic acid.

Diabetes insipidus—Increased water intake and increased urine output resulting from inadequate secretion of antidiuretic hormone (ADH) by the posterior pituitary or by failure of the kidney tubules to respond to ADH; underlying causes can be tumor, surgery, trauma, infection, radiation injury, or congenital anomaly.

Diabetes mellitus—Disease caused by insufficient insulin secretion by the pancreas or insulin resistance by body tissues causing excess glucose in the blood and deranged carbohydrate, fat, and protein metabolism.

Diabetic neuropathy—Degeneration of peripheral nerves occurring in diabetes; possible causes are microscopic changes in blood vessels or metabolic defects in nerve tissue.

Diacetic acid—A ketone body found in the urine; can be due to the excessive breakdown of stored body fat.

Diagnostic—Relating to scientific and skillful methods to establish the cause and nature of a sick person's illness.

Dialysate—In renal failure, the fluid used to remove or deliver compounds or electrolytes that the failing kidney cannot excrete or retain in proper concentrations.

Dialysis—The process of diffusing blood across a semipermeable membrane to remove toxic materials and to maintain fluid, electrolyte, and acid–base balances in cases of impaired kidney function or absence of the kidneys.

Dialysis dementia—A neurological disturbance seen in clients who have been on dialysis for a number of years.

Diastolic pressure—Pressure exerted against the arteries between heartbeats; the lower number of a blood pressure reading.

Dietary fiber—Material in foods, mostly from plants, that the human body cannot break down or digest.

Dietary recall, 24-hour—Description of what a person has eaten for the previous 24 hours.

Dietary Reference Intake (DRI)—Four nutrient-based reference values that can be used for assessing and planning diets for the healthy general population; refer to average daily intakes for 1 or more weeks; include Estimated Average Requirements (EARs), Recommended Dietary Allowances (RDAs), Adequate Intakes (AIs), and Tolerable Upper Intake Levels (ULs).

Dietary status—Description of what a person has been eating; his or her usual intake.

Digestion—The process by which food is broken down mechanically and chemically in the gastrointestinal tract into forms simple enough for intestinal absorption.

Diglyceride—Two fatty acids joined to a glycerol molecule.

Dilutional hyponatremia—Low serum sodium due not to an absolute lack of sodium but to an excess of water.

Diplopia—Double vision.

Disaccharide—A simple sugar composed of two units of $C_6H_{12}O_6$ joined together; examples include sucrose, lactose, maltose.

Disulfide linkage—Specific chemical bond joining amino acids; in hair, skin, and nails, holds amino acids in their distinct shapes.

Diverticulitis—Inflammation of a diverticulum.

Diverticulosis—Presence of one or more diverticula.

Diverticulum—A sac or pouch in the walls of a tubular organ; pl., diverticula.

DNA—*See* Deoxyribonucleic acid.

Docosahexaenoic acid (DHA)—A polyunsaturated omega-3 fatty acid found in fish oils.

Dopamine—Catecholamine synthesized by the adrenals; immediate precursor in the synthesis of norepinephrine.

Double-blind—Technique of scientific investigation in which neither the investigator nor the subject knows what treatment, if any, the subject is receiving.

Double bond—A type of chemical connection in which, for example, a fatty acid has two neighboring carbon atoms, each lacking one hydrogen atom.

Drink—An alcoholic beverage; *see* Standard drink.

Dual-energy x-ray absorptiometry (DEXA)—Diagnostic test using two x-ray beams to determine body composition; used to measure bone mineral density as an indicator of osteopenia and osteoporosis.

Duct—A structural tube designed to allow secretions to move from one body part to another body part.

Dumping syndrome—A condition in which the contents of the stomach empty too rapidly into the duodenum; mostly occurs in patients who have had gastric resections.

Duodenum—The first part of the small intestine between the stomach and the jejunum.

Durable power of attorney—A document in which the client gives another person power to make medical treatment and related personal care decisions for him or her.

Dysgeusia—Abnormal taste.

Dysphagia—Difficulty swallowing; component of many diseases from Alzheimer disease and other neurological disorders to tumors of the head and neck.

Dysphoria—A speech disorder characterized by hoarseness.

Dyspnea—Difficulty breathing.

Eclampsia—An obstetrical emergency involving hypertension, proteinuria, and convulsions appearing after the 20th week of pregnancy.

Eczema—Skin inflammation, acute or chronic; caused by external (chemical irritation or microbial invasion) or internal (genetic or psychological) factors.

Edema—The accumulation of excessive amounts of fluid in interstitial spaces.

Edentulous—The state of having no teeth.

Efferent—Directed away from a center; used to describe arteries, veins, lymphatic vessels, and nerves.

Efferent arteriole—Small blood vessel by which blood leaves the nephron.

Efficacy—Ability of a drug or treatment to achieve the desired effect.

Eicosapentaenoic acid (EPA)—Omega-3 fatty acid found in fish oils.

Electrocardiogram (ECG)—A graphic record produced by an electrocardiograph that shows the electrical activity of the heart.

Electroencephalogram (EEG)—The record obtained from an electroencephalograph that shows the electrical activity of the brain.

Electrolyte—An element or compound that when dissolved in water separates (dissociates) into ions that are capable of conducting an electrical current; acids, bases, and salts are common electrolytes.

Element—A substance that cannot be separated into simpler parts by ordinary means.

Elemental and semielemental formula—Formula that contains either totally or partially hydrolyzed nutrients.

Embolus—A circulating mass of undissolved matter in a blood or lymphatic vessel; may be composed of tissues, fat globules, air bubbles, clumps of bacteria, or foreign bodies, including pieces of medical devices.

Embryo—A developing infant in the prenatal period between the second and eighth weeks inclusive.

Empty kilocalories—Refers to a food that contains kilocalories and almost no other nutrients.

Emulsification—The physical breaking up of fat into tiny droplets.

Emulsifier—A molecule that attracts both water- and fat-soluble molecules.

Emulsion—One liquid evenly distributed in a second liquid, with which it usually does not mix.

Encephalopathy—Generalized brain dysfunction with varying degrees of impairment of speech, cognition, orientation, and arousal.

Endemic—The constant presence of a disease or infectious agent within a given geographic area; the usual prevalence of a given disease within such an area.

Endogenous—Produced within or caused by factors within the organism.

Endoscope—A device consisting of a tube and an optical system for observing the inside of a hollow organ or cavity.

Endothelium—Flat cells lining blood and lymphatic vessels, the heart, and various body cavities; produce compounds affecting vascular lumen and platelets.

End-stage renal disease (ESRD)—A state in which the kidneys have lost most or all of their ability to maintain internal homeostasis and produce urine.

Energy—The capacity to do work.

Energy balance—A situation in which kilocaloric intake equals kilocaloric output.

Energy expenditure—The amount of fuel the body uses for a specified period.

Energy imbalance—Situation in which kilocalories eaten do not equal the number of kilocalories used for energy.

Energy nutrients—The chemical substances in food that are able to supply fuel; refers collectively to carbohydrate, fat, and protein.

Enrichment—The addition of nutrients previously present in a food but removed during food processing or lost during storage.

Enteral nutrition—Nutrition provided through the gastrointestinal tract via a tube, catheter, or stoma that delivers nutrients distal to the oral cavity.

Enteric-coated—A type of drug preparation designed to dissolve in the intestine rather than in the stomach.

Enteritis—Inflammation of the intestines, particularly the small intestine.

Enzyme—Complex protein produced by living cells that acts as a catalyst.

EPA—*See* Eicosapentaenoic acid.

Epidemic—Affecting or tending to affect a disproportionately large number of individuals within a population, community, or region at the same time; excessively prevalent or widespread.

Epilepsy—Disease marked by repetitive abnormal electrical discharges within the brain; signs and symptoms vary with type: partial, generalized, or unclassified.

Epinephrine—Hormone of the adrenal gland; produces the fight-or-flight response.

Epigenetics—The process that regulates how and when genes are turned on and off.

Epithelial tissue—A type of tissue that forms the outer layer of skin and lines body surfaces opening to the outside; functions include protection, absorption, and secretion.

Ergocalciferol—Vitamin D_2 formed by the action of sunlight on plants.

Ergot poisoning—Poisoning resulting from excessive use of the drug ergot or from the ingestion of grain or grain products infected with the *Claviceps purpurea* fungus.

Erikson, Erik—Psychologist who devised a theory of human development consisting of eight stages of life, each with a psychosocial developmental task to be mastered.

Erosion—Destruction of the surface of a tissue, either on the external surface of the body or internally.

Erythropoietin—Hormone released by the kidney to stimulate red blood cell production.

Esophagostomy—A surgical opening in the esophagus.

Esophagus—A muscular canal extending from the mouth to the stomach.

Essential amino acid—One of the amino acids that cannot be manufactured by the human body; must be obtained from food or artificial feeding.

Essential (primary) hypertension—Elevated blood pressure that develops without apparent cause.

Essential nutrient—A substance found in food that must be present in the diet because the human body lacks the ability to manufacture it in sufficient amounts for optimal health.

Estimated Average Requirement (EAR)—Intake that meets the estimated nutrient need of 50% of the individuals in a life-stage and gender group; used to set the Recommended Dietary Allowance (RDA) and to assess or plan the intake of groups.

Ethanol—Grain alcohol; ounces of ethanol in beverages can be estimated with the conversion factors of 0.045 for beer, 0.121 for wine, and 0.409 for liquor.

Ethnocentrism—Belief that one's own culture and worldview is superior to anyone else's.

Etiology—The cause of a disease.

Evaporative water loss—Insensible water loss through the skin.

Exchange—A defined quantity of food on the Academy of Nutrition and Dietetics Exchange List for Diabetes or on another exchange list.

Exchange List—A food guide used in clinical practice to aid in meal planning.

Excretion—The elimination of waste products from the body in feces, urine, exhaled air, and perspiration.

Exogenous—Outside the body.

External muscle layer—Muscle layer of the alimentary canal.

External water loss—Water lost to the outside of the body.

Extracellular fluid—Fluid found between the cells and within the blood and lymph vessels.

Extrinsic factor—Vitamin B_{12}, necessary for proper red blood cell development.

Failure to thrive (FTT)—Medical diagnosis for infants who fail to gain weight appropriately or who lose weight; also applied to elderly who lose ability to care for themselves.

Fasting—The state of having had no food or fluid enterally or no parenteral nutrition.

Fasting blood sugar (FBS)—Blood glucose measured in the fasting state; normal values are 70 to 100 mg per deciliter.

Fat-free mass—Lean body mass plus nonfat components of adipose tissue.

Fatty acid—Part of the structure of a fat.

Fatty liver—Accumulation of lipids in the liver cells; may be reversible if the cause, of which there are many, is removed.

Feedback cycle—Control system of many bodily functions involving the interaction between a stimulus and an effect; in positive feedback, the effect increases the stimulus as uterine contractions increasing oxytocin secretion; in negative feedback, the effect decreases the stimulus as blood levels of thyroid hormone decrease secretion of thyroid-stimulating hormone.

Ferric iron—Oxidized iron, which is less absorbable from the gastrointestinal tract than ferrous iron; abbreviated Fe^{3+}.

Ferritin—An iron–phosphorus–protein complex formed in the intestinal mucosa by the union of ferric iron with apoferritin; the form in which iron is stored in the tissues, mainly in liver, spleen, and bone marrow cells.

Ferrous iron—The more absorbable form of iron for humans; abbreviated Fe^{2+}.

Fetal alcohol syndrome (FAS)—A condition characterized by mental and physical abnormalities in an infant caused by the mother's consumption of alcohol during pregnancy.

Fetus—The human child in utero from the third month until birth; also applicable to the later stages of gestation of other animals.

Fiber, dietary—Material in foods, mostly from plants, that the human body cannot break down or digest.

Fibrin—Insoluble protein formed from fibrinogen by the action of thrombin; forms the meshwork of a blood clot.

Fibrinogen—Protein in blood essential to the clotting process; also called Factor I; *see* Fibrin.

Filtration—The process of removing particles from a solution by allowing the liquid to pass through a membrane or other partial barrier.

First-degree relatives—An individual's parents, siblings, or children.

First pass effect—Process whereby drugs are extensively metabolized by the small intestine or liver enzymes; result is that less drug reaches the systemic circulation.

Flatus—Gas in the digestive tract, averaging 400 to 1,200 milliliters per day.

Flavonoids—Nonnutritive antioxidant compounds that occur naturally in certain foods such as onions, apples, tea, and red wine; inhibit oxidation of low-density lipoprotein in laboratory experiments.

Flow phase—The second phase in the stress response; marked by pronounced hormonal changes.

Fluorosis—Condition due to excessive prolonged intake of fluoride; tissues affected are teeth and bones.

FODMAPs—Fermentable Oligosaccharides, Disaccharides, Monosaccharides, And Polyols; carbohydrates that are known to cause symptoms in patients with irritable bowel syndrome because of their poor absorption, osmotic activity, and rapid fermentation.

Folate—B vitamin necessary for DNA formation and proper red blood cell formation; form occurring in foods and body tissues.

Folic acid—B vitamin necessary for DNA formation and proper red blood cell formation; oxidized form used to fortify foods and in supplements.

Food acceptance record—A checklist that indicates food items accepted or rejected by the client.

Food allergy—Sensitivity to a food that does not cause a negative reaction in most people.

Food faddism—An unusual pattern of food behavior enthusiastically adapted by its adherents.

Food frequency—A usual food intake or a description of what an individual usually eats during a typical day.

Food infection—Infection acquired through contact with food or water contaminated with disease-producing microorganisms.

Food insecurity—Limited or uncertain availability of nutritionally adequate and safe foods; uncertain ability to acquire food either sometimes or always.

Food intoxication—An illness caused by the consumption of a food in which bacteria have produced a poisonous toxin.

Food quackery—The promotion for profit of a medical scheme or remedy that is unproven or known to be false.

Food record—A diary of a person's self-reported food intake.

Fortification—Process of adding nutritive substances not naturally occurring in the given food to increase its nutritional value; for example, milk fortified with vitamins A and D.

Free radicals—Atoms or molecules that have lost an electron and vigorously pursue its replacement; in doing so, free radicals can damage normal cell constituents.

Fructose—A monosaccharide found in fruits and honey; a simple sugar.

Functional disease—One for which anatomic abnormality is not apparent; opposite of organic disease.

Functional foods—Foods or food components that have additional health or physiological benefits over and above the normal nutritional value they provide.

Fundus—Larger part of a hollow organ; the part of the stomach above its attachment to the esophagus.

Galactose—A monosaccharide derived mainly from the breakdown of the sugar in milk, lactose; a simple sugar.

Galactosemia—Lack of an enzyme needed to metabolize galactose; absolute contraindication to breastfeeding.

Gallbladder—A pear-shaped organ on the underside of the liver that concentrates and stores bile.

Gastric bypass—A surgical procedure that routes food around the stomach.

Gastric lipase—An enzyme in the stomach that aids in the digestion of fats.

Gastric residual volume (GRV)—The volume of unabsorbed enteral feeding in the stomach.

Gastric stapling—A surgical procedure on the stomach to induce weight loss by reducing the size of the stomach; also known as gastroplasty.

Gastrin—A hormone secreted by the gastric mucosa; stimulates the secretion of gastric juice.

Gastritis—Inflammation of the stomach.

Gastroesophageal reflux (acid-reflux disorder) (GERD)—Regurgitation of stomach contents into the esophagus.

Gastroparesis—Partial paralysis of the stomach.

Gastrostomy—A surgical opening in the stomach.

Gene—Basic unit of heredity; linear segment of deoxyribonucleic acid (DNA) that occupies a specific location on a specific chromosome; provides the instructions for protein synthesis.

Generativity—The seventh of Erikson's developmental stages, in which the middle-aged adult guides the next generation.

Generic name—The name given to a drug by its original developer; usually the same as the official name given to it by the Food and Drug Administration.

Genetic code—Hereditary instructions for building proteins; analogous to software that dictates the processing of information by the computer.

Genetic susceptibility—Likelihood of an individual developing a given trait as determined by heredity.

Genomics—The study of an organism's complete set of DNA; regarding nutrition, the study of how different foods may interact with specific genes to increase the risk of common chronic diseases.

Genotype—Total of the hereditary information present in an organism whether or not expressed in the individual's phenotype (*see* Phenotype).

Geriatrics—Branch of medicine involved in the study and treatment of diseases of the elderly.

Gestation—Time from fertilization of the ovum until birth; in humans, the length of gestation is usually 38 to 42 weeks.

Gestational diabetes (GDM)—Hyperglycemia and altered carbohydrate, protein, and fat metabolism related to the increased physiological demands of pregnancy.

Globin—The simple protein portion of hemoglobin.

Glomerular filtrate—The fluid that has been passed through the glomerulus.

Glomerular filtration rate (GFR)—An index of kidney function; the amount of filtrate formed each minute in all the nephrons of both kidneys.

Glomerulonephritis—Inflammation of the glomeruli.

Glomerulus—The network of capillaries inside the Bowman capsule.

Glossitis—Inflammation of the tongue.

Glucagon—A hormone secreted by the alpha cells of the pancreas; increases the concentration of glucose in the blood.

Gluconeogenesis—The production of glucose from noncarbohydrate sources such as amino acids and glycerol.

Glucose—A monosaccharide (simple sugar) commonly called the blood sugar; the same as dextrose.

Glucose tolerance test—A test of blood and urine after the patient receives a concentrated dose of glucose; used to diagnose abnormalities of glucose metabolism.

Gluteal-femoral obesity—Excess body fat centered around an individual's buttocks, hips, and thighs.

Gluten—A type of protein found in wheat, rye, and barley; may contaminate oats through processing.

Gluten-sensitive enteropathy (celiac disease)—An intestinal disorder caused by an abnormal response following the consumption of gluten.

Glycemic index—A measure of how much the blood glucose level increases after consumption of a particular food that contains a given amount of carbohydrate.

Glycerol—The backbone of a fat molecule; pharmaceutical preparation is glycerin.

Glycogen—The form in which carbohydrate is stored in liver and muscle.

Glycogenolysis—The breakdown of glycogen.

Glycosuria—Glucose in the urine.

Glycosylated hemoglobin—Hemoglobin to which a glucose group is attached; in diabetes mellitus, if the blood glucose level has not been controlled over the previous 120 days, the glycosylated hemoglobin level is elevated.

Goiter—Enlargement of the thyroid gland characterized by pronounced swelling in the neck.

Goitrogens—Substances that block the absorption of iodine, thereby causing goiter; found in cabbage, rutabaga, and turnips, but only related to goiter in cassava.

Gout—A hereditary metabolic disease that is a form of acute arthritis and is marked by inflammation of the joints.

GRAS List—Food additives categorized by the U.S. Food and Drug Administration to be **G**enerally **R**ecognized **A**s **S**afe.

Growth—Progressive increase in size of a living thing that entails the synthesis of new protoplasm and multiplication of cells.

Gut failure—Impaired absorption due to structural damage to the small intestine; symptoms include diarrhea, malabsorption, and unsuccessful absorption of oral food.

Halal—Pertaining to food prepared and served according to Islamic dietary laws.

Half-life—In drug therapy, time required by the body to metabolize or inactivate half the amount of a substance.

Harris–Benedict equation—A formula commonly used to estimate resting energy expenditure in a stressed client.

Health—The state of complete physical, mental, and social well-being, not just the absence of disease or infirmity.

Healthy body weight (HBW)—Estimate of a weight suitable for an individual based on frame size and height and weight tables.

Heart failure—Inability of heart to circulate blood sufficiently to meet body's needs; peripheral edema is an early sign of right-sided failure usually due to lung disease; difficulty breathing is an early sign of left-sided failure usually a consequence of myocardial infarction.

Hematemesis—Vomiting blood.

Hematocrit—Percentage of total blood volume that is red blood cells; normal levels are 40% to 54% for men, 37% to 47% for women.

Hematuria—Blood in the urine.

Heme—The iron-containing portion of the hemoglobin molecule.

Heme iron—Iron bound to hemoglobin and myoglobin in meat, fish, and poultry; 10% to 30% of the iron in these foods is absorbed.

Hemochromatosis—A genetic disease of iron metabolism in which iron accumulates in the tissues.

Hemodialysis—A method for cleansing the blood of wastes by circulating blood through a machine that contains tubes made of synthetic semipermeable membranes.

Hemoglobin—The iron-carrying pigment of the red blood cells; carries oxygen from the lungs to the tissues.

Hemolysis—Rupture of red blood cells releasing hemoglobin into the plasma; causes include bacterial toxins, chemicals, inappropriate medications, vitamin E deficiency.

Hemolytic anemia—An abnormal reduction in the number of red blood cells due to hemolysis.

Hemosiderin—An iron oxide–protein compound derived from hemoglobin; a storage form of iron.

Hemosiderosis—Condition resulting from excess deposits of hemosiderin, especially in the liver and spleen; caused by destruction of red blood cells, which occurs in diseases such as hemolytic anemia, pernicious anemia, and chronic infection.

Heparin—A chemical, found naturally in many tissues, that inhibits blood clotting by preventing the conversion of prothrombin to thrombin; also given as an anticoagulant medication.

Hepatic portal circulation—A subdivision of the vascular system in which blood from the digestive organs and spleen circulates through the liver before returning to the heart.

Hepatitis—Inflammation of the liver, caused by viruses, drugs, alcohol, or toxic substances.

Hepcidin—Hormone synthesized by the liver that regulates iron metabolism; released in response to high body iron levels to inhibit iron transport in the duodenum and to prevent release of stored iron.

Heterozygous—Having dissimilar pairs of genes, one from each parent, for any hereditary characteristic; genes, one from each parent, governing a particular trait; the dominant gene will produce the given trait in the individual.

Hiatal hernia—A protrusion of part of the stomach into the chest cavity.

High-density lipoprotein (HDL)—A plasma protein that carries fat in the bloodstream to the tissues or to the liver to be excreted; elevated blood levels are associated with a decreased risk of heart disease.

High-fructose corn syrup (HFCS)—Corn syrup that has been enzymatically processed to convert some of its glucose into fructose to produce a desired sweetness; principal sweetener used in processed foods and beverages because it costs less than sucrose.

Hives (urticaria)—Sudden swelling and itching of skin or mucous membranes, often caused by allergies; if the respiratory tract is involved, may be life-threatening.

Homeostasis—Tendency toward balance in the internal environment of the body, achieved by automatic monitoring and regulating mechanisms.

Homozygous—Having two identical genes, one from each parent, governing a particular trait; necessary condition to produce a disease caused by a recessive gene, such as sickle cell anemia.

Hormone—A substance produced by cells of the body that is released into the bloodstream and carried to target sites to regulate the activity of other cells and organs.

Human immunodeficiency virus (HIV)—The virus that causes AIDS.

Humoral immunity—Development of antibodies to specific antigens by the B-lymphocytes, some of which retain the ability to recognize the antigen if it is encountered again; basis of immunizations.

Humulin—Exact duplicate of human insulin manufactured by altering bacterial DNA.

Hunger—The sensation resulting from a lack of food, characterized by dull or acute pain around the lower part of the chest; in global context, insufficient quantity of food where minimum kilocalorie intake is not met.

Hydrochloric acid (HCl)—Strong acid secreted by the stomach that aids in protein digestion.

Hydrogenation—The process of adding hydrogen to a fat to make it more highly saturated.

Hydrolysis—A chemical reaction that splits a substance into simpler compounds by the addition of water; in hydrolyzed infant formulas, whole proteins are split into smaller pieces.

Hydrostatic pressure—The pressure created by the pumping action of the heart on the fluid in the blood vessels.

Hyperbilirubinemia—Excessive bilirubin in the blood; bilirubin is produced by the breakdown of red blood cells.

Hypercalcemia—A serum calcium level that is too high; in adults, more than 5.5 milliequivalents per liter.

Hypercholesterolemia—Excessive cholesterol in the blood.

Hyperemesis gravidarum—Severe nausea and vomiting persisting after the fourteenth week of pregnancy of unknown etiology.

Hyperglycemia—An elevated level of glucose in the blood; fasting value above 110 milligrams per deciliter, depending on measuring technique used.

Hyperglycemic hyperosmolar nonketotic syndrome (HHNS)—Life-threatening complication of non–insulin-dependent diabetes (NIDDM) characterized by blood glucose levels greater than 600 milligrams per deciliter, absence of or slight ketosis, profound cellular dehydration, and electrolyte imbalances.

Hyperkalemia—Excessive potassium in the blood; greater than 5.0 milliequivalents per liter of serum in adults.

Hyperlipoproteinemia—A group of acquired and inherited disorders causing increased lipoproteins and lipids in the blood; also referred to as hyperlipidemia.

Hypermetabolism—An abnormal increase in the rate at which fuel or kilocalories are burned.

Hypernatremia—An excess of sodium in the blood; greater than 145 milliequivalents per liter of serum in adults.

Hyperparathyroidism—Excessive secretion of parathyroid hormone, causing changes in the bones, kidney, and gastrointestinal tract.

Hyperphosphatemia—Excessive amount of phosphates in the blood; in adults, greater than 4.7 milligrams per 100 milliliters of serum.

Hypertension—Condition of elevated blood pressure readings on 2 to 3 separate occasions; diagnosed if blood pressure is greater than 120/80 mm Hg (elevated blood pressure); a systolic reading of 130 to 139 mm Hg, or a diastolic reading of 80 to 89 mm Hg (high blood pressure stage 1); or a systolic reading greater than 140 mm Hg, or a diastolic reading greater than 90 mm Hg (high blood pressure stage 2).

Hypertensive disorders of pregnancy—Blood pressure greater than 140 mm Hg systolic or greater than 90 mm Hg diastolic occurring in pregnancy; subcategories are chronic hypertension, gestational hypertension, preeclampsia, and eclampsia.

Hypertensive kidney disease—A condition in which vascular or glomerular lesions cause hypertension but not total renal failure.

Hyperthyroidism—Oversecretion of thyroid hormones, which increases the metabolic rate above normal.

Hypertonic—A solution that contains more particles and exerts more osmotic pressure than the plasma.

Hypervitaminosis—Condition caused by excessive intake of vitamins.

Hypocalcemia—A depressed level of calcium in the blood; less than 4.5 milliequivalents per liter of serum in adults.

Hypoglycemia—A depressed level of glucose in the blood; less than 70 milligrams per deciliter.

Hypokalemia—Potassium depletion in the circulating blood; less than 3.5 milliequivalents per liter of serum in adults.

Hyponatremia—Too little sodium per volume of blood; less than 135 milliequivalents per liter of serum in adults.

Hypophosphatemia—Too little phosphate per volume of blood; in adults, less than 2.4 milligrams per 100 milliliters of serum.

Hypothalamus—A portion of the brain that helps to regulate water balance, thirst, body temperature, carbohydrate and fat metabolism, and sleep.

Hypothyroidism—Undersecretion of thyroid hormones; reduces the metabolic rate.

Hypotonic—A solution that contains fewer particles and exerts less osmotic pressure than the plasma does.

Iatrogenic malnutrition—Excessive or deficit intake of one or more nutrients induced by the oversight or omissions of health-care workers.

Ideal body weight—Person's projected healthy weight based on height, frame, and gender; for information about MetLife's development of the tables, see http://www.halls.md/ideal-weight/met.htm.

Identity—The fifth developmental task in Erikson's theory, in which the adolescent decides on an appropriate role.

Idiopathic—Without a recognizable cause.

Ileocecal valve—The valve between the ileum and cecum.

Ileostomy—Surgical procedure in which an opening to the small intestine (ileum) is constructed on the abdomen.

Ileum—The lower portion of the small intestine.

Immune—Produced by, involved in, or concerned with resistance or protection against a specified disease.

Immune system—The organs in the body responsible for fighting off substances interpreted as foreign.

Immunity—The state of being protected from a particular disease, especially an infectious disease.

Immunoglobulin—Blood proteins with known antibody activity; five types of immunoglobulins have been identified: IgA, IgD, IgE, IgG, and IgM.

Immunosuppressive agent—Medication that interferes with the body's ability to fight infection.

Impaired glucose tolerance (IGT)—A type of classification for hyperglycemia; for persons who have a glucose intolerance but do not meet the criteria for classification as having diabetes.

Implantation—Embedding of the fertilized egg in the lining of the uterus 6 or 7 days after fertilization.

Incidence—The frequency of occurrence of any event or condition over a given time and in relation to the population in which it occurs.

Incomplete protein—Protein lacking one or more of the essential amino acids that humans need; found primarily in plant sources such as grains and vegetables; gelatin is an animal product but is an incomplete protein.

Incubation period—The time it takes to show disease symptoms after exposure to the causative organism.

Indication—A circumstance that indicates when a treatment should or can be used.

Indoles—Compounds found in vegetables of the cruciferous family that activate enzymes to destroy carcinogens.

Industry—The fourth stage of development in Erikson's theory in which the school-age child learns to work effectively.

Infant botulism—Neurological toxicity caused by ingestion of *Clostridium botulinum* spores from honey or soil-contaminated foods; infant's intestinal tract flora cannot suppress the spores; also called intestinal botulism.

Infection—Entry and development of parasites or entry and multiplication of microorganisms in the bodies of persons or animals; may or may not cause signs and symptoms.

Inflammatory response—The metabolic response of the immune system to infection or injury.

Initiation—The first step in the cell's becoming cancerous, when physical forces, chemicals, or biologic agents permanently alter the cell's DNA.

Initiative—The third stage of development in Erikson's theory in which the preschooler learns to set and achieve goals.

Insensible water loss—Water that is lost invisibly through the lungs and skin.

Insoluble—Incapable of being dissolved in a given substance.

Insulin—Hormone secreted by the beta cells of the pancreas in response to an elevated blood glucose level.

Insulin resistance—A disorder characterized by elevated levels of both glucose and insulin; thought to be related to a lack of insulin receptors.

Intact feeding—A feeding consisting of nutrients that have not been predigested.

Intact nutrients—Nutrients that have not been predigested.

Integrity—The final stage of Erikson's theory of psychosocial development, in which the older adult learns to look back on his or her life as worthwhile.

Intermittent feeding—Giving a 4- to 6-hour volume of a tube feeding over 20 to 30 minutes.

Intermittent peritoneal dialysis—Method of dialysis treatment in which the dialysate remains in a patient's abdominal cavity for about 30 minutes and then drains from the body by gravity.

International normalized ratio (INR)—Measure of standardized prothrombin time; used to monitor anticoagulation effects of warfarin; normal individual = 1; therapeutic range for anticoagulation = 2 to 3, meaning client's blood takes 2 to 3 times as long as normal to clot.

International unit (IU)—Individually scaled measure of vitamins A, D, and E agreed to by a committee of scientists; also used for some hormones, enzymes, and biologicals such as vaccines.

Interstitial fluid—Extracellular fluid located between the cells.

Intimacy—The sixth stage of development in Erikson's theory, in which the young adult builds reciprocal, caring relationships.

Intracellular fluid—Fluid located within the cells.

Intravascular fluid—Fluid found in the blood and lymph vessels.

Intravenous—Through a vein.

Intrinsic factor—Specific protein-binding factor secreted by the stomach, necessary for the absorption of vitamin B_{12}.

Invisible fat—Dietary fats that cannot be seen easily; hidden fats in foods such as baked goods, peanut butter, emulsified milk, and so forth.

Ion—An atom or group of atoms carrying an electrical charge; an ion with a positive charge is called a cation; an ion with a negative charge is called an anion.

Ionic bond—A chemical bond formed between atoms by the loss and gain of electrons.

Iron deficiency—State of inadequate iron stores measured by laboratory tests such as serum ferritin and transferrin saturation; may progress to anemia when the person's hemoglobin value drops.

Irrigation—Flushing a prescribed solution through a tube or cavity.

Irritable bowel syndrome—Diarrhea or alternating constipation-diarrhea with no discernible organic cause.

Islet cell antibody—A protein found to be elevated in a person with insulin-dependent diabetes mellitus.

Islets of Langerhans—Clusters of cells in the pancreas, including alpha, beta, and delta cells; alpha cells produce glucagon, beta cells produce insulin, and delta cells produce somatostatin.

Isotonic—A solution that has the same osmotic pressure as blood plasma.

Isotretinoin—Vitamin A metabolite used to treat severe acne, requiring strict contraceptive protocols in fertile women because the metabolite can cause birth defects.

Jaundice—Yellowing of skin, whites of eyes, and mucous membranes due to excessive bilirubin in the blood; causes may be obstructed bile duct, liver disease, or hemolysis of red blood cells.

Jejunoileal bypass—A surgical procedure that removes a portion of the small intestine, bypassing about 90% of it.

Jejunostomy—A surgical opening into the jejunum.

Jejunum—The second portion of the small intestine.

Joule—A measurement of energy; amount of energy needed to raise the temperature of 1 gram of cool, dry air by 1.8°F (1.0°C).

Kaposi sarcoma—A type of cancer often related to the immunocompromised state that accompanies AIDS; characterized by multiple areas of cell proliferation, initially in the skin and eventually in other body sites.

Keshan disease—Deterioration of the heart due to selenium deficiency, but heart failure not reversible by supplementation; named for the province of Keshan, China; fatality rate as high as 80%; in mice, linked to a mutation of an avirulent virus to a virulent one producing myocardial disease; virulent strain then caused heart disease in mice not selenium deficient.

Keto acid—Amino acid residue left after deamination.

Ketoacidosis—Acidosis due to an excess of ketone bodies.

Ketone—Any of a class of organic compounds characterized by a carbonyl group attached to two carbon atoms; example: acetone, used in nail polish remover and paint remover.

Ketone body—Any of the three compounds (acetoacetic acid, acetone, and B-hydroxybutyric acid) that are normal intermediates in lipid metabolism; accumulate in blood and urine in abnormal amounts in conditions of impaired metabolism.

Ketonuria—The presence of ketone bodies in the urine.

Ketosis—Accumulation of ketone bodies in the blood; result of incomplete metabolism of fatty acids, generally from carbohydrate deficiency or malfunctioning carbohydrate metabolism.

Kilocaloric density—The kilocalories contained in a given volume of a food.

Kilocalorie (Kcal)—A measurement unit of energy; the amount of heat required to raise 1 kilogram of water 1.8°F (1°C); on food labels: Calorie.

Kilocalorie:nitrogen ratio—A mathematical relationship expressed as the number of kilocalories per gram of nitrogen provided in a feeding.

Kilojoule—A measurement unit of energy required to move a mass of 1 kilogram with an acceleration of one meter per second; one kilocalorie equals 4.184 kilojoules.

Konzo—An irreversible paralytic disease of the lower extremities caused by consumption of inadequately processed cassava roots that contain cyanide along with a diet deficient in sulphur-based amino acids.

Korsakoff psychosis—Amnesia, often seen in chronic alcoholism, caused by degeneration of the thalamus due to thiamin deficiency; characterized by loss of short-term memory and inability to learn new skills.

Kosher—Pertaining to food prepared and served according to Jewish dietary laws.

Krebs cycle—A complicated series of reactions that results in the release of energy from carbohydrates, fats, and proteins, also known as the TCA (tricarboxylic acid) cycle.

Kussmaul respirations—Pattern of rapid and deep breathing due to the body's attempt to correct metabolic acidosis by eliminating carbon dioxide through the lungs.

Kwashiorkor—Severe protein deficiency in child after weaning; symptoms include edema, pigmentation changes, impaired growth and development, and liver pathology.

Lactalbumin—Simple soluble protein found in greater concentration in human breast milk than in cow's milk; easily absorbed by the infant.

Lactase—An intestinal enzyme that converts lactose into glucose and galactose.

Lactational amenorrhea—Absence of menstrual cycle in a mother who is fully breastfeeding.

Lacteal—The central lymph vessel in each villus.

Lactose—A disaccharide found mainly in milk and milk products.

Large intestine—The part of the alimentary canal that extends from the small intestine to the anus.

LCAT deficiency—A lack of LCAT (lecithin-cholesterol acyltransferase), an enzyme that transports cholesterol from the tissues to the liver for removal from the body.

Lean body mass—Also called fat-free mass; the weight of the body minus the fat content but including essential fats that are associated with the central nervous system, the viscera, the bone marrow, and cell membranes.

Legumes—Plants that have nitrogen-fixing bacteria in their roots; a good alternative to meat as a protein source; examples: dried beans, lentils.

Lesion—Area of diseased or injured tissue.

Leukopenia—Abnormal decrease in the number of white blood corpuscles; usually below 5,000 per cubic millimeter.

Life expectancy—The probable number of years that persons of a given age may be expected to live.

Limiting amino acid—Particular essential amino acid lacking or undersupplied in a food that classifies the food as an incomplete protein.

Linoleic acid—An essential fatty acid.

Lipectomy—Surgical removal of adipose tissue.

Lipid—Any one of a group of fats or fat-like substances that are insoluble in water; includes true fats (fatty acids and glycerol), lipoids, and sterols.

Lipoid—Substances resembling fats but containing groups other than glycerol and fatty acids that make up true fats; example: phospholipids.

Lipolysis—The breakdown of adipose tissue for energy.

Lipoprotein—Combination of a protein with lipid components such as cholesterol, phospholipids, and triglycerides.

Lipoprotein lipase—An enzyme that breaks down chylomicrons.

Liposuction—Surgical removal of adipose tissue through a vacuum hose.

Listeriosis—Bacterial infection caused by *Listeria monocytogenes* that is particularly virulent for fetuses; transmitted from the mother to the fetus in utero or through the birth canal; outbreaks associated with raw or contaminated milk, soft cheeses, contaminated vegetables, and ready-to-eat meats; others at risk include the elderly, those with impaired immune systems, and farm workers.

Liver—A digestive organ that aids in the metabolism of all the energy nutrients, screens toxic substances from the blood, manufactures blood proteins, and performs many other important functions.

Locus, loci (pl.)—In genetics, the site of a gene on a chromosome.

Loop of Henle—The segment of the renal tubule that follows the proximal convoluted tubule.

Low birth weight (LBW)—Characterizing an infant that weighs less than 2,500 g (5.5 lb) at birth.

Low-density lipoprotein (LDL)—A plasma protein containing more cholesterol and triglycerides than protein; elevated blood levels are associated with increased risk of heart disease.

Luminal effect—Drug-induced changes within the intestine that affect the absorption of nutrients and drugs without altering the intestine.

Lycopene—A red pigmented carotenoid with powerful antioxidant functions but no provitamin A activity; found in tomatoes and various berries and fruits.

Lymph—A body fluid collected from the interstitial fluid all over the body and returned to the bloodstream via the lymphatic vessels.

Lymphatic system—All the structures involved in the transportation of lymph from the tissues to the bloodstream.

Lysine—Amino acid often lacking in grains.

Macrocytic anemia—Anemia in which the red blood cells are larger than normal; one characteristic of pernicious anemia also found in folic acid deficiency.

Macrophage—Monocyte that has left the circulation and settled in a tissue such as the spleen, lymph nodes, and tonsils; with neutrophils, major phagocytic cells of immune system.

Major minerals—Those present in the body in quantities greater than 5 grams (approximately 1 teaspoonful); humans need at least 100 milligrams daily (approximately 1/50 teaspoonful); also called macrominerals.

Malabsorption—Inadequate movement of digested food from the small intestine into the blood or lymphatic system.

Malignant—Tumor that infiltrates surrounding tissue and spreads to distant sites of the body.

Malnutrition—Poor nutrition; results when the body's cells receive either an excess or a deficiency of one or more nutrients.

Maltase—An intestinal enzyme that converts maltose into glucose.

Maltose—A disaccharide produced when starches are broken down by the body into simpler units; two units of glucose joined together.

Marasmus—Malnutrition due to a protein and kilocalorie deficit.

Mastication—The process of chewing.

Mechanical digestion—The digestive process that involves the physical breaking down of food into smaller pieces.

Median—Statistical measure of central tendency; in a ranked set, value above which and below which are an equal number of values.

Medical foods—Foods formulated to be consumed or administered enterally under the supervision of a physician intended for the specific dietary management of a disease or condition, which have distinctive nutritional requirements.

Medical Nutrition Therapy (MNT)—Provision of nutrient, dietary, and nutrition education based on a comprehensive nutritional assessment by a registered dietitian (RD); can offer cost-effective health benefits in disease management and medication optimization.

Megadose—Dose providing 10 times or more of the recommended dietary allowance.

Megaloblastic anemia—Anemia characterized by large immature red blood cells in the bloodstream that cannot carry oxygen properly; occurs in folic acid deficiency and pernicious anemia.

Melatonin—Hormone produced from the amino acid tryptophan by the pineal gland in the brain; stimulates the onset and duration of sleep; used to treat sleep disorders and jet lag.

Melena—dark, sticky feces containing blood

Menaquinone—Vitamin K that is synthesized by intestinal bacteria; also called vitamin K_2.

Meninges—Three membranes covering the brain and spinal cord; from the outside named the dura, arachnoid, and pia maters.

Meningocele—Congenital protrusion of the meninges through a defect in the skull or the spinal column.

Meningoencephalocele—Protrusion of the brain and its coverings through a defect in the skull.

Menkes disease—Metabolic defect blocking the absorption of copper in the gastrointestinal tract.

Meta-analysis—Statistical procedure for combining data from a number of studies to analyze therapeutic effectiveness.

Metabolic syndrome—Combination of atherosclerotic risk factors, including dyslipidemia, insulin resistance, obesity, and hypertension, that produces an increased risk for coronary artery disease.

Metabolism—The sum of all physical and chemical changes that take place in the body; the two fundamental processes involved are anabolism and catabolism.

Metabolite—Any product of metabolism; 4,229 human serum metabolites commonly detected and quantified (with today's technology) in the human serum metabolome have recently been cataloged for use by researchers.

Metastasis—The "seeding" of cancer cells to distant sites of the body; spread via blood or lymph vessels or by spilling into a body cavity.

Methionine—Sulfur-containing amino acid often lacking in legumes.

Microalbuminuria—Small amounts of protein in the urine. Detected by a laboratory using methods more sensitive than traditional urinalysis.

Microbiota—Gut microflora

Microflora—Resident bacteria in the intestinal tract; functions include assisting in the development of the immune system and protecting the host from foreign microbes.

Microgram—One-millionth of a gram or one-thousandth of a milligram; abbreviated mcg.

Micronize—To pulverize a substance into very tiny particles.

Microvilli—Microscopic, hairlike rodlets (resembling bristles on a brush) covering the edge of each villus.

Midarm circumference—Measure of the distance around the middle of the upper arm; used to assess body protein stores.

Milliequivalent (mEq)—Unit of measure used for determining the concentration of electrolytes in solution; expressed as milliequivalents per liter.

Milling—The process of grinding grain into flour.

Milliosmole—Unit of measure for osmotic activity.

Mineral—An inorganic element or compound occurring in nature; in the body, some minerals help regulate bodily functions and are essential to good health.

Mixed malnutrition—The result of a deficiency or excess of more than one nutrient.

Modified diet—A term used in healthcare institutions to mean that the food served to a client has been altered or changed from that served to clients on regular diets, usually by physician order.

Modular supplement—A nutritional supplement that contains a limited number of nutrients, usually only one.

Mold—Any of a group of parasitic or other organisms living on decaying matter; fungi.

Molecule—The smallest quantity into which a substance may be divided without loss of its characteristics.

Monoamine oxidase inhibitor (MAOI)—A class of drugs that may have critical interactions with foods.

Monocyte—White blood cell that circulates in the bloodstream for about 24 hours before settling into tissues to become a macrophage; with macrophages, provide a defense against foreign antigens.

Monoglyceride—One fatty acid joined to a glycerol molecule.

Monosaccharide—A simple sugar composed of one unit of $C_6H_{12}O_6$; examples: glucose, fructose, galactose.

Monounsaturated fat—A lipid in which the majority of fatty acids contain one carbon-to-carbon double bond.

Morbid obesity—Body mass index (BMI) greater than 39.

Morbidity—The state of being diseased; number of cases of disease in relation to population.

Mortality—State of being subject to death; the death rate; number of deaths per unit of population.

Motility—Power to move spontaneously.

Mucosa—A mucous membrane that lines body cavities.

Mucosal effect—Drug-induced changes within the intestine that affect the absorption of drugs or nutrients by damaging the tissues.

Mucus—A thick fluid secreted by the mucous membranes and glands.

Multiparous—Having borne more than one child.

Mutation—Permanent transmissible change in a gene; natural mutation produces evolutionary change in organisms; induced mutation results from exposure to environmental influences such as physical forces, chemicals, or biologic agents.

Mycotoxin—A substance produced by mold growing in food that can cause illness or death when ingested by humans or animals.

Myelin sheath—Fatty covering surrounding the long appendages of some nerves; serves to increase the transmission speed of impulses.

MyPlate—U.S. Department of Agriculture food guide using the visual cues of a divided plate and a glass to represent the proportions of healthy foods for consumers.

Myocardial infarction (MI)—Area of dead heart muscle; usually the result of coronary occlusion.

Myocardium—The heart muscle.

Myoglobin—A protein located in muscle tissue that contains and stores oxygen.

Myxedema—A condition that occurs in older children and adults, resulting from hypofunction of the thyroid gland characterized by a drying and thickening of the skin and slowing of physical and mental activity.

Narcolepsy—A chronic condition consisting of recurrent attacks of drowsiness and sleep.

Nasoduodenal tube (ND tube)—A tube inserted via the nose into the duodenum.

Nasogastric tube (NG tube)—A tube inserted via the nose into the stomach.

Nasojejunal tube (NJ tube)—A tube inserted via the nose into the jejunum.

Necrotizing enterocolitis—A condition in premature infants in which intestinal cells die and fall off.

Neonate—Infant from birth to age 28 days.

Neoplasm—A new and abnormal formation of tissue (tumor) that grows at the expense of the healthy organism.

Nephritis—General term for inflammation of the kidneys.

Nephron—The structural and functional unit of the kidney.

Nephropathy—A kidney disease characterized by inflammation and degenerative lesions.

Nephrosclerosis—A hardening of the renal arteries; may be caused by arteriosclerosis of the kidney arteries.

Nephrotic syndrome—The end result of a variety of diseases that cause the abnormal passage of plasma proteins into the urine.

Neuropathy—Any disease of the nerves.

Neural tube defects—A birth defect of the brain, spine, or spinal cord; includes spina bifida and anencephaly.

NHANES—National Health and Nutrition Examination Survey, a nationally representative cross-sectional survey of civilian noninstitutionalized population of the United States; conducted by the Centers for Disease Control and Prevention's National Center for Health Statistics; the interview includes demographic, socioeconomic, dietary, and health-related questions; the examination component consists of medical, dental, and physiological measurements, as well as laboratory tests.

Niacin—A B vitamin that functions as a coenzyme in the production of energy from glucose; obtained from meat or produced from the amino acid tryptophan, present in milk, eggs, and meat; also called nicotinic acid.

Niacin equivalent (NE)—Measure of niacin activity; equal to 1 milligram of preformed niacin or 60 milligrams of tryptophan.

Night blindness—Vision that is slow to adapt to dim light; caused by vitamin A deficiency or hereditary factors or, in the elderly, by poor circulation.

Nitrogen—Colorless, odorless, tasteless gas forming about 80% of Earth's air.

Nitrogen balance—The difference between the amount of nitrogen ingested and that excreted each day; when intake is greater, a positive balance exists; when intake is less, a negative balance exists.

Nitrogen-fixing bacteria—Organisms that absorb nitrogen from the air, which, upon the death of the bacteria, is released for legume plants to use in the anabolism of protein.

Nomogram—A chart that shows a relationship between numerical values.

Nonessential—In nutrition, refers to a chemical substance or nutrient the body normally can manufacture in sufficient amounts for health.

Nonessential amino acid—Any amino acid that can normally be synthesized by the body in sufficient quantities.

Nonheme iron—Iron that is not bound to hemoglobin or myoglobin; all the iron in plant sources.

Norwalk virus norovirus—A causative organism that is responsible for more than 50% of the reported cases of epidemic viral gastroenteropathy. The incubation period ranges from 18 to 72 hours, and the outbreaks are usually self-limiting; influenzalike intestinal symptoms last for 24 to 48 hours.

NSAID—Nonsteroidal anti-inflammatory drug; examples: aspirin, ibuprofen, naproxen, as well as agents available by prescription.

Nulliparous—Never having borne a child.

Nursing action (intervention)—Specific care to be administered, including physical and psychological care, teaching, counseling, and referring.

Nursing-bottle syndrome—A condition in which an infant has many dental caries caused by drinking milk or other sweet liquids during sleep.

Nutraceutical—Food component used for medicinal purposes; examples: vitamins, minerals, amino acids; regulated under Dietary Supplement Health Education Act of 1994 (see Chapter 15).

Nutrient—Chemical substance supplied by food that the body needs for growth, maintenance, and/or repair.

Nutrient density—The concentration of nutrients in a given volume of food compared with the food's kilocalorie content.

Nutrigenetics—Detection of gene variants within an individual to identify environmental factors that trigger dysfunction or disease; part of the initiation of food allergies and **celiac disease**.

Nutrigenomics—Study of the interaction between one's diet and his or her genes in order to alter susceptibilities to disease and responses to foods.

Nutrition—Science of food and its relationship to health; processes of taking in and utilizing nourishment.

Nutrition support service—A team service for clients on enteral and parenteral feedings that assesses, monitors, and counsels these clients.

Nutritional assessment—The evaluation of a client's nutritional status based on a physical examination, anthropometric measurements, laboratory data, and food intake information.

Nutritional status—Condition of the body as it relates to the intake and use of nutrients.

Obese—Body mass index (BMI) of 30 kg/m² or more; muscular person may exceed BMI of 30 kg/m² but not be obese.

Obesity—Excessive amount of fat on the body; for women, a fat content greater than 30%; for men, a fat content greater than 25%.

Obesogens—Chemical in the environment that may have an effect on obesity.

Objective data—Findings verifiable by another through physical assessment or diagnostic tests, also termed signs.

Obligatory excretion—Minimum amount of urine production necessary to keep waste products in solution, amounting to 400 to 600 milliliters per day.

Oliguria—A decreased output of urine.

Oncogene—Carcinogenic gene that stimulates excessive reproduction of the cell.

Opportunistic infection—Infection caused by normally nonpathogenic organisms in a host with decreased resistance.

Opsin—A protein that combines with vitamin A to form rhodopsin, a chemical in the retina necessary for vision.

Optic nerve—The second cranial nerve, which transmits impulses for the sense of sight.

Oral cavity—The cavity in the skull bounded by the mouth, palate, cheeks, and tongue.

Oral rehydration solution—Oral fluid that prevents or treats dehydration.

Organ—Somewhat independent body part having specific functions; examples: stomach, liver.

Orthostatic hypotension—A drop in blood pressure producing dizziness, fainting, or blurred vision when arising from a lying or sitting position or when standing motionless in a fixed position.

Osmolality—Measure of osmotic pressure exerted by the number of dissolved particles per weight of liquid; usually reported clinically as mOsm/kg.

Osmolarity—Measure of osmotic pressure exerted by the number of dissolved particles per volume of liquid; usually reported clinically as mOsm/L.

Osmosis—The movement of water across a semipermeable cell membrane from an area with fewer particles to one with more particles.

Osmotic demyelinating disease—Brain pathology caused by too rapid correction of hyponatremia resulting in motor nerve dysfunction, including quadriplegia; more common in malnourished and debilitated clients.

Osmotic pressure—The pressure that develops when a concentrated solution is separated from a less-concentrated solution by a semipermeable membrane.

Osteoarthritis—Progressive deterioration of the cartilage in the joints; risk factors are aging, obesity, occupational or athletic abuse of joints, and trauma.

Osteoblasts—Bone cells that build bone.

Osteocalcin—Vitamin K–dependent protein; second most abundant protein in bone but its function is not yet clearly defined.

Osteoclasts—Bone cells that break down bone.

Osteodystrophy—Defective bone formation.

Osteomalacia—Adult form of rickets.

Osteopenia—Bone mineral density 1 to 2.5 standard deviations below the mean of healthy young adults.

Osteoporosis—Bone mineral density more than 2.5 standard deviations below the mean of young adults.

Ostomy—A surgically formed opening to permit passage of urine or bowel contents to the outside.

Overnutrition—The result of an excess of one or more nutrients in the diet.

Overweight—Body mass index from 25 to 29.99 kg/m².

Ovum—The egg cell that, after fertilization by a sperm cell, develops into a new individual.

Oxalates—Salts of oxalic acid found in some plant foods; bind with the calcium in the plant, making it unavailable to the body.

Oxidation—The process in which a substance is combined with oxygen.

Oxidative stress—Cellular damage caused by oxygen-derived free radical formation; potential damage can be decreased by antioxidants.

Oxytocin—A hormone produced by the posterior pituitary gland in the brain; effects are uterine contractions and release of milk.

Pancreas—An abdominal gland that secretes enzymes important in the digestion of carbohydrates, fats, and proteins; also secretes the hormones insulin and glucagon.

Pancreatic lipase—An enzyme produced by the pancreas; used in fat digestion.

Pancreatitis—Inflammation of the pancreas.

Pantothenic acid—A B-complex vitamin found in almost all foods; deficiencies from lack of food have not been documented.

Paralytic ileus—A temporary cessation of peristalsis that causes an intestinal obstruction.

Paralytic shellfish poisoning—Disease caused by the consumption of poisonous clams, oysters, mussels, or scallops.

Parasite—An organism that lives within, upon, or at the expense of a living host.

Parathyroid hormone (PTH)—Hormone secreted by the parathyroid glands; regulates calcium and phosphorus metabolism in the body.

Parenteral feeding—Administration of nutrients by a route other than the gastrointestinal tract, such as subcutaneously, intravenously, intramuscularly, or intradermally.

Parenteral nutrition (PN)—Provision of nutrients through a vein (intravenously) into a large diameter vein (see Chapter 14).

Paresthesia—Abnormal or unpleasant sensation resulting from nerve injury; described as a feeling of numbness, prickliness, stinging, or burning.

Parietal—Two bones that form the sides and roof of the skull; also two lobes of the cerebrum lying roughly under those bones.

Parity—Condition of having carried a pregnancy to viability (20 weeks or

500-gram birth weight) regardless of whether resulted in a live birth; nulliparous—never carried a child to viability; multiparous—more than once.

Parotid glands—One of the salivary glands of the mouth, located just below and in front of the ears; the mumps virus causes infectious parotitis.

Pathogen—Any disease-producing agent, especially a virus, bacterium, fungus, or other microorganism.

Pectin—Purified carbohydrate obtained from peel of citrus fruits or apple pulp; gels when cooked with sugar at correct pH to thicken jelly and jam; contained in mashed raw apple, applesauce, firm banana; recommended for diarrhea to contribute firmness to stools.

Pellagra—Deficiency disease due to lack of niacin and tryptophan; characterized by the three D's: dermatitis, diarrhea, and dementia.

Pepsin—An enzyme secreted in the stomach that begins protein digestion.

Pepsinogen—The antecedent of pepsin; activated by hydrochloric acid, a component of gastric juice.

Peptidases—Enzymes that assist in the digestion of protein by reducing the smaller molecules to single amino acids.

Peptide bond—Chemical bond that links two amino acids in a protein molecule.

Percutaneously—Affected through the skin.

Perforated ulcer—Condition in which an ulcer penetrates completely through the stomach or intestinal wall, spilling the organ's contents into the peritoneal cavity.

Perinatal—Period beginning after the 28th week of pregnancy and ending 28 days after birth.

Periodontal disease—Disorder of the gingiva (gums) and the supporting structures of the teeth.

Perioperative immunonutrition—Provision of nutritional support before, during, and after surgery using enteral preparations modified by the addition of specific nutrients, such as arginine, omega-3 fatty acids, and others, which have been shown to upregulate the immune response, to control inflammatory response, and to improve gut function after surgery.

Peripheral parenteral nutrition (PPN)—An intravenous feeding via a vein away from the center of the body, usually in the hand or forearm.

Peristalsis—A wavelike muscular movement that propels food along the alimentary canal.

Peritoneal dialysis—Method of removing waste products from the blood by injecting the flushing solution into a client's abdomen and using the client's peritoneum as the semipermeable membrane.

Peritoneum—The membrane that covers the internal abdominal organs and lines the abdominal cavity.

Peritonitis—Inflammation of the peritoneal cavity.

Pernicious anemia—Inadequate red blood cell formation due to lack of intrinsic factor from the stomach, which is required for the absorption of vitamin B_{12}; leads to neural deterioration.

Pesticides—A chemical used to kill insects or rodents.

Petechiae—Pinpoint, flat, round, red lesions caused by intradermal or submucosal hemorrhage.

P-glycoprotein—Cell membrane pump influencing cellular uptake and release of chemicals; affects relative susceptibility or resistance of cells to drug therapy.

pH—*Potential of hydrogen*; a scale representing the relative acidity or alkalinity of a solution; a value of 7 is neutral, less than 7 is acidic, and greater than 7 is alkaline.

Pharmacodynamics—Study of drugs and their actions on living organisms; the clinical effects of the drugs.

Pharmacokinetics—The study of the action of drugs, emphasizing absorption time, duration of effect, distribution in the body, and method of excretion.

Pharynx—Muscular passage between the oral cavity and the esophagus.

Phenotype—Observable properties of an organism; blood type is completely inherited; other phenotypes can be altered by environmental agents.

Phenylalanine—Essential amino acid, which is indigestible if a person lacks a particular enzyme. Accumulation of phenylalanine in the blood can lead to mental retardation.

Phenylketonuria (PKU)—Hereditary disease caused by the body's failure to convert phenylalanine to tyrosine because of a defective enzyme.

Phlebotomy—Puncturing or surgical opening of a vein to withdraw blood.

Phospholipid—Diglyceride containing phosphorus; primary lipid constituent of cell membranes; examples: lecithin, myelin.

Photosynthesis—Process through which plants containing chlorophyll are able to manufacture carbohydrates from carbon dioxide and water using the sun's energy.

Phylloquinone—Vitamin K_1, found in foods.

Phytic acid—A substance found in grains that forms an insoluble complex with calcium; phytates.

Phytochemicals—Nonnutritive food components that provide medical or health benefits including the prevention or treatment of a disease.

Phytonadione—Synthetic, water-soluble pharmaceutical form of vitamin K_1; can be administered orally or by injection.

Pica—The craving to eat nonfood substances such as dirt and laundry starch.

Pitting edema—Usually of the skin of the extremities; firm pressure by a finger produces an indentation that remains for 5 seconds.

Placebo—Drug or treatment used as inactive control in a test of therapy; "placebo effect" attributed to positive response caused by subject's expectations.

Placenta—The organ in the uterus through which the unborn child exchanges carbon dioxide for oxygen and wastes for nourishment; lay term is *afterbirth*.

Plant sterols—Compounds, structurally similar to cholesterol, that in prescribed amounts interfere with the absorption of cholesterol and thus lower low-density lipoprotein cholesterol levels; marketed as table spreads (butter substitutes) and salad dressings.

Plaque—Accumulation of material; in lining of arteries, obstructs blood flow; on crowns of teeth, forerunner of dental caries and periodontal disease.

Plasma—The liquid portion of the blood including the clotting elements.

Plasma transferrin receptor—Measure of iron status; increases even in mild deficiency; unaffected by inflammation.

Plumbism—Lead poisoning.

Pneumocystis pneumonia—A type of lung infection frequently seen in AIDS patients; caused by the organism *Pneumocystis jiroveci*, formerly called *Pneumocystis carinii*.

Polycythemia—Increase in red blood cells; may be physiologic due to demand for oxygen-carrying capacity or pathologic as in *polycythemia vera*, a chronic, life-shortening disorder of unknown etiology involving hematologic stem cells.

Polydipsia—Excessive thirst.

Polymer—A natural or synthetic substance formed by combining two or more molecules of the same substance.

Polymorphism—Occurrence of more than one form in a life cycle; variation in alleles within a species.

Polypeptide—A chain of amino acids linked by peptide bonds that form proteins.

Polyphagia—Excessive appetite.

Polypharmacy—Concurrent use of a large number of drugs, increasing risk of interactions; especially likely in client with many diseases treated by multiple health-care providers.

Polyphenols—Chemicals found in plant-based foods which may help prevent cell damage in the body.

Polysaccharide—Complex carbohydrates composed of many units of $C_6H_{12}O_6$ joined together; examples important in nutrition include starch, glycogen, and fiber.

Polyunsaturated fat—A fat in which the majority of fatty acids contain more than one carbon-to-carbon double bond; intake is associated with a decreased risk of heart disease.

Polyuria—Excessive urination.

Positive feedback cycle—Situation in which a condition provokes a response that worsens the condition; example: low blood pressure due to a failing heart stimulates the kidney to save sodium and water, increasing fluid retention that further overloads the failing heart.

Postprandial—After a meal.

Potable water—Water that is safe for drinking, free of harmful substances.

Potassium pump—Proteins located in cell membranes that provide an active transport mechanism to move potassium ions across a membrane to their area of greater concentration; moves potassium ions into the cells.

Prebiotic—Nondigestible food ingredients that encourage the growth of favorable intestinal microorganisms.

Precursor—A substance from which another substance is derived.

Preeclampsia—Hypertension and proteinuria, appearing after the twentieth week of pregnancy.

Preformed vitamin—A vitamin already in a complete state in ingested foods, as opposed to a provitamin, which requires conversion in the body to be in a complete state.

Pressure injury—Tissue breakdown from external force impairing circulation.

Prevalence—The number of cases of a disease or condition present in a specified population at a given time.

Primary amenorrhea—Delay of menarche (initial menstrual period) until after age of 16 or absence of secondary sex characteristics after age 14.

Primary malnutrition—A nutrient deficiency due to poor food choices or a lack of nutritious food to eat.

Primary prevention—The implementation of practices that are likely to avert the occurrence of disease; nutrition example: maintaining a healthy body weight.

Principle of complementarity—Combining incomplete-protein foods so that each supplies the amino acids lacking in the other.

Prion—A proteinaceous infectious agent, extremely difficult to destroy; resistant to heat, pressure cooking, ultraviolet light, irradiation, bleach, formaldehyde, and weak acids; even autoclaving at 135°F (57.2°C) for 18 minutes does not eliminate infectivity.

Probiotic—Live microbial food supplements that improve the microbial balance of the intestine, mainly by reinforcing the intestinal mucosal barrier against harmful agents.

Prognosis—Probable outcome of an illness based on client's condition and natural course of the disease.

Promotion—The second step in a cell turning cancerous, through the action of environmental substances on the altered, initiated gene.

Proportionality—A medical treatment is ethically mandatory to the extent that it is likely to confer greater benefits than burdens to the client.

Prostaglandins—Long-chain, unsaturated fatty acids mostly synthesized in the body from arachidonic acid; have hormone-like effects.

Protein—Nutrient necessary for building body tissue; composed of carbon, hydrogen, oxygen, and nitrogen (and sometimes with sulfur, phosphorus, or iron); amino acids represent the basic structure of proteins.

Protein binding sites—Various sites in the body tissues to which drugs may become attached, rendering the drug temporarily inactive.

Protein-calorie malnutrition (PCM)—Condition in which the person's diet lacks both protein and kilocalories.

Protein-energy malnutrition (PEM)—Condition in which the person's diet lacks both protein and kilocalories. Also termed protein-calorie malnutrition (PCM).

Proteinuria—Protein in the urine.

Prothrombin—A protein essential to the blood-clotting process; manufactured by the liver using vitamin K.

Protocol—A description of steps to be followed when performing a procedure or providing care for a particular condition.

Proto-oncogene—Gene that in the normal cell stimulates growth and maintenance; when mutated, becomes an oncogene.

Provitamin—Inactive substance that the body converts to an active vitamin.

Provitamin A—Carotenoids that are precursors of vitamin A, the most powerful of which is beta-carotene.

Proximal convoluted tubule—The first segment of the renal tubule.

Psychology—The science of mental processes and their effects on behavior.

Psychosis—Severe mental disturbance with personality derangement and loss of contact with reality.

Psychosocial development—The maturing of an individual in relationships with others and within himself or herself.

Ptyalin—A salivary enzyme that breaks down starch and glycogen to maltose and a small amount of glucose; also known as salivary amylase.

Puberty—The period of life at which the physical ability to reproduce is attained.

Pulmonary—Concerning or involving the lungs.

Pulmonary edema—The accumulation of fluid in the lungs.

Pulse pressure—The difference between systolic and diastolic blood pressure; normally 30 to 40 mm Hg; narrows in insufficient fluid volume and widens in excessive fluid volume.

Purging—The intentional clearing of food out of the human body by vomiting and/or using enemas, laxatives, and/or diuretics.

Purines—One of the end products of the digestion of some nitrogen-containing compounds.

Pyelonephritis—An inflammation of the central portion of the kidney.

Pyloric sphincter—The sphincter muscle guarding the opening between the stomach and small intestine.

Pyridoxine—Pharmaceutical name for vitamin B_6.

Pyruvate—An intermediate in the metabolism of energy nutrients.

Quality assurance—A planned and systematic program for evaluating the quality and appropriateness of services rendered.

Quetelet index—Body mass index.

Radiologist—Physician with special training in diagnostic imaging and radiation treatments.

Rancid—Having the rank smell and sour taste of stale fat or oil from decomposition.

Rate—The speed or frequency of an event per unit of time.

Rationale—Reason certain actions are likely to achieve a desired outcome; in nursing, ideally based on research indicating a nursing action was effective in similar circumstances.

Rebound scurvy—Vitamin C deficiency produced in a person after cessation of megadosing due to a habitually lessened rate of absorption.

Recessive trait—One that requires two recessive genes for the trait, one from each parent, for the trait to be expressed (to be manifested) in the individual.

Recommended Dietary Allowance (RDA)—Intake that meets the needs of 97% to 98% of the individuals in a life stage and gender group; intended as a goal for daily intake by individuals, not for assessing adequacy of an individual's nutrient intake.

Rectum—The lower part of the large intestine.

Refeeding—The reintroduction of kilocalories and nutrients into a patient either orally or parenterally.

Refeeding syndrome—A detrimental state that results when a previously severely malnourished person is reintroduced to food and/or nutrients and kilocalories improperly.

Regurgitate—To cause to flow backward, as with an infant "spitting up."

Relative risk—In epidemiological studies, the ratio of the frequency of a certain disorder in groups exposed and groups not exposed to a particular hereditary or environmental factor.

Renal—Pertaining to the kidney.

Renal corpuscle—Refers collectively to both Bowman's capsule and the glomerulus.

Renal exchange lists—A specialized type of exchange list for clients with kidney disease who require restriction of one or more of the following: protein, sodium, phosphorus, and potassium.

Renal osteodystrophy—Defective bone development caused by phosphorus retention, a low or normal serum calcium level, and increased parathyroid activity.

Renal pelvis—A structure inside the kidney that receives urine from the collecting tubules.

Renal threshold—The blood glucose level at which glucose begins to spill into the urine.

Renal tubule—The second major portion of the nephron; appears ropelike.

Renin—An enzyme produced by the kidney that catalyzes the conversion of angiotensinogen to angiotensin I.

Rennin—An enzyme that coagulates milk.

Reservoir—Place that an infectious agent normally lives and multiplies so that it can be transmitted to a susceptible host.

Residue—Trace amount of any substance in a product at the time of sale; substance remaining in the bowel after absorption.

Respiration—The exchange of oxygen and carbon dioxide between a living organism and the environment.

Respirator—A machine used to assist respiration.

Respiratory acidosis—Blood pH less than 7.35 caused by pulmonary disease, characterized by a retention of carbon dioxide.

Respiratory alkalosis—Blood pH greater than 7.45 caused by pulmonary disease, characterized by a loss of carbon dioxide.

Resting energy expenditure (REE)—The amount of fuel the human body uses at rest for a specified period of time; often used interchangeably with basal metabolic rate (BMR).

Retina—Inner lining of eyeball that contains light-sensitive nerve cells; corresponds to film in camera.

Retinal—Form of vitamin A specifically required for vision.

Retinoic acid syndrome—Characteristic fetal deformities, including small ears or no ears, abnormal or missing ear canals, brain malformation, and heart defects caused by excessive preformed vitamin A or isotretinoin.

Retinoids—Group of structurally similar compounds possessing the biological activity of all-*trans* retinol, including retinol, retinal, retinoic acid, retinyl ester, and synthetic analogues.

Retinol—One of the active forms of preformed vitamin A.

Retinol Activity Equivalent (RAE)—Measure of vitamin A activity that considers both preformed vitamin A (retinol) and its precursor (carotene); 1 RAE equals 3.3 international units from animal foods or 20 international units from the beta-carotene in plant foods.

Retinopathy—Any disorder of the retina.

Retrolental fibroplasia (RLF)—A disease of the vessels of the retina present in premature infants; often caused by exposure to high postnatal oxygen concentration.

Rhabdomyolysis—Breakdown of muscle fibers resulting in myoglobin in the bloodstream; some components are toxic to kidney and can cause kidney damage.

Rhodopsin—Light-sensitive protein in the retina that contains vitamin A; also called visual purple.

Riboflavin—Coenzyme in the metabolism of protein; also called vitamin B_2.

Ribonucleic acid (RNA)—Nucleic acid that controls protein synthesis in all living cells; HIV/RNA is the genetic material of human immunodeficiency virus.

Rickets—Disease caused by a deficiency of vitamin D that affects the young during the period of skeletal growth, resulting in bones that are abnormally shaped and weak.

Ritter syndrome—An inflammatory skin disease seen in newborns, characterized by pustules that fill with a straw-colored fluid and become encrusted.

Rooting reflex—The infant's natural response to a stroke on its cheek, which turns the head toward that side to nurse.

Rotavirus—Most common cause of infectious enteritis in human infants; survives for long periods on hard surfaces, in contaminated water, and on hands.

Roux-en-Y—A surgical connection between the distal end of the small bowel and another organ such as the stomach.

Rugae—Folds of mucosa of organs such as the stomach.

Salivary amylase—An enzyme that initiates the breakdown of starch in the mouth.

Salivary glands—The glands that secrete saliva into the mouth.

Salmonella—A genus of bacteria responsible for many cases of foodborne illness.

Salmonellosis—A bacterial infection manifested by the sudden onset of headache, abdominal pain, diarrhea, nausea, and vomiting. Fever is almost always present. Contaminated food is the predominant method of transmission.

Sarcoma—A malignant neoplasm that occurs in connective tissue such as muscle or bone.

Sarcopenia—Muscle loss.

Satiety—The feeling after consuming food that enough has been eaten; the sensation of satisfaction.

Saturated fat—A fat in which the majority of fatty acids contain no carbon-to-carbon double bonds.

Scurvy—Disease due to deficiency of vitamin C marked by bleeding problems and, later, by bony skeleton changes.

Seasonal variation—Refers to differences during spring, summer, fall, and winter.

Sebaceous gland—Oil-secreting gland of the skin; most sebaceous glands have a hair follicle associated with them.

Second-degree relative—A relative sharing one-quarter of an individual's genes; examples: grandparent, grandchild, uncle, aunt, nephew, niece, half-sibling.

Secondary diabetes—A World Health Organization classification for diabetes when the hyperglycemia occurs as a result of another disorder.

Secondary hypertension—High blood pressure that develops as the result of another condition.

Secondary malnutrition—A nutrient deficiency due to improper absorption and distribution of nutrients.

Secondary prevention—Institution of monitoring techniques to discover incipient diseases early to enhance the opportunity to control their effects; nutrition example: testing blood glucose levels to diagnose prediabetes.

Secretin—A hormone that stimulates the production of bile by the liver and the secretion of sodium bicarbonate juice by the pancreas.

Self-efficacy—The extent to which a person believes that he or she has the ability to perform a particular task or behavior.

Self-monitoring of blood glucose (SMBG)—A procedure that persons with diabetes follow to test their own blood glucose levels.

Sensible water loss—Visible water loss through perspiration, urine, and feces.

Sensitivity—Characteristic of diagnostic test; the proportion of people correctly identified as having the condition in question; a score of 100% would indicate that all the affected persons were identified by the test.

Sepsis—A condition in which disease-producing organisms are present in the blood.

Sequelae—Conditions following and resulting from a disease; sequel.

Serosa—A serous membrane that covers internal organs and lines body cavities.

Serotonin—A body chemical that assists the transmission of nerve impulses; it produces constriction of blood vessels and is thought to be related to sleep.

Serum—The liquid portion of the blood minus the clotting elements.

Serum transferrin—Globulin in the blood that binds and transports iron; level increases in early iron deficiency, before hemoglobin and hematocrit readings drop.

Shelf life—The duration a product can remain in storage without deterioration.

Shigella—Organisms causing intestinal disease; spread by fecal–oral transmission from a client or carrier via direct contact or indirectly by contaminated food.

SIAD (syndrome of inappropriate antidiuresis)—Dilutional hyponatremia resulting from diverse pathologies (central nervous system disorders, certain lung diseases, some tumors, particular drugs). Formerly called syndrome of inappropriate secretion of antidiuretic hormone (SIADH).

Signs—*See* Objective data.

Simple carbohydrate—Composed of one or two units of $C_6H_{12}O_6$; includes the monosaccharides (glucose, fructose, and galactose) and the disaccharides (sucrose, lactose, and maltose).

Simple fat—Lipids that consist of fatty acids or a simple filler such as a hydroxyl (OH) molecule joined to glycerol.

Small for gestational age (SGA)—Infant weighing less at birth than considered normal for the calculated length of the pregnancy.

Small intestine—The part of the alimentary canal between the stomach and the large intestine, where most absorption of nutrients occurs.

Sodium pump—Proteins located in cell membranes that provide an active transport mechanism to move sodium ions across a membrane to their area of greater concentration; moves sodium ions out of the cells and water follows.

Solubility—The ability of one substance to dissolve into another in solution.

Soluble—Able to be dissolved.

Solute—The substance that is dissolved in a solvent.

Solvent—A liquid holding another substance in solution.

Somatostatin—A hormone produced by the delta cells of the islets of Langerhans that inhibits both the release of insulin and the production of glucagon.

Specific gravity—The weight of a substance compared to an equal volume of a standard substance; usual standard for liquids is water; its specific gravity set at 1.000.

Specificity—Characteristic of diagnostic test; the proportion of people correctly identified as not having the condition in question; a score of 100% would indicate that all of the unaffected persons were identified by the test.

Sphincter—A circular band of muscles that constricts a passage.

Spina bifida—Congenital defect in spinal column whereby the vertebrae fail to close; clinical manifestations may or may not include protrusion of the meninges outside the spinal canal.

Spore—A form assumed by some bacteria that is highly resistant to heat, drying, and chemicals.

Sprue—Chronic form of malabsorption syndrome affecting the small intestine; subcategories: tropical and nontropical.

Standard (polymeric) formula—An oral or enteral feeding that contains all the essential nutrients in a specified volume.

Standard drink—0.5 oz. of alcohol found in 12 oz. of beer, 5 oz. of wine, or 1.5 oz. distilled spirits.

Staphylococcus aureus—One of the most common species of bacteria, which produces a poisonous toxin. The main reservoir is nose and throat discharge. Food can act as a vehicle for transmission, so proper hand washing is an essential means of control.

Starches—Polysaccharides; many units of $C_6H_{12}O_6$ joined together; complex carbohydrates.

Steatorrhea—The presence of greater than normal amounts of fat in the stool, producing foul-smelling, bulky excrement.

Sterol—Substance related to fats and belonging to the lipoids; example: cholesterol.

Stimulus control—The identification of cues that precede a behavior and rearranging daily activities to avoid such cues.

Stoma—A surgically created opening in the abdominal wall.

Stomach—The portion of the alimentary canal between the esophagus and small intestine.

Stomatitis—An inflammation of the mouth.

Stress—Any threat to a person's mental or physical well-being.

Stress factor—A number used to predict how much a client's kilocalorie need has increased as a result of a disease state.

Subcutaneously—Beneath the skin.

Subdural hematoma—Collection of blood under the outermost membrane covering the brain and spinal cord; usually resulting from head injury.

Subjective data—Experiences the client reports, also termed *symptoms*.

Submucosa—Structural layer of the alimentary canal below the mucosa; contains tissues and blood vessels.

Sucrase—An enzyme in the intestinal mucosa that splits sucrose into glucose and fructose.

Sucrose—A disaccharide; one unit of glucose and one unit of fructose joined together; ordinary white table sugar.

Superior vena cava—One of the largest diameter veins in the human body; used to deliver parenteral nutrition.

Supplemental Feeding Program for Women, Infants, and Children (WIC)—Federal program providing nutrition education and supplemental food to low-income pregnant or breastfeeding women and children up to 5 years of age.

Symptoms—*See* Subjective data.

System—An organized grouping of related structures or parts.

Systolic pressure—Pressure exerted against the arteries when the heart contracts; the upper number of the blood pressure reading.

Tapeworm—A parasitic intestinal worm that is acquired by humans through the ingestion of raw seafood or undercooked beef or pork.

Tardive dyskinesia—Neurological syndrome involving involuntary, slow, rhythmic, movements often seen in the mouth and tongue; side effect of psychotropic drugs, especially phenothiazines.

Target heart rate—Seventy percent of maximum heart rate (number of heart beats per minute); a person's target heart rate can be objectively determined by a stress test. Individuals can estimate their target heart rate by subtracting their age from 220 and multiplying the difference by 70%. A person's target heart rate is the rate at which the pulse should be maintained for at least 20 minutes during aerobic exercise.

Telomerase—Enzyme that helps repair cell damage that occurs to the end of the DNA molecule during each cycle of cell division; cancer cells have telomerases that allow infinite repair to the DNA strands, contributing to their immortality.

Teratogenic—Capable of causing abnormal development of the embryo; results in a malformed fetus.

Term infant—One born between the beginning of the 38th week through the 42nd week of gestation.

Tertiary prevention—Use of treatment techniques after a disease has occurred to prevent complications or to promote maximum adaptation; nutrition example: interventions to treat swallowing disorders to maintain nourishment and avoid choking incidents.

Tetany—Muscle contractions, especially of the wrists and ankles, resulting from low levels of ionized calcium in the blood; causes include parathyroid deficiency, vitamin D deficiency, and alkalosis.

Therapeutic index—Maximum tolerated dose of a drug divided by the minimum curative dose; a narrow index indicates greater potential for adverse side effects.

Thermic effect of exercise (TEE)—The number of kilocalories used above resting energy expenditure as a result of physical activity.

Thermic effect of foods (diet-induced thermogenesis, specific-dynamic action)—The energy cost to extract and utilize the kilocalories and nutrients in foods; the heat produced after eating a meal.

Thiamin—Coenzyme in the metabolism of carbohydrates and fats; vitamin B_1.

Thiaminase—An enzyme in raw fish that destroys thiamin.

Third-space losses—Sequestering of fluid in body cavities such as the chest and abdomen; in the abdominal cavity, it produces ascites.

Thoracic—Pertaining to the chest, or thorax.

Threonine—Essential amino acid often lacking in grains.

Thrombus—A blood clot that obstructs a blood vessel; obstruction of a vessel of the brain or heart is among the most serious effects.

Thrush—An infection caused by the organism *Candida albicans*; characterized by the formation of white patches and ulcers in the mouth and throat.

Thymus—Gland in the chest, above and in front of the heart, that contributes to the immune response, including the maturation of T-lymphocytes.

Thyroid-stimulating hormone (TSH)—A hormone secreted by the pituitary gland that stimulates the thyroid gland to secrete thyroxine and triiodothyronine; thyrotropin.

Thyrotropin-releasing factor (TRF)—Stimulates the secretion of thyroid-stimulating hormone; produced in the hypothalamus.

Thyroxine (T_4)—A hormone secreted by the thyroid gland; increases the rate of metabolism and energy production.

Tissue—A group or collection of similar cells and their similar intercellular substance that acts together in the performance of a particular function.

T-lymphocytes (T-cells)—White blood cells that recognize and fight foreign cells such as cancer; thymic lymphocytes.

Tolerable Upper Intake Level (UL)—Highest average daily intake by an individual that is unlikely to pose risks of adverse health effects in 97% to 98% of individuals in specified life-stage and gender group; ordinarily refers to intake from food, fortified food, water, and supplements.

Tolerance level—The highest dose at which a residue causes no ill effects in laboratory animals.

Toxoplasmosis—Infection with the protozoan *Toxoplasma gondii*; when infected in utero, infant may suffer mental retardation, blindness, and epilepsy.

Trace minerals—Those present in the body in amounts less than 5 grams; daily intake of less than 100 milligrams needed; also called microminerals or trace elements.

Traction—The process of using weights to draw a part of the body into alignment.

Transcellular fluid—Located in body cavities and spaces; constantly being secreted and absorbed; examples: cerebrospinal fluid, pericardial fluid, pleural fluid.

Transferrin—Protein in the blood that binds and transports iron.

Trauma—A physical injury or wound caused by an external force; an emotional or psychological shock that usually results in disordered behavior.

Triceps skinfold—Measure of skin and subcutaneous tissue over the triceps muscle in the upper arm; used in body fat assessment.

Trichinella spiralis—A wormlike parasite that becomes embedded in the muscle tissue of pork.

Trichinosis—The infestation of *Trichinella spiralis*, a parasitic roundworm, transmitted by eating raw or insufficiently cooked pork.

Triglyceride—Three fatty acids joined to a glycerol molecule.

Triiodothyronine (T_3)—A hormone secreted by the thyroid gland that increases the rate of metabolism and energy production.

Trousseau sign—Spasms of the forearm and hand upon inflation of the blood pressure cuff; sign of tetany or lack of ionized calcium in the blood.

Trust—First stage of Erikson's theory of psychosocial development, in which the infant learns to rely on those caring for it.

Trypsin—An enzyme formed in the intestine that assists in protein digestion.

Tryptophan—An essential amino acid, often lacking in legumes; serves as provitamin for the production of niacin by the liver.

Tubular reabsorption—The movement of fluid back into the blood from the renal tubule.

Tubule—A small tube or canal.

Tumor suppressor gene—Gene that inhibits growth and division of the cell.

Turgor—Resilience of skin; when pinched, quickly returns to original shape in well-hydrated young person; test for deficient fluid volume that is not reliable for elderly clients.

Type 1 diabetes—Persons with this disorder must take insulin to survive and are prone to ketoacidosis; formerly called insulin-dependent diabetes mellitus (IDDM) and juvenile diabetes.

Type 2 diabetes—Although some persons with this disorder take insulin, it is not necessary for their survival; formerly called non–insulin-dependent diabetes (NIDDM) and adult-onset diabetes mellitus.

Tyramine—A monoamine present in various foods that will provoke a hypertensive crisis in persons taking monoamine oxidase inhibitors (MAOIs).

Ulcer—An open sore or lesion of the skin or mucous membrane.

Ulcerative colitis—Inflammatory disease of the large intestine that usually begins in the rectum and spreads upward in a continuous pattern.

Ultrasound bone densitometer—Machine that uses sound waves to estimate bone density as a screening test.

Uncomplicated starvation—A food deprivation without an underlying stress state.

Undernutrition—The state that results from a deficiency of one or more nutrients.

Underwater weighing—Most accurate measure of body fatness.

Universal precautions—A list of procedures developed by the Centers for Disease Control and Prevention for when blood and certain other body fluids should be considered contaminated and treated as such.

Unsaturated fat—A fat in which the majority of fatty acids contain one or more carbon-to-carbon double bonds.

Urea—The chief nitrogenous constituent of urine; the final product, along with CO_2, of protein metabolism.

Uremia—A toxic condition produced by the retention of nitrogen-containing substances normally excreted by the kidneys.

Ureter—The tube that carries urine from the kidney to the bladder.

Urinary calculus—A kidney stone, or deposit of mineral salts.

Urinary tract infection (UTI)—The condition in which disease-producing microorganisms invade a client's bladder, ureter, or urethra.

USDA Dietary Guidelines—Guidelines for health promotion issued by the U.S. Department of Agriculture and U.S. Department of Health and Human Services; revised in 2010.

U.S. Pharmacopeia (USP)—Compendium of standards of strength and purity for drugs; issued and revised periodically by a national committee.

Usual food intake—A description of what a person habitually eats.

Vaginitis—Inflammation of the vagina, most often caused by an infectious agent.

Vagotomy—Surgical cutting of vagus nerve to reduce gastric acid secretion; achieving similar results by the use of medications is termed medical vagotomy.

Vasopressin—Antidiuretic hormone; abbreviated ADH.

Ventilation—Process by which gases are moved into and out of the lungs;

two aspects of ventilation are inhalation and exhalation.

Very low-calorie diet (VLCD)—Diet that contains less than 800 kilocalories per day.

Very low-density lipoprotein (VLDL)—A plasma protein containing mostly triglycerides with small amounts of cholesterol, phospholipid, and protein; transports triglycerides from the liver to tissues.

Villi—Multiple minute projections on the surface of the folds of the small intestine that absorb fluid and nutrients; plural of villus.

Virus—Very small noncellular parasite that is entirely dependent on the nutrients inside host cells for its metabolic and reproductive needs.

Viscera—Internal organs enclosed in a cavity.

Visible fat—Dietary fat that can be easily seen, such as the fat on meat or in oil.

Vitamin—Organic substance needed by the body in very small amounts; yields no energy and does not become part of the body's structure.

Waist-to-hip ratio (WHR)—Waist measurement divided by hip measurement; if greater than 0.8 in women or greater than 0.95 in men, indicates increased risk of health problems related to obesity.

Warfarin—Anticoagulant that interferes with the liver's synthesis of vitamin K–dependent clotting factors II, VII, IX, and X.

Water intoxication—Excess intake or abnormal retention of water.

Weight cycling—The repeated gain and loss of body weight.

Wernicke–Korsakoff syndrome—A disorder of the central nervous system resulting from thiamine deficiency; often seen in chronic alcoholism; signs and symptoms include motor, sensory, and memory deficits.

Wernicke encephalopathy—Inflammatory, hemorrhagic, degenerative lesions in several areas of the brain resulting in double vision, involuntary eye movements, lack of muscle coordination, and mental deficits; caused by thiamin deficiency, often seen in chronic alcoholism but also in gastrointestinal tract disease and hyperemesis gravidarum.

Whey—Component of milk; in human milk, contains soluble proteins that are easily digested; major whey protein in breast milk is alpha-lactalbumin, with an amino acid pattern much like that of the body tissues.

Whipple procedure—Pancreatoduodenectomy; surgical procedure for cancer of the head of the pancreas; removal of the head of the pancreas, lower portion of common bile duct, most of duodenum, and possibly part of stomach.

WIC—*See* Supplemental Feeding Program for Women, Infants, and Children.

Wilson disease—Rare genetic defect of copper metabolism that permits copper to accumulate in various organs; inherited as an autosomal recessive trait.

Xerophthalmia—Drying and thickening of the epithelial tissues of the eye; can be caused by vitamin A deficiency.

Xerostomia—Dry mouth caused by decreased salivary secretions.

X-linked inheritance—Hereditary pattern involving a gene on the X chromosome; in females, a dominant gene or two recessive genes will cause the trait to be manifested; in males, with only one X chromosome, the trait will be manifested whether the gene is dominant or recessive.

Index

Page numbers followed by "f" denote figures; those followed by "t" denote tables; and those followed by "b" denote boxes

Radura symbol, 225f
Rancid, 38
Reabsorption, tubular, 333, 335f
Reactive hypoglycemia, 313
Recommended Dietary Allowances, 17, 426–427
Rectum, 150
Red meat, 378
Red wine, 328
Reduced body mass, 292–294
Reduced sugar, 26, 26b
Refeeding syndrome, 103, 398–399
Registered dietitians, 11
Registered nurses, 11
Regurgitation, 249
Renal osteodystrophy, 342
Renal system, acid-base balance and, 131
Renal threshold, 299
Renal tubule, 333
Renin, 129
Rennin, 145
Residues, 231
Respiratory acidosis, 397
Respiratory alkalosis, 130, 397
Respiratory failure, 396
Respiratory function, impaired nutritional status and, 397
Respiratory system, acid-base balance and, 130–131
Resting energy expenditure (REE), 62–63, 212
Retina, 73
Retinoic acid syndrome, 164
Retinol, 72
Retinol activity equivalents, 72
Retinopathy, diabetic, 304
Rheumatoid arthritis, 216
Rhodopsin, 73
Riboflavin, 81t, 85
Ribonucleic acid (RNA), 53
Rickets, vitamin D and, 77
Ritonavir, 262
Rotavirus, 192
Roux-en-Y, 290
Rugae, 144
Rule of Nines, 392f

S

Saccharin, 27t
Salivary amylase, 143
Salivary glands, 143
Salmonella infection, 226, 227t
Salmonellosis, 226
Salt intake, hypertension and, 321
Salt substitutes, 268
Saquinavir, 271
Sarcomas, 375
Sarcopenia, 211b
Satiety
  cancer patients and, 382–383
  definition of, 28
  fats and, 39
  fiber and, 28
Saturated fats, 38, 324–325, 342–343
Saturated fatty acids, 37
Saunders, Cicely, 416
Scar tissue, 50b

School foods, 199b
School-age child (ages 6 to 12 years)
  meal patterns and behaviors, 197
  MyPlate serving guidelines and, 198t
  nutrition indications and, 198t
  nutritional needs and concerns, 197–198
  physical growth and development of, 197
  psychosocial development of, 197
  school nutrition for, 197–198, 199b
Scombroid fish poisoning, 230
Screening. *see* Nutrition screening
Scurvy, 81–83
Seafood, toxic, 230
Secondary diabetes, 301
Secondary hypertension, 318
Secondary prevention, 3
Secretion, tubular, 333–334, 335f
Secretions, digestion and, 142
Seizure control, ketogenic diet for, 262
Selenium
  deficiency of, 116
  functions of, 110t
  properties of, 110t
  sources of, 116
  toxicity of, 102t, 116
Self-care, diabetes and, 313
Self-feeding, 246
Self-monitoring
  blood glucose and, 305–306
  weight management and, 290b
Semisolid food introduction, infants and, 186–188
Senior Farmer's Market Nutrition Program, 217
Sensible water losses, 131–133
Sensory system, older adults and, 209
Sepsis, burn patients and, 393
Serotonin syndrome, 271
Serum, 123
Set point theory, obesity and, 288
Shellfish, 168
Sibutramine, 270
Silicon, 118
Simple carbohydrates, 24
Simvastatin, 263
Siraitia grosvenorri, 27t
Skin, vitamin D synthesis by, 77
Slower eating, weight management and, 290b
Small intestine
  absorption in, 148–150
  carbohydrate digestion in, 145–146
  cross-section of, 149f
  fat digestion in, 146–147
  protein digestion in, 147
Smell, older adults and, 209
Smoking, 323
SOAP format, 18
Social consequences, obesity and, 284–285
Social workers, 11
Sodium
  abnormal levels of, 105t
  in beverages, 329t
  calcium balance and, 98
  deficiency of, 104
  dietary reference intakes of, 104
  fluids and lithium and, 268
  in fresh and processed foods, 105t

functions of, 96t
hypernatremia and, 104
hyponatremia and, 104
kidney disease and, 340
kidney failure and, 336–337
mean intake of, 104f
properties of, 96t
table salt, 104
toxicity of, 101t, 104
Sodium pumps, 127
Sodium-controlled diets, 328–330, 329t
Soft cheeses, 168
Soft diets, 242
Solubility, 28
Soluble fiber, 28
Solutes, 124
Somatostatin, 302
Sorbitol, 409
Soy protein, 186, 326, 328
Spare body protein, 29
Special diets, 242
Special formulas, 185–186
Specific dynamic action, 63
Specific gravity, 135
Speech pathologists, 11
Sphincters, 141
Spina bifida, 163b
Spores, 182
St. John's wort, 271
Standard feedings, 248
Standard formulas, 247
Staph infection, 228
Staphylococcus aureus, 228
Starches, 24, 27, 31
Starvation
  critical care and, 389–390
  fuel consumption during, 390f
  gluconeogenesis and, 389
  glycogenolysis and, 389
  ketosis and, 389
  lipolysis and, 389
  prolonged, 390
  refeeding syndrome and, 398–399
  uncomplicated, 389
Steatorrhea, 98, 153, 409
Sterols, 36
Steviol glycosides, 27t
Stimulus control, weight management and, 290b
Stoma, 364
Stomach
  cancer of, 376
  delayed gastric emptying, 355–356
  dumping syndrome, 357, 358t
  food pathway and, 144–145
  gastritis, 355, 355f
  peptic ulcers, 356–357
  postprandial hypotension, 357
  vitamin B_{12} deficiency and, 88
Stomatitis, 337, 383, 419b
Stretching exercises, 65
Stroke, 319–320, 330
Subjective data, of nutritional assessment, 12, 12t
Sucralose, 27t
Sucrase, 146
Sucrose, 25